Minimally Invasive Surgery: A Comprehensive Approach

Minimally Invasive Surgery: A Comprehensive Approach

Edited by Philip Rudolf

hayle medical
New York

Hayle Medical,
750 Third Avenue, 9th Floor,
New York, NY 10017, USA

Visit us on the World Wide Web at:
www.haylemedical.com

ISBN: 978-1-63241-773-2

The publisher's policy is to use permanent paper from mills that operate a sustainable forestry policy. Furthermore, the publisher ensures that the text paper and cover boards used have met acceptable environmental accreditation standards.

Printed in China.

Cataloging-in-Publication Data

Minimally invasive surgery : a comprehensive approach / edited by Philip Rudolf.
p. cm.
Includes bibliographical references and index.
ISBN 978-1-63241-773-2
1. Endoscopic surgery. 2. Endoscopy. 3. Microsurgery. 4. Surgery, Operative. I. Rudolf, Philip.
RD33.53 .M56 2019
617.05--dc23

Table of Contents

Preface

The surgical procedures which limit the size of incisions required and consequently reduce the pain, wound healing time, and the risk of infection are known as minimally invasive surgeries. The advancement in technology has resulted in advanced techniques of minimally invasive surgery. One such example is remote-control manipulation of instruments with indirect observation through a large scale display panel. Minimally invasive direct coronary artery bypass is an example of minimally invasive surgery. It is a type of surgical procedure for coronary heart disease. It is often known as "keyhole" heart surgery because in this surgery, the operation is analogous to operating through a keyhole. This book provides comprehensive insights into the field of minimally invasive surgery. It includes some of the vital pieces of work being conducted across the world, on various topics related to minimally invasive surgery. The extensive content of this book provides the readers with a thorough understanding of the subject.

This book unites the global concepts and researches in an organized manner for a comprehensive understanding of the subject. It is a ripe text for all researchers, students, scientists or anyone else who is interested in acquiring a better knowledge of this dynamic field.

I extend my sincere thanks to the contributors for such eloquent research chapters. Finally, I thank my family for being a source of support and help.

Editor

1

From the Idea to Its Realization: The Evolution of Minimally Invasive Techniques in Neurosurgery

P. Grunert

Neurosurgical Department, University of Saarland, 66424 Homburg, Germany

Correspondence should be addressed to P. Grunert; peter.grunert@uks.eu

Academic Editor: John Y. K. Lee

Minimally invasive techniques in neurosurgery evolved in two steps. Many minimally invasive concepts like neuronavigation, endoscopy, or frame based stereotaxy were developed by the pioneers of neurosurgery, but it took decades till further technical developments made the realization and broad clinical application of these early ideas safe and possible. This thesis will be demonstrated by giving examples of the evolution of four minimally invasive techiques: neuronavigation, transsphenoidal pituitary surgery, neuroendoscopy and stereotaxy. The reasons for their early failure and also the crucial steps for the rediscovery of these minimally invasive techniques will be analysed. In the 80th of the 20th century endoscopy became increasingly applied in different surgical fields. The abdominal surgeons coined as first for their endoscopic procedures the term minimally invasive surgery in contrast to open surgery. In neurrosurgery the term minimally invasive surgery stood not in opposiotion to open procedures but was understood as a general concept and philosophy using the modern technology such as neuronavigation, endoscopy and planing computer workstations with the aim to make the procedures less traumatic.

1. Introduction

> *Despite success in surgical technique permitting to perform hemicraniotomy for removing a small intracranial lesion, one cannot but admits, both a priori and from clinical experience, the necessity to minimize surgical injury and approve all methods of precise localization of a cerebral lesion. GI Rossolimo, J Neuropath Psych Korsakow 1907; 7: p 640.*

This statement of Rossolimo, one of the leading Russian neurologists at the beginning of the 20th century, shows that the idea of minimally invasive neurosurgery was already appreciated by the pioneers of this discipline.

Atraumatic operative techniques were considered from the beginning in neurosurgery due to the disastrous possible functional complications inherent to manipulations on the central nervous system. However due to technical limitations most of the promising projects and concepts had to be postponed at the end of the 19th and beginning of 20th century and had to wait sometimes even many decades till technical developments, necessary diagnostic radiological imaging, and the appropriate operative instruments made a safe clinical application of these nearly forgotten ideas in the second half of the 20th century possible. An example for an extreme long time-lag between an idea and its technical realization may serve the development of automata and robots. The main concept of these devices was already described in the Iliad of Homer 2700 years ago. Thetis, the mother of Achilles, arrived in the smithy of the God Hephaistos and asked for the new armour for her son. She was filled with wonder about two types of marvellous machines there. The one called automata were vehicles on three wheels driven by themselves and bringing food and drinks intelligently to the Olympic deities [1]. The others were beautiful female robots in form of androids from gold which were able to speak and sing and which supported God Hephaistos in his smithy [2]. After 2700 years, the present advanced computer technology and progress in artificial intelligence realized this ancient human dream and concept.

In this paper, I will demonstrate my thesis of a two-step development of minimally invasive neurosurgical techniques giving examples from four neurosurgical fields:

(1) localization of intracerebral lesions and eloquent cortical areas,

(2) transsphenoidal approach to the pituitary tumours,

(3) endoscopic treatment of hydrocephalus,

(4) functional stereotaxic neurosurgery.

2. Localization of Intracerebral Lesions and Eloquent Cortical Areas

The existence and the localization of specific cognitive functions of cortical areas such as movement, speech, or vision were of great importance for the pioneers of neurosurgery to omit severe postoperative side effects such as hemiparesis or aphasia in the mid 19th century. At this time not only the precise localization of brain functions in particular the higher cognitive functions but even their morphological existence was an open question. Some experimental studies spoke in favour of the localization theory; others such as the results of the biologist Jean Pierre Flourens (1794–1867) performed on rabbits and pigeons were compatible with a global representation of cognitive functions distributed over the whole cortex [3].

A precursor of the localization of eloquent cortical areas constituted the phrenology developed by the Viennese physician Franz Joseph Gall (1758–1828) at beginning of 19th century [4]. Gall subdivided the cortex initially in 27 and later his pupil Johannes Spurzheim (1776–1832) in 37 separated independently functioning areas which were responsible for different faculties (Figure 1). Besides cognitive functions such as intelligence, memory, or the ability to recognize the size of the objects, Gall associated in a very speculative way based on anatomy of the skull also personality features such as parental love, belief in religion, idealism, or benevolence with distinct cortical areas. He was convinced that pronounced features or the character of a person had a strict morphologic correlate leading to a hypertrophy of the corresponding cortical area and the skull beyond [4]. He believed also that in reverse by palpation of the external bony bumbs on the hypertrophy of specific functional cortical areas and thus on the personality and character of the person can be concluded. Phrenology spread with Spurzheim to UK and to the United States and became an amusing subject in the salons of the upper class society in the first half of the 19th century. Despite the fact that from our present scientific point of view this theory is obsolete, it has to be admitted in favour of Gall that he was one of the first physicians who again underlined the significance of the brain and who initiated further study on the localization of the higher cognitive brain functions. However at the academic level, the location of brain functions in particular the higher cognitive abilities remained an unsolved issue in that time. Over time an increasing opposition against phrenology arouse from scientists in particular by Flourens [3] who was asked by the French academy of sciences to investigate scientifically the propositions of Gall's theory. Challenged by Gall's assumptions and due to increasing withdrawing from a romantic natural philosophy toward measurable objective science of nature, an intense study of cortical functions with anatomical, histological, and electrophysiological methods started to develop in the mid 19th century. It is not surprising therefore that also pioneers of neurosurgery among others such as Victor Horsley (1857–1916) participated in this research themselves and investigated experimentally the localization of cognitive functions.

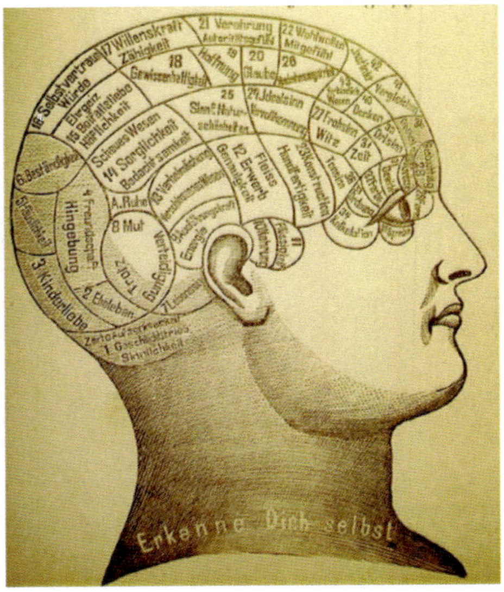

FIGURE 1: Gall's phrenology: the cortex is subdivided in several independent areas with particular functions of cognition and behavior.

The first breakthrough in favour of the localization theory was the observations of the French anatomist, surgeon, and anthropologist Paul Broca (1824–1880) who was able to demonstrate that patients with a severe speech disturbance have a lesion in their frontoopercular cortical area in the left dominant hemisphere. First, he described this finding, 1861 after dissection of the brain of a patient known as Tan who died in the hospital where Broca was working as an appointed surgeon. During his life time this patient suffered from a severe speech disturbance and was able only to say the word Tan [5]. In the following years Broca confirmed his initial result on additional 12 patients [6]. His findings were supported in London by the neurologist John Hughlings Jackson (1835–1911) who published a similar case as Broca (1864) [7]. Carl Wernicke (1848–1905), a neurologist and psychiatrist in Breslau, described in his influential work in 1874 "*The aphasic symptoms: a psychological study based on anatomy*" the critical area for understanding the language in the upper temporal gyrus: the sensory speech area [8]. More detailed histological studies of the cortical areas followed by Camillo Golgi (1843–1926) who developed the first staining of neurons [9] and their arborisation. This silver impregnation method enabled Santiago Ramon y Cajal (1852–1934) to investigate in detail the pattern of axonal and dendrite connections of the neuronal tissue [10]. For this work, both scientists were honoured with the Nobel Prize in 1906. The married couple Oscar and Cecilie Vogt (1870–1959 and 1875–1962, resp.) established the first institute dedicated entirely to neuroscience in Berlin where they integrated cytoarchitectonical and electrophysiological techniques for studies of the brain cortex [11]. Korbinian Brodmann (1868–1918) worked at that institute and classified there in the first decade of 20th century the whole cortex into 45 distinct areas based on morphologic characteristics of the grey matter [12]. Besides the pathoanatomical studies, experiments with electrical stimulation became increasingly important for the understanding of cortical function. The first experimental electrical stimulation of the cortex of dogs was performed in 1870 by the two German neuroscientists Julius Eduard Hitzig (1838–1907) and Gustav Theodor Fritsch (1838–1927) [13]. They observed by stimulation of the frontal cortical areas involuntary movements in the contralateral extremities. The experimental Scotch neurologist David Ferrier (1843–1928) published a detailed map of motor functions obtained by stimulation of brain cortex in different animal species in 1876. He published his results under the title "*The function of the brain*" [14]. The significance of these results for neurosurgery was picked by one of the pioneers of neurosurgery in London, Victor Horsley (1857–1916), who already published back in 1887 a map of motor cortical representation based on his experimental study on animals and partly intraoperative studies on humans [15]. Neurosurgery was a unique opportunity to study cortical function intraoperatively also in humans and to obtain important data almost as side effect during the intervention. At the beginning of 20th century the neurophysiologist and later Nobel laureate Charles Scott Sherrington (1857–1952) performed experiments to delineate the motor and the sensory cortex [16]. His map in opposition to previous studies was only a narrow strip on both sides of the Rolandic sulcus [17]. In 1900, Sherrington while working in Liverpool was attended during his experiments for 3 weeks by the promising young American neurosurgeon Harvey Cushing (1869–1939) who was on his educational journey leading him through many important European medical centres. Back home in Baltimore, Cushing applied the cortical stimulation technique on humans during neurosurgical interventions and published a map of sensory cortex in 1908 [18, 19]. Cortical stimulation had also practical implications in neurosurgery and became increasingly important during epilepsy surgery. Fedor Krause (1857–1937), the pioneer of the German neurosurgery, and the neurologist and neurosurgeon Otfrid Foerster (1873–1941) from Breslau, Germany, used the cortical electric stimulation to localize intraoperatively the epileptic foci by provoking an aura or a typical epileptic fit [20–22]. This electrical stimulation was superior to focus localization based merely on anatomical landmarks.

The knowledge of the localization of the eloquent cortical areas had also a very practical consequence for neurosurgery. At the end of the 19th century, two Swiss professors of surgery Rudolf Ulrich Krönlein (1847–1910) [23, 24] in Zurich and Theodor Kocher (1841–1917) [25, 26] in Bern developed independently a method to localize the underneath situated central sulcus and the Sylvian fissure on the scalp. Krönlein used for this a construction of two parallel horizontal and three vertical supporting lines which were based on external bony landmarks (Figure 2) [23]. These lines allowed defining

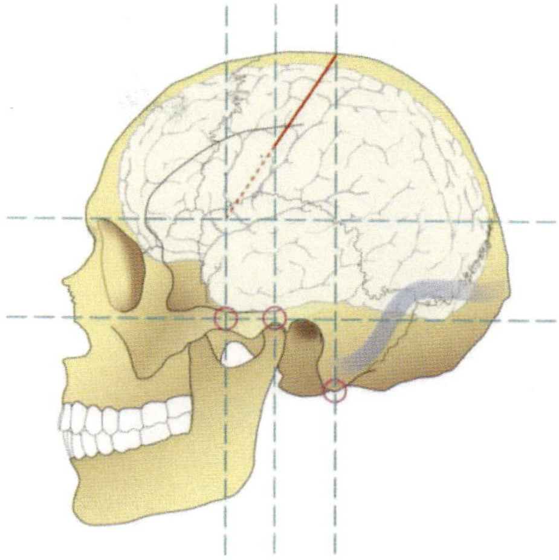

Figure 2: Krönlein's construction of the central region and the Sylvian fissure based on external anatomical landmarks. The horizontal inferior orbitomeatal line is the base line. The parallel supraorbital line marks the inferior border of the central region and the Sylvian fissure. By means of additional three perpendicular vertical lines, first at the anterior zygomatic bone, second at the level through the temporomandibular joint, and the last immediately behind the mastoid, the position of the central region can be drawn into X-ray images or on the head of the patient.

and localizing the position and extension of the central sulcus on the scalp or on the sagittal X-ray image. These supporting lines and the lines representing the central sulcus and the Sylvian fissure in form of ribbons could be also pulled over the head. They marked on the scalp the position of these intracranial structures [24]. The device was called craniometer. In contrast to Krönlein, Kocher's craniometer was based on cadaver studies and consisted of elastic ribbons which were arranged and fixed on the head in a way that the ribbons were just beyond the central sulcus. The elasticity of this craniometer had the advantage that the ribbons preserved their relative position independently of the size of the head. Kocher already described this method in 1892 in his book Lessons in Operative Surgery [25, 26].

A more general approach to the problem of localization of cortical structures was developed by the anatomist Dimitri Zernov (1843–1917) [27] and his pupil Nikolay Altukhov [28] at the end of the 19th century in Russia. Zernov called his device an encephalometer. It was a head ring, which was fixed to the patients skull [29, 30]. The basic idea was to understand the head approximately as a terrestrial globe (Figure 3). Every point at the surface of the head was defined similar to the globe by polar coordinates expressed in degrees of latitude and longitude. The position of the globe was in a way that the poles of the globe corresponded to the nose and the protuberantia occipitalis, the zero meridian to the mid sagittal plane along the falx, and the equator to the frontal plane perpendicular to the mid sagittal plane. Thus, the equator was around the central region and divided the head in the frontal plane into two halves. A 2-dimensional map of the brain surface with gyri and sulci with appropriate graticule of meridians and parallels corresponding to a geographical

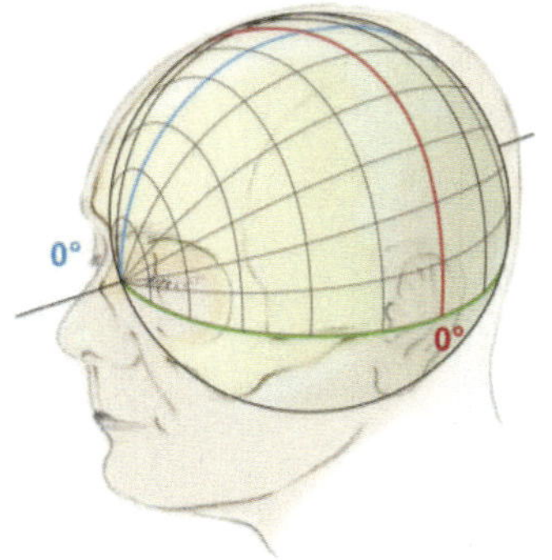

FIGURE 3: By analogy with a terrestrial globe the superficial coordinates on the head are defined by polar coordinate system by degrees of longitude and latitude. The poles correspond to the nose anterior and to the protuberantia occipitalis posterior, respectively. The (blue) zero meridian is running in the midline from anterior to posterior, dividing the head into a right and a left hemisphere, and the (red) equator divides the head into an anterior and posterior half and is running near the central region.

atlas was drawn. The localizations of the cortical structures were established as a mean from measurements of several "normal" cadaver brains. To localize the deep brain structures accurately, a third variable coordinate denoting the distance from the arc centre to the target would be necessary. Since this was not possible with the encephalometer, this apparatus was suitable only for superficially situated lesions. To localize the desired target at the head the frame was equipped with additional two arcs which allowed gliding a stamp like pointer along the meridians and the parallels to set the desired geodetic coordinates on the scalp.

Altukhov published two patients whose central sulcus was successfully localized by this method, and an abscess in this region was subsequently removed in 1891. In a third case the system was used in an inverse modus. The pointer of the encephalometer was set over a visible displaced frontal skull fraction and the geodetic coordinates were read and transferred into the 2D cortical map to identify the affected gyrus [28–30]. Furthermore, the encephalometer was not developed for neurosurgical purposes only. Altukhov used it also for comparative studies to demonstrate possible differences of brains regarding sex, age, and race [28].

Grigorii Ivanovich Rossolimo (1860–1928) [31] from Odessa and Professor of neurology in Moscow, who was one of the founders of paediatric neurology and psychiatry, developed a more sophisticated instrument in 1907 [32]. It was based on the same mathematical principle as the encephalometer, but, instead of a head ring with arcs, it consisted of a helmet in form of a sphere which was fixed to the patient's head and resembled in its mechanical construction the later developed helmet of gamma knife for stereotactic external irradiation. The helmet had in constant distances small holes, arranged along meridians and parallels. It allowed marking with a pointer any target on the scalp without being restricted by the limited movement of the arcs. Rossolimo called this instrument a brain topographer.

However at this stage of neurosurgical development, a broader applicability of these devices was restricted due to insufficient diagnostic imaging capabilities. At that time only a plane X-ray of the head in anterior-posterior and lateral projection was available. Ventriculography was introduced by Walter Dandy (1886–1946) in 1918 [33] and the angiography by the Portuguese neurosurgeon and Nobel Prize laureate Egas Moniz (1874–1955) in 1927 [34]. Therefore, before availability of these two imaging techniques the localization of the lesions was determined entirely by neurologic symptoms of the patient. This circumstance made it necessary to perform the craniotomy large enough to find the lesion at the cortical surface by direct vision or in the subcortical region by palpation with a digit along the brain surface feeling different brain consistence over the lesion. Probably these practical limitations restricted at that time a minimally invasive approach to the lesions and made the application of a brain topographer or encephalometer with few exceptions not practicable. Therefore this original and ingenious method never achieved a general acceptance and fell for many decades into oblivion.

In the 70th and 80th, the diagnostic neuroradiological tools such as CT and MRI were so far advanced that also small intracerebral lesions could be detected inside the intracranial space. The additional fast development of computer technology raised the question whether it is possible to use this computer technology also for real time localization of lesions during neurosurgical interventions without the accurate but time consuming classical frame based stereotaxy. The stereotactic frame restricted additionally the surgical operating field and the mechanical construction of the stereotactic system allowed only limited approaches. The idea to outline in the operating theatre a small craniotomy just above the lesion and to localize the tumour precisely during the intervention without imposing restrictions to the neurosurgeon was finally realized at the end of 80th with the development of neuronavigation devices. These instruments were equipped with a pointer, whose tip could be precisely localized in the space and mapped simultaneously into the corresponding CT/MRI images in real time. The basic mathematics and technology were at this time already extant and used in form of robots [35–38] and GPS navigation and had only to be adapted for the surgical requirements. However robots were already used in neurosurgery some years before neuronavigation systems were applied to neurosurgical localization [39–41].

Robots and global positioning system (GPS) were originally developed by the US army. The robots were developed after the World War II with the aim of working up at distance without human contact radioactively contaminated material, and the GPS was introduced originally for the US navy to navigate ballistic missiles in 1973.

The robotic technology inspired the development of arm-based navigation systems. They calculate their own position in space in a relative homogeneous coordinates system independently of a fixed external point (Figure 4). This is done in real time by evaluation of the angulation in each joint measured by means of encoders integrated in the joint and

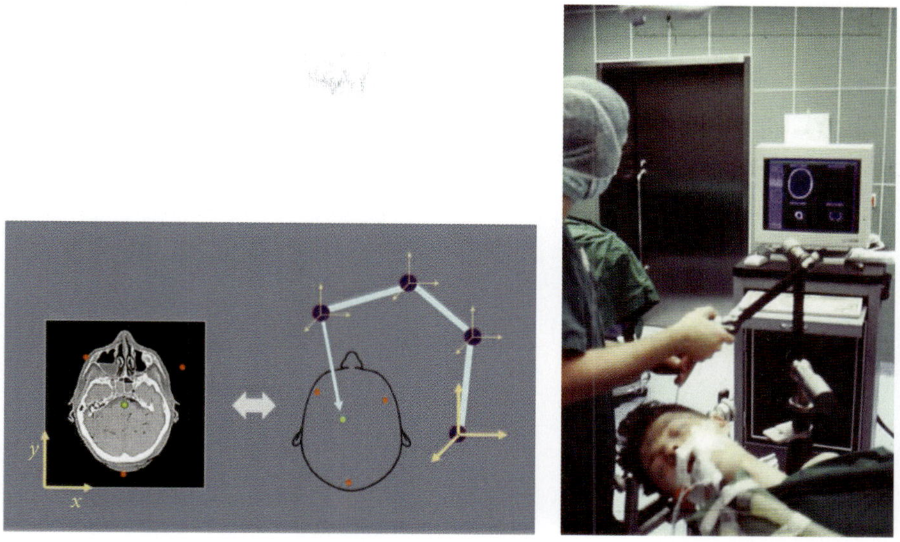

(a) (b)

Figure 4: (a) Principle of an arm-based navigation system with calculation of the position from the length of each arm and the angulation of the joints. (b) Arm-based navigation system during intraoperative calibration.

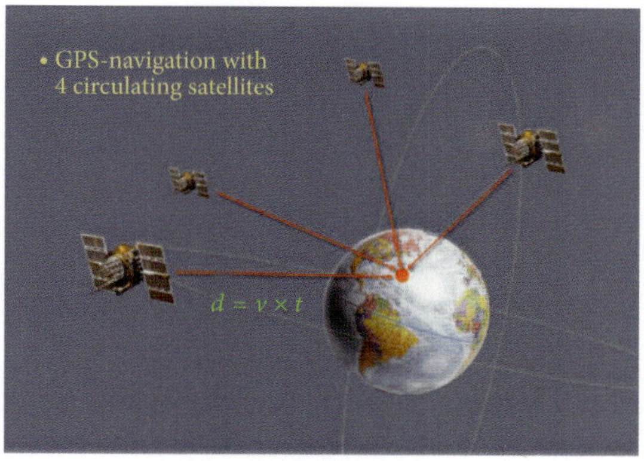

Figure 5: GPS navigation with satellites circulating in an orbit around the earth. From the distances of at least 4 satellites to the receiver, the localization of the receiver can be calculated as the crossing point of spheres with the radius being the distance to the receiver from each satellite.

the a priori known length of each arm between two adjacent joints [42–44].

The armless navigation systems on the other hand were inspired by the GPS. The GPS enables by circulating satellites around the globe the localization of every position at the earth. The principle of the localization consists in measurement of the distances from several satellites to the receiver. Every distance can be understood as a diameter of a sphere. The intersection of these spheres defines the position of the receiver (Figure 5). Each distance is calculated from the known velocity of the electromagnetic wave and the time to reach the receiver. The GPS replaced local navigation systems operating since the World War II by receiving radio signals from fixed navigation beacons. First, satellites were sent into the orbit in 1978, and the full operational capability for the GPS with 24 satellites was reached in 1995. The accuracy of GPS under optimal conditions is about 8 m and is much better than the accuracy of local navigation systems with 180 m. To be not misused by enemies, the accuracy of GPS was till the year 2000 for the public use artificially deteriorated to about 100 m. Thereafter, the undisturbed signal and accuracy were available also for the civil purposes. The GPS was implemented in cars, boots aircrafts, and recently even in cell phones.

The present advanced armless pointer-based neuronavigation systems can be understood as a miniature GPS [45–47]. Like the GPS system, the neuronavigation device calculates distances from several emitting sources whose intersection defines the position in space. The other possibility is to calculate the distance by triangulation technique using at least two fixed cameras (Figure 6). The technical accuracy of the navigation devices to calculate its own position in space is less than 0.5 mm. The emitting sources use either ultrasound infrared light or electromagnetic waves. In GPS system, the position is mapped into a 2D atlas and similarly the calculated position of the pointer tip in the neuronavigation system is transferred into CT/MR image to show in real time the position of the pointer tip during surgery in relation to the anatomical structures visible in the images. To map the pointer tip into the image space, a registration has to be performed first before application. This is done either by paired point registration with touching several corresponding points on the patient and in the image or by matching the skin surface of the image with that of the patient. The serial production and clinical application of neuronavigation devices started in the 90th [45–47]. The operating microscope was also integrated and adapted to be used as an navigation device [48, 49]. Due to the simple handling, the armless pointer based navigation systems gained a general acceptance. They are in the present neurosurgery

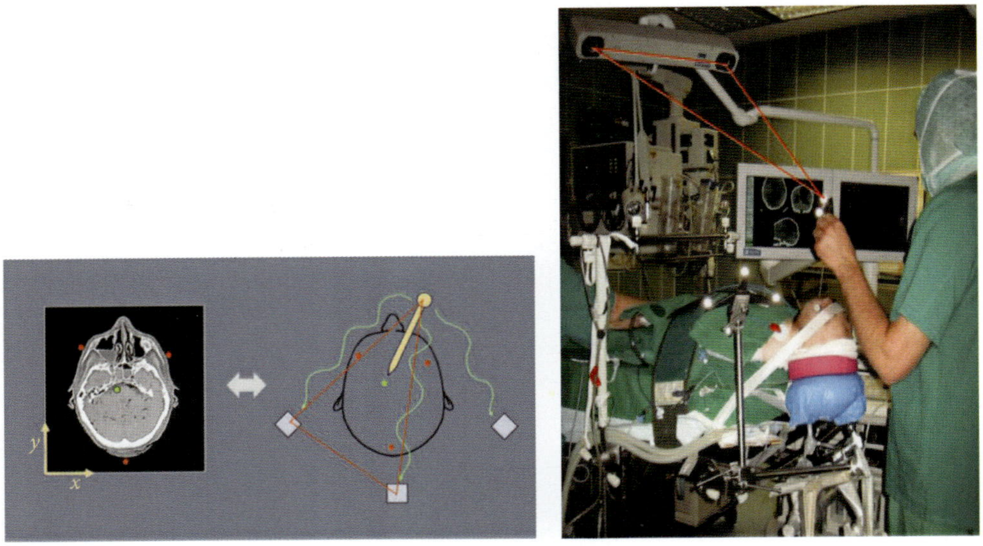

(a) (b)

Figure 6: (a) Principle of armless navigation system with emitting infrared diodes on the pointer and a three-camera system as receiver. (b) Armless navigation system with a two-infrared camera system and emitting diodes on the pointer during intraoperative registration. The localization of the pointer is calculated by triangulation method.

an indispensable tools for localization of intracranial lesions and minimally invasive craniotomies, exactly as Rossolimo demanded 100 years ago.

3. Transsphenoidal Approach to the Hypophysis

Transsphenoidal pituitary surgery is a further example of a minimally invasive operative technique which was introduced already at the very beginning of the treatment of this pathology, but which became a generally accepted method only in the last 30 years.

At the end of the 19th century endocrinologic disorders started to be related also to the pituitary gland. The French neurologist Pierre Marie (1853–1940) follower of Jean-Martin Charcot in the Hopital Salpetrier in Paris described two patients with acromegaly due to a pituitary tumour in 1886 [50]. Joseph Babinski (1857–1932) [51], a Polish stemming French neurologist in Paris, and the Viennese neurologist and pharmacologist Alfred Fröhlich (1871–1953) [52] published independently of each other two separate cases of an endocrinologically inactive pituitary tumour associated with adipositas and underdeveloped sexual organs later known as dystrophia adiposogenitalis in 1900 and in 1901, respectively. In 1939, Fröhlich fled from the Nazi regime in Austria to the USA and continued his research on the neurovegetative system in Cincinnati, Ohio.

First operations of pituitary tumours were performed by Victor Horsley through a frontal approach in London in 1889, and later in 1904, he described a temporal transcranial approach [53–55]. Fedor Krause (1857–1937) proposed a subfrontal approach in 1905 [55]. His approach was further improved in the United States by Frazier, Heuer, Cushing and Dandy and became the standard transcranial approach in the following years. As an alternative to the transcranial route the transsphenoidal approach was developed simultaneously in the first decade of the 20th century in the United States and in Europe, in particular in the Austrian monarchy. One reason that Vienna became the cradle for minimally invasive approach to pituitary tumours using an endonasal transsphenoidal approach was among others due to the basic and detailed anatomical studies of the paranasal sinuses performed in Vienna by the Austrian anatomist and Violin virtuoso Emil Zuckerkandl (1849–1910). His main work "*On normal and pathological anatomy of the paranasal sinus and its pneumatic adnexes*" in 1882 was the anatomical presupposition for the Viennese ENT surgeons to successfully develop minimally invasive endonasal approaches to pituitary tumours [56] (Figure 7).

The first transsphenoidal approach to the hypophysis in humans was elaborated in Innsbruck, Austria, by the surgeon Hermann Schloffer in 1906 [57]. He reported on the success of this operation in 1907 [58]. In his original work, he used a very traumatic and cosmetically unfavourable superior transsphenoidal approach with nose flected to the side and removing all endonasal bony structures (Figure 8). Modifications of this very invasive and mutilating method with the aim of reducing the operative trauma were performed by Anton von Eiselsberg (1860–1939), Head of the First Surgical Department at the University of Vienna in 1907. von Eiselsberg reported on his experience with this approach at the influential North American Surgical Society Meeting in 1910 [59]. He had the greatest surgical experience with this approach with 36 patients. His counterpart Julius Hochenegg (1859–1940), Head of the Second Surgical Department at the same University of Vienna, used this approach in 1909 to treat successfully the first case of acromegaly [60]. In the same year, Theodor Kocher (1841–1917) reported on his experience with the first operated case of a pituitary tumour using

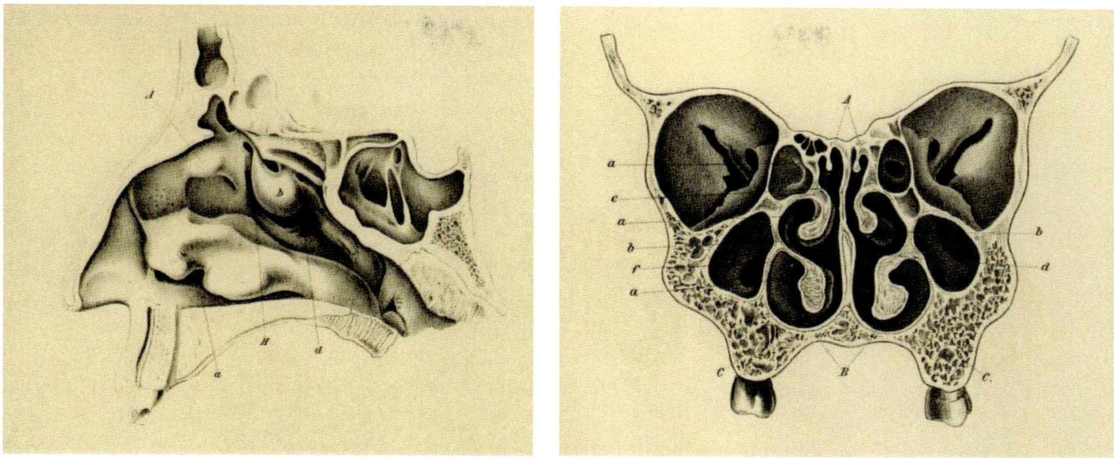

(a) (b)

FIGURE 7: Paranasal sinuses from the publication of Emil Zuckerkandl in 1882: (a) sagittal section through the nose, (b) frontal section through the nose and the maxillary sinuses.

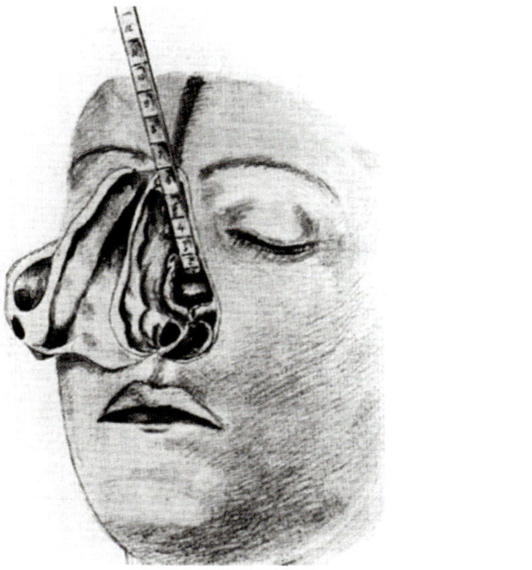

FIGURE 8: Superior transsphenoidal approach as used in the first transsphenoidal operation by Herman Schloffer 1907 with nose flected to the side.

a submucous transseptal transsphenoidal approach preserving the middle turbinate and the ethmoidal cells [61]. At that time, Kocher was the head of the surgery in Bern, Switzerland, and obtained the Nobel Prize for his contributions to physiology and surgery of the thyroid gland in 1905. From our present point of view, all these superior transsphenoidal approaches were so destructive that—despite their principal extracranial route through the nose—they cannot be called minimally invasive.

The first transsphenoidal approach which deserves to be named minimally invasive was developed again at the University of Vienna—but this time by ENT surgeons. Forerunner of the endonasal transsphenoidal approach to the pituitary tumours was the Hungarian stemming Markus Hajek (1861–1941). With his publication "*Pathology and therapy of inflammatory diseases of the nose and paranasal sinuses*" in 1899, he belongs to the founders of rhinology. Hajek published an endonasal approach to treat abscesses in the sphenoidal sinus and the posterior ethmoidal cells in 1904 [62]. With the outbreak of the Second World War, he was forced to leave Austria due to his Jewish origin in 1939, and he died in exile in London in 1941. For Oskar Hirsch (1877–1965) working in Vienna at the same department as Hajek, it was then only a small step to extend Hajek's approach through the sphenoidal sinus also into the sella turcica. Hirsch presented in an anatomical study this approach for treatment of pituitary tumours during a session of the Viennese medical society 1909 [63]. Later he modified the approach and used an endonasal submucosal rhino-septal route. He performed the first operation 1910 under local anesthesia in several sessions. The first report with two successful operations was published by him in 1910 [64] and the results of 12 operated patients in 1911 [65]. Later he performed the operations in one single step, and he completed the treatment in case of inaccessible tumour remnats by local radiation therapy. Hirsch fled from the Nazis to Boston in 1939 and worked there as a consultant for ENT surgery at the Massachusetts General Hospital. He comprised his surgical experience with pituitary tumours in his late publications with a review of 277 operations in 1952 [55] and of 413 operated pituitary tumours in 1956 [66].

Simultaneously to Austria in the first decade of the 20th century, there was also a great interest in pituitary surgery in the United States. Harvey Cushing (1869–1939) studied the physiology and the anatomy of the pituitary gland in the Hunterian Laboratory at John Hopkins University in Baltimore since 1904.

The first operation of a pituitary tumour in the States was performed by Allen Buckner Kanavel (1874–1938) in Chicago at the Northwest University introducing the inferior transsphenoidal approach to the pituitary through a skin incision under the nose in 1909 [67]. One of the operated patients was suffering from a pituitary tumour and the second from a malignant tumour at the skull base. Samuel Jason Mixter (1855–1926), working as a surgeon at the Harvard Medical School in Boston, operated by the same method as Kanavel on a man with pituitary tumour and clinical signs of infantilism in 1910 [68, 69]. Samuel Mixter became known also for the first posterior interbody fusion at C1/C2. Later he and his son William Jason Mixter (1880–1953) worked together as neurosurgeons at the Harvard Medical School. The son became later known for the first endoscopic ventriculostomy and the first description of disc herniation. The first who applied a cosmetically satisfactory sublabial oronasal transsphenoidal approach was William Stuart Halstead in 1910 [70]. Halstead (1852–1922) was one of the outstanding surgical personalities in the United States of America at the turn of the 19th century. He spent two years till 1880 in Europe at the beginning of his academic carrier. He was impressed there with the basic medical sciences and the medical education. He had contact there to the most known anatomists, pathologists, and surgeons of that time such as Emil Zuckerkandl, Theodor Billroth, Jan Mikulcz-Radecki, and Hans Chiari. Back in the States, he realized his concept of surgery, science, and education at the John Hopkins University in Baltimore where he was one of the four founders of the medical faculty in 1892. He was the first to establish an educational program for surgeons in the States. Outstanding neurosurgeons like Harvey Cushing (1869–1939) and Walter Dandy (1886–1946) absolved their residency and the surgical training in the John Hopkins hospital and worked there in the Hunterian laboratory—Cushing in the field of endocrinology from 1904 till 1912 and Dandy thereafter performing basic work on CSF circulation. The first operative results from the United States and from Europe were vividly discussed at the American Surgical Society Meeting in 1910, and this discussion of papers of von Eiselsberg, Halstead, Mixter, and Quackenboss was believed to be so important that it was published by Cushing and Kanavel in the same year [71]. Cushing performed by chance in the same month as Oskar Hirsch in Vienna the first sublabial transsphenoidal approach to the pituitary in 1910. Initially Cushing used a modified superior transsphenoidal approach, later the inferior transsphenoidal approach, and finally he gave up the transsphenoidal approach at all and turned to the subfrontal transcranial approach because of less complications less recurrences, and better visual control [72, 73]. At that time, the handling of CSF leakages was problematic and the lack of antibiotics worsened the outcome of patients operated on by a transsphenoidal route. The authority of Harvey Cushing brought about that the transsphenoidal approach to the pituitary tumours was more or less given up for many decades. Only Norman Dott (1897–1973) [74] in Edinburgh, a pupil of Cushing equipped with a light at the speculum tip, and Gerard Guiot (1912–1998) [75] in Paris, using fluoroscopy for better orientation and cisternal pneumography to visualize intraoperatively the suprasellar tumour contours, continued with the transsphenoidal approach to pituitary tumours.

The turning point toward a modern era of transsphenoidal hypophysis surgery started with the application of the microscope to this surgery by the Canadian Neurosurgeon Jules Hardy in 1965 [76, 77]. Microsurgery with improved light also in narrow spaces, such as nasal cavities, contributed essentially to a reintroduction and broader application of the transsphenoidal approach. By means of the microscope a separation of tumour from pituitary gland became possible [78], and Hardy proposed the concept of a microadenoma instead of diffuse hyperplasia of the pituitary gland. In 1968 Hardy enlarged the operative indications and performed a selective anterior hypophysectomy in the treatment of diabetic retinopathy [79]. He developed also suitable instruments in bayonet shape to work with despite coaxial light transmission. The last step consisted in the introduction of endoscopic technique for this procedure by Jho and Carrau in Philadelphia [80] and Cappabianca [81] in Naples which enabled even better illumination and superior control in the deep nasal cavity than with a microscope. Beyond that, the endoscopic technique made it possible to look around the corner in the cavernous sinus and behind the carotid artery with application of angled optics. Since the initial introduction, many different groups all over the world popularized the endonasal technique more and more. The further development of this technique is still ongoing. In this paper only an overview about the history of pituitary surgery is possible. For more detailed information on history of pituitary surgery, I refer the reader to the excellent historical papers on this topic by Liu et al. [82], Lanzino and Laws Jr. [83], and Landolt [54].

4. Endoscopic Treatment of Hydrocephalus

In the second half of the 19th century, Maximilian Nitze, a German physician, developed an endoscope which was serially produced and used as cystoscope in urology at the beginning of the 20th century [84–88]. Nitze's endoscopes had an optical system based on the principle of a Keppler telescope (Figure 9) which produced a virtual, zoomed, and upside down image. The light source was a platinum wire on the tip of the endoscope and required a special cooling system to prevent burning. Nitze developed the first prototype 1866 in Vienna together with the instrument maker Joseph Leiter in the department of surgery under the chairman von Dittel who was deeply intersted in the application of endoscopes in urology [89].

This endoscopic technology was brought across the Atlantic by the German instrument maker Wappler who founded the American Cystoscope Makers Incorporation (ACMI) in 1890. Thus, slightly improved Nitze-type endoscopes with an additional lens to reverse the upside down view were available at the beginning of the 20th century at the American universities. They were mainly applied in urology, gynaecology, and abdominal surgery. In 1910 at the Northwestern University in Chicago, the urologist and founder of andrology Victor Darwin L'Espinasse (1878–1946) and the neurosurgeon Allen Buckner Kanavel (1874–1938) performed the first endoscopic treatment of hydrocephalus by fulguration of the choroid plexus in the lateral ventricle [90]. However, they gave up this procedure after the second child died immediately after the the operation. Simultaneously in 1922 and 1923, Walter Edward Dandy (1886–1946) at John Hopkins

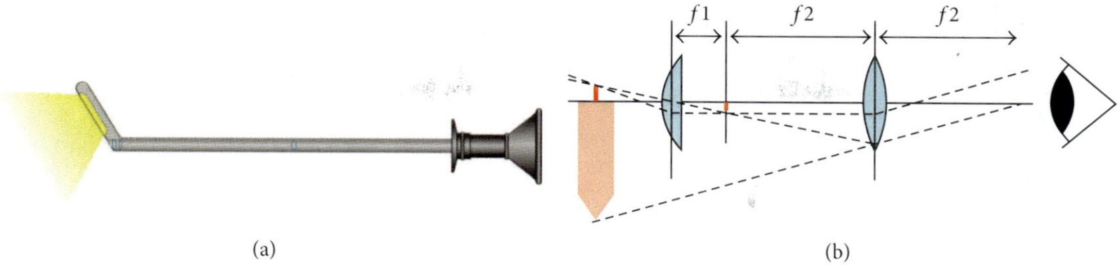

FIGURE 9: Nitze endoscope. (a) Nitze endoscope with a light source at the tip of the instrument and lenses at the tip and approximately at the middle of the shaft. (b) Principle of the Nitze endoscope. The optic is a Keppler telescope producing a virtual zoomed upside down image.

University in Baltimore, Temple Fay (1895–1963) with Francis Clark Grant (1891–1967) at the Temple University in Philadelphia, and William Jason Mixter (1880–1958) in Massachusetts General Hospital in Boston made their first experiences with the endoscope in the treatment of hydrocephalus. Dandy called the endoscope due to its neurosurgical application a ventriculoscope [91]. He recognized the potential of this new technology for neurosurgery but because of technical limitations of the available endoscopes he preferred an open surgical approach to treat hydrocephalus [92–94]. Fay performed only an inspection of the ventricles in one single case and performed photographs of the ventricles. During the procedure he had however to switch to an open procedure. He published his experience with the endoscope and discussed the potentials and the limitations of this method [95]. Mixter performed the first endoscopic ventriculocisternostomy with the same method as it is performed today in 1923 [96]. All of these neurosurgeons gave the endoscopic procedure up due to technical limitations after few trials. Only John Edwin Scarff (1898–1978) who was resident in Baltimore with Dandy continued later at the Columbia University in New York with the neurosurgeon Byron Stookey (1887–1966) to treat hydrocephalus in case of obstructive hydrocephalus by ventriculocisternostomy and in case of malresorptive hydrocephalus by endoscopic fulguration of the choroid plexus [97–99]. The success rate of endoscopic fulguration of the plexus was about 50% and the mortality between 5%–15%. Thus, as soon as shunt system became available in the 50th, the implantation of these valves became the preferred method in the treatment of any type of hydrocephalus. Endoscopic techniques were given up for decades.

The key turning point in the application of endoscopy in neurosurgery was the development of optically improved endoscopes by Harold Horaz Hopkins (1918–1994). Hopkins was Professor of physics at the University of Reading, UK [100, 101]. At the beginning of the 50th, he met at a dinner party a physician complaining about the restricted flexibility of the endoscopes [102]. Hopkins had the idea to use bundles of glass fibres for light conduction by total reflection. This guaranteed a propagation of the light over a longer distance. For this purpose the glass fibres had to be cladded by a material with lower refraction than the glass. Hopkins published the prototype in 1954 in the journal Nature [103] (Figure 10). However his invention found no interest, and he had no money to develop the flexible endoscope to the final product. Hopkins' idea was picked up by the

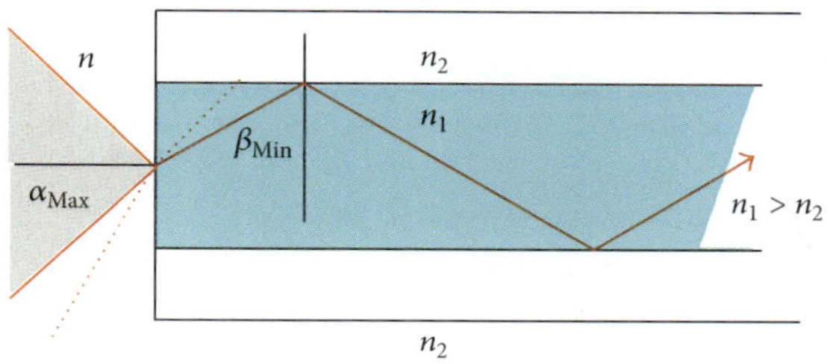

FIGURE 10: Flexible Hopkins fiberscope. The light is propagated in every fiber by total reflection due to the higher refraction of the glass fiber in relation to its cladding isolation.

gastroenterologist Basil Hirschowitz from Ann Arbor, USA, who improved the flexible endoscope and presented it for the first time at a gastroenterological meeting in Colorado in 1957 [104]. Due to the negative experience from the previous invention, Hopkins hesitated to give his consent when he was asked to improve the image quality of rigid endoscopes in 1960. Finally, he agreed to this project, and he constructed 1961 a rigid endoscope with improved image quality, which allowed 80 times better light transmission than the standard endoscopes of that time. This could be achieved by replacing the standard lense with rod lenses which reversed the proportion of air to glass and thus increased nine fold the light transmission (Figure 11). A special cladding of the lenses contributed additionally to a better light conduction. The presentation of this endoscope during a urological meeting in Rio de Janeiro in 1961 was followed again by the same ignorance as his first invention. In 1964, Hopkins was invited to Düsseldorf, Germany, where he presented again the images of his rigid endoscope. This time Karl Storz, the Head and Founder of the Karl Storz Company, Tuttlingen, Germany, attended the meeting, and he realized immediately the great potential of Hopkins invention. A fruitful cooperation began. Storz contributed with an external "cold light" to the final product. The serial production of these endoscopes started in 1967.

In neurosurgery, the advanced endoscopes were used first for diagnostic purposes in the ventricles. Pioneers of the application of the advanced endoscopes in neurosurgery were Gerard Guiot (1912–1998) in Paris [105], Takanori Fukushima in Japan and later in Raleigh, US [106], and Hugh Griffith (1930–1993) in Bristol, UK [107]. In the 80th, endoscopic ventriculostomies were performed by few neurosurgeons

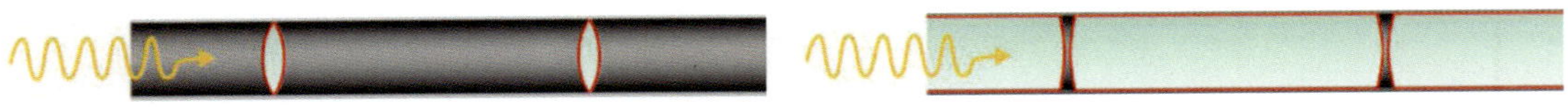

FIGURE 11: Principle of a rigid endoscope. (a) Standard rigid endoscope with high air to glass ratio. (b) Rod lens Hopkins endoscope. The reverse relation of glass to air and better coating of the lenses improves the light transmission 80-fold in comparison to the standard endoscope.

scattered around the whole world—Nigel Jones and Charles Teo in Australia [108, 109], Kim Manwaring and Patric Kelly in the United States [110], and Christian Saint-Rose in Paris [111]. A strong impetus towards a common indication, technical development, with comparable experience and clinical results came at the beginning of the 90th from 3 centres in Germany: from Mainz around Axel Perneczky (1945–2009) [112–114], from Marburg by Dieter Hellwig and Berhard Bauer [115], and from Greifswald by Michael Robert Gaab, Henry Schröder, and Joachim Oertel [116] and from two Benelux countries by Andre Grotenhuis from Nijmegen [117] and by Jaque Caemaert from Ghent [118]. These centres successfully integrated endoscopy as a surgical tool in the concept of the minimally invasive neurosurgery. It is at present a recognized neurosurgical technique to treat obstructive hydrocephalus and further some lesions in or around the ventricles and in combination with microsurgery to check during the procedure the anatomy also around the corner.

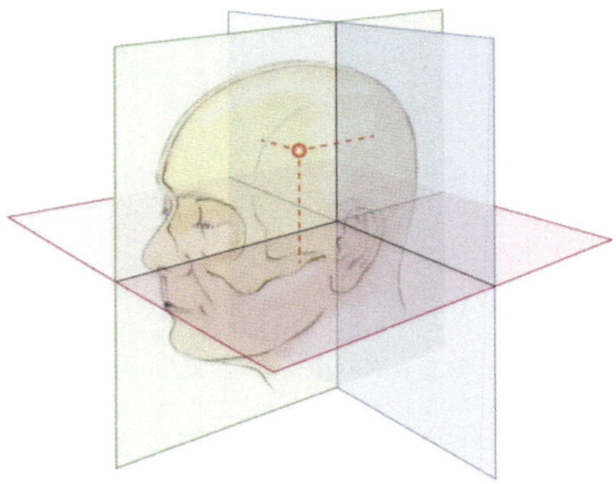

FIGURE 12: Clarke's concept of Cartesian localization. Every point is defined as a distance to three perpendicular planes. Horizontal plane defined as inferior orbital plane running through both acoustic meatus. The frontal plane is perpendicular to the horizontal plane and running through both acoustic meatus. Sagittal plane is perpendicular to the two other planes and divides the head in the midline in two equal parts.

5. Functional Stereotaxy

Originally stereotaxy was developed by the physician Robert Henry Clarke (1850–1926) who worked together with the pioneer of British Neurosurgery Victor Horsley (1857–1916) at the University College in London since 1880. Both scientists were interested at the beginning of the 20th century in the contribution of the cerebellum and the deep cerebellar nuclei to movement. For this purpose, they intended to place electrodes into these deep cerebellar nuclei in apes for electrical stimulation and then to set a precise electrolytic lesion without collateral injury at the target to control the localization. Clarke and Horsley started their project in the Laboratory of Pathological Chemistry at University College in London in 1903. It turned out that a precise placement of the electrodes was difficult due to lacking anatomical landmarks, due to the curvature of the skull, and due to the variable depth which depended additionally on the various thicknesses of the bone and the integument beyond. Clarke developed a method which was independent of these disturbing factors. The idea was to create an intersection of three perpendicular planes and to measure from each plane the distance to the target point (Figure 12).

His long-winded formulation corresponds exactly to the concept of coordinates x, y, and z in a rectangular Cartesian coordinate system. Each distance from a plane coincides exactly with one of the three coordinates. Clarke was not a mathematician and he never used the term coordinates in his publication. In Clarke's formulation each point was in one of the 8 subspaces which were created by intersection of 3 perpendicular planes. A triple of 3 distances from each plane defined the position of the target. The planes had a constant way of construction. The first transversal plane was defined running from the low orbital line through each internal acoustic meatus. The second frontal or coronal plane was perpendicular to the transverse plane and was also running through each acoustic meatus. The third mid sagittal plane was perpendicular to the transverse and the frontal plane diving the head in the middle along the falx. The three distances to the anatomical structures could be read of from an atlas of the apes which were dissected exactly along the three perpendicular planes whose construction was described previously. To reach the target, a rectangular frame was constructed which was fixed to the skull prohibiting head movements during electrode introduction (Figure 13). The frame served also as a stable holder and carrier for the implanted electrodes. Electrolytic lesioning was performed with anodal current. The method was published first as a short report by Clarke as author in 1906 [119] and in detail as coauthor of Horsley in Brain in 1908 [120]. They called this method stereotaxis derived from the ancient Greek words stereos and taxis. Stereos means originally hard or solid but was also used as a technical term in the ancient mathematics to denote a special class of geometrical solids and also the third root of a number because in the ancient mathematics the third root could be visualized geometrically as a diagonal in a three-dimensional cube. Later stereos was

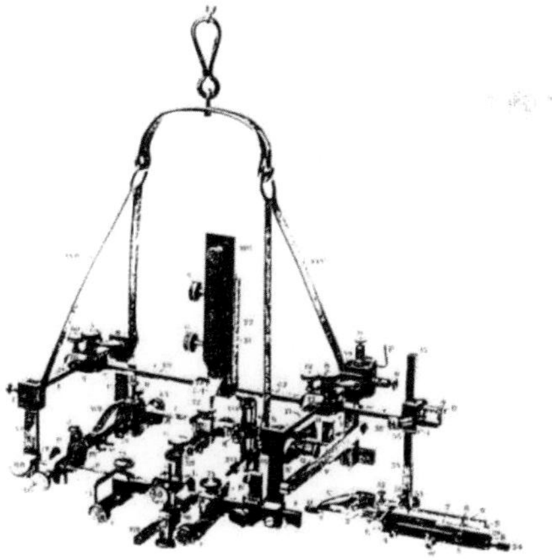

FIGURE 13: Clarke's stereotaxic apparatus for introduction of electrodes into deep nuclei for neurophysiological studies. The frame is fixed to the head and serves as a stable coordinate system and holder for the electrodes.

used to denote spatial and three dimensional in general. Taxis means positioning or placement. Thus, stereotaxis should mean positioning in the 3-dimensional space. Clarke had also the idea to use this method in humans, but this did not occur before 1947. Clarke's idea was picked up by the Canadian anatomist and neurophysiologist Aubrey Mussen who worked with Clarke in London in the first decade of the 20th century. He bought also in London Clarke's stereotaxic system and used it for experimental studies on animals back in the Neurological Institute of McGill University in Montreal, Canada. Mussen's interest was in the anatomy of the brain stem and in particular the anatomy and physiology of the red nucleus and the cerebellum [121]. Mussen constructed also a stereotactic frame for human applications based on Clarke's principle [122]. However, this frame was never used. The stereotactic method had not gained a general acceptance for the application in humans before the Second World War. Although neurophysiologists such as Clarke or Mussen had the idea and also disposed of the necessary knowhow to perform stereotaxic operations in humans, but they did not have the corresponding surgical partners at that time to realize their ideas. The long standing surgical partner of Clarke, Victor Horsley, who would be able to perform a stereotaxic intervention, died in World War I in Mesopotamia in 1916. Mussen developed already a stereotaxic frame for human requirements but he could not convince a surgeon and a neurologist of the method to perform this operation with him. However, retrospectively it has to be admitted that due to the variability of the human skull in comparison to the animals the accuracy of Clarke's calculation method using only external bony reference structures would not have been sufficient for human applications. It is necessary to have additionally at least one internal reference point in the brain, and at that time, the imaging X-ray technique did not allow localizing intracerebral structures.

Ernst Adolf Spiegel (1895–1985), who introduced the human stereotaxy, used an additional internal reference point—at the beginning just the calcified pineal body. Later, he used the posterior commissure as reference point because the pineal body was not always calcified and thus not always visible in radiographic images [123]. The visualization of the posterior commissure required a lateral image of the ventricles through ventriculography. This was achieved initially with air and later with diluted contrast media. Spiegel was originally born in Vienna in 1895. About his time in Austria is not much known. A publication on Hemitetanus in 1920 testifies his residency at the Neurological Institute in Vienna. In 1938, just before the occupation of Austria, he was a lecturer for physiology, neurology, and psychiatry at the University of Vienna. In 1939, he was forced to escape from the Nazis and fled to the United States where he worked at Temple University in Philadelphia as a neurologist. In his historical review on stereotaxy, Spiegel reported that he attended an open psychosurgical intervention in form of a lobotomy in 1947, and he was shocked with regard to the destructiveness of the procedure. He was convinced that this procedure with the same functional effect can be performed much less traumatically by a precise circumscribed lesion in the medial thalamic nucleus. In Philadelphia, Spiegel found in the neurosurgeon Henry Wycis (1911–1972) a skilful surgical partner who was able to realize this minimally invasive stereotaxic method for treatment of functional disorders [124–126]. It comprised the treatment of intractable pain, extrapyramidal movement disorders, epilepsy, and certain psychiatric disorders by means of accurate small circumscribed lesions of pathways or deep seated nuclei of thalamus, basal ganglia, or midbrain. These lesions were very effective and were much less invasive than open procedures in this region. At this time, the knowledge of anatomy, neurophysiology, and imaging technique with pneumoencephalography was so far advanced that an operation in these very eloquent areas seemed sufficiently accurate and safe. As the first stereotaxic operation, a lobotomy was performed with a modified Clarke's frame and the head as additionally fixed with a cast in 1947 (Figure 14) [123]. Only one year later, Spiegel and Wycis performed the first stereotactic operation on a patient with Parkinson's disease. Till the discovery of L-DOPA medication at the end of the 60th, the stereotaxic procedure constituted the only effective therapy of Parkinson disease.

Basically, the functional stereotaxic operations can be understood as procedures in the field of applied neurophysiology. Therefore, these procedures require a deep neurophysiological understanding of stimulation effects besides sophisticated mechanical equipment, good imaging technology, and knowledge of topographical anatomy. Therefore, stereotaxy started to flourish in neurosurgical departments where a close cooperation between a neurosurgeon, a neurologist, a neurophysiologist, a physicist, and an instrument maker was possible to establish.

In Paris, it was the team around the neurosurgeon Jean Talairach (1911–2007) and the Neurophysiologist Jean Bancaud (1921–1993) who introduced stereotaxy in the L'Hôpital St. Anne in 1949 [127]. Talairach showed in his basic stereotactic research work in 1954 that Spiegel's calculations were only accurate for targets close to the reference point of the

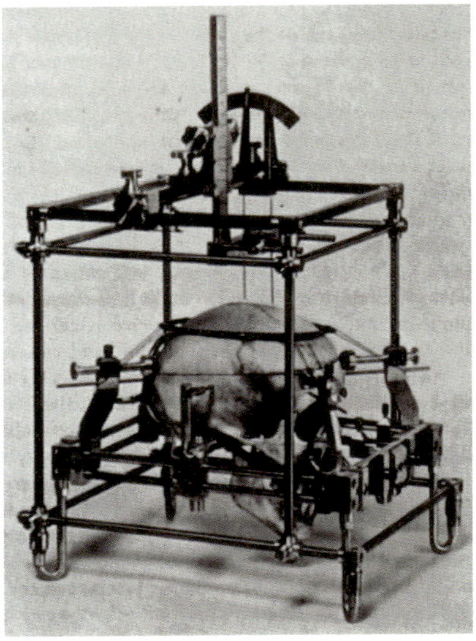

FIGURE 14: Stereotaxic apparatus of Spiegel and Wycis used during the first stereotactic procedures in humans.

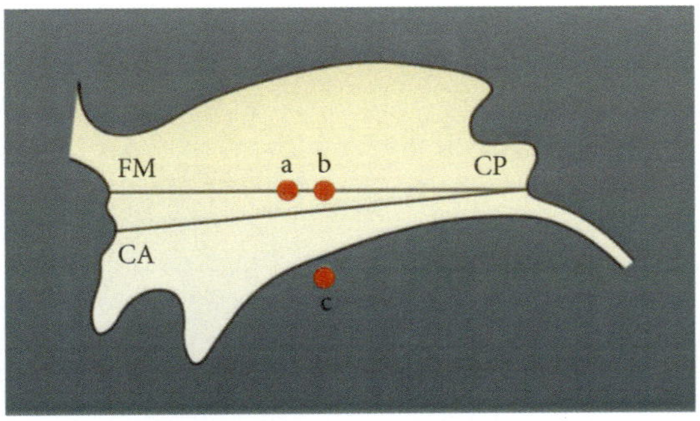

FIGURE 15: Third ventricle in lateral view with the stereotactic baselines for calculation: anterior-posterior commissure (CA-CP) line and the Foramen Monroi-posterior commisure (FM-CP) which was used in case the commissura anterior was not clearly visible. The red points mark the target points in relation to the baselines CA-CP and FM-CP. a: v.o.a. nucleus of thalamus for treating the rigor, b: v.o.p. nucleus of thalamus for treating tremor, c: Forel H field.

posterior commissure and became increasingly inaccurate the more the target was anterior to this reference point. Talairach introduced therefore in addition to the posterior commissure the anterior commissure. The distance connecting these two reference points—the CACP distance—became the stereotactic baseline for localization of deep brain structures independent of individual size and shape (Figure 15) [128]. Also in Paris, Gerard Guiot (1912–1998) established at the L'Hôpital Foch a stereotactic unit in 1958 where he worked together with Madame Denise Albe-Fessard (1916–2003) who was one of the most recognized specialists in neurophysiology of the thalamus and the basal ganglia. They introduced successfully 1961 during stereotaxic operations microelectrode recordings in the thalamus and were able to record tremor sensitive cells intraoperatively in Parkinson patients and thus to delineate the best target for treatment of tremor in the ventrointermediate nucleus (VIM) of the thalamus in [129]. Lars Leksell (1907–1986) at Karolinska Institute working under Herbert Olivecrona developed a target centred stereotactic frame in 1949. It enabled by positioning the target into the isocenter of the frame the surgeon to reach the target from any angle leading to a higher degree of flexibility for the trajectory [130]. In cooperation with Uppsala University cyclotron, he developed with the physicist Borje Larson the first stereotactic irradiation apparatus in 1951 [131]. He called this device due to its precision in Swedish language a "stralkniven" (ray knife). It was a prototype of the later gamma knife, which was developed in 1968 and is a sphere with fixed radiation sources whose gamma rays from all directions cross in the geometrical isocenter. By placing the target area into the isocenter, high dose local radiation can be applied which spares the surrounding brain tissue because the radiation is distributed through about 200 single radiation sources.

In Germany, the centre for stereotactic surgery became Freiburg starting in the 50th of the last century. Trautgott Riechert (1905–1983), the head of the neurosurgery, developed with the physicist and instrument maker Wolff a prototype in 1951 [132] and an advanced version of a very precise stereotactic system based on a polar coordinate system in 1953. The latter was additionally equipped with a phantom to check the coordinates and the trajectory [133]. This system was, due to its mechanical accuracy and the manually subtle instruments and electrodes, the most often used stereotaxic system worldwide till the 80th. The success of the Freiburg group would not be possible without the contribution of Rolf Hassler (1914–1984). He was a neuroanatomist and a specialist in the anatomy of the thalamus. Based on his anatomical knowledge a precise subdivision of thalamic nuclei was elaborated. Due to his work, the thalamus instead, of the basal ganglia, became more and more important for functional stereotaxy—particularly in the treatment of Morbus Parkinson [134]. Later he switched to basic research and was heading a laboratory for the study of Morbus Parkinson at the Max Plank Institute in Frankfurt.

Across the pacific, Spiegel's technique was picked up by Hirotaro Narabayashi (1922–2001) in Japan who developed with Uchimura a stereotactic frame based on the drawings of the stereotactic apparatus of Horsley and Clarke in Tokyo in 1949 [135]. The first successful stereotactic pallidotomy was performed by him in 1951. At this time, he was an Associate Professor of psychiatry at the Jutendo University in Tokyo. Later, he became Chairman of the Department of Neurology at the University of Tokyo. In 1957, he established a private clinic for stereotactic surgery which became a well-known research centre for movement disorders.

At this time, the topographical anatomy for stereotaxic procedures was supported by atlases of the deep brain structures. First atlas for stereotaxic applications was published by Spiegel and Wycis in 1952 [125] and 1962 [126]. Most known and used by the stereotaxic neurosurgeons became the Schaltenbrand-Bailey atlas published by the German neurologist from Würzburg Georg Schaltenbrand (1897–1979) and the pioneer of neuropathology and neurosurgery from Chicago Percival Bailey (1892–1973) in 1959 [136, 137]. A revised and enlarged version of this atlas was published

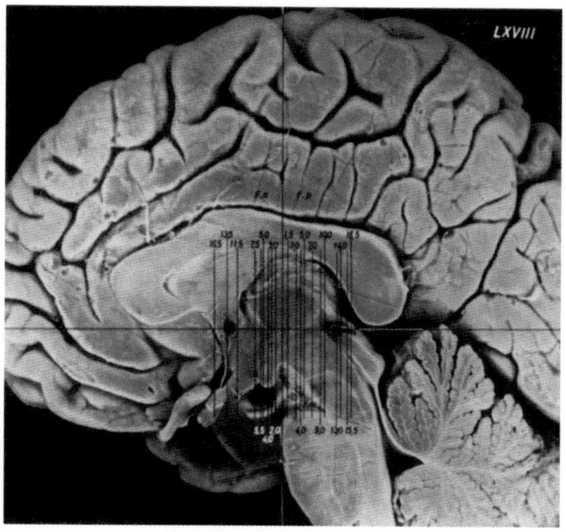

FIGURE 16: Schaltenbrand-Bailey Atlas. Lateral view with scout view of coronal sections of thalamus perpendicular to the stereotactic baseline (anterior-posterior commissure).

together with Waldemar Wahren in 1977. The atlas was based on a cadaver study and consisted of 1–1.5 mm thin sections through the thalamus and the basal ganglia aligned to the CACP line in horizontal, sagittal, and frontal sections. The nomenclature of the detailed thalamic nuclei was influenced by the work of the German neuroscientist Rolf Hassler (1914–1984). The atlas was used by generation of stereotactic neurosurgeons to determine the coordinates of the desired targets in relation to the CACP line (Figure 16).

After the introduction of L-DOPA medication in the 70th the stereotactic surgery lost its most important clientele and the functional stereotactic operations were mostly given up except in few centres. However, 10 years later adverse effects of the drug therapy emerged such as on-off phenomena. Other extrapyramidal diseases such as essential tremor was also only partly treatable by drug medication. Therefore, since the 80th the stereotaxic treatment became again more and more popular. Instead of performing lesions, nondestructive treatment with chronic electrodes for stimulation was successfully introduced into the treatment of movement disorders using the same targets as for lesional stereotaxy. This deep brain stimulation (DBS) was in the 70th and mid 80th primarily used for the treatment of intractable pain. Alim Louis Benabid in Grenoble introduced DBS in 1987 in the VIM nucleus of thalamus for treatment of Morbus Parkinson [138], and Jean Siegfried in Zürich applied this technique in 1994 bilaterally in the pallidum [139]. Due to it effectiveness on tremor rigor and akinesia the Nucleus subthalamicus STN became, due to the work of Benabid in 1994, the preferred target for this disease [140].

6. Towards a Common Philosophy of Minimally Invasive Neurosurgery MIN

The advanced endoscopic technology was primarily applied for diagnostic purposes by gastroenterologists, urologist, orthopaedist, and abdominal surgeons. 1976 these disciplines organized themselves in the US as "surgical study group for endoscopy and ultrasound."

During the 80th, endoscopic procedures were increasingly applied in the abdominal surgery. The indication comprised inguinal herniations, appendectomies, cholecystectomies, and also tumors of the digestive tract. This new endoscopic surgery required the development of new surgical instruments and required an operative technique which was very different from the standard open operations regarding the visual control using only a screen and have an image distortion with a fisheye effect. The different handling of the instruments required a special training. This caused the endoscopic surgery to become increasingly recognized as an independent discipline. The British surgeon John EA Wickham coined for these procedures in 1984 the term minimally invasive surgery. He published his philosophy of this type of surgery in the British Medical Bulletin 1986 [141]. He understood the endoscopic surgery as a new minimally invasive method in opposition to the standard open operative procedures. In neurosurgery, the term minimally invasive neurosurgery acquired a slightly different interpretation. In neurosurgery as I showed in this paper in four examples from different neurosurgical fields, endoscopy was not the single technical development which contributed to making of a surgical procedure less traumatic and invasive. In neurosurgery converged with endoscopy, the neuronavigation, the stereotaxy, the 3D planning computer workstations, and the planning of individual microsurgical approaches based on the anatomical peculiarities and details of the pathology in all fields of neurosurgery toward a common philosophy of minimally invasive neurosurgery. The endoscope became only a useful tool during a part of the microsurgical procedure.

The neurosurgeon who deserves the greatest merits in developing and popularizing the minimally invasive technique for neurosurgery was at the end of the 80th Axel Perneczky (1945–2009), a Hungarian stemming consultant of neurosurgery at the University of Vienna. In Vienna he was at that time a recognized neurosurgeon in the field of vascular microsurgery. The philosophy of minimally invasive surgery suited very much his general neurosurgical concept. His ambition was to minimize as much as possible the intraoperative trauma for the patient respecting also the cosmetic aspects. This could be achieved by careful and thorough preoperative planning of the best approach which was based on a detailed analysis of individual anatomy and topographic relationships of the lesion visible in the radiological images. The lowest functional intraoperative trauma required sometimes new and unusual approaches such as the contralateral approach to the suprasellar region or through the lateral ventricle. The new approaches required detailed knowledge of topographic anatomy, which he acquired while working as demonstrator at the anatomical institute in Vienna and in the late 70th while working at the laboratory of Gazi Yasargil in Zurich. Perneczky understood neurosurgery as applied neuroanatomy. In 1988, Perneczky became Chairman of the Neurosurgery at the Johannes Gutenberg University in Mainz. There, he organized a team of neurosurgeons which started to realize his idea of minimally invasive neurosurgery. The clinical application preceded work in basic research. With his friend Manfred Tschabitscher, anatomist at the University of Vienna, Perneczky studied the anatomy of the ventricles and the basal cisterns from an endoscopic view [142]. The neurosurgeon Klaus Resch completed in Mainz the anatomical study by postmortem endoscopic inspections. He convinced also Perneczky of the superiority of rigid endoscopes over flexible endoscopes for neurosurgery due to the much better image quality. Additionally, a laboratory was established for anatomical studies on cadavers. The first meeting in Mainz in 1989 on the subject of minimally invasive neurosurgery was too early and not successful. The breakthrough of this new technique in neurosurgery was the international meeting in Wiesbaden in 1993 for minimally invasive neurosurgery. This meeting, organized by Perneczky, gathered for the first time all neurosurgeons involved worldwide in neuroendoscopy and was also attended by many internationally recognized neurosurgeons. Their basic approval of this new method had a stimulating effect for the irradiation of these new techniques and philosophy around the whole world. During this meeting a society for minimally invasive neurosurgery (MIN) was established with international conferences every 2 years and a journal with the same name. The spark of minimally invasive neurosurgery spread also to the industry and with Minop1 and Minop2 projects for development of minimally invasive technology, instruments became supported and sponsored by many companies. For Perneczky minimally invasive neurosurgery comprised not only endoscopy. The endoscope was only a tool during the operation or a part of the operation. Minimally invasive neurosurgery comprised all surgical instruments or devices and operative techniques which helped to diminish the intraoperative trauma including 3-D operation planning workstations, navigation devices, and endoscopes. He demonstrated that by the key hole effect also huge deep seated brain tumours can be satisfactorily controlled and removed through a small craniotomy [143, 144].

As I could show in this paper Perneczky was not the founder of minimally invasive methods in neurosurgery. These ideas started to be realized even by the pioneers of the neurosurgery. Interestingly, the great historic neurosurgical personalities were usually creative spirits not only in one but also in several neurosurgical fields. However, Perneczky deserves the merit of bundling and further developing all the new technical developments existent in the late 80th under a common neurosurgical concept of minimally invasive neurosurgery. Although Perneczky was one of the protagonists of this new philosophy, he would not be successful if not other neurosurgical centres in Europe and in other continents had at the same time simultaneously similar ideas and intentions. In particular in Germany it was the neurosurgery in Greifswald with Michael Gaab, Henry Schöder, and Joachim Oertel, in Marburg with Bernhard Bauer and Dieter Hellwig, and in the Benelux countries by Andre Grotenhuis, a close friend of Perneczky in Nijmegen and Jaque Caemmaert in Ghent who also essentially contributed to the development and promotion of this new surgical philosophy and technology in neurosurgery. All these groups exchanged their experiences during frequent international endoscopic, navigation, and keyhole surgery courses which were performed with the intention of education and hands-on training for neurosurgeons interested in this new field.

Acknowledgment

The author thanks Stefan Kindel for the excellent graphical contributions.

References

[1] Homer, *Iliad*, vol. 18, Harvard university press, London, UK, pp. 372–378, 1974.

[2] Homer, *Iliad*, vol. 18, Harvard university press, London, UK, pp. 416–420, 1974.

[3] J. P. M. Flourens, *Recherches Experimenteles sur les Proprieties e les Fonctions du Système Nerveux dans les Animaux Vertébrés*, Chez Crevot, Paris, France, 1st edition, 1824.

[4] F. Gall, *Sur les Fonctions du Cerveau et sur celles de Chacune de ses Parties*, Schoell, Paris, France, 1822.

[5] P. Broca, "Perte de la parole, ramollissement chronique et destruction partielle du lobe antérieur gauche," *Bulletin De La Société D'Anthropologie*, vol. 2, pp. 235–238, 1861.

[6] P. Broca, "Localisations des fonctions cérébeles. Siège de la faculté du langage articulé," *Bulletin De La Société D'Anthropologie*, vol. 4, pp. 200–208, 1863.

[7] J. H. Jackson, "Loss of speech," *Clinical Lecture and Reports of London Hospital*, vol. 1, article 459, 1864.

[8] C. Wernicke, *Der Aphasische Komplex. Eine Psychologische Studie Auf Anatomischer Basis*, Cohn and Weigert, Breslau, Poland, 1874.

[9] C. Golgi, "Sulla struttura della sostanza grigia del cervello," *Gazzetta Medica Italiana*, vol. 33, pp. 244–246, 1873.

[10] S. Ramon y Cajal and L. Azoulay, *Les Nouveles Idée Sur la Structure du Système Nerveux chez l'Homme et chez les Vertébrés*, 1894.

[11] C. Vogt and O. Vogt, "Die vergleichend-architektonische und die vergleichend-reizphysiologische Felderung der Großhirnrinde unter besonderer Berücksichtigung der menschlichen," *Die Naturwissenschaften*, vol. 14, no. 50-51, pp. 1190–1194, 1926.

[12] K. Brodmann, "Vergleichende Lokalisationslehreder Großhirnrinde," in *Ihren Principien Dargestellt Auf Grund Des Zellaufbaues*, Ja Barth, Leipzig, Germany, 1909.

[13] G. Fritsch and E. Hitzig, "Über die elektrische Erregbarkeit des Grosshirns," *Archiv Fur Anatomie, Physiologie Und Wissenschaftliche Medicin*, vol. 37, pp. 300–332, 1870.

[14] D. Ferrier, *The Functions of the Brain*, Smith Elder and Co, London, UK, 1876.

[15] V. Horsley, "Discussion on cerebral localization," *Transactions of the Congress of American Physicians and Surgeons*, vol. 1, pp. 34–35, 1888.

[16] C. S. Sherrington, *The Integrative Action of the Nervous System*, Cambridge University press, 1906.

[17] A. Leyton and C. S. Sherrington, "Observations on the excitable cortex of chimpanzee, Orang-Utan and gorilla," *Experimental Physiology*, vol. 11, pp. 135–222, 1917.

[18] H. Cushing, "A note upon the faradic stimulation of the postcentral gyrus in conscious patients," *Brain*, vol. 32, no. 1, pp. 44–53, 1909.

[19] S. Uematsu, R. P. Lesser, and B. Gordon, "Localization of sensorimotor cortex: the influence of Sherrington and Cushing on the modern concept," *Neurosurgery*, vol. 30, no. 6, pp. 904–912, 1992.

[20] F. Krause, *Chirurgische Operationslehre Des Kopfes*, vol. 2, Berlin, Germany, 1912.

[21] F. Krause, *Chirurgische Operationslehre Des Kopfes*, vol. 2, Berlin, Germany, 1914.

[22] O. Foerster, "Zur Pathogenese und chirurgischer Behandlung der Epilepsie," *Zentrblattfiir Chirurgie*, vol. 52, pp. 513–560, 1925.

[23] R. U. Krönlein, "Zur cranio cervikalen Topographie Beiträge," *Zeitschrift Fur Klinik Chirurgie*, vol. 22, pp. 364–370, 1898.

[24] G. Hildebrandt, M. N. Stienen, J. Patzer, and W. Surbeck, "Neurosurgical contributions of the Swiss surgeon, Rudolf Ulrich Krönlein: a further pioneer in Swiss neurosurgery," *Acta Neurochirurgica*, vol. 154, no. 10, pp. 1923–1933, 2012.

[25] T. Kocher, *Chirurgische Operationslehre*, Fischer Verlag, Jena, Germany, 1892.

[26] G. Hildebrandt, W. Surbeck, and M. N. Stienen, "Emil Theodor Kocher: the first Swiss neurosurgeon," *Acta Neurochirurgica*, pp. 1–11, 2012.

[27] D. Zernov, "Entsefalometr-ustroistvo dlya mozgovych strictur u zhivogo choloveka. Predvaritel'noe soobshenie," *Trudi Fiziko-Meditsinskogo Obshestva Moskovskogo Universiteta*, vol. 2, pp. 70–80, 1889.

[28] N. Altukhov, *EntsefalometrIya Mozga CholoveKa v OtnoshenII K Polu, vo Zrastu I Cherepnomu Ukazatelyu*, Isdatelstvo Moscovskogo Universiteta, Moscow, Russia, 1891.

[29] E. I. Kandel and Y. V. Schavinsky, "Stereotaxic apparatus and operations in Russia in the 19th century," *Journal of Neurosurgery*, vol. 37, no. 4, pp. 407–411, 1972.

[30] B. L. Lichterman, "Roots and routes of Russian neurosurgery (from surgical neurology towards neurological surgery)," *Journal of the History of the Neurosciences*, vol. 7, no. 2, pp. 125–135, 1998.

[31] R. Satran, "G.I. Rossolimo (1860-1928)," *Journal of Neurology*, vol. 252, pp. 1423–1424, 2005.

[32] G. I. Rossolimo, "Mozgovoi topograf," *Zhurnal Nevropatologii I Psikhiatrii Imeni Korsakova*, vol. 7, no. 24, pp. 640–644, 1907.

[33] W. E. Dandy, "Ventriculography following the injection of air into the cerebral ventricles," *American Journal of Roentgenology*, vol. 174, no. 1, p. 201, 2000.

[34] E. Moniz, "L'encephalographie arterielle son importance dans la localization des tumeurs cerebrales," *Revue Neurologique*, vol. 2, pp. 72–90, 1927.

[35] J. Denavit and R. S. Hartenberg, "A kinematic notion for lower-paired mechanisms based on matrices," *Journal of Applied Mechanics*, vol. 22, pp. 215–221, 1955.

[36] L. G. Roberts, "Machine perception of three-dimensional solids," Tech. Rep. 315, Lincoln Laboratory, Massachustts Intitute of Technology, 1963.

[37] L. G. Roberts, "Homogenous matrix representation and manipulation of N-dimensional constructs," Tech. Rep. MS1045, Lincoln Laboratory Massachusetts Institute of Technology, 1965.

[38] D. L. Pieper, "The kinematics of manipulators under computer control," AIM 72, Standford Artificial Intelligece Laboratory, Standford University, 1968.

[39] Y. S. Kwoh, J. Hou, E. A. Jonckheere, and S. Hayati, "A robot with improved absolute positioning accuracy for CT guided stereotactic brain surgery," *IEEE Transactions on Biomedical Engineering*, vol. 35, no. 2, pp. 153–160, 1988.

[40] J. M. Drake, M. Joy, A. Goldenberg, and D. Kreindler, "Computer- and robot-assisted resection of thalamic astrocytomas in children," *Neurosurgery*, vol. 29, no. 1, pp. 27–31, 1991.

[41] A. L. Benabid, S. Lavallee, D. Hoffmann, P. Cinquin, J. Demongeot, and F. Danel, "Computer-driven robot for stereotactic neurosurgery. Computers in stereotactic surgery," *Blackwell Scientific Boston*, pp. 330–642, 1992.

[42] G. Schlöndorff, D. Meyer-Ebrecht, R. Mösges, W. Krybus, and L. Adams, "CAS: computer assisted surgery," *Archives of Otolaryngology*, vol. 2, article 45, supplement, 1987.

[43] E. Watanabe, T. Watanabe, and S. Manaka, "Three-dimensional digitizer (neuronavigator): new equipment for computed tomography-guided stereotaxic surgery," *Surgical Neurology*, vol. 27, no. 6, pp. 543–547, 1987.

[44] J. M. Drake, J. T. Rutka, and H. J. Hoffman, "ISG Viewing Wand System," *Neurosurgery*, vol. 34, no. 6, pp. 1094–1097, 1994.

[45] H. Reinhardt, H. Meyer, and E. Amrein, "A computer-assisted device for the intraoperative CT-correlated localization of brain tumors," *European Surgical Research*, vol. 20, no. 1, pp. 51–58, 1988.

[46] A. Kato, T. Yoshimine, T. Hayakawa et al., "A frameless, armless navigational system for computer-assisted neurosurgery: technical note," *Journal of Neurosurgery*, vol. 74, no. 5, pp. 845–849, 1991.

[47] L. J. Zamorano, L. Nolte, A. M. Kadi, and Z. Jiang, "Interactive intraoperative localization using an infrared-based system," *Neurological Research*, vol. 15, no. 5, pp. 290–298, 1993.

[48] D. W. Roberts, J. W. Strohbehn, and J. F. Hatch, "A frameless stereotaxic integration of computerized tomographic imaging and the operating microscope," *Journal of Neurosurgery*, vol. 65, no. 4, pp. 545–549, 1986.

[49] B. Westermann, M. Trippel, and H. Reinhardt, "Optically-navigable operating microscope for image-guided surgery," *Minimally Invasive Neurosurgery*, vol. 38, no. 3, pp. 112–116, 1995.

[50] M. Pierre, "Sur deux cas d'acromegalie hypertrophie singuliere non congenital des extremiteties superiores inferieures et cephalic," *Review of Medicine*, vol. 6, pp. 297–333, 1886.

[51] J. Babinski, "Tumeur du corps pituitair sans acromegalie et avec arret de development des organs genitaux," *Revue Neurologique*, vol. 8, pp. 531–533, 1900.

[52] A. Fröhlich, "Ein Fall von Tumor der Hypophyse ohne Acromegalie," *Wien Klin Wochenschr*, vol. 15, pp. 883–886, 1901.

[53] J. R. Pollock, J. Akinwunmi, F. Scaravilli et al., "Transcranial surgery for pituitary tumors performed by Sir Victor Horsley," *Neurosurgery*, vol. 52, no. 4, pp. 914–926, 2003.

[54] A. M. Landolt, "History of pituitary surgery," in *A History of Neurosurgery in Its Scientific and Professional Contexts*, pp. 373–400, Greenblatt, 1997.

[55] O. Hirsch, "Symptoms and treatment of pituitary tumors," *Acta Oto-Laryngologica*, vol. 55, pp. 268–306, 1952.

[56] E. Zuckerkandl, *Normale und pathologische Anatomie der Nasenhöhlen und ihrer pneumatisierten Anhänge*, Braumüller, Vienna, Austria, 1882.

[57] H. Schloffer, "Zur Frage der Operation an der Hypophyse," *Beiträge zur klinischen Chirurgie*, vol. 50, pp. 767–817, 1906.

[58] H. Schloffer, "Erfolgreiche operation an der hypophyse auf nasalem Weg," *Wien Klin Wochenschr*, vol. 20, pp. 621–624, 1907.

[59] A. H. von Eiselsberg, "My experience about operation upon the hypophysis," *Annals of Surgery*, vol. 52, pp. 1–14, 1910.

[60] J. Hochenegg, "Zur Therapie von Hypophysentumoren," *Deutsche Zeitschrift für Chirurgie*, vol. 100, no. 1, pp. 317–326, 1909.

[61] T. Kocher, "Ein Fall von Hypophysis-Tumor mit operativer Heilung," *Deutsche Zeitschrift für Chirurgie*, vol. 100, no. 1, pp. 13–37, 1909.

[62] M. Hajek, "Diagnose und intranasale Chirurgie in der Behandlung von Eiterungen der Keilbeinhöhle und des hinteren Siebbeinlabyrinthes," *Archives of Oto-Rhino-Laryngology*, vol. 16, pp. 105–143, 1904.

[63] O. Hirsch, "Eine neue Methode der endonasalen Operation von Hypophysentumoren," *Wien Klin Wochenschr*, vol. 59, pp. 578–580, 1909.

[64] O. Hirsch, "Endonasal method of removal of hypophyseal tumors. With a report of two successfully operated cases," *JAMA*, vol. 55, pp. 772–774, 1910.

[65] O. Hirsch, "Über endonasale Operationsmethode bei Hypophysentumoren mit Bericht über 12 Fälle," *Berl Klin Wochenschr*, vol. 48, pp. 1933–1935, 1911.

[66] O. Hirsch, "Pituitary tumors A borderland between cranial and transsphenoidal surgery," *The New England Journal of Medicine*, vol. 254, pp. 937–939, 1956.

[67] A. B. Kanavel, "The removal of tumours of the pituitary body by an infranasal route. A proposed operation with a description of the technique," *JAMA*, vol. 53, pp. 1704–1707, 1909.

[68] S. J. Mixter and A. Quackenboss, "Tumor of the hypopysis (with infantililism)," *Annals of Surgery*, vol. 52, pp. 15–22, 1910.

[69] S. J. Mixter and A. Quackenboss, "Tumor of hypophysis," *Transactions of the American Surgical Association*, vol. 28, pp. 94–109, 1910.

[70] A. E. Halstead, "Remarks on the operative treatment of tumors of the hypophysis with a report of two cases operated on by an oro-nasal method," *Transactions of the American Surgical Association*, vol. 28, pp. 73–93, 1910.

[71] H. Cushing, A. B. Kanavel, and D. Lewis, "Discussion of papers by von Eiselsberg, Halstead, Mixter and Quackenboss," *Transactions of the American Surgical Association*, vol. 28, pp. 110–115, 1910.

[72] H. Cushing, "The Weir Mitchell lecture. Surgical experiences with pituitary disorders," *JAMA*, vol. 63, pp. 1515–1525, 1914.

[73] H. Cushing, *Intracranial tumours. Notes upon a series of two thousand verified cases with surgical mortality percentage*, Charles Thomas, Springfield, Ill, USA, 1932.

[74] N. M. Dott and P. S. Bailey, "A consideration of the hypophyseal adenomata," *British Journal of Surgery*, vol. 13, pp. 699–707, 1925.

[75] G. Guiot and B. Thibaut, "L'extirpation des adénomes hypophysaires par voie trans-sphenoidale," *Neurochirurgia*, vol. 1, pp. 133–150, 1959.

[76] J. Hardy and S. M. Wigser, "Trans-sphenoidal surgery of pituitary fossa tumors with televised radiofluoroscopic control," *Journal of Neurosurgery*, vol. 23, no. 6, pp. 612–619, 1965.

[77] J. Hardy, "La chirurgie de l'hypophyse par voie transsphenoidale. Etude comparative de deux modalités techniques," *Annales De Chirurgie*, vol. 21, pp. 1011–1022, 1967.

[78] J. Hardy, "Transphenoidal microsurgery of the normal and pathological pituitary," *Clinical neurosurgery*, vol. 16, pp. 185–217, 1969.

[79] J. Hardy and I. S. Ciric, "Selective anterior hypophysectomy in the treatment of diabetic retinopathy. A transsphenoidal microsurgical technique," *Journal of the American Medical Association*, vol. 203, no. 2, pp. 73–78, 1968.

[80] H.-D. Jho and R. L. Carrau, "Endoscopy Assisted Transsphenoidal Surgery for Pituitary Adenoma: Technical Note," *Acta Neurochirurgica*, vol. 138, no. 12, pp. 1416–1425, 1996.

[81] P. Cappabianca, A. Alfieri, and E. De Divitiis, "Endoscopic endonasal transsphenoidal approach to the sella: Towards functional endoscopic pituitary surgery (FEPS)," *Minimally Invasive Neurosurgery*, vol. 41, no. 2, pp. 66–73, 1998.

[82] J. K. Liu, A. A. Cohen-Gadol, E. R. Laws Jr., C. D. Cole, P. Kan, and W. T. Couldwell, "Harvey Cushing and Oskar Hirsch: Early forefathers of modern transsphenoidal surgery," *Journal of Neurosurgery*, vol. 103, no. 6, pp. 1096–1104, 2005.

[83] G. Lanzino and E. R. Laws Jr., "Key personalities in the development and popularization of the transsphenoidal approach to pituitary tumors: An historical overview," *Neurosurgery Clinics of North America*, vol. 14, no. 1, pp. 1–10, 2003.

[84] J. Shah, "Endoscopy through the ages," *BJU International*, vol. 89, no. 7, pp. 645–652, 2002.

[85] D. Schultheiss and F. Moll, *Die Geschichte Der Urologie in Dresden*, Springer, Berlin, Germany, 2009.

[86] A. B. Verger-Kuhnke, M. A. Reuter, and M. L. Beccaría, "The biography of Maximilian Nitze (1848-1906) and its contribution to the urology," *Actas Urologicas Espanolas*, vol. 31, no. 7, pp. 697–704, 2007.

[87] C. Netzhat, "The era Nitze chapter chapter 11(b) History of Endoscopy," 2005, http://laparoscopy.blogs.com/endoscopyhistory/chapter_11/.

[88] M. Nitze, *Lehrbuch Der Kystoskopie. Technik Und Klinische Bedeutung*, Von Bergmann, Wiesbaden, Germany, 1889.

[89] J. Leiter, *Elektro-Endoskopische Instrumente. Beschreibung und Instruction durch M. Nitze und J. Leiter*, Wilhelm Braunmüller und Söhne Wien, 1880.

[90] Northwestern university Feinberg School of medicine. Department of history, http://www.feinberg.northwestern.edu/neurosurgery/residency/history.

[91] W. Hsu, K. W. Li, M. Bookland, and G. I. Jallo, "Keyhole to the brain: Walter Dandy and neuroendoscopy. Historical vignette," *Journal of Neurosurgery*, vol. 3, no. 5, pp. 439–442, 2009.

[92] W. E. Dandy and K. D. Blackfan, "An experimental and clinical study on internal hydrocephalus," *JAMA*, vol. 61, pp. 2216–2217, 1913.

[93] W. E. Dandy and K. D. Blackfan, "Internal hydrocephalus. An experimental clinical and pathological study," *The American Journal of Diseases of Children*, vol. 8, pp. 406–482, 1914.

[94] W. E. Dandy, *Practice of Surgery*, chapter 1, WF Prior Company, Hagerstown, Md, USA, 1932.

[95] T. Fay and F. C. Grant, "Ventriculoscopy and intraventricular photography in internal hydrocephalus," *JAMA*, vol. 80, pp. 461–463, 1923.

[96] W. J. Mixter, "Ventriculoscopy and puncture of the floor of the third ventricle," *Boston Medical and Surgical Journal*, vol. 188, pp. 277–278, 1923.

[97] J. E. Scarff, "Endoscopic treatment of hydrocephalus: description of the ventriculoscope and primary report of cases," *Archives of Neurology and Psychiatry*, vol. 35, pp. 853–861, 1936.

[98] J. E. Scarff and B. Stookey, "Treatment of obstructive hydrocephalus by third ventriculostomy. Report of two cases," *Archives of Neurology*, vol. 36, pp. 1400–1411, 1936.

[99] J. E. Scarff, "Treatment of obstructive hydrocephalus by puncture of the lamina terminalis and floor of the third ventricle," *Journal of neurosurgery*, vol. 8, no. 2, pp. 204–213, 1951.

[100] H. H. Hopkins and H. J. Tiziani, "A theoretical and experimental study of lens centring errors and their influence on optical image quality," *British Journal of Applied Physics*, vol. 17, no. 1, article no. 303, pp. 33–54, 1966.

[101] H. H. Hopkins, *Wave Theory of Aberrations*, Oxford university press, 1950.

[102] C. W. Mc Combie and J. Smith, "Harold Horaz Hopkins. 6. December 1918-22. October 1994," *Biographical Memories Fellows of the Royal Sociaty*, vol. 44, pp. 239–252, 1998.

[103] H. H. Hopkins and N. S. Kapany, "A flexible fibrescope, using static scanning," *Nature*, vol. 173, no. 4392, pp. 39–41, 1954.

[104] B. I. Hirschowitz, L. E. Curtis, C. W. Peters, and H. M. Pollard, "Demonstration of a new gastroscope: the fiberscope," *Gastroenterology*, vol. 35, no. 1, pp. 50–53, 1958.

[105] G. Guiot, J. Rougerie, M. Fourestier et al., "Intracranial endoscopic explorations," *La Presse Médicale*, vol. 71, pp. 1225–1228, 1963.

[106] T. Fukushima, B. Ishijima, and K. Hirakawa, "Ventriculofiberscope: a new technique for endoscopic diagnosis and operation: technical note," *Journal of Neurosurgery*, vol. 38, no. 2, pp. 251–256, 1973.

[107] H. B. Griffith, "Endoneurosurgery: endoscopic intracranial surgery," in *Advances and Technical Standards in Neurosurgery*, L. Symon, Ed., vol. 14, pp. 3–24, Springer, 1986.

[108] R. F. C. Jones, B. C. T. Kwok, W. A. Stening, and M. Vonau, "The current status of endoscopic third ventriculostomy in the management of non-communicating hydrocephalus," *Minimally Invasive Neurosurgery*, vol. 37, no. 1, pp. 28–36, 1994.

[109] C. Teo and R. Jones, "Management of hydrocephalus by endoscopic third ventriculostomy in patients with myelomeningocele," *Pediatric Neurosurgery*, vol. 25, no. 2, pp. 57–63, 1996.

[110] P. J. Kelly, S. Goerss, B. A. Kall, and D. B. Kispert, "Computed tomography-based stereotactic third ventriculostomy: technical note," *Neurosurgery*, vol. 18, no. 6, pp. 791–794, 1986.

[111] C. Sainte-Rose, "Third ventriculostomy," in *Neuroendoscopy*, H. K. Manwaring and K. R. Crone, Eds., Mary Ann Lieber, New York, NY, USA, 1992.

[112] A. Perneczky, A. Cohen, B. George, and T. Kanno, *MinimallyInvasive Neurosurgery*, vol. 37, article 1, 1994.

[113] A. Perneczky and G. Fries, "Endoscope-assisted brain surgery. Part 1: evolution, basic concept, and current technique," *Neurosurgery*, vol. 42, no. 2, pp. 219–225, 1998.

[114] P. Grunert, A. Perneczky, and K. Resch, "Endoscopic procedures through the foramen interventriculare of Monro under stereotactical conditions," *Minimally Invasive Neurosurgery*, vol. 37, no. 1, pp. 2–8, 1994.

[115] D. Hellwig and B. L. Bauer, "Minimally invasive neurosurgery by means of ultrathin endoscopes," *Acta Neurochirurgica, Supplement*, vol. 54, pp. 63–68, 1992.

[116] M. R. Gaab and H. W. S. Schroeder, "Neuroendoscopic approach to intraventricular lesions," *Journal of Neurosurgery*, vol. 88, no. 3, pp. 496–505, 1998.

[117] J. A. Grotenhuis and T. Been, "The role of endoscopic third ventriculostomy in the treatment of hydrocephalus associated with myelomeningocele," *Minimally Invasive Neurosurgery*, vol. 42, pp. 161–162, 1999.

[118] J. Caemaert, J. Abdullah, L. Calliauw, D. Carton, C. Dhooge, and R. Van Coster, "Endoscopic treatment of suprasellar arachnoid cysts," *Acta Neurochirurgica*, vol. 119, no. 1–4, pp. 68–73, 1992.

[119] R. H. Clarke and V. Horsley, "On a method of investigating the deep ganglia and tracts of the central nervous system (cerebellum)," *Clinical Orthopaedics and Related Research*, vol. 463, pp. 1799–1800, 2007.

[120] V. Horsley and R. H. Clarke, "The structure and functions of the cerebellum examined by a new method," *Brain*, vol. 31, no. 1, pp. 45–124, 1908.

[121] A. T. Mussen, *Cerebellum and the Red Nucleus: Anatomy and Physiology*, Haffner, New York, NY, USA, 1967.

[122] C. Picard, A. Olivier, and G. Bertrand, "The first human stereotaxic apparatus. The contribution of Aubrey Mussen to the field of stereotaxis," *Journal of Neurosurgery*, vol. 59, no. 4, pp. 673–676, 1983.

[123] E. A. Spiegel, H. T. Wycis, and H. W. Baird, "Studies in Stereoencephalotomy. I. Topical relationships of subcortical structures to the posterior commissure," *Confinia Neurologica*, vol. 12, no. 3, pp. 121–133, 1952.

[124] E. A. Spiegel, H. T. Wycis, M. Marks, and A. J. Lee, "Stereotaxic apparatus for operations on the human brain," *Science*, vol. 106, no. 2754, pp. 349–350, 1947.

[125] E. A. Spiegel and H. T. Wycis, *Stereoencephalotomy Part I*, Grune and Stratton, New York, NY, USA, 1952.

[126] E. A. Spiegel and H. T. Wycis, *Stereoencephalotomy Part II*, Grune and Stratton, New York, NY, USA, 1962.

[127] J. Talairach, H. Hecaen, and M. David, "Recherches sur la coagulation therapeutique des structures sous-cortical chez l'home," *Revue Neurologique*, vol. 81, pp. 4–24, 1949.

[128] J. Talairach, "Les explorations radiologique stereotaxique," *Revue Neurologique*, vol. 90, pp. 556–584, 1954.

[129] G. Guiot, J. Hardy, and D. Albe-Fessard, "Delimination precise des structures souscorticales et identification de noyuax thalamique chez l'homme par l'electrophysiologie stereotaxique," *Neurochirugia*, vol. 5, pp. 1–18, 1961.

[130] L. Leksell, "A stereotactic apparatus for intracerebral surgery," *Acta Chirurgica Scandinavica*, vol. 99, pp. 229–233, 1949.

[131] L. Leksell, "The stereotaxic method and radiosurgery of the brain," *Acta chirurgica Scandinavica*, vol. 102, no. 4, pp. 316–319, 1951.

[132] T. Riechert and M. Wolff, "Über ein neues Zielgerät zur intrakraniellen elektrischen Ableitung und Ausschaltung," *Archiv für Psychiatrie und Nervenkrankheiten*, vol. 186, no. 2, pp. 225–230, 1951.

[133] T. Riechert and M. Wolff, "Die technische Durchführung von gezielten Hirnoperationen," *Archiv für Psychiatrie und Nervenkrankheiten*, vol. 190, no. 4, pp. 297–316, 1953.

[134] R. Hassler and T. Riechert, "Indications and localization of stereotactic brain operations," *Der Nervenarzt*, vol. 25, no. 11, pp. 441–447, 1954.

[135] Y. Uchimura and H. Narabayashi, "Stereoencephalotomy," *Psychiatry and Neurology*, vol. 52, pp. 265–270, 1951.

[136] G. Schaltenbrand and P. Bailey, *Introduction to Stereotaxis with an Atlas of the human Brain*, Georg Thieme Stuttgart, 1959.

[137] G. Schaltenbrand and W. Wahren, *Atlas for Stereotaxy of the Human Brain*, Georg Thieme Stuttgart, 1977.

[138] A. L. Benabid, P. Pollak, A. Louveau, S. Henry, and J. De Rougemont, "Combined (thalamotomy and stimulation) stereotactic surgery of the VIM thalamic nucleus for bilateral Parkinson disease," *Applied Neurophysiology*, vol. 50, no. 1–6, pp. 344–346, 1987.

[139] J. Siegfried, B. Lippitz, R. A. E. Bakay, and P. J. Kelly, "Bilateral chronic electrostimulation of ventroposterolateral pallidum: a new therapeutic approach for alleviating all parkinsonian symptoms," *Neurosurgery*, vol. 35, no. 6, pp. 1126–1130, 1994.

[140] A. L. Benabid, P. Pollak, C. Gross et al., "Acute and long-term effects of subthalamic nucleus stimulation of Parkinson's disease," *Stereotactic and Functional Neurosurgery*, vol. 62, no. 1–4, pp. 76–84, 1994.

[141] J. E. Wickham, "The new surgery," *British Medical Journal*, vol. 295, no. 6613, pp. 1581–1582, 1987.

[142] A. Perneczky, M. Tschabitscher, and K. D. M. Resch, *Endoscopic Anatomy For Neurosurgery*, Thieme, 1993.

[143] A. Perneczky, W. Müller-Forell, and E. van Lindert, *Keyhole Concept in Neurosurgery: With Endoscope Assisted Microsurgery and Case Studies*, Thieme, 1999.

[144] A. Perneczky, R. Reisch, and S. Kindel, *Keyhole Approaches in Neurosurgery. Vol. 1: Concept and Surgical Technique*, Springer, 2008.

2

Minimally Invasive Treatment of the Thoracic Spine Disease: Completely Percutaneous and Hybrid Approaches

Tamburrelli Francesco Ciro, Scaramuzzo Laura, Genitiempo Maurizio, and Proietti Luca

Department of Spinal Surgery, Catholic University of Rome, lg A. Gemelli 8, 00135 Rome, Italy

Correspondence should be addressed to Tamburrelli Francesco Ciro; f.tamburrelli@tiscali.it

Academic Editor: Casey M. Calkins

The aim of the study was to evaluate the feasibility of a limited invasive approach for the treatment of upper thoracic spine disease. Seven patients with type-A thoracic fractures and three with tumors underwent long thoracic stabilization through a minimally invasive approach. Four patients underwent a completely percutaneous approach while the other three underwent a modified hybrid technique, a combination of percutaneous and open approach. The hybrid constructs were realized using a percutaneous approach to the spine distally to the spinal lesion and by open approach proximally. In two patients, the stabilization was extended proximally up to the cervical spine. Clinical and radiographic assessment was performed during the first year after the operation at 3, 6, and 12 months. No technically related complications were seen. The postoperative recovery was rapid even in the tumor patients with neurologic impairment. Blood loss was irrelevant. At one-year follow-up there was no loosening or breakage of the screws or failure of the implants. When technically feasible a completely percutaneous approach has to be taken in consideration; otherwise, a combined open-percutaneous approach could be planned to minimize the invasivity of a completely open approach to the thoracic spine.

1. Introduction

Although widely used in the lumbar and lower thoracic spine, the minimally invasive approach is still limited in the treatment of the upper thoracic spine disease. The principal issue regarding treatment of thoracic spinal disorders through a minimally invasive approach is the potential for resulting neurologic injuries. The high risk of devastating complications is probably the primary roadblock to a wider use of the percutaneous approach to the thoracic spine.

Anatomic peculiarities and difficult clear visualization under fluoroscopy of the pedicles of the upper thoracic spine make percutaneous screw fixation a demanding procedure especially when multilevel thoracic fixation is required.

In order to limit the invasiveness of completely open surgery and to verify the feasibility of this demanding procedure, we began using a minimally invasive approach to the thoracic spine according to the following strategy. A completely percutaneous approach was carried out in well-selected cases in which the fluoroscopic visualization of the pedicles was optimal, while in cases where a completely percutaneous procedure was unfeasible, a combined, open-percutaneous approach to the thoracic spine was then performed. The surgical strategy we developed consists in percutaneous placement of pedicle screws in the lower and mid thoracic spine and conventional open pedicle screw insertion at the proximal portion of the fixation constructs.

We report our preliminary experience in treating thoracic spinal disorders requiring long stabilization. Four procedures were performed using a completely percutaneous technique and six through a combined, open-percutaneous approach.

2. Materials and Methods

We performed a long thoracic construct through an open-percutaneous combined approach (OPCA) in 6 patients (2 males, 4 females) and an entirely percutaneous approach in 4 patients (2 male, 2 female) (Table 1) using the minimally invasive PathFinder (Zimmer Spine) (Figure 1) and Viper system

Table 1: Details of the patients. In the table are recorded the levels affected and the levels instrumented by completely percutaneous or combined (open-percutaneous) approach.

Pt no.	Sex/age	Fracture	Tumor	OPCA	Completely percutaneous	Other sites fractures	Comorbidities	Head injury	Neurologic deficit
1	M/41	T4, 5, 6	—	—	T2, 3/T8, 9	Sternum	Lung contusion	—	—
2	F/59	T4, 5	—	—	T2, 3/T6/T9, 10	Ribs, spinous apophysis	Lung contusion	—	—
3	M/54	T5, 6, 7	—	—	T3, 4/T8/T10, 11	—	—	Y	—
4	M/71	T4, 5	—	C5, 6/T1, 2 open T6/T8, 9 percutaneous	—	Wrists, C6, C7, ribs, spinous processes	Lung contusion	Y	—
5	M/65	T4, 5	—	T2, 3 open T6/T9, 10 percutaneous	—	Ribs	Pneumothorax	—	—
6	F/63	T4, 5	—	T2, 3 open T6/T8, 9 percutaneous	—	—	—	—	—
7	F/52	T5, 7	—	T3, 4 open T6/T8, 9 percutaneous	—	—	—	—	—
8	F/71	—	T4 myeloma	T1, 2/T5 open T9, 10 percutaneous	—	—	—	—	Y
9	F/65	—	T2, 3, 4 metastasis of breast cancer	C6, 7, T1 open T6/T8, 9 percutaneous	—	—	—	—	Y
10	F/57	—	T6, 7 metastasis of breast cancer	—	T4, 5/T11, 12	—	—	—	—

OPCA: open-percutaneous combined approach.

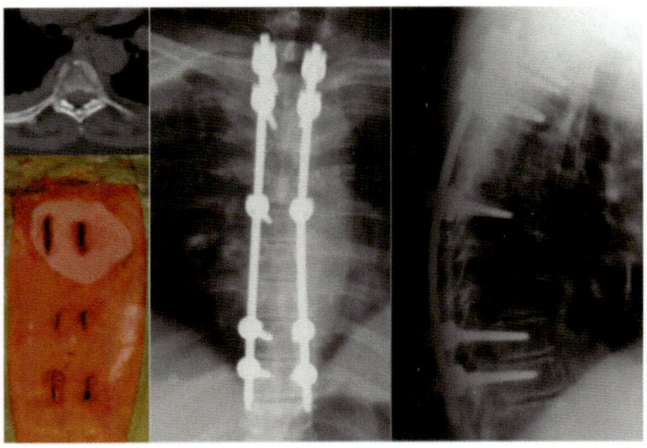

Figure 1: A 59-year-old female with fractures of T4 and T5, multiple, bilateral rib fractures, fractures of the spinous processes of T4/5/6/7, and lung contusion, treated surgically by posterior fixation with long instrumentation carried out percutaneously with screws implanted in T2-3/T6/T9-10.

(DePuy Synthes Spine) (Figure 2). Seven patients (4 males and 3 females; minimum age, 41 years; maximum age, 71 year's) had traumatic thoracic A3 fractures according to Magerl's classification, while the other three patients (all females) were affected by spinal tumors (Figures 3 and 4). T4 and T5 vertebral bodies were involved 5 and 7 times, respectively, T6 and T7 were involved in 2 cases. The most caudal pedicle screws were implanted in T12 while the most proximal were implanted in the lateral masses of C5. Associated bony lesions included multiple rib fractures, spinous processes fractures, fractures of the costotransverse joints, and bilateral fractures of the wrists in one case. The most severe associated lesions were lung contusion in three cases with slight impairment of respiratory function, traumatic pneumothorax in one case, and head injury in two cases.

Two of the OPCA constructs were extended proximally because of concomitant cervical lesions. One of these two patients had articular mass fractures of C6 and C7 with unilateral joint displacement requiring reduction and stabilization (Figure 5). Extension to the cervical spine in the other was necessary to ensure adequate anchorage proximal to neoplastic osteolysis of T2 (Figure 3). In both cases a specifically modified double diameters rod was used (Mountaineer, DePuy Synthes Spine).

In four cases (three fractures and one tumor) the implant was performed completely percutaneous. A very long construct was realized to obtain a more solid implant, able to better share loads of a long segment of the spine. The implant was extended from T2-3 proximally till T8-9-10 distally in case of fractures involving T4-5-6 vertebral bodies (Figures 1 and 2), while in the case affected by tumor, the neoplasia was localized at T6-7 vertebral bodies and the stabilization was carried out from T4 proximally to T12 distally.

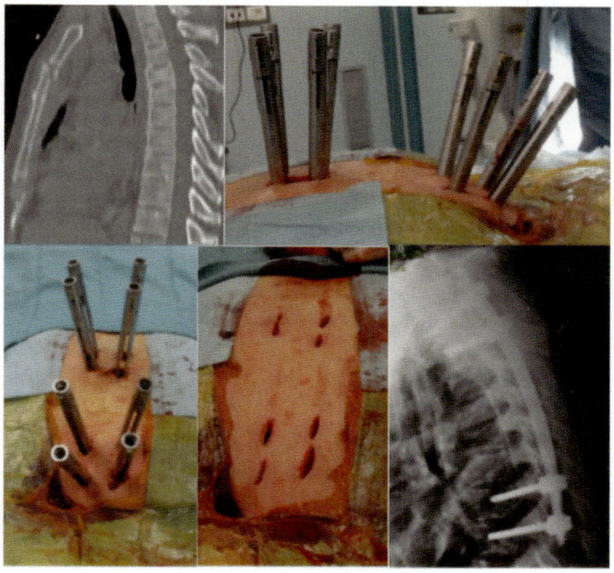

Figure 2: A 41-year-old man with traumatic fractures of T4-T5-T6 and fracture of the sternum. A completely percutaneous long fixation was carried out from T2-T3 till T8-T9. The patient was discharged from the hospital on the third postoperative day.

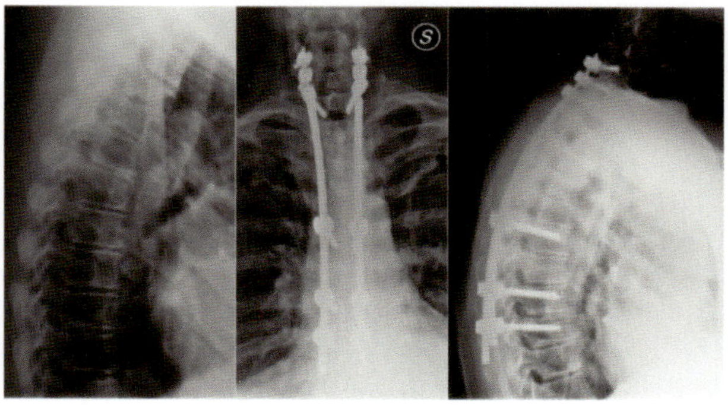

Figure 3: A 65-year-old female. Metastasis of breast cancer of T2-T3-T4. To limit the invasiveness of a completely open surgical approach, a hybrid long construct was carried out (percutaneous from T9-8 to T6 and open from T1, C7-6) using a double diameter rod.

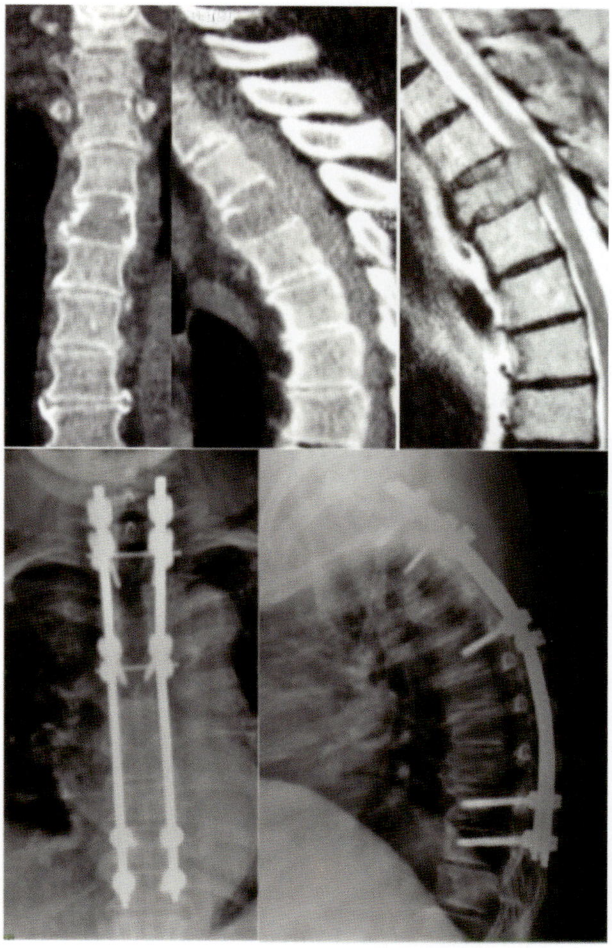

Figure 4: CT scan and MRI of a 71-year-old, obese female (120 Kg) with osteolysis of the T4. Hybrid construct performed percutaneously in the lower tract (T9-10) and by open approach in upper part (T1-2/5). No failure of the implant at 1-year follow-up X-rays.

One patient with tumor lesions had a long history of severe axial pain due to vertebral insufficiency before the onset of mild neurologic impairment (Figure 4). In this patient, who had multiple myeloma, computed tomography (CT) showed extensive destruction of the vertebral body and right pedicle of T4, while magnetic resonance imaging (MRI) showed tumor compression of the spinal cord at the same level. The other patient underwent surgery for breast cancer 5 years previously. During the last 2 months she experienced gradual onset of pain in the upper thoracic spine and minor neurologic impairment in the lower limbs. MRI showed neoplastic osteolysis of T2, T3, and T4 with compromise of the canal and mild cord compression. As a palliative procedure, we decided to decompress and stabilize the spine through an OPCA (Figure 3). Finally the third patient belonging to the tumoral group was admitted to our institution due to severe dorsal pain. She had history of breast cancer treated few years before. The preoperative MRI and CT scan demonstrated severe osteolysis of the T6 and T7 vertebral body. The fixation was carried out completely percutaneous except for a small incision focused on the lesion for taking samples for histological examination.

In 3 of 6 cases of OPCA the open exposure was extended distally to the level of the lesion either to allow autologous bone grafting in fractures or for spinal cord decompression in the tumor patients. Both of these procedures are unfeasible in a totally percutaneous way.

The surgical technique does not differ a lot from what we previously reported for long instrumentation of the thoracolumbar spine [1]. A crucial step at the beginning of the operation is the careful check of the optimal fluoroscopic view of the pedicles. The upper thoracic pedicles are generally better recognizable in anteroposterior (AP) views with the C-arm rotated in the craniocaudal plane according to the degree of kyphosis. Shoulders and soft tissues, especially in obese patients, frequently hinder visualization on lateral views. A

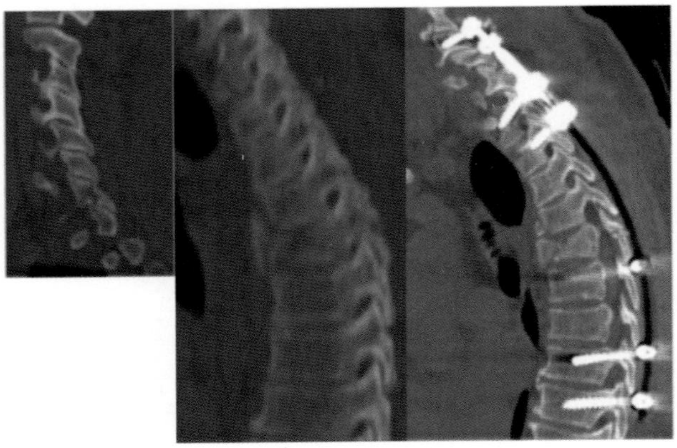

FIGURE 5: A 71-year-old man with traumatic fracture of the lower cervical spine and the T4-T5 vertebral bodies. A long fixation was carried out with hybrid procedure utilizing a double diameter rod. Pedicle screws of T6, T8, and T9 were implanted percutaneously.

second important technical feature is the right contouring of the rods before their implantation to preserve sagittal alignment, which varies substantially from patient to patient. This variability of thoracic kyphosis sometimes increased the difficulty of the procedure. Some patients had hyperkyphosis or worsening of preexisting pronounced kyphosis due to the vertebral lesion. Clinical assessment and implant surveillance were performed at 1, 3, 8, and 12 months. The accuracy of the pedicle screw placement was assessed at first postoperative control by means of CT scan with very thin slices in the three planes of the space and evaluated according to Youkilis's method [2]. Of 92 screws implanted, 84 were positioned inside the thoracic pedicles of which 22 by open and 62 by percutaneous approach. Eight screws were placed in the lateral masses of the cervical spine. The survival of the construct was assessed with standard X-rays at the subsequent controls till the first 1 y postoperative end-point, checking the failure of the implant, screw breakages or the presence of radiolucencies around the screws, signs of an impending loosening.

3. Results

No complications related to the surgical technique were observed and all patients showed satisfactory clinical outcome after a minimum 1-year follow-up. None of the patients had excessive intraoperative bleeding estimated maximum 250 cc and 100 cc for OPCA and completely percutaneous, respectively. Concerning the accuracy of the screws placement we observed that 22 of 24 open screws were good positioned and 2 were acceptable (more than 2 mm cortical violation) while 63 of 70 percutaneous screws were good positioned and 5 were acceptable. No infection or delayed wound healing was observed, including an obese patient (120 Kg), where the limited extension of the open approach facilitated mostly the postoperative nursing. No implant failed or loosened during follow-up. Patients treated for fractures started to walk in second day after the operation and were discharged from the hospital in 3–5 day postoperatively. Two patients belonging to the tumoral group were transferred to another hospital for postoperative rehabilitation because of the neurologic impairment. Both the neurologic patients had full recovery and all the patients because of the very limited approach were very quickly enrolled in the chemotherapy protocol treatment and oncologic clinical surveillance. At 1-year follow-up, they were still alive, able to walk without any external aids, and completely autonomous.

4. Discussion and Conclusions

Major thoracic spine fractures are generally caused by high-energy trauma, and, for this reasons, they are frequently associated with rib fractures and pulmonary contusions with severe impairment of respiratory function. The primary goal in treating patients with thoracic lesions is the rapid improvement of respiratory function to avoid sequelae and potentially fatal pulmonary complications. To obtain this goal, it is mandatory to stabilize the spinal injuries as soon as possible and in the less invasive way. The decision to stabilize with long instead of short constructs in the present series of patients was determined either by the association of multiple thoracic spinal fractures or the necessity of stabilizing vertebral structures compromised by cancer. When extensive instrumentation is required for proper support of thoracic vertebral lesions, there is necessarily a tradeoff between the desired mechanical efficacy and the debilitating procedures employed to obtain this efficacy. Until few years ago, it would have been unthinkable to use minimally invasive techniques to manage thoracic lesions because of the anatomical peculiarities of the region and the high risk of devastating complications [3]. With the advent of reliable percutaneous pedicle screw fixation systems, some surgeons recently tried to use this method in the treatment of thoracic fractures to minimize the invasiveness of an entirely open approach [4, 5]. Certainly the availability of the method relates to many aspects; the most important is the perfect visualization of the pedicle under fluoroscopy and its size and morphology. It is clear that the percutaneous approach allows consistent savings in terms of blood loss, recovery of the patient, and postoperative morbidity such as infection when compared to an open approach. Of course there are technical problems that need to be addressed, such as perfect visualization of the pedicle. Using fluoroscopically guided percutaneous insertion of thoracic pedicle screws, we relied more on AP views with the C-arm rotated in the sagittal plane according to the patient's kyphosis than on lateral views, where the shoulders, in the upper thoracic spine, tend to reduce detection of the vertebral bodies and pedicles. Perfect visualization of the pedicle, checked before starting the procedure, is essential for the insertion of the screw. On the AP view the pedicle appears as an oval within the limits of the vertebral body. This was the landmark we used for percutaneous pedicle screw placement. To ensure satisfactory purchase in the pedicle, we introduced the tip of the screw slightly medially without exceeding the medial border of the oval to avoid spinal canal encroachment and far from the superior edge of the vertebral body to avoid penetration of the disc space. The lateral view was limited to check the length of the screw. With this technique we did not experience major complications related to wrong screw placement except for a small incidence of uneventful violation of the cortical of the pedicle (2 for open and 4 for percutaneous). Park et al. using similar fluoroscopic guided technique reported very low screw malpositioning rates in their series of 172 screws postoperatively verified by CT [6]. If the tip of the screw remains lateral to the medial pedicle wall until the engagement of the vertebral body, it is highly improbable that it can cause a canal encroachment.

It may be argued that various navigation systems have been developed to reduce pedicle screws misplacement. Lieberman et al. reported that the use of robot guidance system increases the accuracy of percutaneous pedicle screw placement thereby reducing radiation exposure and procedure time [7], compared to the control group. They concluded that this advanced technology might also allow inclusion of patients with complicated anatomic deformities. Kakarla et al. treated percutaneously six patients affected by thoracic fractures (five acute unstable thoracic fracture and one osteoporotic burst fracture) with the assistance of intraoperative Iso-C C-arm fluoroscopy [8]. Accuracy of screw placement was investigated by postoperative CT scan according to the method of Youkilis et al. [2]. They concluded positively about the feasibility of percutaneous stabilization of complex spinal fracture with the aid of neuronavigation.

Undoubtedly the accuracy of the screw-navigated placement is higher in comparison with other "free-hand" techniques, but unfortunately the cost of navigation systems is often prohibitive. Even without a sophisticated pedicle screw-navigation system, neither our percutaneous technique nor our open "free-hand" technique was associated with intraoperative complications. Open "free-hand" pedicle screw insertion, guided by recognizable anatomical landmarks, is widely used at present, particularly for spinal deformities, even in the upper thoracic spine given the superiority of these constructs over hook constructs in terms of coronal and axial correction [9]. In the present series we experienced no difficulty using this technique in the upper thoracic spine, where percutaneous screw insertion would have been less feasible and more dangerous.

Although the limits of this work are the low number of patients and the short time of the outcome, we believe that they do not represent, however, a major limitation. In fact, the main purpose of our study was to verify the possibility to extend to the thoracic spine the advantages of minimally invasive procedure in the treatment of instability diseases in the same way we do in the lower spine. In this first phase of the study, we selected a limited number of patients that were eligible for less invasive approach with long stabilization. In particular, in the three cases of cancer it was important to assess the long-term outcome although it was mainly related to the underlying disease but the more important was to evaluate the possibility of achieving a good stabilization of the spine with fewer early and late complications. Given the impossibility to realize a completely percutaneous approach, an OPCA was carried out with the specific aim to reduce to the least the morbidity of the surgery in highly debilitated patients. Although palliative, the operation allowed a good general recovery and a strong support of the spine. Completely percutaneous approach in two cases of multiple fractures showed good clinical recovery of the patients with very fast discharge from the hospital 3 days after the operation. In two cases, we utilized an OPCA procedure limiting the proximal opening only to the segments chosen for pedicle screwing. In one case, the proximal approach was limited to the lower cervical spine and to the first two thoracic segments to allow the screwing of the cervical lateral masses and placement of the screws in the pedicles of T1 and T2. In the other case, the incision was prolonged to the fracture site to allow bone grafting. The need of posterior arthrodesis in the treatment of fractures is still a matter of discussion [10]. However, an OPCA can allow local bone grafting by distal extension of the proximal open approach. In conclusion, although a higher number of series with long-term outcome are needed to prove the reliability of the mininvasive techniques in the treatment of thoracic spine diseases, our series showed promising results at one-year follow-up with no complications technique-related.

References

[1] C. A. Logroscino, L. Proietti, and F. C. Tamburrelli, "Minimally invasive spine stabilisation with long implants," *European Spine Journal*, vol. 18, supplement 1, pp. S75–S81, 2009.

[2] A. S. Youkilis, D. J. Quint, J. E. McGillicuddy, and S. M. Papadopoulos, "Stereotactic navigation for placement of pedicle screws in the thoracic spine," *Neurosurgery*, vol. 48, no. 4, pp. 771–779, 2001.

[3] C. Schaefer, P. Begemann, I. Fuhrhop et al., "Percutaneous instrumentation of the cervical and cervico-thoracic spine using pedicle screws: preliminary clinical results and analysis of accuracy," *European Spine Journal*, vol. 20, no. 6, pp. 977–985, 2011.

[4] B. Blondel, S. Fuentes, P. Tropiano, P. Roche, P. Métellus, and H. Dufour, "Systems for long-segment percutaneous spinal fixation: technical feasibility for various indications," *Acta Neurochirurgica*, vol. 153, no. 5, pp. 985–991, 2011.

[5] H. Roldan, L. Perez-Orribo, M. Spreafico, and M. Ginoves-Sierra, "Long constructs in the thoracic and lumbar spine with a minimally invasive technique," *Minimally Invasive Neurosurgery*, vol. 54, no. 2, pp. 100–103, 2011.

[6] D. H. Park, A. O. Thomas, and S. St Clair, "Percutaneous lumbar and thoracic pedicle screws, a trauma experience," *Journal of Spinal Disorders*, 2012.

[7] I. H. Lieberman, M. A. Hardenbrook, J. C. Wang, and R. D. Guyer, "Assessment of pedicle screw placement accuracy, procedure time, and radiation exposure using a miniature robotic guidance system," *Journal of Spinal Disorders & Techniques*, vol. 25, no. 5, pp. 241–248, 2011.

[8] U. K. Kakarla, A. S. Little, S. W. Chang, V. K. H. Sonntag, and N. Theodore, "Placement of percutaneous thoracic pedicle screws using neuronavigation," *World Neurosurgery*, vol. 74, no. 6, pp. 606–610, 2010.

[9] A. F. Samdani, A. Ranade, D. M. Sciubba et al., "Accuracy of free-hand placement of thoracic pedicle screws in adolescent idiopathic scoliosis: how much of a difference does surgeon experience make?" *European Spine Journal*, vol. 19, no. 1, pp. 91–95, 2010.

3

Endoscopic Transforaminal Thoracic Foraminotomy and Discectomy for the Treatment of Thoracic Disc Herniation

Hong-Fei Nie[1] and Kai-Xuan Liu[2]

[1] *Department of Orthopaedic Surgery, West China Hospital, Sichuan University, Chengdu, Sichuan 610041, China*
[2] *Atlantic Spine Center, 475 Prospect Avenue, Suite 110, West Orange, NJ 07052, USA*

Correspondence should be addressed to Kai-Xuan Liu; doc@atlanticspinecenter.com

Academic Editor: Peng Hui Wang

Thoracic disc herniation is a relatively rare yet challenging-to-diagnose condition. Currently there is no universally accepted optimal surgical treatment for symptomatic thoracic disc herniation. Previously reported surgical approaches are often associated with high complication rates. Here we describe our minimally invasive technique of removing thoracic disc herniation, and report the primary results of a series of cases. Between January 2009 and March 2012, 13 patients with symptomatic thoracic disc herniation were treated with endoscopic thoracic foraminotomy and discectomy under local anesthesia. A bone shaver was used to undercut the facet and rib head for foraminotomy. Discectomy was achieved by using grasper, radiofrequency, and the Holmium-YAG laser. We analyzed the clinical outcomes of the patients using the visual analogue scale (VAS), MacNab classification, and Oswestry disability index (ODI). At the final follow up (mean: 17 months; range: 6–41 months), patient self-reported satisfactory rate was 76.9%. The mean VAS for mid back pain was improved from 9.1 to 4.2, and the mean ODI was improved from 61.0 to 43.8. One complication of postoperative spinal headache occurred during the surgery and the patient was successfully treated with epidural blood patch. No other complications were observed or reported during and after the surgery.

1. Introduction

Thoracic disc herniation is an uncommon condition. Although conservative treatment works well for many patients with thoracic disc herniation, surgical treatment is needed for patients suffering from myelopathy and/or neurological deficit caused by thoracic disc herniation. In the past decade, quite a few surgical procedures have been reported in the literature, and each of them has its own advantages and disadvantages [1–14]. Currently there is no universally accepted optimal surgical treatment for symptomatic thoracic disc herniation.

Minimally invasive spine surgery has proven safe and effective in treating lumbar and cervical herniations [15–24]. The advantages of minimally invasive techniques have compelled many physicians to explore the feasibility of using minimally invasive techniques in treating thoracic disc herniation, and a number of authors have reported encouraging primary results [14, 25–28]. Based on our extensive experience with treating lumbar and cervical disc herniation using minimally invasive techniques, we have developed an endoscopic transforaminal foraminotomy and discectomy technique for treating thoracic disc herniation. The purposes of this paper are to describe the technique and to report the results of a series of cases.

2. Materials and Methods

Between January 2009 and January 2012, 13 patients with symptomatic thoracic disc herniation were treated with percutaneous endoscopic thoracic foraminotomy and discectomy. The surgical procedures were performed under local anesthesia at our outpatient surgical center. All patients had soft thoracic disc herniation confirmed with magnetic resonance imaging (MRI). Symptoms related to the herniation were confirmed using discography. After a mean of 17 months of followup (range: 6–41 months), we analyzed the clinical

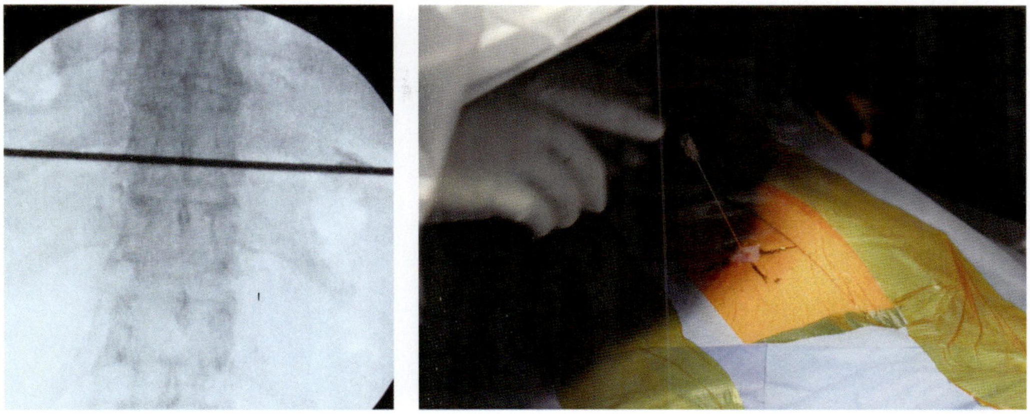

(a) (b)

FIGURE 1: The target disc was identified under fluoroscopic guidance (a), and the entry point between the rib head and the facet was marked on the skin (b).

outcomes using the visual analogue scale (VAS), MacNab classification, and Oswestry disability index (ODI).

2.1. Diagnosis and Patient Selection. Considering that patients with thoracic disc herniation may have varied symptoms, some of which may be similar to symptoms of other medical conditions, we made the diagnosis by reviewing the patients' medical history, performing physical examination, and analyzing radiographic findings. Patients qualified for our surgical procedure met the following criteria. First, the patient had middle back pain with or without radiation. Second, conservative pain treatments had failed to alleviate the pain. Third, magnetic resonance imaging (MRI) revealed soft thoracic disc herniation. And finally discography confirmed painful disc before the surgical procedure.

Patients with calcified discs or hard disc herniations were not treated with this procedure.

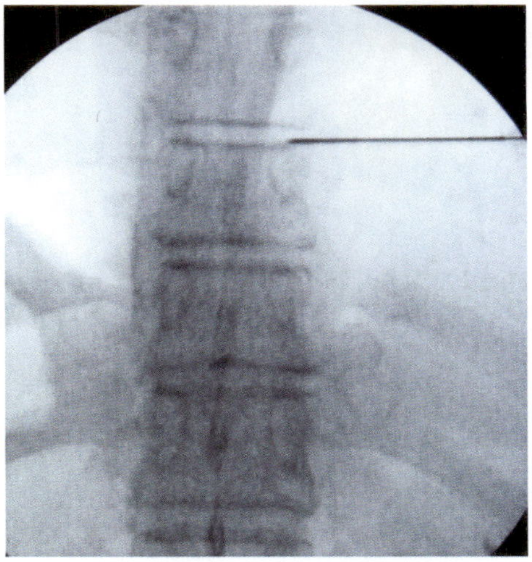

FIGURE 2: Discography was performed to confirm the target disc and to help identify the location of the herniation; the needle was parallel to the upper endplate of the lower vertebral body.

2.2. Tools. During the surgical procedure, a burr, a bone shaver, and the Holmium-YAG laser were used to undercut the facet and rib head for foraminotomy. Discectomy was achieved by using a grasper, radiofrequency, and the Holmium-YAG laser. The surgical procedures were performed with the assistance of an 8 mm (outer diameter) Wolf endoscope (Richard Wolf Medical Instruments Corporation, Vernon Hills, IL, USA).

2.3. Surgical Technique. The procedures were performed under local anesthesia with the patient in a prone position on a radiolucent table. The target disc was identified under fluoroscopic guidance (Figure 1(a)), and the entry point between the rib head and the facet (on oblique view) was marked on the skin (Figure 1(b)). Discography was performed to confirm the target disc and to help identify the location of the herniation. The 18 G needle inserted to perform discography was parallel to the upper endplate of the lower vertebral body (Figure 2). The tip of the needle reached posterior disc margin (on the lateral view) and was situated between midline and medial pedicle line (on the AP view). The surgical region was anesthetized with a combination of 0.5% lidocaine and epinephrine.

After discography, a guiding wire was inserted through the needle, and a 10 mm skin incision was subsequently made. The needle was removed, and a sequential dilator was then inserted over the wire towards the posterolateral margin of the facet (Figure 3(a)). Once the tip of the dilator reached the surface of the annulus, the guiding wire was removed and the dilator was further inserted into the target foramen. A working cannula was then guided to the extraforaminal region over the dilator (Figure 3(b)). At this juncture, the dilator was removed and the endoscope was placed to assist with visualization.

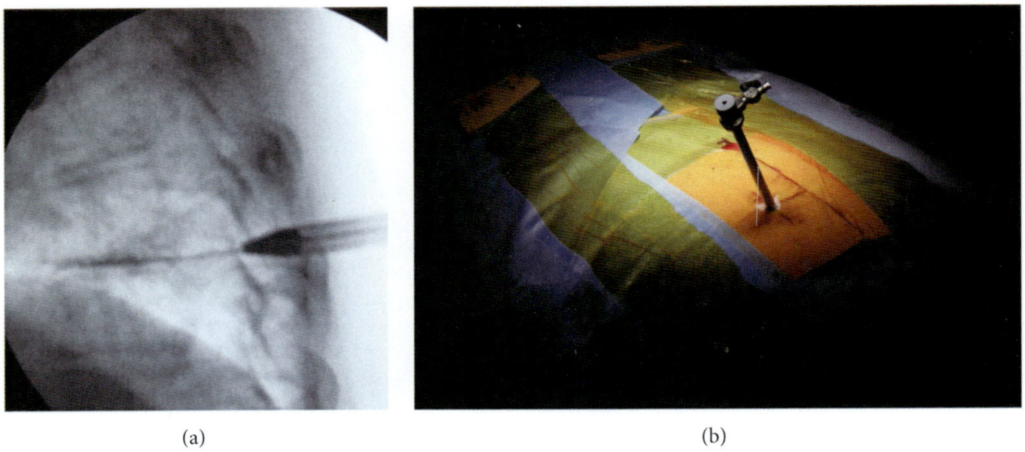

FIGURE 3: A sequential dilator was then inserted over the wire towards the posterolateral margin of the facet (a). A working cannula was guided to the extraforaminal region over the dilator (b).

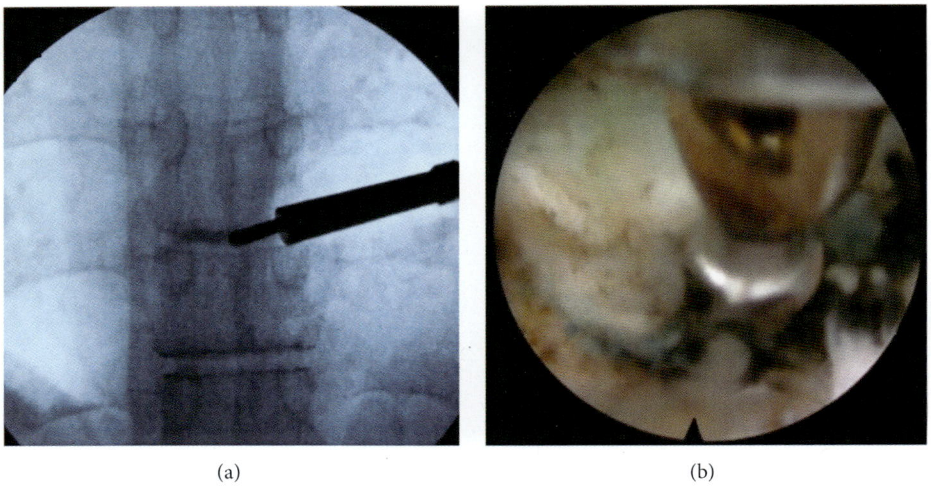

FIGURE 4: An Ellman radiofrequency probe (a) and a shaver (b) were used to expose the foraminal structure.

To perform foraminotomy, we first titled the cannula to expose the foraminal epidural space. We then used an Ellman radiofrequency probe (Ellman International, New York, USA) and a shaver to expose the facet medially and rib head laterally (Figure 4). The radiofrequency, as well as the Holmium-YAG laser, was used to remove scar tissue, when needed. A burr, bone shaver (Richard Wolf Medical Instruments Corporation, Vernon Hills, IL, USA), and the Holmium-YAG laser were used to undercut the facet and rib head, when necessary, to enlarge the foramen so the working cannula could be easily advanced to the inner foraminal zone. Once adequate foraminotomy was achieved, the inferior pedicle, disc, epidural space, and exiting spinal nerve root were exposed. Herniated disc material was then removed using a grasper, radiofrequency, and the laser (Figure 5). At the end of the procedure, free movement of the thecal sac was visible. After satisfactory decompression had been achieved, the endoscope was removed, and the wound was covered with a sterile strip.

3. Results

The treated disc levels included T5-6 (1), T6-7 (3), T7-8 (4), T8-9 (2), T9-10 (2), and T12-L1 (2). One patient had herniation at T6-7 and T7-8. The chief complain of these patients was mid back pain with or without radiation (Table 1).

The patients (male: 7; female: 6; age: 40–69) were followed up for more than 6 months. At the final followup (mean: 17 months; range: 6–41 months), patient self-reported satisfactory rate (excellent and good results) was 76.9%. The mean VAS for mid back pain was improved from 9.1 to 4.2, and the mean ODI was improved from 61.0 to 43.8 (Table 1). The average operation time for each herniated disc was about 50 minutes. Blood loss during the surgery was minimal to none. Only one complication of postoperative spinal positional headache occurred and the patient was successfully treated with epidural blood patch. No other complications were observed or reported during or after the surgery. One patient

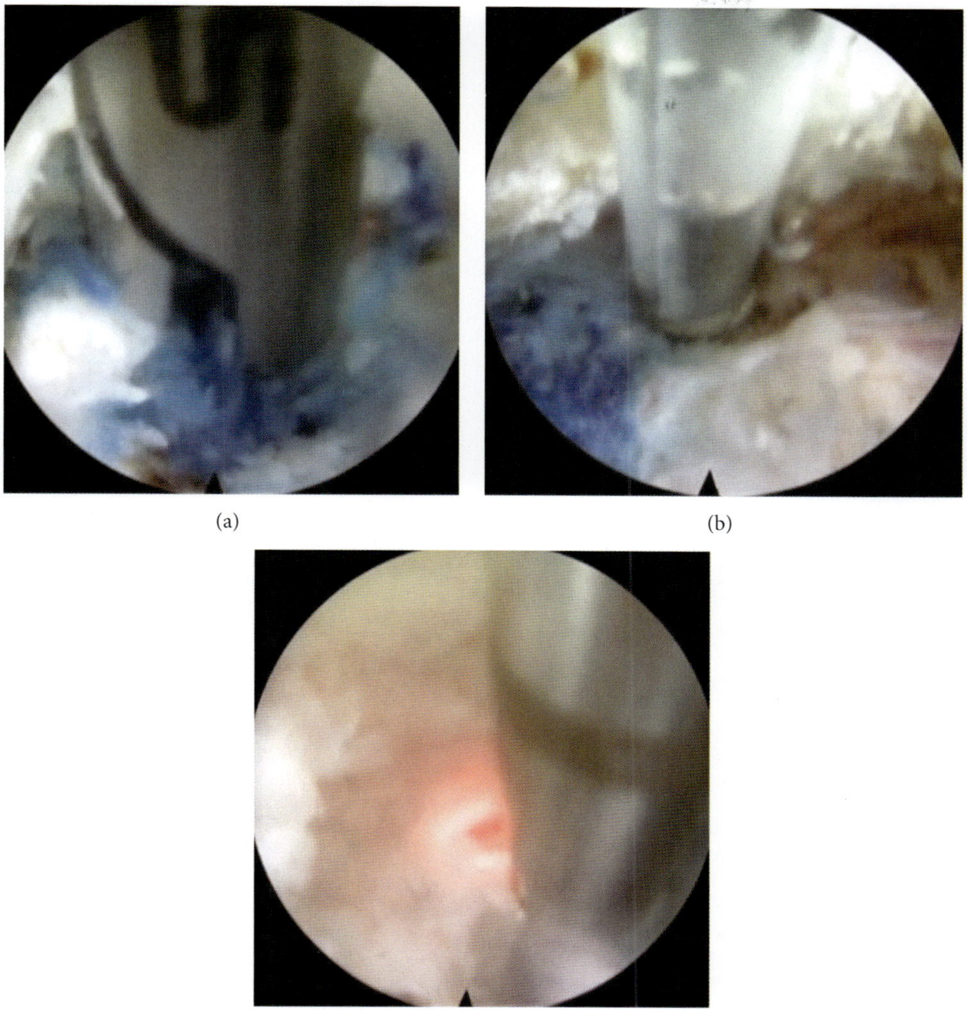

(a) (b) (c)

FIGURE 5: The herniated disc material was removed using a grasper (a), radiofrequency (b), and the Holmium-YAG laser (c).

had recurrent thoracic disc herniation 8 months after the initial surgery. None of the patients experienced worsening of symptoms. When asked if they would undergo the same procedure again if needed in the future, 12 of the 13 patients said yes.

Adequate decompression of the spinal cord was confirmed by postoperative MRI (Figure 6).

4. Discussion

Surgical treatment for thoracic herniation has evolved from the posterior approach to posterolateral and anterior approaches and from open surgery to minimally invasive surgery. To reduce access-induced complications and to improve surgical outcomes, various surgical techniques have been developed over the years. The literature review shows that minimally invasive techniques assisted with endoscopic or microscopic visualization have gained tremendous popularity in recent years. An analysis of a national database showed that utilizing minimally invasive techniques to treat thoracic disc herniation has become a new trend [29]. Despite the advancement in surgical instruments and techniques, surgically treating thoracic herniation remains a challenge because of the anatomical characteristics of the thoracic spine. Currently there are still no universally agreed upon indications for surgery, and the optimal type of decompression method is still controversial. Until a gold standard treatment is established, surgeons worldwide will employ different surgical techniques to treat thoracic disc herniations. And the choice of the technique will be dependent on the surgeon's training background, clinical experience, and personal preference.

Techniques using transforaminal approaches to treat thoracic disc herniation have a few advantages. The techniques generally need to remove only a small, lateral part of the facet joint to gain access for surgical and visualization instruments, and they generally do not require the resection of the unilateral facet joint and the caudal pedicle. Compared with posterior and anterior approaches, transforaminal approaches preserve postoperative spinal stability by avoiding resection

TABLE 1: Patient baseline characteristics and clinical outcomes.

Case number	Age	Sex	Level	Main symptoms	Follow-up (M)	Pre-VAS	Post-VAS	Pre-ODI	Post-ODI	MacNab
1	59	F	T12-L1	Low back and mid back pain, leg pain	33.5	10	5	42	52	Good
2	43	F	T9-10	Mid back pain	32.5	10	7	56	88	Fair
3	40	M	T9-10 (R)/T9-10 (L)	Mid back pain	18	10	2	42	12	Excellent
4	56	F	T6-7	Mid back pain	13	7	4	60	52	Good
5	48	F	T6-7	Mid back pain	13	9	0	66	6	Excellent
6	52	M	T8-9	Mid back pain, upper back pain	13	10	5	92	62	Good
7	57	F	T5-6	Mid back pain, low back pain, and neck pain	12	10	9	70	58	Good
8	69	F	T7-8	Mid back pain, right chest pain	11.5	9	6	58	54	Poor
9	48	M	T7-8	Mid back pain, right chest pain radiates to abdomen	6.5	9	5	60	66	Excellent
10	32	M	T8-9	Mid back pain radiates to shoulder blade	6	6	4	36	18	Good
11	59	M	T6-7, T7-8	Mid back pain radiates to chest	15	10	6	62	54	Fair
12	54	M	T12-L1	Mid back pain	41	8	1	78	32	Excellent
13	51	M	T7-8	Mid back pain radiates to left side chest and rib	6	10	1	70	16	Excellent

VAS: visual analog scale, ODI: Oswestry Disability Index, Pre: preoperative, Post: postoperative.

of posterior vertebral elements and significantly reduce operative blood loss and postoperative pain by avoiding soft tissue dissection.

In our case series, thoracic disc herniations occurred at a wide range of disc levels (from T5-6 to T12-L1). Severe mid back pain with or without radiation was the chief complaint among all the patients treated. All patients reported immediate pain relief after the surgery, and at the final followup, the majority of the patients were still satisfied with the surgical outcome. This encouraging result suggests that our surgical technique is effective in improving the symptoms of thoracic herniations at different disc levels. When using a similar technique to treat soft thoracic disc herniations, Choi et al. also achieved satisfying results [28], which indicates the technique is reproducible.

In our study, at the final followup, 3 of the 13 patients (patients 1, 2, and 9 in Table 1) reported worsened functionality, as assessed by ODI scores. However, the worsened scores were most likely caused by factors unrelated to the original thoracic surgery. Before undergoing the thoracic discectomy at our center, patient number 1 had lumbar discectomy at L4-5 and L5-S1 levels. At the time when the patient answered the ODI questionnaire for our final followup assessment, the patient was suffering from recurrent L4-5 and L5-S1 herniations, which might be the reason that the patient gave poor ODI scores. Patient number 2 gave positive feedback right after the thoracic surgery, but she developed lumbar spondylolisthesis later. And at the time when the patient answered the ODI questionnaire, she was suffering from a broken ankle, which resulted in a loss of feeling in the foot. Patient number 9 had another herniation at T6-7, for which she was suggested to have another surgery. Despite the poor ODI scores at the final followup, when asked if they would consider the same surgery again if necessary in the future, all of the three patients said yes. This suggests that our technique is well accepted by the patients.

Compared with traditional surgical treatment, our endoscopic transforaminal technique offers a few advantages. Small incision and minimal bone removal reduce postoperative pain and ensure fast recovery. Local anesthesia enhances safety and further shortens the recovery. And excellent visualization provided by the endoscope ensures adequate decompression of the nerve. Moreover, same-day surgery with no need for hospital stay significantly reduces the total treatment cost. The low complication rate (0.08%, 1 of 13) and high patient self-reported satisfactory rate (76.9%) suggest that the technique is safe and effective in treating symptomatic soft thoracic disc herniation.

However, like all other surgical techniques, our technique also has limitations. First, the technique is not indicated for sequestrated thoracic disc herniation. And it is extremely challenging to remove large central herniations in patients with severe spinal stenosis. Patients with these conditions are generally referred to surgeons specializing in performing

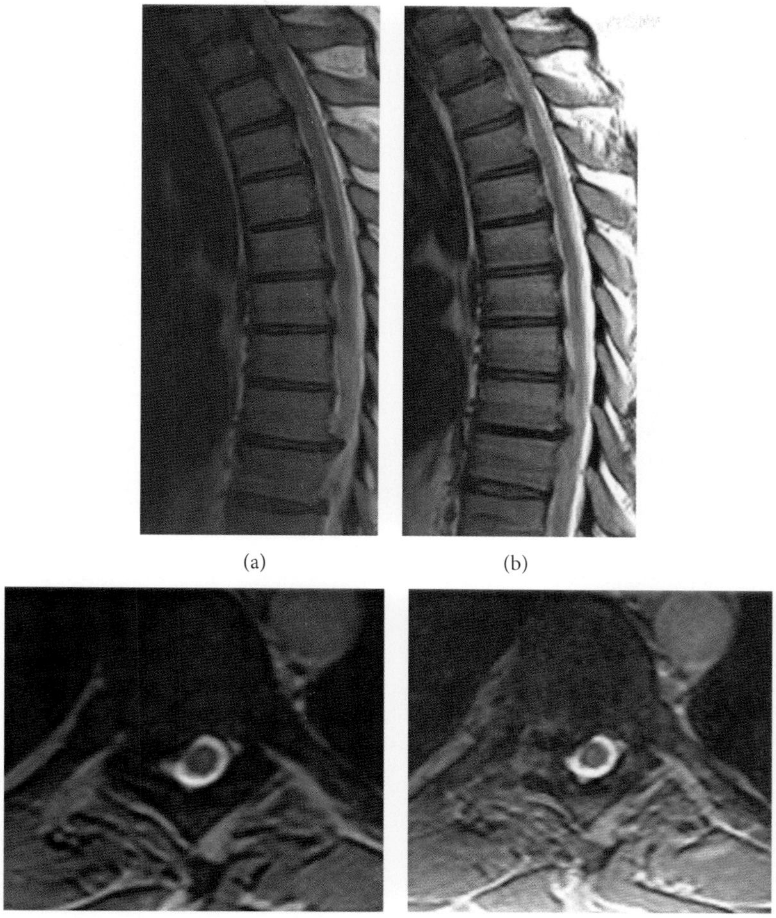

(a) (b)

(c) (d)

FIGURE 6: Preoperative MRI images of a T8-9 disc herniation compressing the spinal cord, which caused the patient to have mid back pain radiating to the shoulder blade ((a) and (b)). Postoperative MRI images showing removal of the extruded disc material ((c) and (d)).

traditional open spine surgery, or thoracotomy. Because the thoracic spinal cord is highly susceptible to injury due to the anatomical nature of the thoracic spine, our technique requires the surgeon to have great surgical skills and considerable amount of experience with endoscopic surgery.

5. Conclusions

For carefully selected patients, endoscopic transforaminal thoracic discectomy and foraminotomy is a safe and effective treatment option for symptomatic soft thoracic disc herniation.

Acknowledgment

The authors thank Dr. Yanni Wang for assisting in revising the paper.

References

[1] T. Aizawa, T. Sato, H. Sasaki et al., "Results of surgical treatment for thoracic myelopathy: minimum 2-year follow-up study in 132 patients," *Journal of Neurosurgery*, vol. 7, no. 1, pp. 13–20, 2007.

[2] D. J. Maiman, S. J. Larson, E. Luck, and A. El-Ghatit, "Lateral extracavitary approach to the spine for thoracic disc herniation: report of 23 cases," *Neurosurgery*, vol. 14, no. 2, pp. 178–182, 1984.

[3] U. K. Debnath, J. R. McConnell, D. K. Sengupta, S. M. H. Mehdian, and J. K. Webb, "Results of hemivertebrectomy and fusion for symptomatic thoracic disc herniation," *European Spine Journal*, vol. 12, no. 3, pp. 292–299, 2003.

[4] K. D. Kim, J. D. Babbitz, and J. Mimbs, "Imaging-guided costotransversectomy for thoracic disc herniation," *Neurosurgical Focus*, vol. 9, no. 4, article e7, 2000.

[5] C. B. Stillerman, T. C. Chen, J. D. Day, W. T. Couldwell, and M. H. Weiss, "The transfacet pedicle-sparing approach for thoracic disc removal: cadaveric morphometric analysis and preliminary clinical experience," *Journal of Neurosurgery*, vol. 83, no. 6, pp. 971–976, 1995.

[6] P. D. Le Roux, M. M. Haglund, A. B. Harris, and R. H. Patterson, "Thoracic disc disease: experience with the transpedicular

approach in twenty consecutive patients," *Neurosurgery*, vol. 33, no. 1, pp. 58–66, 1993.

[7] M. J. Perez-Cruet, B. Kim, F. Sandhu, D. Samartzis, and R. G. Fessler, "Thoracic microendoscopic discectomy," *Journal of Neurosurgery*, vol. 1, no. 1, pp. 58–63, 2004.

[8] Z. Lidar, J. Lifshutz, S. Bhattacharjee, S. N. Kurpad, and D. J. Maiman, "Minimally invasive, extracavitary approach for thoracic disc herniation: technical report and preliminary results," *Spine Journal*, vol. 6, no. 2, pp. 157–163, 2006.

[9] R. E. Isaacs, V. K. Podichetty, F. A. Sandhu et al., "Thoracic microendoscopic discectomy: a human cadaver study," *Spine*, vol. 30, no. 10, pp. 1226–1231, 2005.

[10] H. Sheikh, D. Samartzis, and M. J. Perez-Cruet, "Techniques for the operative management of thoracic disc herniation: minimally invasive thoracic microdiscectomy," *Orthopedic Clinics of North America*, vol. 38, no. 3, pp. 351–361, 2007.

[11] H. Jho, "Endoscopic microscopic transpedicular thoracic discectomy: technical note," *Journal of Neurosurgery*, vol. 87, no. 1, pp. 125–129, 1997.

[12] M. H. Coppes, N. A. Bakker, J. D. Metzemaekers, and R. J. Groen, "Posterior transdural discectomy: a new approach for the removal of a central thoracic disc herniation," *European Spine Journal*, vol. 21, pp. 623–628, 2012.

[13] U. Quint, G. Bordon, I. Preissl, C. Sanner, and D. Rosenthal, "Thoracoscopic treatment for single level symptomatic thoracic disc herniation: a prospective followed cohort study in a group of 167 consecutive cases," *European Spine Journal*, vol. 21, pp. 637–645, 2012.

[14] J. S. Uribe, W. D. Smith, L. Pimenta et al., "Minimally invasive lateral approach for symptomatic thoracic disc herniation: initial multicenter clinical experience: clinical article," *Journal of Neurosurgery*, vol. 16, no. 3, pp. 264–279, 2012.

[15] A. T. Yeung and P. M. Tsou, "Posterolateral endoscopic excision for lumbar disc herniation: surgical technique, outcome, and complications in 307 consecutive cases," *Spine*, vol. 27, no. 7, pp. 722–731, 2002.

[16] S. Ruetten, M. Komp, and G. Godolias, "An extreme lateral access for the surgery of lumbar disc herniations inside the spinal canal using the full-endoscopic uniportal transforaminal approach-technique and prospective results of 463 patients," *Spine*, vol. 30, no. 22, pp. 2570–2578, 2005.

[17] S. Ruetten, M. Komp, and G. Godolias, "A new full-endoscopic technique for the interlaminar operation of lumbar disc herniations using 6-mm endoscopes: prospective 2-year results of 331 patients," *Minimally Invasive Neurosurgery*, vol. 49, no. 2, pp. 80–87, 2006.

[18] G. Choi, S. Lee, A. Bhanot, P. P. Raiturker, and Y. S. Chae, "Percutaneous endoscopic discectomy for extraforaminal lumbar disc herniations: extraforaminal targeted fragmentectomy technique using working channel endoscope," *Spine*, vol. 32, no. 2, pp. E93–E99, 2007.

[19] A. T. Yeung and C. A. Yeung, "Minimally invasive techniques for the management of lumbar disc herniation," *Orthopedic Clinics of North America*, vol. 38, no. 3, pp. 363–372, 2007.

[20] T. Hoogland, K. van den Brekel-Dijkstra, M. Schubert, and B. Miklitz, "Endoscopic transforaminal discectomy for recurrent lumbar disc herniation: a prospective, cohort evaluation of 262 consecutive cases," *Spine*, vol. 33, no. 9, pp. 973–978, 2008.

[21] J. Nellensteijn, R. Ostelo, R. Bartels, W. Peul, B. van Royen, and M. van Tulder, "Transforaminal endoscopic surgery for symptomatic lumbar disc herniations: a systematic review of the literature," *European Spine Journal*, vol. 19, no. 2, pp. 181–204, 2010.

[22] S. Ruetten, M. Komp, H. Merk, and G. Godolias, "Full-endoscopic anterior decompression versus conventional anterior decompression and fusion in cervical disc herniations," *International Orthopaedics*, vol. 33, no. 6, pp. 1677–1682, 2009.

[23] Y. Ahn, S. H. Lee, S. E. Chung, H. S. Park, and S. W. Shin, "Percutaneous endoscopic cervical discectomy for discogenic cervical headache due to soft disc herniation," *Neuroradiology*, vol. 47, no. 12, pp. 924–930, 2005.

[24] J. C. Chiu, T. J. Clifford, M. Greenspan, R. C. Richley, G. Lohman, and R. B. Sison, "Percutaneous microdecompressive endoscopic cervical discectomy with laser thermodiskoplasty," *Mount Sinai Journal of Medicine*, vol. 67, no. 4, pp. 278–282, 2000.

[25] T. G. Burke and A. J. Caputy, "Treatment of thoracic disc herniation: evolution toward the minimally invasive thoracoscopic technique," *Neurosurgical Focus*, vol. 9, no. 4, article e9, 2000.

[26] J. C. Chiu, T. J. Clifford, and R. Sison, "Percutaneous microdecompressive endoscopic thoracic discectomy for herniated thoracic discs," *Surgical Technology International*, vol. 10, pp. 266–269, 2002.

[27] G. J. Regev, K. Salame, E. Behrbalk, O. Keynan, and Z. Lidar, "Minimally invasive transforaminal, thoracic microscopic discectomy: technical report and preliminary results and complications," *The Spine Journal*, vol. 12, pp. 570–576, 2012.

[28] K. Y. Choi, S. S. Eun, S. H. Lee, and H. Y. Lee, "Percutaneous endoscopic thoracic discectomy; transforaminal approach," *Minimally Invasive Neurosurgery*, vol. 53, no. 1, pp. 25–28, 2010.

[29] A. Mesfin, A. Jain, and E. N. Menga, "National trends in the treatment of thoracic disc herniation with and without myelopathy," *The Spine Journal*, vol. 12, article S12, 2012.

4

Complications of Minimally Invasive, Tubular Access Surgery for Cervical, Thoracic, and Lumbar Surgery

Donald A. Ross[1,2]

[1] *Section of Neurological Surgery, Operative Care Division, Portland Veterans Administration Hospital, Portland, OR, USA*
[2] *Department of Neurological Surgery, Oregon Health & Science University, 3303 SW Bond Avenue, CH8N, Portland, OR 97239, USA*

Correspondence should be addressed to Donald A. Ross; rossdo@ohsu.edu

Academic Editor: Stephen Kavic

The object of the study was to review the author's large series of minimally invasive spine surgeries for complication rates. The author reviewed a personal operative database for minimally access spine surgeries done through nonexpandable tubular retractors for extradural, nonfusion procedures. Consecutive cases ($n = 1231$) were reviewed for complications. There were no wound infections. Durotomy occurred in 33 cases (2.7% overall or 3.4% of lumbar cases). There were no external or symptomatic internal cerebrospinal fluid leaks or pseudomeningoceles requiring additional treatment. The only motor injuries were 3 C5 root palsies, 2 of which resolved. Minimally invasive spine surgery performed through tubular retractors can result in a low wound infection rate when compared to open surgery. Durotomy is no more common than open procedures and does not often result in the need for secondary procedures. New neurologic deficits are uncommon, with most observed at the C5 root. Minimally invasive spine surgery, even without benefits such as less pain or shorter hospital stays, can result in considerably lower complication rates than open surgery.

1. Introduction

Minimal access spinal surgery is a rapidly developing set of techniques, which have compared favorably with open surgeries in the recent literature (see review in Wong et al., 2012) [1–4]. In addition to reduced blood loss, shorter operative time, reduced postoperative pain, earlier discharge, rapid return to normal activities, and other reported advantages of minimally invasive surgery, [5] a decreased complication rate associated with these surgeries has also been noted, particularly with respect to wound infections [6]. The author reports experience on management of a large series of minimally invasive spine procedures.

2. Methods

2.1. Patient Population. The author began using the Metrx Tubular Retraction System (Medtronic, Minneapolis) in 2001. This report constitutes a retrospective review of all consecutive spine cases done using this system from that time to the present. Information was obtained from the author's personal surgeries database. This report does not include intentionally intradural procedures or fusion procedures. This series does not include the use of expandable tubes or other minimal access retractor systems other than a tubular system. Procedures reported here were for laminectomy and/or foraminotomy for spondylotic diseases such as discectomy or stenosis, for epidural masses such as metastases, abscesses, or synovial cysts, or for spinal cord stimulator paddle electrode implantation.

2.2. Surgical Approach. In each procedure, the patient was positioned prone on a Jackson Table (Mizuho OSI, Union City, CA). Care was taken not to hyperextend the cervical spine. Neuromuscular blockade was not used after induction of anesthesia. Nerve root/spinal cord monitoring was not routinely used. A single dose of preoperative antibiotic was used, usually weight adjusted cefazolin or vancomycin in the case of contraindication to cephalosporins. Ioban (3M, St. Paul, MN) drapes were used in all cases except in cases of iodine allergy. Placement of the tubular retractor system was done according to standard procedure, using first anterior-posterior fluoroscopy for initial placement followed by lateral fluoroscopy for final positioning of the tube. The tubes were affixed to the table mount. For tubes of up to 6 cm in length, an 18 mm diameter tube was used. As the depth increased beyond 6 cm, 20 or 22 mm tubes were used to increase the degree of freedom at depth.

A paramedian approach was used for lumbar laminectomy or discectomy and for cervical laminectomy or foraminotomy. A far lateral approach was used for lumbar foraminotomy or far lateral discectomy, with the incision lateral to the pars interarticularis. Bilateral canal decompression was performed by angling the tube toward the contralateral side after removal of some of the base of the spinous process. For spondylotic stenosis, attention was paid to directing the tube to the site of maximal canal stenosis, usually just below the disc space where the ligamentum flavum is most compressive of the thecal sac.

The microscope was used for visualization throughout the procedure. No monopolar coagulation was ever used during these procedures. A 5 mm diamond drill under continuous automatic irrigation was used for bone removal. Hemostasis was obtained with low power bipolar coagulation, bone wax, and NuKnit (Ethicon). Copious irrigation was done with lactated ringers without antibiotic. Multilevel cervical procedures were done by wanding the tube to redirect it to another level without removing it. Two-level lumbar procedures were performed by removing the tube and redirecting it through the same incision to the additional levels. Three-level lumbar procedures were done through two incisions, using one incision for two levels and a second incision for the third. In these cases, an 8-French-red-rubber tube was left in at the initial level as a suction drain to prevent epidural hematoma accumulation and then removed at the end of the procedure. Rarely, a 3/32 Hemovac (Zimmer, Warsaw, IN) drain was left in place for a few hours postoperatively if hemostasis was not perfect. Fluoroscopic verification of the rostrocaudal extent of decompression was always obtained using a nerve hook and a ball hook to define the points of maximal rostral and caudal canal decompression.

When a durotomy occurred, if possible, suture repair was performed using a 4-0 silk suture on a very small round needle using the micropituitary forceps from the Metrx set as the needle holder. Instrumentation is now available to facilitate dural closure (Haque et al., 2013; [7] Scanlan International, St. Paul). In some cases, a small piece of NuKnit (Ethicon) or dural substitute was placed intradurally such that it was pushed flat up against the internal side of the dura by the arachnoid to prevent nerve root herniation through the durotomy. Fibrin glue (Tisseel, Baxter) was placed over the durotomy prior to closure. The wound closure was not altered from that described below. Lumbar patients were kept in 3 degrees of Trendelenburg for 6–12 hours postoperatively and then mobilized if a 2-hour test period of sitting up 30 degrees did not produce a postural headache.

After obtaining hemostasis at the dural level, the retractor tube was slowly withdrawn under the microscope, and hemostasis was assured in the muscle layers. The lumbodorsal, thoracodorsal, or cervical fascia and Scarpa's layer were independently closed with 2-0 absorbable suture on a curved urology needle. In some obese patients, the fascia could not be reached for closure and only Scarpa's layer could be closed. The dermis was closed with inverted 3-0 absorbable suture. No skin suture was used. Mastisol and a single longitudinal Steri-strip (3 M) were used for the skin. A simple band-aid was placed. Patients were allowed to shower 48 hours postoperatively. Patients were instructed that a bump would be visible at the incision for several months before resolving. All patients were seen postoperatively at 4 weeks and 3 months after the procedure. If the patient was doing well, no further follow-up was performed after that time. Patients with ongoing problems were followed until a therapeutic endpoint was reached. The author has been in practice in the State of Oregon for 15 years and patients in need of further care have been able to contact him continuously throughout that time.

3. Results

In the 12-year period from 2001 to 2013, 1231 cases were performed using Metrx tubes, excluding fusion procedures and intentionally intradural procedures such as intradural tumors, vascular malformations, or hematomas. Case distribution is detailed in Table 1: 262 cases were cervical, 40 cases were thoracic, and 929 cases were lumbar. Patient age ranged from 16 to 95 years (mean 53 ± 18 years; standard deviation). No patient was excluded from this type of surgery based upon weight.

There were no direct nerve root or spinal cord injuries or new motor neurologic deficits after surgery with the exception of the C5 root. Three patients of a total of 53 foraminotomy patients operated at the C5 level (5.7%) developed delayed C5 weakness within a few days of surgery. Two patients made complete recoveries within three months and one never regained function of the C5 root. For comparison, during the author's career, 46 patients had an anterior cervical surgery including the C5 root level for radiculopathy and 76 patients for myelopathy. One of these 122 patients had a transient C5 palsy (0.8%). Thus, for this entire series of 1231 procedures, there were 3 motor deficits (0.24%) and one permanent motor deficit (0.08%). Two patients noted increased sensory deficits in the dermatomal distribution of the operated cervical nerve root (one C6 and one C8), both of which resolved over 2 months. One patient early in the series developed a symptomatic epidural hematoma at the first level of a two-level lumbar laminectomy which required evacuation the night of surgery. There were no neurologic sequelae of this event, but the author began using the red rubber drain as noted above after this event. Another patient early in the series developed pain after a durotomy resulted in a nerve root herniation requiring reexploration from the contralateral side to reduce this. The use of NuKnit or artificial dura to prevent nerve root herniation has prevented this from happening again (see above). Overall, there were 33 durotomies in 1231 patients (2.7%).

There were 295 first time lumbar discectomies, one two-level lumbar discectomy, and 55 redo discectomies. There were 88 procedures for lumbar far lateral discectomies and 11 for redo far lateral discectomies. 186 procedures were performed for lumbar spinal stenosis at a single level, 59 for two-level decompressions (one of which was done at

TABLE 1: Surgical case distribution.

Surgery	Procedure	Number (n)	Durotomy (n)
Lumbar	Paramedian discectomy	295	12
	Redo discectomy	55	3
	Two-level discectomy	1	0
	Far lateral discectomy	88	1
	Redo far lateral discectomy	11	0
	Stenosis, single level	186	7
	Stenosis, multilevel	59	6
	Stenosis, redo	1	0
	Synovial cyst	44	1
	Epidural abscess	15	0
	Other	3	0
	Foraminotomy, single level	149	1
	Foraminotomy, multilevel	21	1
	Foraminotomy, bilateral	1	0
	Total lumbar	**929**	**32**
Cervical	Foraminotomy, single level	160	0
	Foraminotomy, two-level	72	0
	Foraminotomy, bilateral	1	0
	Foraminotomy, discectomy	11	0
	Foraminotomy, redo	9	0
	Laminectomy for stenosis	6	0
	Laminectomy for tumor	1	0
	Laminectomy for epidural hematoma	1	0
	Laminectomy for synovial cyst	1	0
	Total cervical	**262**	**0**
Thoracic	Discectomy	7	1
	Laminectomy for stenosis	5	0
	Laminectomy for biopsy	4	0
	Laminectomy for abscess	1	0
	Laminectomy for tumor	3	0
	Laminotomy for electrode	20	0
	Total thoracic	**40**	**1**

nonadjacent levels), and 2 for three-level decompressions. Forty-four lumbar procedures were for resection of synovial cysts. Lumbar epidural abscesses were drained in 15 cases. Two procedures were for lumbar epidural metastatic tumor resections and one was for a spontaneous lumbar epidural hematoma. 149 procedures were for single-level lumbar foraminotomy, 21 were for two-level lumbar foraminotomy, and one was for bilateral foraminotomy at the same level.

In total, there were 929 lumbar procedures. There were no infections in these patients during the 3-month postoperative follow-up and no delayed infections that have been brought to the author's attention. There were no neurologic injuries in these patients. A single patient early in the series undergoing a two-level lumbar laminectomy for stenosis developed a symptomatic epidural hematoma at the first level several hours after surgery requiring evacuation with no permanent sequelae. There have been no further events since the use of drains during the second level procedure as described above. There were 12 durotomies in the 295 (4.1%) first time lumbar discectomies, 3 durotomies in the 55 (5.5%) redo lumbar discectomies, 7 durotomies in the 186 (3.8%) single-level lumbar laminectomies for stenosis, 6 durotomies in the 59 (10.1%) multilevel lumbar laminectomies, 1 durotomy in the 44 (2.3%) synovial cyst resections, 2 durotomies in the 171 (1.2%) lumbar foraminotomies, and one durotomy in the 99 (1%) far lateral discectomies. Thus, over the entire 929 patients, there were 32 durotomies (3.4%). No patient developed postural headaches, CSF leaks, symptomatic pseudomeningocele, or requirement for any additional intervention for CSF leak in the 3-month minimum period of follow-up after surgery.

There were 160 first time single-level cervical foraminotomies. There were 72 two-level cervical foraminotomies, 9 redo cervical foraminotomies, and one bilateral cervical foraminotomy. Six cervical laminectomies were performed for canal stenosis, one for epidural tumor, one for synovial cyst, and one for an acute epidural hematoma.

In total, there were 262 cervical procedures. There were no infections in these patients. Two patients noted transient increased hypesthesia in the dermatomal distribution of an operated nerve root after surgery, but these both resolved within 2 months. There were no motor deficits other than C5 as noted above. There were no durotomies in these patients.

There were 7 thoracic discectomies, 6 thoracic laminectomies for stenosis, 4 thoracic biopsies, 3 thoracic epidural tumor resections, and one drainage procedure for a thoracic epidural abscess. Twenty spinal cord stimulator paddle electrodes were implanted. In total, there were 40 thoracic procedures. There were no wound infections, new neurologic deficits, and one durotomy. One paraplegic patient developed fatal staphylococcal sepsis 6 weeks after surgery, presumed to be due to one of many decubitus ulcers, with no evidence of wound infection at the time of his demise.

4. Discussion

While there is accumulating data supporting minimally invasive spine surgery techniques, recent reviews still suggest the need for more Level I and II data to demonstrate benefit over open surgery [3]. Reduced complication rates as a benefit of tubular retractor based surgeries may factor into the decision of when to use these techniques.

There were no wound infections in this series of 1231 cases. Without any infections, it was not possible to assess the role of diabetes, obesity, timing of perioperative antibiotics, or anterior versus posterior approaches in infection, but these have been reported to be risk factors by others [8, 9]. Wound infection rates after open spine surgery have been reported to be in the range of 0.7 to 16% [6]. In O'Toole et al.'s review [6] of 1338 cases performed by three surgeons through tubular retractors, which included fusions and intradural procedures, there were 2 superficial wound infections (both in fusion procedures) and one deep infection, discitis in a decompressive laminectomy in a 90-year-old patient. This patient had suffered from streptococcal cellulitis and urinary tract infection 2 months postoperatively and grew the same organism from his disc space at needle biopsy, presumably by hematogenous spread and not by direct contamination at surgery. The infection rate for decompression only was 0.1%, for fusion 0.74%, and overall 0.22%. They concluded that minimally invasive techniques may reduce postoperative wound infection by as much as 10-fold compared with modern series of open procedures. Ikuta et al. [10] reported on 114 consecutive patients undergoing minimally invasive lumbar decompression for stenosis. There were no surgical site infections noted. Summing these series with the present data, there were 1039 plus 114 plus 1231 = 2384 noninstrumented, extradural procedures with only a single deep wound infection which is likely to have been due to secondary hematogenous seeding from an unrelated source.

O'Toole et al. [6] speculate on four potential reasons for the low surgical site infection rate: (1) reduced tissue exposure as much of the wound is covered by the tubular retractor, (2) minimal exposure of the skin to the wound, with little opportunity for instruments or the surgeons hands to contact the skin, (3) smaller wounds which are more likely to heal rapidly, and (4) reduction in dead space with resulting hematoma and seromas which can serve as the nidus for infection.

The author agrees and adds (5) lack of use of monopolar coagulation which minimizes devitalized tissue in the wound, another potential source of infection, (6) symmetric distribution of retraction forces which minimizes the risk of tissue ischemia and necrosis, (7) the incision which is made in a single stroke, as the number of knife passes has been shown to increase the infectability of experimental wounds, [11] and (8) the absence of skin sutures, which may allow an avenue of access to the wound.

Postoperative C5 root palsy is an enigmatic entity. It has been reported to occur in 5.1% of all cervical cases including the C5 level and 8.7% of posterior decompressions at the C5 level [12]. Another study reported an incidence of 12% in 98 patients undergoing either anterior or posterior approaches without foraminotomy [13]. This study found that the likelihood of a postoperative palsy was higher in patients with narrower spinal canal anterior posterior diameter, with narrower foraminal diameter, and with increases in the cord lamina angle at the operated level [13]. The use of cooled saline during drilling has been reported to reduce the incidence of new neurologic deficits after cervical laminoplasty, [14] but if heating related to drilling was the cause of root palsy, then C5 would not be the only affected root. Therefore, there remains something unique to the C5 root's vulnerability [13].

New neurologic deficit after elective spinal surgery has been reported based upon the Scoliosis Research Society database [15]. Of 108,419 cases, new neurologic deficits were documented for 1064 (1.0%), including 662 nerve root injuries, 74 cauda equine injuries, and 293 spinal cord injuries (deficit type was not specified for 35 cases). The rate of new neurologic deficits for cases with implants was more than twice that for cases without implants (1.15% versus 0.52%). Therefore, the lower rate of 0.52% is more comparable with the current series and indicates that minimally invasive surgery can be performed with acceptable neurologic complication rates when compared to such a large database.

Durotomy is a common complication of spinal surgery. In 1014 procedures for 1261 levels of lumbar spinal stenosis, Takahashi et al. [16] reported durotomy in 4% of cases and 3.3% of operated levels. Durotomy was highest with juxtafacet cysts (18.2%) and spondylolisthesis (9%). In the SPORT analysis, [17] 9% of 409 patients undergoing first time open laminectomy had a durotomy. Durotomy prolonged surgery time, blood loss, and inpatient stay, but there was no difference in primary outcomes at follow-up [17]. In the United Kingdom, prospective data on 1549 cases showed an incidence of durotomy to be 3.5% for primary discectomy, 8.5% for spinal stenosis surgery, and 13.2% for revision discectomy [18]. Durotomy appears to be less common during tubular retraction based surgery than that reported in these open surgical series and the consequences of such appear to be reduced. With no wound cavity in which to accumulate a pseudomeningocele and no easy route of egress from the wound, delayed complications of CSF leakage appear to be reduced by tubular retraction surgery.

Minimally access spinal surgery using tubular retractors, in properly selected cases, does appear to result in a reduced rate of wound infection, durotomy, symptomatic CSF leak, and new neurologic deficit. In turn, this may result in reduced costs of health care.

5. Conclusion

In the author's experience, minimally invasive spine surgery undertaken through tubular retractors shows a low wound infection rate when compared to open surgery. Durotomy is no more common than open procedures and does not result in the need for secondary procedures. New neurologic deficits are uncommon; however, when present, they are most common at the C5 root.

Study Limitations

This study was undertaken in an effort to describe the author's personal experience. The retrospective review exposes the study to inherent observational bias. The author has however made every effort to provide an accurate account of the data available.

Acknowledgment

The author thanks Shirley McCartney, Ph.D., for editorial assistance.

References

[1] C. D. Lawton, Z. A. Smith, S. K. Lam, A. Habib, R. H. Wong, and R. G. Fessler, "Clinical outcomes of microendoscopic foraminotomy and decompression in the cervical spine," *World Neurosurgery*, vol. 81, no. 2, pp. 422–427, 2014.

[2] P. Lee, J. C. Liu, and R. G. Fessler, "Perioperative results following open and minimally invasive single-level lumbar discectomy," *Journal of Clinical Neuroscience*, vol. 18, no. 12, pp. 1667–1670, 2011.

[3] Z. A. Smith and R. G. Fessler, "Paradigm changes in spine surgery-evolution of minimally invasive techniques," *Nature Reviews Neurology*, vol. 8, no. 8, pp. 443–450, 2012.

[4] A. P. Wong, Z. A. Smith, R. R. Lall, L. E. Bresnahan, and R. G. Fessler, "The microendoscopic decompression of lumbar stenosis: a review of the current literature and clinical results," *Minimally Invasive Surgery*, vol. 2012, Article ID 325095, 11 pages, 2012.

[5] P. Shih, A. P. Wong, T. R. Smith, A. I. Lee, and R. G. Fessler, "Complications of open compared to minimally invasive lumbar spine decompression," *Journal of Clinical Neuroscience*, vol. 18, no. 10, pp. 1360–1364, 2011.

[6] J. E. O'Toole, K. M. Eichholz, and R. G. Fessler, "Surgical site infection rates after minimally invasive spinal surgery: clinical article," *Journal of Neurosurgery: Spine*, vol. 11, no. 4, pp. 471–476, 2009.

[7] R. M. Haque, S. Z. Hashmi, Y. Ahmed, O. Uddin, A. T. Ogden, and R. Fessler, "Primary dural repair in minimally invasive spine surgery," *Case Reports in Medicine*, vol. 2013, Article ID 876351, 6 pages, 2013.

[8] M. A. Olsen, J. J. Nepple, K. D. Riew et al., "Risk factors for surgical site infection following orthopaedic spinal operations," *Journal of Bone and Joint Surgery*, vol. 90, no. 1, pp. 62–69, 2008.

[9] M. A. Olsen, J. Mayfield, C. Lauryssen et al., "Risk factors for surgical site infection in spinal surgery," *Journal of Neurosurgery*, vol. 98, no. 2, pp. 149–155, 2003.

[10] K. Ikuta, O. Tono, T. Tanaka et al., "Surgical complications of microendoscopic procedures for lumbar spinal stenosis," *Minimally Invasive Neurosurgery*, vol. 50, no. 3, pp. 145–149, 2007.

[11] T. K. Hunt and H. W. Hopf, "Wound healing and wound infection: what surgeons and anesthesiologists can do," *Surgical Clinics of North America*, vol. 77, no. 3, pp. 587–606, 1997.

[12] V. M. Bhalodia, D. M. Schwartz, and A. K. Sestokas, "Efficacy of intraoperative monitoring of transcranial electrical stimulation-induced motor evoked potentials and spontaneous electromyography activity to identify acute-versus delayed-onset C-5 nerve root palsy during cervical spine surgery: clinical article," *Journal of Neurosurgery: Spine*, vol. 19, no. 4, pp. 395–402, 2013.

[13] D. Lubelski, A. Derakhshan, A. S. Nowacki et al., "Predicting C5 palsy via the use of preoperative anatomic measurements," *The Spine Journal*, 2013.

[14] S. Takenaka, N. Hosono, Y. Mukai, T. Miwa, and T. Fuji, "The use of cooled saline during bone drilling to reduce the incidence of upper-limb palsy after cervical laminoplasty: clinical article," *Journal of Neurosurgery: Spine*, vol. 19, no. 4, pp. 420–427, 2013.

[15] D. K. Hamilton, J. S. Smith, C. A. Sansur et al., "Rates of new neurological deficit associated with spine surgery based on 108,419 procedures: a report of the scoliosis research society morbidity and mortality committee," *Spine*, vol. 36, no. 15, pp. 1218–1228, 2011.

[16] Y. Takahashi, T. Sato, H. Hyodo et al., "Incidental durotomy during lumbar spine surgery: Risk factors and anatomic locations: Clinical article," *Journal of Neurosurgery: Spine*, vol. 18, no. 2, pp. 165–169, 2013.

[17] A. Desai, P. A. Ball, K. Bekelis et al., "SPORT: does incidental durotomy affect long-term outcomes in cases of spinal stenosis?" *Neurosurgery*, vol. 69, no. 1, pp. 38–44, 2011.

[18] S. I. Tafazal and P. J. Sell, "Incidental durotomy in lumbar spine surgery: Incidence and management," *European Spine Journal*, vol. 14, no. 3, pp. 287–290, 2005.

5

Laparoscopic Hernia Repair versus Open Herniotomy in Children

Rafik Shalaby,[1] Refaat Ibrahem,[1] Mohamed Shahin,[2] Abdelaziz Yehya,[1] Mohamed Abdalrazek,[1] Ibrahim Alsayaad,[2] and Maged Ali Shouker[3]

[1] *Pediatric Surgery Unit, Al-Azhar University Hospitals, Cairo, Egypt*
[2] *Pediatric Surgery Unit, Al-Azhar University Hospitals, Damietta, Egypt*
[3] *Diagnostic Imaging Department, Al-Azhar University Hospitals, Cairo, Egypt*

Correspondence should be addressed to Rafik Shalaby, rafikshalaby@yahoo.com

Academic Editor: Othmar Schöb

Background. Laparoscopic hernia repair in infancy and childhood is still debatable. The objective of this study is to compare laparoscopic assisted hernia repair versus open herniotomy as regards operative time, hospital stay, postoperative hydrocele formation, recurrence rate, iatrogenic ascent of the testis, testicular atrophy, and cosmetic results. *Patients and Methods.* Two hundred and fifty patients with inguinal hernia were randomized into two equal groups. Group A was subjected to laparoscopic inguinal hernia repair. Group B was subjected to open herniotomy. The demographic data were matched between both groups. Assessment of the testicular volume and duplex assessment in preoperative, early, and late postoperative periods were done. *Results.* All cases were completed successfully without conversion. The mean operative time for group A was 7.6 ± 3.5 minutes, 9.2 ± 4.6 minutes and 11.4 ± 2.7 minutes, for unilateral hernia, unilateral hernia in obese child, and bilateral hernia, respectively. The recurrence rate was 0.8% in group A, whereas in group B the recurrence rate was 2.4%. *Conclusion.* Laparoscopic hernia repair by RN is an effective line of hernia repair. It resulted in marked reduction of operative time, low rate of recurrence, no testicular atrophy, no iatrogenic ascent of the testis, and excellent cosmetic results.

1. Introduction

Inguinal hernia (IH) repair is one of the most frequently performed surgical procedures in infants and children. Open herniotomy is its standard treatment against which all alternative modalities of treatment are evaluated. It is credited with being easy to perform, having a high success rate, and low rate of complications. However, recently, many centers routinely perform laparoscopic hernia repair in children and there have been numerous reports describing various laparoscopic techniques rather than the traditional open approach [1–4].

Reported advantages of laparoscopic hernia repair include excellent visual exposure, minimal dissection, less complications, comparable recurrence rates, and improved cosmetic results compared with the traditional open approach. In addition, laparoscopic hernia repair also allows contralateral patent process vaginalis (PPV) hernias to be defined and repaired in the same operation [5–7].

Randomized control study of laparoscopic hernia repair versus OH in pediatrics is rare in the literature [8–10]. This paper presents a big series and describes a new technique which is the use of Reverdin Needle (RN) in laparoscopic hernia repair in comparison with OH, to the best of our knowledge, this technique has not been reported before. So, this prospective randomized controlled study was conducted to compare laparoscopic assisted hernia repair by RN with OH in infancy and childhood as regards operative time, hospital stay, postoperative hydrocele formation, recurrence rate, iatrogenic ascent of the testis, testicular atrophy, and cosmetic results.

2. Patients and Methods

A prospective randomized controlled study was carried out in the Pediatric Surgery Unit of Al-Azhar University Hospitals and 2 private hospitals, over four-year period.

TABLE 1: The demographic data for the two groups.

Groups	Group A		Group B		Total	P value
	Number	%	Number	%		
Sex						
(i) Male	38	30.4	92	73.6	179 (71.6%)	0.48**
(ii) Female	87	69.6	33	26.4	71 (28.4%)	
Age/month						
(i) 1–12	58	46.4	50	40	95 (38%)	
(ii) 12–24	45	36	55	44	113 (45.2%)	0.80**
(iii) 24<	22	17.6	20	16	42 (16.8%)	
Presentation						
(i) Unilateral in obese child	25	20	28	22.4	53 (21.2%)	
(ii) Bilateral	44	35.2	48	38.4	52 (20.8%)	
(iii) Recurrent inguinal hernia	12	9.6	15	12	27 (10.8%)	0.18**
(iv) Inguinal hernia with umbilical hernia	18	14.4	22	17.6	40 (16%)	
(v) Inguinal hernia with questionable other side	26	20.8	12	9.6	38 (15.2%)	

** Insignificant.

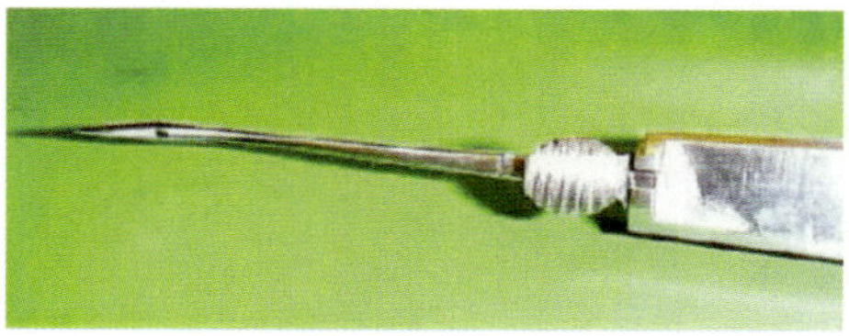

(a)

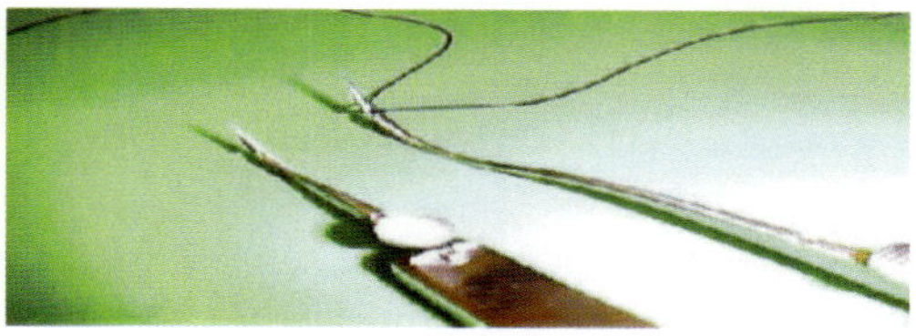

(b)

FIGURE 1: Reverdin needle.

The study was approved by our ethical committee. Two hundred and fifty patients with IH were randomized into two equal groups by a random-number table sequence after a written informed parental consent was obtained. Group A ($n = 125$) was subjected to laparoscopic assisted inguinal hernia repair by RN (Figure 1) (Martin Medizin Technik, Tuttlingen, Germany). Group B ($n = 125$) was subjected to open herniotomy (OH). The demographic data were matched between both groups (Table 1). Inclusion criteria included bilateral inguinal hernia, recurrent hernia, hernia in obese child, inguinal hernia with umbilical hernia and hernia on ipsilateral with questionable contralateral side. Exclusion criteria included unilateral inguinal hernia in nonobese child and hernia with undescended testicles. The main outcome measurements were operative time, hospital stay, postoperative hydrocele formation, recurrence rate, iatrogenic ascent of the testis, testicular atrophy, and cosmetic results. All children were subjected to full history taking, thorough clinical examination, routine laboratory investigations, and inguinoscrotal U/S. Testicular size and perfusion of male cases ($n = 179$) were evaluated in the preoperative, early postoperative (within 48 hours of surgery), and late postoperative periods (6 months after surgery) using Gray-scale ultrasonography, and Doppler ultrasound (DUS) (both duplex and power Doppler mode). (Sonoline Antaris, Siemens, Medical Corporation U/S Erlangen, Germany). The patients were examined with a 7.5 MHz linear, phased-array transducer. Both testes were scanned in transverse and longitudinal planes while the patient was in the supine position, and sedation was used when required in the form of paracetamol suppository. The testis on the unaffected side (in unilateral cases) was scanned first to optimize the Doppler settings for assessment of slow blood flow in the testis.

The volume of testis on both sides was calculated using the ellipsoid formula (volume = $0.523 \times D_1 \times D_2 \times D_3$), where D_1, D_2, and D_3 were the maximally measured longitudinal, anteroposterior, and transverse diameters.

The ratio v was defined as v = testicular volume of the operated side (postoperatively)/testicular volume of the same side (preoperatively). Volume of the testis and the ratio v were calculated during the preoperative and late postoperative examinations.

Criteria of testicular atrophy were defined as 75% reduction in estimated testicular volume, ratio v less than 75%, and resistive index (RI) more than 0.7.

All operations were done by the first three authors, and a senior resident holds the camera. In group A, after induction of general endotracheal tube anesthesia, the patient was placed supine in Trendelenburg's position. Insertion of the main umbilical port was accomplished by the open method. Pneumoperitoneum was established to a pressure of 8 to 12 mm Hg.

Laparoscopy was used for initial visualization of the pelvis and IIRs on both sides. Laparoscopic hernia repair was done according to the technique described by Shalaby et al., 2006, with some modifications [11]. A 3 mm Maryland

TABLE 2: Distribution of the studied groups according to operative time.

Groups	Group A (mean SD)	Group B (mean SD)	P value
Unilateral and recurrent unilateral	7.6 ± 3.5 minutes	12.8 ± 4.5 minutes	<0.001*
Hernia in obese child	9.2 ± 4.6 minutes	14.3 ± 3.6 minutes	<0.001*
Bilateral	11.4 ± 2.7 minutes	21.9 ± 7.2 minutes	<0.001*

* Significant.

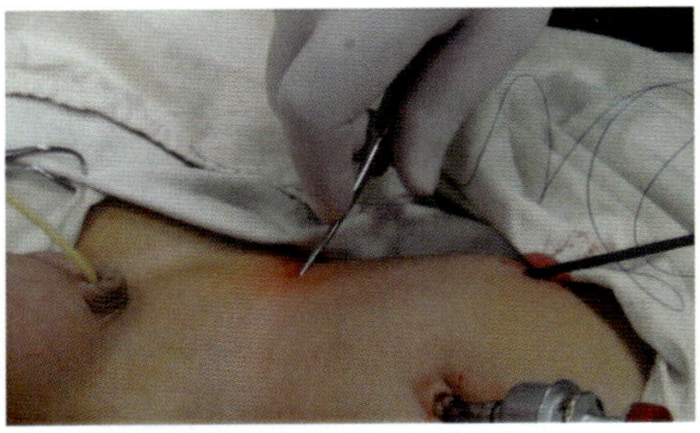

FIGURE 2: Insertion of RN on the right side.

forceps, holding the tip of a 3/0 Prolene thread, was inserted into the abdomen without trocar at the lateral border of the rectus muscle just above the level of the umbilicus leaving the long end of the thread outside the abdomen (Figure 2).

A stab incision of the skin was done 2 cm above and lateral to the IIR on the right side, and 2 cm above and medial to the IIR on the left side and RN was inserted into the abdominal cavity (Figure 2). The needle was manipulated to pierce the peritoneum at 3 O'clock on IIR and was advanced to pass through the lower margin of IIR under the peritoneum and in front of the spermatic vessels and vas to pierce the peritoneum at 9 O'clock on the IIR. Care was taken to avoid injury of the spermatic vessels, and vas by grasping and lifting the peritoneum away from the vas and vessels and the RN was seen all the time beneath the peritoneum (needle sign). Then, the side of the hole of RN was opened and the thread hold by Maryland was inserted inside it. Then, the side of the hole of RN was closed, and the needle was withdrawn backward in the same path till reaching the starting point at 3 O'clock. Then, RN mounted by the thread was reinserted again at 3 O'clock and was advanced along the upper margin of the IIR beneath the peritoneum and fascia transversalis to come out from the same opening at 9 O'clock where the short end of the thread was withdrawn out of RN and pulled outside the abdominal cavity for extracorporeal suture tie. Before tightening the knot, the scrotum was squeezed and the intraperitoneal pressure was released to expel the gas in the hernial sac.

A contralateral internal ring with a patent processus vaginalis (more than 2 mm) was regarded as a possible cause of developing clinical hernia and repaired at the same time [7]. The skin incisions were closed with Steri-strips.

In group B, OH was done through an inguinal skin crease incision. High ligation of the sac was performed using 4/0, 3/0 absorbable (Monocryl) suture. The distal sac was slit open to prevent postoperative hydrocele formation. The wound was closed in layers, using absorbable suture.

All patients were followed up in the out-patient clinic after 7 days, 2 weeks, 6 months, 1 year, and 2 years. Parents were advised to contact the department of pediatric surgery, if there were any concerns in the immediate postoperative period.

3. Statistical Analysis

The collected data were organized, tabulated, and statistically analyzed using Statistical Package for Social Science (SPSS) version 16 (SPSS Inc., USA). Qualitative data, frequency, and percent distribution were calculated, and Chi square test was used for comparison between groups. Quantitative data, mean, standard deviation (SD), and range were calculated, and for comparison between two groups, the independent samples (t) test was used. For interpretation of results, $P < 0.05$ was considered significant.

4. Results

Two hundred and fifty patients with IH were operated upon by 2 different techniques. Group A ($n = 125$) was subjected to laparoscopic assisted inguinal hernia repair by RN. Group B ($n = 125$) was subjected to OH. They were 179 males and 71 females. The youngest was 5 months and the oldest was 96 months, given an overall mean age of 61.56 ± 28.32 months. All procedures of group A were completed laparoscopically without any conversion. No intraoperative complications occurred during this study.

In group A the patients resumed normal activities within 6 hours after surgery, whereas in patients of group B they resumed normal activities within 10 hours. All patients had uneventful postoperative recoveries and were discharged on the same day of admission. The mean hospital stay was 5 ± 3.23 hours with no significant difference between both groups. There is significant statistical difference between the studied groups as regards operative time (Table 2). Three cases developed hydrocele in the early postoperative follow-up period in group A, while in group B, postoperative hydrocele was reported in 5 cases. However, all cases responded well to conservative management within 3 weeks (Table 3). Over a mean follow-up period of 24 months (range of 16–30 months), the recurrence rate was 0.8% (one case) in group A, whereas in group B recurrence rate was 2.4% (3 cases) (Table 3).

In group A, there were no cases of iatrogenic ascent of the testis, while in group B 4 cases (4.35%) developed iatrogenic ascent of the testis.

The early cosmetic results for bilateral cases were excellent (Figures 3(a) and 3(b)). At a follow-up examination more than 6 months later, there were practically no visible scars in group A, while in group B 5 cases had ugly scars as

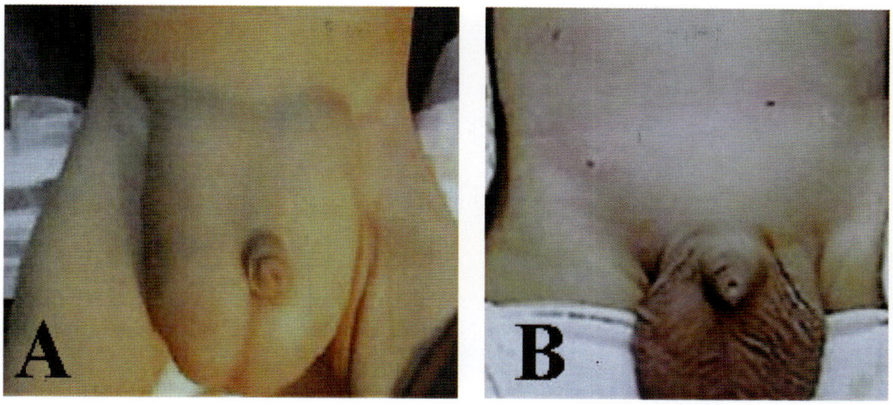

(a) (b)

Figure 3: (a) Bilateral huge inguinal hernia. (b) Postoperative view.

Table 3: Postoperative complications in the studied groups.

Groups	Group A		Group B		*P* value
	Number	%	Number	%	
Hydrocele	3/87	2.4%	5/92	5.4%	0.52**
Recurrence	1/125	0.8%	3/125	2.4%	0.31**
Iatrogenic ascent of the testis	0/87	0%	4/92	4.35%	0.049*
Testicular atrophy	0/87	0%	3/92	3.3%	0.089**
Ugly scar	0/125	0%	5/125	4.0%	0.024*

* Significant, ** insignificant.

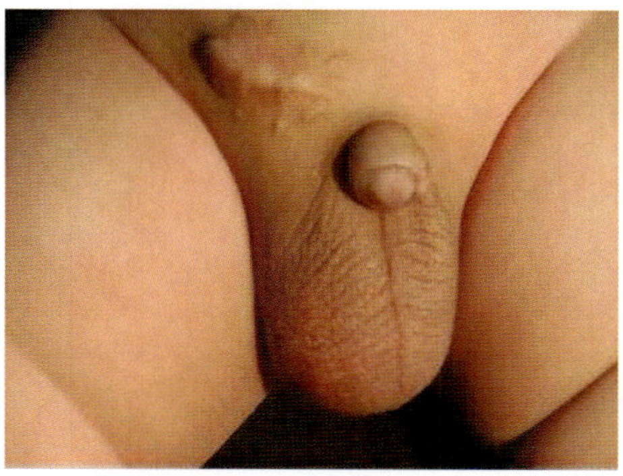

Figure 4: Right inguinal hernia postoperative view with ugly scar.

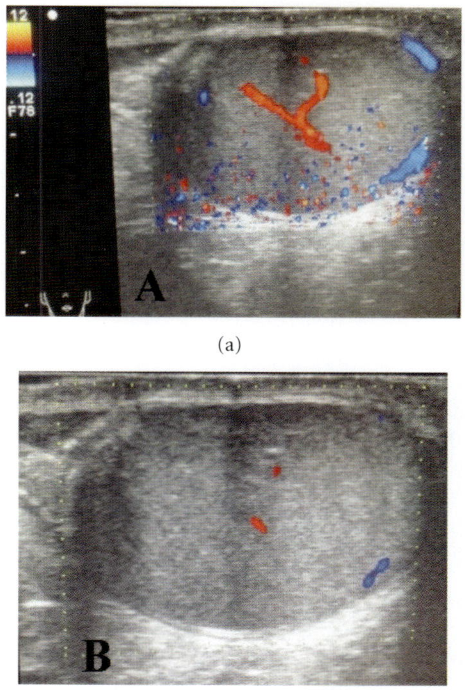

(a)

(b)

Figure 5: (a) Testicular Doppler U/S showed no signs of ischemia with good blood flow. (b) Testicular Doppler U/S showed poor blood flow.

reported by parents (Figure 4). The umbilical scars were not visible in all of the patients of group A.

Concerning the outcome of imaging assessment, in group A, there was no significant difference in values of perfusion and size of the testis between preoperative, early postoperative, and late postoperative periods (Figure 5(a)). While in group B; 3 cases (3.3%) had significant diminution of testicular perfusion and size, indicating atrophy (Figure 5(b)).

Duplex scan was performed for all male cases preoperatively and postoperatively for detection of significant changes of testicular blood flow. RI index was calculated, using paired *t*-test, and *P* values were obtained in group A.

Table 4 clearly shows that there are significant differences (increase of testicular volume) between preoperative and late postoperative volumes of testis units on the operated side in group A, while in group B it clearly shows that there are significant differences (decrease of testicular volume) between preoperative and late postoperative volumes of testis units on the operated side.

The ratio v was more than 75% in all cases of group A. RI was less than 0.7 in all cases of group A (no atrophy) as shown in Table 5. The ratio v was less than 75% in 3 cases of group B. RI was more than 0.7 in 3 cases of group B (atrophy) as shown in Table 5.

Table 4: Evaluation of volume of testis in males of both groups.

Groups	Group A ($n = 87$)			Group B ($n = 92$)		
	Mean volume	Volume range	SD	Mean volume	Volume range	SD
Preoperative	1.34	1.01–1.41	0.03*	1.35	0.89–1.49	0.05*
Late postoperative	1.36	1.21–1.86	0.05*	1.31	0.22–1.56	0.12*
Statistics	Paired (t) = 4.73, P value < 0.001*			Paired (t) = 6.36, P value < 0.001*		

* Significant.

Table 5: Duplex evaluation of centripetal artery in males of both groups.

Groups	Group A ($n = 87$)			Group B ($n = 92$)		
	Mean (RI)	RI range	SD	Mean (RI)	RI range	SD
Preoperative	0.48	0.41–0.52	0.03*	0.48	0.41–0.52	0.029
Early postoperative	0.47	0.40–0.52	0.031*	0.47	0.40–0.52	0.031
Late postoperative	0.46	0.40–0.49	0.032*	0.50	0.40–0.78	0.037
Statistics	Paired (t) = 75.0, P value < 0.001*			Paired (t) = 3.02, P value = 0.003*		

* Significant.

5. Discussion

In children, the standard surgical treatment of IH is limited to division and ligation of the hernial sac at the IIR without narrowing the ring [5]. The internal ring normally is reached by dissecting the hernial sac from the cord structures. Open herniotomy is an excellent method of repair in the pediatric population. However, it has the potential risk of injury of the spermatic vessels or vas deferens, hematoma formation, wound infection, iatrogenic ascent of the testis, testicular atrophy, and recurrence of hernia. It also carries the potential risk of tubal or ovarian damage which may cause infertility [12–14].

Laparoscopic approach is rapidly gaining popularity with more and more studies validating its feasibility, safety, and efficacy [5, 15].

Advantages of laparoscopic inguinal hernia repair include excellent visual exposure, the ability to evaluate the contralateral side, minimal dissection and avoidance of access trauma to the vas deferens and testicular vessels, iatrogenic ascent of the testis, and decreased operative time especially in recurrent and obese cases [3, 5]. However, Alzahem claimed that he is unable to identify any clear benefit of laparoscopic inguinal herniotomy over OH apart from reduction in metachronous hernia development and shorter operative time for bilateral cases [16].

Laparoscopic hernia repair in children is known to take longer operative time than OH. Many reports showed that it ranged from 20 to 74 minutes [5, 17–19]. However, the operative time is reduced with experience. It is well documented that the limiting step in laparoscopic hernia repair is the intracorporeal suturing of the IIR [2, 5]. In OH, time is consumed in gaining access, obtaining adequate exposure, in localizing and isolating the sac from the cord structures. In laparoscopic surgery, approaching the hernial defect from within the abdomen, makes the area of interest bloodless, and the magnification renders anatomy very clear, making surgery precise [13, 15, 20]. With growing experience and use of refinements, such as hydrodissection and needle sign, operative time does come down. Chan and Tam found that laparoscopic surgery is marginally quicker (5 min), but this difference appears insignificant, both statistically and in practice [18].

In our series the operative time is less than that reported in the literature as we use an easy simple and rapid technique for repair of IH using RN which can be done with far great ease in a very short time. Also, we used the extracorporeal suture ligation which is less time consuming [21].

Different laparoscopic techniques for repair of IH in children were reported in the literature. Schier (1998) used 2 mm instruments without a trocar for intra-abdominal suturing of the open inguinal rings in 25 girls by the placement of two Z-sutures with good results [17]. Bharathi et al. stated that SEAL resulted in marked reduction of operative time than TNH technique (unilateral, 15 versus 25 minutes, and bilateral, 25 versus 40 minutes). They added that avoiding the vas deferens and testicular vessels during SEAL repair in males may leave a small gap at the internal ring as well as leaving the hernial sac in situ, which has the potential to contribute to a higher incidence of hydrocele and recurrence in male patients [8, 21]. Yang et al. reported that laparoscopic herniorrhaphy is superior to open herniotomy in the repair of bilateral IH and lower rate of metachronous contralateral hernia, with similar operative time for unilateral hernias, length of hospital stay, recurrence, and complication rates [22]. Endo and Ukiyama introduced the Endoneedle that is designed specifically for laparoscopic extraperitoneal closure of the patent processus vaginalis [23]. Lee and Liang performed microlaparoscopic high ligation in 450 patients with good results. They reported no complications of the surgery and a remarkably low recurrence rate (0.88%) [5].

Marte et al. stated that the incision of the peritoneum lateral to the internal inguinal ring and the W-shaped suture, compared to the sole W-shaped suture, is safe and effective in preventing hernia recurrence [24].

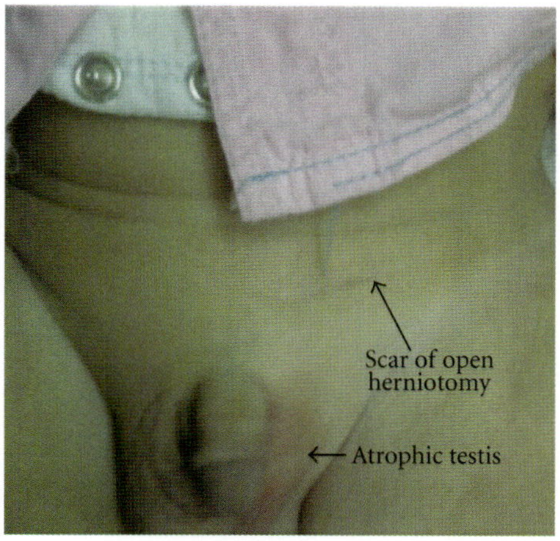

FIGURE 6: Left testicular atrophy after open herniotomy.

Open herniotomy in children has been reported to have recurrence rates of 0.8–3.8% [8]. While in laparoscopic hernia repair it is ranged from 0.7% to 4.5%. That is may be due to the presence of skip areas during placement of purse-string sutures as well as the tension resulting from intracorporeal knotting particularly in closure of large defects. The critical steps of hernia sac neck transaction at the IIR were not achieved in many laparoscopic procedures unlike during OH. Thus, transient or persistent hydrocele was unavoidable after these laparoscopic techniques. Tsai et al. and others dissected and transected the neck of the sac at IIR to be followed by a suture closure, with this being a faithful reproduction of the inguinal approach [24–26]. They claimed that leaving the hernial sac in continuity without disconnection at IIR may be the cause of subsequent recurrence and hydrocele formation. Ozgediz et al. and Bharathi et al. stated that avoiding the vas deferens and gonadal vessels during subcutaneous endoscopically assisted ligation repair in males may leave a small gap at IIR as well as leaving the hernia sac in situ, which has the potential to contribute to a higher incidence of recurrence in male patients [15, 21]. Technical modifications including injection of saline to lift up the peritoneum, the placement of single suture with complete encirclement of the sac, and disconnection of the hernial sac at IIR have been proposed to reduce the recurrence rates [27].

Yang et al. [22] in their meta-analysis stated that the recurrence rate of laparoscopic hernia repair was higher than OH in 2 studies [9, 28], lower in 3 studies [8, 29, 30], and equal (zero) in 2 studies [3, 10]. In the present study, recurrence rate was 0.8% in group A at one-year followup, while in group B the recurrence rate was 2.4%. The recurrence rate in the group A is lower than that reported in the literature that is because we started laparoscopic hernia repair in our unit after gaining good experiences in different laparoscopic procedures. Complete encirclement of the neck of the sac at the IIR with piercing of the peritoneum twice by RN may add fixation of the suture at this level which prevents migration of the suture distally preventing recurrence. It also, may result in creation of adhesions of the sac minimizing hydrocele formation. Laparoscopic approach was conducted for all recurrent hernias in this study as recommended by others [13, 31].

The natural history of the PPV in infants remains a controversial topic. Prior studies indicate that 40% of PPVs close spontaneously by two months of age and 60% by 2 years of age; however, the risk of incarceration is highest during infancy [32]. While in some other series PPVs less than 2 mm were not closed [6]. Our approach has been to ligate all PPVs to avoid the development of metachronous hernia. However, more studies are needed to clarify this point.

For many years, the possible risks of testicular atrophy (0.7–13%), spermatic vessel injury (1.6%), and nerve injury (5–15%) with routine contralateral exploration and repair of PPV in children who have primary unilateral inguinal hernia have been debated [33]. However, in this laparoscopic era, routine exploration and repair of PPV could be a new concept of IH treatment for the following reasons. First, the advantage of laparoscopic hernia repair is the clear and direct view of the vital cord structures that makes dissection of these structures safe and easy. In addition, the incidence of testicular atrophy is so rare in laparoscopic hernia repair because of the multiple collateral circulations of the testis, which makes dissection at IIR level extremely safe even in patients with previous inguinal surgery [34, 35]. Second, the well-known complications with open repair such as iatrogenic cryptorchidism, tethering of the testis and wound infection are almost not seen with laparoscopic repair. Surana and Puri stated that the incidence of iatrogenic ascent of the testis after groin exploration for inguinal herniotomy is 1.2% [36]. A total of 173 boys with previous unilateral inguinal herniotomy were subjected to clinical and U/S examination after a mean postoperative period of 31.68 months. One boy (0.58%) had a more than 50% and 10 boys (5.8%) had a more than 25% decrease in testicular volume on the operated side when compared with the nonoperated side [37].

In our study, no single case of testicular atrophy or iatrogenic ascent of the testis was reported in group A, while in group B 3 cases of testicular atrophy were reported (Figures 5 and 6). Regarding iatrogenic ascent of the testis, no single case was reported in group A, while in group B, 4 cases developed iatrogenic ascent of the testis and the difference is statistically significant. Nagraj et al. reported six cases (2.7%) of testicular atrophy after OH (four of the six patients presented with an incarcerated hernia). There were six cases of iatrogenic ascent of the testis requiring subsequent orchidopexy (2.7%) [38]. Barqawi et al. reported testicular atrophy in 2 cases (1%) after open surgery [34].

Cosmoses, five-millimeter and 3 mm incisions in group A were, indeed, cosmetically more appealing compared with 2 cm incisions in OH group B (Figures 3 and 4). All parents were satisfied with the cosmetic results of group A.

6. Conclusion

Our series supports the finding of other series that laparoscopic assisted inguinal hernia repair by RN is feasible safe and rapid technique. It resulted in marked reduction of operative time, low rate of recurrence, no testicular atrophy, no iatrogenic ascent of the testis, and excellent cosmetic results. Complications are minimal though long-term followup will be needed to determine the validity of these results.

References

[1] M. G. Schwöbel, H. Schramm, and C. A. Gitzelmann, "The infantile inguinal hernia—a bilateral disease?" *Pediatric Surgery International*, vol. 15, no. 2, pp. 115–118, 1999.

[2] T. E. Lobe and K. P. Schropp, "Inguinal hernias in pediatrics: initial experience with laparoscopic inguinal exploration of the asymptomatic contralateral side," *Journal of Laparoendoscopic Surgery*, vol. 2, no. 3, pp. 135–140, 1992.

[3] R. Saranga Bharathi, M. Arora, and V. Baskaran, "Pediatric inguinal hernia: laparoscopic versus open surgery," *Journal of the Society of Laparoendoscopic Surgeons*, vol. 12, no. 3, pp. 277–281, 2008.

[4] D. A. Lloyd and R. J. Rintala, "Inguinal hernia and hydrocele," in *Pediatric Surgery*, J. A. O'Neill Jr., Ed., pp. 1071–1086, Mosby, St. Louis, Mo, USA, 1998.

[5] Y. Lee and J. Liang, "Experience with 450 cases of micro-laparoscopic herniotomy in infants and children," *Pediatric Endosurgery and Innovative Techniques*, vol. 6, no. 1, pp. 25–28, 2002.

[6] F. Schier, P. Montupet, and C. Esposito, "Laparoscopic inguinal herniorrhaphy in children: a three-center experience with 933 repairs," *Journal of Pediatric Surgery*, vol. 37, no. 3, pp. 395–397, 2002.

[7] F. Schier, "Laparoscopic surgery of inguinal hernias in children; initial experience," *Journal of Pediatric Surgery*, vol. 35, no. 9, pp. 1331–1335, 2000.

[8] Y. C. Tsai, C. C. Wu, and S. S. D. Yang, "Open versus minilaparoscopic herniorrhaphy for children: a prospective comparative trial with midterm follow-up evaluation," *Surgical Endoscopy*, vol. 24, no. 1, pp. 21–24, 2010.

[9] A. L. Koivusalo, R. Korpela, K. Wirtavuori, S. Piiparinen, R. J. Rintala, and M. P. Pakarinen, "A single-blinded, randomized comparison of laparoscopic versus open hernia repair in children," *Pediatrics*, vol. 123, no. 1, pp. 332–337, 2009.

[10] K. L. Chan, W. C. Hui, and P. K. H. Tam, "Prospective randomized single-center, single-blind comparison of laparoscopic vs open repair of pediatric inguinal hernia," *Surgical Endoscopy*, vol. 19, no. 7, pp. 927–932, 2005.

[11] R. Y. Shalaby, M. Fawy, S. M. Soliman, and A. Dorgham, "A new simplified technique for needlescopic inguinal herniorrhaphy in children," *Journal of Pediatric Surgery*, vol. 41, no. 4, pp. 863–867, 2006.

[12] R. Shalaby, M. Ismail, A. Dorgham et al., "Laparoscopic hernia repair in infancy and childhood: evaluation of 2 different techniques," *Journal of Pediatric Surgery*, vol. 45, no. 11, pp. 2210–2216, 2010.

[13] F. Schier, "Laparoscopic inguinal hernia repair—a prospective personal series of 542 children," *Journal of Pediatric Surgery*, vol. 41, no. 6, pp. 1081–1084, 2006.

[14] C. Cam, C. Celik, A. Sancak, C. Iskender, and A. Karateke, "Inguinal herniorrhaphy in childhood may result in tubal damage and future infertility," *Archives of Gynecology and Obstetrics*, vol. 279, no. 2, pp. 175–176, 2009.

[15] D. Ozgediz, K. Roayaie, H. Lee et al., "Subcutaneous endoscopically assisted ligation (SEAL) of the internal ring for repair of inguinal hernias in children: report of a new technique and early results," *Surgical Endoscopy*, vol. 21, no. 8, pp. 1327–1331, 2007.

[16] A. Alzahem, "Laparoscopic versus open inguinal herniotomy in infants and children: a meta-analysis," *Pediatric Surgery International*, vol. 27, no. 6, pp. 605–612, 2011.

[17] F. Schier, "Laparoscopic herniorrhaphy in girls," *Journal of Pediatric Surgery*, vol. 33, no. 10, pp. 1495–1497, 1998.

[18] K. L. Chan and P. K. H. Tam, "Technical refinements in laparoscopic repair of childhood inguinal hernias," *Surgical Endoscopy*, vol. 18, no. 6, pp. 957–960, 2004.

[19] A. Darzi and C. C. Nduka, "Endoscopically guided percutaneous repair of inguinal hernia through a 2-cm incision: minihernia repair," *Surgical Endoscopy*, vol. 11, no. 7, pp. 782–784, 1997.

[20] H. Takehara, S. Yakabe, and K. Kameoka, "Laparoscopic percutaneous extraperitoneal closure for inguinal hernia in children: clinical outcome of 972 repairs done in 3 pediatric surgical institutions," *Journal of Pediatric Surgery*, vol. 41, no. 12, pp. 1999–2003, 2006.

[21] R. S. Bharathi, A. K. Dabas, M. Arora, and V. Baskaran, "Laparoscopic ligation of internal ring—three ports versus single-port technique: are working ports necessary?" *Journal of Laparoendoscopic and Advanced Surgical Techniques A*, vol. 18, no. 6, pp. 891–894, 2008.

[22] C. Yang, H. Zhang, J. Pu, and H. Mei, "Laparoscopic vs open herniorrhaphy in the management of pediatric inguinal hernia: a systemic review and meta-analysis," *Journal of Pediatric Surgery*, vol. 46, no. 9, pp. 1824–1834, 2011.

[23] M. Endo and E. Ukiyama, "Laparoscopic closure of patent processus vaginalis in girls with inguinal hernia using a specially devised suture needle," *Pediatric Endosurgery and Innovative Techniques*, vol. 5, no. 2, pp. 187–191, 2001.

[24] A. Marte, M. D. Sabatino, M. Borrelli, and P. Parmeggiani, "Decreased recurrence rate in the laparoscopic herniorraphy in children: comparison between two techniques," *Journal of Laparoendoscopic and Advanced Surgical Techniques A*, vol. 19, no. 2, pp. 259–262, 2009.

[25] Y. C. Tsai, C. C. Wu, and S. S. D. Yang, "Minilaparoscopic herniorrhaphy with hernia sac transection in children and young adults: a preliminary report," *Surgical Endoscopy*, vol. 21, no. 9, pp. 1623–1625, 2007.

[26] S. Giseke, M. Glass, P. Tapadar, L. Matthyssens, and P. Philippe, "A true laparoscopic herniotomy in children: evaluation of long-term outcome," *Journal of Laparoendoscopic and Advanced Surgical Techniques A*, vol. 20, no. 2, pp. 191–194, 2010.

[27] Y. H. Tam, K. H. Lee, J. D. Y. Sihoe et al., "Laparoscopic hernia repair in children by the hook method. A single-center series of 433 consecutive patients," *Journal of Pediatric Surgery*, vol. 44, no. 8, pp. 1502–1505, 2009.

[28] M. E. Hassan and A. R. Mustafawi, "Laparoscopic flip-flap technique versus conventional inguinal hernia repair in children," *Journal of the Society of Laparoendoscopic Surgeons*, vol. 11, no. 1, pp. 90–93, 2007.

[29] M. Endo, T. Watanabe, M. Nakano, F. Yoshida, and E. Ukiyama, "Laparoscopic completely extraperitoneal repair of inguinal hernia in children: a single-institute experience with 1,257 repairs compared with cut-down herniorrhaphy," *Surgical Endoscopy*, vol. 23, no. 8, pp. 1706–1712, 2009.

[30] A. Niyogi, A. S. Tahim, W. J. Sherwood et al., "A comparative study examining open inguinal herniotomy with and without hernioscopy to laparoscopic inguinal hernia repair in a pediatric population," *Pediatric Surgery International*, vol. 26, no. 4, pp. 387–392, 2010.

[31] M. V. Shcheben'kov, "The advantages of laparoscopic inguinal herniorrhaphy in children," *Vestnik khirurgii imeni I. I. Grekova*, vol. 156, no. 1, pp. 94–96, 1997.

[32] S. Stylianos, N. N. Jacir, and B. H. Harris, "Incarceration of inguinal hernia in infants prior to elective repair," *Journal of Pediatric Surgery*, vol. 28, no. 4, pp. 582–583, 1993.

[33] Y. C. Tsai, C. C. Wu, and S. S. Yang, "Transinguinal laparoscopy for a pediatric inguinal hernia: the inability to predict the occurrence of a contralateral metachronous inguinal hernia," *Journal of the Taiwan Urological Association*, vol. 19, no. 2, pp. 94–97, 2008.

[34] A. Barqawi, P. Furness III, and M. Koyle, "Laparoscopic palomo varicocelectomy in the adolescent is safe after previous ipsilateral inguinal surgery," *BJU International*, vol. 89, no. 3, pp. 269–272, 2002.

[35] M. Riccabona, J. Oswald, M. Koen, L. Lusuardi, C. Radmayr, and G. Bartsch, "Optimizing the operative treatment of boys with varicocele: sequential comparison of 4 techniques," *The Journal of Urology*, vol. 169, no. 2, pp. 666–668, 2003.

[36] R. Surana and P. Puri, "Iatrogenic ascent of the testis: an under-recognized complication of inguinal hernia operation in children," *British Journal of Urology*, vol. 73, no. 5, pp. 580–581, 1994.

[37] W. Y. M. Leung, M. Poon, T. W. Fan et al., "Testicular volume of boys after inguinal herniotomy: combined clinical and radiological follow-up," *Pediatric Surgery International*, vol. 15, no. 1, pp. 40–41, 1999.

[38] S. Nagraj, S. Sinha, H. Grant, K. Lakhoo, R. Hitchcock, and P. Johnson, "The incidence of complications following primary inguinal herniotomy in babies weighing 5 kg or less," *Pediatric Surgery International*, vol. 22, no. 6, pp. 500–502, 2006.

6

Retrograde Intrarenal Surgery in Patients Who Previously Underwent Open Renal Stone Surgery

Erdal Alkan,[1] Ali Saribacak,[2] Ahmet Oguz Ozkanli,[3] Mehmet Murad Başar,[1] Oguz Acar,[1] and Mevlana Derya Balbay[1]

[1]*Department of Urology, Memorial Sisli Hospital, Okmeydani, Sisli, 34385 Istanbul, Turkey*
[2]*Department of Urology, Izmit Konak Hospital, Kocaeli, 41100 Izmit, Turkey*
[3]*Department of Anesthesiology, Memorial Sisli Hospital, Okmeydani, Sisli, 34385 Istanbul, Turkey*

Correspondence should be addressed to Erdal Alkan; eralkan@hotmail.com

Academic Editor: David Lee

Purpose. To ascertain whether retrograde intrarenal surgery (RIRS) is as effective in patients treated previously with open renal stone surgery (ORSS) on the same kidney as in patients with no previous ORSS. *Methods.* There were 32 patients with renal stones who had previous ORSS and were treated with RIRS in the study group (Group 1). A total of 38 patients with renal stones who had no previous ORSS and were treated with RIRS were selected as the control group (Group 2). Recorded data regarding preoperative characteristics of the patients, stone properties, surgical parameters, outcomes, SFRs (no fragments or small fragments <4 mm), and complications between groups were compared. *Results.* Mean age, mean BMI, mean hospital stay, and mean operative time were not statistically different between groups. Mean stone size (10.1 ± 5.6 versus 10.3 ± 4.2; $p = 0.551$) and mean stone burden (25.4 ± 14.7 versus 23.5 ± 9.9; $p = 0.504$) were also similar between groups. After the second procedures, SFRs were 100% and 95% in groups 1 and 2, respectively ($p = 0.496$). No major perioperative complications were seen. *Conclusion.* RIRS can be safely and effectively performed with acceptable complication rates in patients treated previously with ORSS as in patients with no previous ORSS.

1. Introduction

The surgical techniques in the treatment of stone disease have dramatically changed in the last 20 years [1]. There has been a significant decrease in the number of patients requiring open renal stone surgery (ORSS) due to the technological developments in the field of urologic surgery. Nowadays shock wave lithotripsy (SWL) and percutaneous nephrolithotomy (PNL) are recommended as the first line treatment modalities in the management of renal stones <20 mm and >20 mm, respectively [2]. However, ORSS has been performed in 0.47–2% in select patients [1].

Since stone recurrence rate within 5 years is about 50%, multiple interventions may be needed for patients with stone disease [3]. Reoperation in patients with previous open renal stone surgery (ORSS) would be difficult due to retroperitoneal scarring around the kidney and distortion of the pelvicaliceal anatomy. Eventually, reoperation may be associated with a longer operative time, higher complication, and lower success rates. There are many studies about PNL in patients who previously underwent ORSS [4–7]. But there is only one study on retrograde intrarenal surgery (RIRS) in patients who previously underwent ORSS in the English literature [8]. In order to ascertain whether RIRS is as effective in patients treated previously with ORSS on the same kidney as in patients with no previous ORSS, we retrospectively compared our groups including stone properties, operative parameters, and postoperative results.

2. Materials and Methods

This study was designed as a retrospective controlled study and included patients who underwent RIRS between December 2007 and January 2015. There were 32 patients with renal stones who had previous ORSS and treated with RIRS in the study group (Group 1). A total of 38 patients with renal stones who had no previous ORSS and treated with RIRS were selected as the control group (Group 2). First 4-5 patients from each year (2008–2015) who were treated with RIRS but did not undergo ORSS were picked out and put together to form the control group. Patients with renal stones together with ureteral stones were also included in this study. All patients were preoperatively evaluated by CT scan with stone protocol to define the total stone burden and collecting system anatomy. Stone burden was calculated by measuring the maximum stone dimension in cases with single stone or sum of dimensions in cases of multiple stones. Recorded data regarding preoperative characteristics of the patients (gender, age), stone properties (stone number, size, and burden), surgical parameters (operative time, use of stents, and basket), outcomes, Stone Free Rates (SFRs), and perioperative complications were collected. Prior to the procedure, informed consent was obtained from all patients.

All procedures were done in a standard lithotomy position under general anesthesia. In patients with intrarenal stones and concomitant middle or lower ureteral stones, a semirigid ureteroscope (8/9.8F Olympus, Tokyo, Japan) was used first for the treatment of ureteral stones. RIRS was performed by three experienced surgeons (each surgeon performed at least 100 RIRS procedures) using URF P-5 flexible ureteroscope (Olympus, Tokyo, Japan) or Cobra flexible dual-channel ureteroscope (Richard Wolf, Knittlingen, Germany) according to its availability. A ureteral access sheath (Flexor ureteral access sheath 12/14F 35 cm; Cook Medical, Bloomington, IN, USA) was used routinely in order to access to the collecting system easily and decrease the intrarenal pressure. In cases where the ureteral access sheath or flexible ureteroscope without access sheath could not be advanced due to ureteral pathologies such as ureteral stricture, a ureteral stent was inserted into the ureter and the procedure delayed for 2 or 3 weeks. Holmium YAG laser (Sphinx, Lisa Laser, 30 watts, Katlenburg, Germany) in combination with a 200 μm (Litho Fib, Lisa Laser, Katlenburg, Germany) or 272 μm (Flexi Fib, Lisa Laser, Katlenburg, Germany) laser fibers was set at an energy level of 0.6–2.2 J and at a rate of 5–12 Hz. This is the only available laser source at our hospital. Holmium laser was used for stone fragmentation in all cases. All stones were fragmented until roughly all get smaller $\leqslant$4 mm in size, and relatively larger fragments were removed with a nitinol basket (Ngage nitinol stone extractor 2,2F 115 cm basket; Cook Medical, Bloomington, IN, USA) according to surgeon's discretion. Endoscopically, intraoperative success was defined as extraction of all stone fragments or laser lithotripsy of all stones to less than 4 mm fragments. At the end of the operation, an internal stent (usually 4.8F 26 cm) was inserted according to surgeon's discretion, which was removed under local anesthesia using a flexible ureteroscope in about 1 month of surgery. Residual fragments were assessed with noncontrast CT two months after internal stent removal. Success rate was defined as no fragments or the presence of clinically insignificant residual fragments (CIRF) smaller than 4 mm in the urinary system [2, 9]. All postoperative complications were recorded according to the Clavien-Dindo classification system [10].

2.1. Statistical Analysis. All analyses were performed using SPSS version 16.0 (Statistical Package for Social Sciences for windows; Chicago, IL, USA). The measurement data were expressed as mean ± standard derivation. Age, BMI, stone number, stone size, stone burden, operative times, and hospitalization times were compared by using Mann-Whitney *U* test. Additionally, use of ureteral access sheath and basket catheter, internal stent placement, SFR, and complication rates were compared by using Pearson Chi- Square test. p value of <0.05 was considered statistically significant.

3. Results

A total of 41 RIRS procedures performed on 32 patients were included in group 1. While 27 of 32 (85%) patients required a single procedure, 3 (9%) patients were treated with 2 procedures. Two (6%) more patients with bilateral renal stones required a total of 8 procedures (two procedures for each kidney) in group 1. On the other hand, RIRS was performed in 34 of 38 (90%) patients as a single procedure in group 2. Additionally second-session RIRS was performed in 2 (5%) patients, and bilateral RIRS was done in another 2 (5%) patients. As a result, a total of 41 and 42 RIRS procedures performed on 32 and 38 patients were included in groups 1 and 2, respectively. RIRS were performed due to back pain (54%), renal colic (23%), recurrent urinary tract infections (11%), persistent hematuria (9%), and patient preference (3%). Lower ureteral stones together with renal stones were present in 3 and 5 patients in groups 1 and 2, respectively. These stones were treated at the same session. Patient demographics and preoperative stone characteristics are shown in Table 1.

Intraoperative and postoperative comparisons between groups are summarized in Table 2. A ureteral access sheath could be placed in all patients but 2 in group 1. RIRS was successfully completed without access sheath in these cases. However, although a ureteral access sheath could be placed in another 2 patients in group 1, renal stones could not be reached due to concomitant ureteropelvic stenosis. Endopyelotomy and internal stent placement were performed in these patients and RIRS was successfully done after 30 days. A ureteral access sheath could not be placed in 5 (12%) patients in group 2. While 3 patients were treated without access sheath, 2 patients were stented and RIRS was delayed for 15 days. After all procedures, SFRs were 100% and 95% in groups 1 and 2, respectively (χ^2 = 1.747; p = 0.496). Although 24 (71%) and 30 (75%) renal units were truly stone free in groups 1 and 2, there were CIRF in 10 (29%) and 8 (20%) renal units in groups 1 and 2, respectively.

No major perioperative complications were seen. Some minor complications were recorded in 7 patients in each group (Table 2). Minor ureteral trauma occurred in 1 and 2 patients in groups 1 and 2, respectively. Intraoperative hemorrhage was seen in 1 case in each group. The procedures were not cancelled due to intraoperative complications and the operations were completed without any difficulty. Renal colic was detected in 3 and 2 patients in groups 1 and 2. Four patients with renal colic were treated with

TABLE 1: Patient demographics and preoperative stone characteristics.

	Group 1 (study group)	Group 2 (control group)	p value
Gender (M/F)	24/08	26/12	0.603
Mean age (year)	40.5 ± 12.8 (20–72)	45.5 ± 12.6 (23–74)	0.110
Mean BMI (kg/m^2)	28.1 ± 5.3 (19–42)	26.7 ± 4.1 (19–41)	0.217
Mean stone number (n)	2.7 ± 1.5 (1–7)	2.5 ± 1.3 (1–8)	0.544
Mean stone size (mm)	10.1 ± 5.6 (3–30)	10.3 ± 4.2 (3–21)	0.551
Mean stone burden (mm)	25.4 ± 14.7 (7–58)	23.5 ± 9.9 (6–60)	0.504
Total stone number (n)	106	101	
Localization (per procedure)			
Upper ureter	6 (5%)	10 (10%)	
Upper calyx	14 (13%)	11 (11%)	
Middle calyx	23 (22%)	18 (18%)	
Lower calyx	36 (34%)	42 (41%)	
Renal pelvis	27 (26%)	20 (20%)	
Lateralization (per patient)			
Right side	17 (53%)	13 (34%)	
Left side	13 (41%)	23 (61%)	
Bilateral	2 (6)	2 (5)	

TABLE 2: Intraoperative and postoperative comparisons between groups.

	Group 1 (study group)	Group 2 (control group)	p value
Mean operative time (min)	79.5 ± 37.8 (25–165)	76.1 ± 35.9 (30–150)	0.463
Use of ureteral access sheath	95% (39/41)	88% (37/42)	0.433
Use of basket catheter	56% (23/41)	52% (22/42)	0.827
Ureteral stent placement	71% (29/41)	67% (28/42)	0.814
Mean duration of ureteral stent (day)	30.3 ± 26.6 (2–120)	22.1 ± 9.2 (3–30)	0.127
Mean hospital stay (hour)	23.7 ± 8.0 (6–48)	25.6 ± 6.4 (18–48)	0.258
SFR (%)			
First procedure	82% (28/34)	90% (36/40)	0.497
Second procedure	100% (34/34)	95% (38/40)	0.496
Complication rates	17% (7/41)	17% (7/42)	0.596
(1) Intraoperative	5%	7%	
Ureteral trauma	1	2	
Hemorrhage	1	1	
(2) Postoperative	12%	10%	
Renal colic	3	2	
Prolonged hematuria	1	1	
Urinary tract infection	1	1	

parenteral medications in the emergency setting in groups 1 and 2 (Clavien 2). On the other hand, internal stent was placed in one patient with renal colic in group 2 due to hydroureteronephrosis (Clavien 3b). Prolonged hematuria that lasted longer than a week was seen in one patient in each group and treated conservatively without any transfusion (Clavien 1). Urinary tract infection (UTI) was seen in one patient in each group. The patient with pyelonephritis was treated with parenteral medications after hospitalization in group 1 (Clavien 2). Another patient with UTI was treated with appropriate antibiotics in the outpatient setting (Clavien 2).

4. Discussion

Since urolithiasis is a recurrent disease, multiple interventions are often needed in these patients [3]. In the past, ORSS was commonly performed in the treatment of urinary stone disease. However, with the recent technological development, ESWL, PNL, and RIRS have replaced open surgery. Eventually PNL and RIRS are being utilized more commonly instead of open surgery in the treatment of many patients who had a previous ORSS because of secondary urolithiasis. While PNL is an effective treatment option performed for the management of large and complex calculi, it is more invasive, with a significant rate of major complications especially in secondary cases [4–6, 11]. According to the European Association of Urology (EAU) guidelines, although RIRS or ESWL is recommended as the first line treatment in the management of kidney stones <10 mm or 10–20 mm, RIRS is not recommended as a first line therapy for kidney stones >20 mm since SFRs are low and staged procedures may become necessary [2, 12]. However, RIRS can be successfully performed by experienced hands at high volume centers [13, 14]. Moreover recent studies have demonstrated that RIRS can be effective and safe as an alternative treatment option for relatively larger, multiple, bilateral, and ESWL refractory renal stones [15–18].

Although a lot of studies have addressed the specific issues regarding PNL in a kidney previously operated on, there is only one study specifically addressing RIRS after ORSS [4–8]. RIRS was performed in 53 patients who previously underwent ORSS by Osman and associates [8]. In their study, mean patient age, mean stone size, and mean stone number were 51 years (18–65), 14.3 mm (5–32), and 3.0 (2–8), respectively. This study mentioned that RIRS after previous ORSS had some challenges. First, accessing the kidney stone may be difficult because of fibrosis and distortion of the collecting system as a result of ORSS. Second, accessing the upper urinary system may be technically challenging because of bilharziasis, causing inflammatory distortion of the bladder and ureters, which is endemic in their country [8]. We did not detect any serious bladder or lower ureteral pathologies in our series. Access sheath was used in the 39 (95%) of 41 procedures. Flexible ureteroscopy without access sheath was done in the remaining 2 (5%) patients, who had mild ureteral stenosis. On the other hand, renal stones could have not been reached due to ureteropelvic stenosis in 2 patients who were successfully treated at 2 separate sessions: in the first session, endopyelotomy and internal stent placement were performed and in the second session flexible ureteroscopy and laser lithotripsy were performed. We encountered that there were infundibular strictures and distortions in the intrarenal collecting system and the stone was covered with fibrotic tissue in one patient. This patient was treated with two separate sessions: fibrotic tissue vaporization and partial laser fragmentation were performed in the first session; the remaining stone fragment was broken in the second session.

In the study by Osman et al., mean operative time, use of ureteral access sheath, and internal stent placement were 82 minutes (20–130), 41 (77%) patients, and 53 (100%) patients, respectively [8]. Their success rates were 79.2% and 92.4% after the first- and second-session RIRS. Our study was different only in internal stent placement rates compared with the above-mentioned study. All patients in their study received internal stent placement to prevent ureteral strictures since bilharziasis is endemic in their country. In our series, internal stent placement was done in 71% (29/41) cases in the study group. Moreover overall SFRs after first- and second-session procedures were 82% and 100% and 90% and 95% for study and control groups, respectively ($p = 0.496$). The success rates in both studies were similar to each other and to the previously published RIRS series [15–17]. Consequently, these two studies demonstrated that RIRS is an effective and safe option in the management of patients with renal stones who previously underwent ORSS.

According to the recent published literature the overall complication rates of RIRS are between 6% and 23% [8, 16–19]. Ureteral traumas, access problems, intraoperative hematuria, prolonged hematuria, urinary tract infections, and renal colic are the most encountered complications [16–18]. Osman and collages reported that overall complication rate after RIRS in patients who underwent ORSS previously was 20.7% [8]. They reported two intraoperative complications (ureteral perforation and bleeding); both were treated conservatively. Additionally, some postoperative complications including febrile UTI (Clavien 2), hematuria (Clavien 1), stone street (Clavien 3b), and anuria in the solitary kidney (Clavien 3b) were also reported in their study [8]. In our study, overall complication rates in both groups were 17% ($p = 0.596$) and were similar to the current literature. All complications but 1 ($n = 7$) in group 1 were conservatively treated at the outpatient setting. Pyelonephritis (Clavien 2) was observed in one patient who was treated with parenteral medication after being hospitalized. On the other hand, only one patient with renal colic (Clavien 3b) in group 2 was treated with internal stent placement. Our study showed that the complication rates and types of complication did not change after RIRS in patients with previous ORSS compared with that of the primary RIRS procedure.

Our study has some limitations. First, it is a retrospective, nonrandomized study from a single center. Second, there were small numbers of patients. In spite of these limitations, our study is the second study on RIRS in the treatment of patients who underwent ORSS previously.

5. Conclusion

RIRS in patients treated previously with ORSS can be safely and effectively performed with acceptable complication rates as in patients with no previous ORSS by the hands of experienced surgeons when essential endourological pieces of equipment are available.

Disclosure

This study was presented in the poster session at the 11th National Endourology Congress in Turkey.

References

[1] P. Honeck, G. Wendt-Nordahl, P. Krombach et al., "Does open stone surgery still play a role in the treatment of urolithiasis? Data of a primary urolithiasis center," *Journal of Endourology*, vol. 23, no. 7, pp. 1209–1212, 2009.

[2] C. Türk, T. Knoll, A. Petrik et al., *Guidelines on Urolithiasis*, EAU, 2014, http://www.uroweb.org/gls/pdf.

[3] M. S. Parmar, "Kidney stones," *British Medical Journal*, vol. 328, no. 7453, pp. 1420–1424, 2004.

[4] D. Margel, D. A. Lifshitz, V. Kugel, D. Dorfmann, D. Lask, and P. M. Livne, "Percutaneous nephrolithotomy in patients who previously underwent open nephrolithotomy," *Journal of Endourology*, vol. 19, no. 10, pp. 1161–1164, 2005.

[5] M. Sofikerim, D. Demirci, I. Gülmez, and M. Karacagil, "Does previous open nephrolithotomy affect the outcome of percutaneous nephrolithotomy?" *Journal of Endourology*, vol. 21, no. 4, pp. 401–403, 2007.

[6] B. Lojanapiwat, "Previous open nephrolithotomy: does it affect percutaneous nephrolithotomy techniques and outcome?" *Journal of Endourology*, vol. 20, no. 1, pp. 17–20, 2006.

[7] R. Gupta, A. Gupta, G. Singh, A. Suri, S. K. Mohan, and C. L. Gupta, "PCNL A comparative study in nonoperated and in previously operated (open nephrolithotomy/pyelolithotomy) patients—a single surgeon experience," *International Brazilian Journal of Urology*, vol. 37, no. 6, pp. 739–744, 2011.

[8] M. M. Osman, W. M. Gamal, M. M. Gadelmoula, A. S. Safwat, and M. A. Elgammal, "Ureteroscopic retrograde intrarenal surgery after previous open renal stone surgery: initial experience," *Urological Research*, vol. 40, no. 4, pp. 403–408, 2012.

[9] M. M. Osman, Y. Alfano, S. Kamp et al., "5-Year-follow-up of patients with clinically insignificant residual fragments after extracorporeal shockwave lithotripsy," *European Urology*, vol. 47, no. 6, pp. 860–864, 2005.

[10] D. Dindo, N. Demartines, and P.-A. Clavien, "Classification of surgical complications: a new proposal with evaluation in a cohort of 6336 patients and results of a survey," *Annals of Surgery*, vol. 240, no. 2, pp. 205–213, 2004.

[11] S. C. Kim, R. L. Kuo, and J. E. Lingeman, "Percutaneous nephrolithotomy: an update," *Current Opinion in Urology*, vol. 13, no. 3, pp. 235–241, 2003.

[12] S. Albanis, H. M. Ather, A. G. Papatsoris et al., "Inversion, hydration and diuresis during extracorporeal shock wave lithotripsy: does it improve the stone-free rate for lower pole stone clearance?" *Urologia Internationalis*, vol. 83, no. 2, pp. 211–216, 2009.

[13] H. Danuser, R. Müller, B. Descoeudres, E. Dobry, and U. E. Studer, "Extracorporeal shock wave lithotripsy of lower calyx calculi: how much is treatment outcome influenced by the anatomy of the collecting system?" *European Urology*, vol. 52, no. 2, pp. 539–546, 2007.

[14] O. M. Aboumarzouk, M. Monga, S. G. Kata, O. Traxer, and B. K. Somani, "Flexible ureteroscopy and laser lithotripsy for stones >2cm: a systematic review and meta-analysis," *Journal of Endourology*, vol. 26, no. 10, pp. 1257–1263, 2012.

[15] H. Jung, B. Nørby, and P. J. Osther, "Retrograde intrarenal stone surgery for extracorporeal shock-wave lithotripsy-resistant kidney stones," *Scandinavian Journal of Urology and Nephrology*, vol. 40, no. 5, pp. 380–384, 2006.

[16] A. Breda, O. Ogunyemi, J. T. Leppert, J. S. Lam, and P. G. Schulam, "Flexible ureteroscopy and laser lithotripsy for single intrarenal stones 2 cm or greater—is this the new frontier?" *The Journal of Urology*, vol. 179, no. 3, pp. 981–984, 2008.

[17] E. Alkan, O. Ozkanli, E. Avci et al., "Effectiveness of flexible ureterorenoscopy and laser lithotripsy for multiple unilateral intrarenal stones smaller than 2 cm," *Advances in Urology*, vol. 2014, Article ID 314954, 5 pages, 2014.

[18] E. Alkan, E. Avci, A. O. Ozkanli, O. Acar, and M. D. Balbay, "Same-session bilateral retrograde intrarenal surgery for upper urinary system stones: safety and efficacy," *Journal of Endourology*, vol. 28, no. 7, pp. 757–762, 2014.

[19] K. Stav, A. Cooper, A. Zisman, D. Leibovici, A. Lindner, and Y. I. Siegel, "Retrograde intrarenal lithotripsy outcome after failure of shock wave lithotripsy," *Journal of Urology*, vol. 170, no. 6 I, pp. 2198–2201, 2003.

7

National Trends in the Adoption of Laparoscopic Cholecystectomy over 7 Years in the United States and Impact of Laparoscopic Approaches Stratified by Age

Anahita Dua,[1,2] Abdul Aziz,[3] Sapan S. Desai,[4] Jason McMaster,[1] and SreyRam Kuy[1]

[1] *Department of Surgery, Medical College of Wisconsin, Milwaukee, WI 53226, USA*
[2] *Department of Surgery, Center for Translational Injury Research, University of Texas-Houston, Houston, TX 77030, USA*
[3] *Department of Surgery, Queens Medical Centre, Nottingham NG7 2UH, UK*
[4] *Department of Surgery, Duke University, Durham, NC 27710, USA*

Correspondence should be addressed to Anahita Dua; anahita.dua@uth.tmc.edu

Academic Editor: Casey M. Calkins

Introduction. The aim of this study was to characterize national trends in adoption of laparoscopic cholecystectomy and determine differences in outcome based on type of surgery and patient age. *Methods*. Retrospective cross-sectional study of patients undergoing cholecystectomy. Trends in open versus laparoscopic cholecystectomy by age group and year were analyzed. Differences in outcomes including in-hospital mortality, complications, discharge disposition, length of stay (LOS), and cost are examined. *Results*. Between 1999 and 2006, 358,091 patients underwent cholecystectomy. In 1999, patients aged ≥80 years had the lowest rates of laparoscopic cholecystectomy, followed by those aged 65–79, 64–50, and 49–18 years (59.7%, 65.3%, 73.2%, and 83.5%, resp., $P < 0.05$). Laparoscopic cholecystectomy was associated with improved clinical and economic outcomes across all age groups. Over the study period, there was a gradual increase in laparoscopic cholecystectomy performed among all age groups during each year, though elderly patients continued to lag significantly behind their younger counterparts in rates of laparoscopic cholecystectomy. *Conclusion*. This is the largest study to report trends in adoption of laparoscopic cholecystectomy in the US in patients stratified by age. Elderly patients are more likely to undergo open cholecystectomy. Laparoscopic cholecystectomy is associated with improved clinical outcomes.

1. Introduction

It is well established that open cholecystectomy has worse outcomes than laparoscopic cholecystectomy [1–3]. In 1993, the National Institutes of Health (NIH) Consensus Conference on gallstones and laparoscopic cholecystectomy reported lower mortality, decreased disability, shorter LOS, and less patient discomfort with laparoscopic cholecystectomy in the general population and recommended laparoscopic cholecystectomy as the preferred surgical approach [2, 3]. It has been previously demonstrated that elderly patients are more likely to have more complex biliary disease and nearly six times greater odds of mortality following cholecystectomy than their younger counterparts [1–4]. As the proportion of population >65 years old is predicted to rise from 12% to 20% [1] over the next several decades, gallstone disease among the elderly will represent a major surgical burden. However, few studies have examined differences in rates of adoption of laparoscopic cholecystectomy among elderly patients compared with their younger counterparts.

Few studies have examined differences in the adoption of laparoscopic cholecystectomy among elderly patients compared with their younger counterparts. The objective of this study was to characterize national trends in adoption of laparoscopic cholecystectomy performed in the United States (US) and determine differences in outcomes based on laparoscopic or open type procedures by age group.

2. Methods

This was a retrospective cross-sectional analysis of inpatient hospitalizations from 1999 to 2006, utilizing the Health Care Utilization Project-Nationwide Inpatient Sample (HCUP-NIS) database, which is a stratified 20% sample of all inpatient admissions to nonfederal, acute care hospitals maintained by the Agency for Healthcare Research and Quality (AHRQ). This is the largest all-payer inpatient database in the U.S., with records from approximately eight million hospital stays each year. Records were limited to adults aged 18–100 years old hospitalized with a diagnosis of cholecystitis, as identified by ICD-9 codes and Clinical Classifications Software (CCS). ICD-9 procedure codes were used to identify all patients who underwent cholecystectomy as the primary procedure during hospitalization (open versus laparoscopic). Patients were stratified into four age groups, aged 18–49, 50–64, 65–79, and ≥80 years. Patient comorbidity was calculated using ICD-9 codes and the Charlson Comorbidity Index.

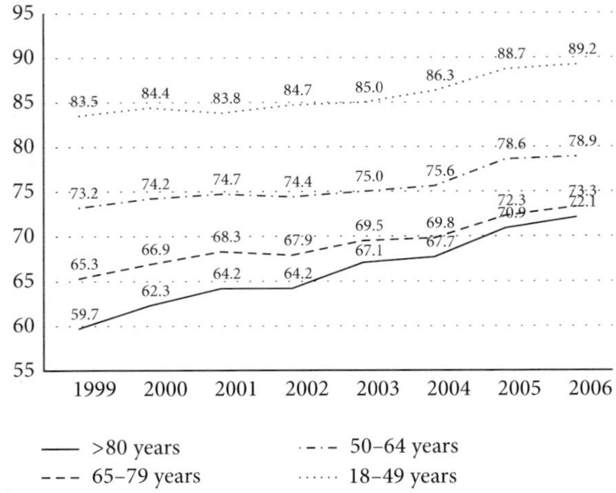

FIGURE 1: Yearly trends in adoption of laparoscopic cholecystectomy by age group (1999–2006).

2.1. Independent Variables. Type of procedure (open versus laparoscopic cholecystectomy) was the primary independent variable of interest. For this study, only those patients who carried a diagnosis of cholecystitis and had cholecystectomy as the primary procedure performed during that hospitalization were included.

2.2. Outcome Variables. The primary outcome examined was rate of laparoscopic cholecystectomy by year and age group. Outcomes by type of cholecystectomy (open versus laparoscopic) examined were mortality; in-hospital complications; discharge disposition (routine discharge to home versus discharge with home health care or discharge to a short-term hospital, intermediate care facility, or skilled nursing facility), mean length of stay (LOS); and mean total inpatient hospital costs.

Surgical complications were identified using ICD-9 codes and categorized as cardiac, postoperative shock, gastrointestinal, hematologic, renal, pulmonary, infection, thrombosis or embolism, and bile duct injury or repair. Surgical complications were treated as dichotomous variables (none versus ≥1). Mean total inpatient hospital costs were calculated using the HCUP-NIS hospital-specific cost-to-charge ratios (available for 2001–2006) and were standardized to 2006 dollars utilizing the Bureau of Labor Statistics Medical Consumer Price Index [5]. The NIS charge information represents the amount that hospitals were billed for services but does not reflect the actual amount hospital services cost or the specific amounts that hospitals received in payment. In order to see how much to calculate how the hospital charges translate into actual costs, the NIS Cost-to-Charge Ratio Files in the database enable this conversion. Each file contains hospital-specific cost-to-charge ratios based on all-payer inpatient cost for each hospital in the corresponding NIS databases. For this study, cost information was obtained by the NIS database from the hospital accounting reports collected by the Centers for Medicare and Medicaid Services and merged with the appropriate file to the corresponding NIS databases by the data element hospital identification number. Using the merged data elements from the cost-to-charge ratio files and the total charges reported in the NIS databases, the hospital total charge data was converted to cost estimates by multiplying total charges with the appropriate cost-to-charge ratio. Then, using the US Bureau of Labor Statistics Medical Consumer Price Index, they were standardized to 2006 dollars [5].

2.3. Statistical Analysis. Bivariate analysis of the independent variables by outcomes was performed using χ^2 tests for categorical variables and analysis of variance (ANOVA) for continuous variables. Data analysis and management were performed using SAS version 9.1 (Cary, NC, USA). Statistical significance was set at a probability value of $P \leq 0.05$.

3. Results

Of the 1,332,195 adult admissions for biliary disease in the HCUP-NIS database between 1999 and 2006, cholecystectomy was performed as the primary procedure during hospitalization in 145,675 patients aged 50–64 years, 149,855 patients aged 65–79 years, and 62,561 patients aged ≥80 years. In 1999, representing the start of the study period, laparoscopic cholecystectomy was performed most frequently in patients aged between 18 and 49 years (83.5%) (Figure 1).

In contrast, laparoscopic cholecystectomy was performed less often as the age groups ascended: 50–64 years (73.2%), 65–79 years (65.3%) and >80 years (59.7%). During each year, there was a gradual increase in patients undergoing laparoscopic surgery across all age groups. By the end of the study period in 2006, 89.2% of patients aged 18–49 underwent laparoscopic cholecystectomy. There was also an increase in frequency for patients aged 50–64 years (78.9%) and 65–79 years (73.3%). Interestingly, patients aged >80 years witnessed a marked increase from 59.7% to 72.1%. This represented the biggest increase, of 12.4%, compared to all other age groups.

3.1. Outcomes. The mortality rate in the study population undergoing open cholecystectomy increased significantly with advancing age (0.5%, 1.6%, 4.0%, and 8.3%; $P < 0.001$) (Table 1).

However, mortality rates were lower in all age groups with laparoscopic cholecystectomy (0.1%, 0.3%, 0.9%, and 2.3%; $P < 0.001$). Patients aged ≥80 years experienced a significant reduction in mortality following laparoscopic cholecystectomy (open = 8.3% versus laparoscopic = 2.3%; $P < 0.001$) when compared to an open procedure. There was a lower overall rate of surgical complications when comparing laparoscopic to open cholecystectomy between age groups. This was most evident for patients aged 65–79 years (open = 50% versus laparoscopic = 26.3%; $P < 0.001$) and ≥80 years (open = 61.1% versus laparoscopic = 37.2%; $P < 0.001$). The trend in adoption of laparoscopic cholecystectomy was also associated with lower LOS (mean days) when compared to open cholecystectomy among all age groups. In particular, patients aged 65–79 years had significantly shorter LOS (open = 10.29 days versus laparoscopic = 5.01 days; $P < 0.001$) resulting in lower hospital costs (open = $24, 060 versus laparoscopic = $12, 451; $P < 0.001$). Improved outcomes were also observed in patients ≥80 years with respect to LOS (open = 11.91 versus laparoscopic = 6.77; $P < 0.001$) and hospital costs (open = $26, 342 versus laparoscopic = $15, 030; $P < 0.001$). In addition, among patients aged ≥80 years, there was a significant increase in these patients being successfully discharged home directly from the hospital (open = 37.0% versus laparoscopic = 63.2%; $P < 0.001$).

4. Discussion

Gallstone disease is the most common indication for abdominal surgery in the United States. Prevalence of gallstone disease is known to increase with age. An increasing life expectancy means that, over the next several decades, the proportion of the population aged over 65 years is expected to rise from 12% to 20% resulting in more patients presenting with gallstone disease requiring surgery [1]. Evaluating national trends to decipher the optimum surgical approach for these patients is important.

This large cross-sectional study of hospitalized patients undergoing cholecystectomy found a steady increase in the adoption of laparoscopic cholecystectomy from 1999 to 2006 among all age groups. Although older patients clearly benefited from laparoscopic cholecystectomy than open cholecystectomy, they are significantly less likely than younger patients to undergo laparoscopic cholecystectomy. However, there was an increasing trend among elderly patients (65–79 years and ≥80 years) undergoing toward laparoscopic cholecystectomy over the study period. Compared to younger patients, elderly patients experienced more adverse outcomes overall, but this was reduced with the adoption of laparoscopic surgery. This is important given that elderly patients tend to present with more complex biliary disease and multiple diagnoses that may increase their surgical risk [3]. Elderly patients are also more likely to require further procedures such as cholecystostomy decompression, endoscopic retrograde cholangiopancreatography (ERCP), common bile duct exploration, and intraoperative cholangiogram [3, 4]. Among the elderly, laparoscopic cholecystectomy, compared with open cholecystectomy, is associated with lower mortality rates, surgical complications, LOS, hospital costs, and better discharge deposition overall, supporting laparoscopic cholecystectomy as the procedure of choice in this population.

In previous studies, the mortality rates in elderly patients undergoing laparoscopic cholecystectomy are reported between 0 and 1% [6–8]. However, these studies defined elderly as patients between the ages of 65 to 79 years only. In direct comparison, we observed a comparable mortality rate of 0.9% in the same age group. In our study cohort of patients aged ≥80 years, the mortality rate was 2.3% among those undergoing laparoscopy compared to 8.3% among those undergoing an open procedure.

This study also observed lower rates in morbidity among elderly patients undergoing laparoscopic compared with open cholecystectomy. Compared to younger patients, the rates were higher in the elderly population overall. However, rates significantly declined when comparing open versus laparoscopic cholecystectomy in the aged-matched elderly groups. Clinically, this translated to reduced LOS and decreased disability, reflected by the fact that more patients were primarily discharged home directly from hospital. Legner et al. [9] reported that elderly patients discharged to an institutional care facility following abdominopelvic surgery had a 4-fold increase in 1-year mortality [9]. Based on this finding, it would appear that elderly patients undergoing laparoscopic compared with open cholecystectomy may also have improved 1-year outcomes given that higher numbers of these patients were discharged directly to their homes.

To our knowledge, this is the largest, comprehensive study of its kind examining the trends in adoption of laparoscopic cholecystectomy among elderly patients and outcomes of laparoscopic cholecystectomy in this population. Other studies examining outcomes of laparoscopic cholecystectomy in the elderly population have been limited to single institutions [10–16]. The findings from such studies are comparable to our study describing decreased morbidity and mortality, LOS, and surgical complications among elderly patients undergoing laparoscopic cholecystectomy. Our study validates these single institutional findings using a large generalizable sample from across the US. While current literature supports the role of laparoscopic cholecystectomy in elderly patients, it should also be acknowledged that elderly patients more commonly present with complex biliary disease resulting in increased complication rates and mortality regardless of procedure choice (open or laparoscopic).

Limitations. This was a retrospective study of a large database and hence limitations inherent to any administrative database such as HCUP-NIS are noted. A limitation of this study was the fact that there is no ICD-9 code for conversion from laparoscopic to open cholecystectomy; hence, we were unable to calculate the rate of conversion. However, HCUP-NIS is

Table 1: Outcomes by type of cholecystectomy procedure (laparoscopic versus open).

Patient outcomes	≥80 years old			65–79 years old			45–64 years old			18–44 years old		
	Laparoscopic (%)	Open (%)	*P* value	Laparoscopic (%)	Open (%)	*P* value	Laparoscopic (%)	Open (%)	*P* value	Laparoscopic (%)	Open (%)	*P* value
Surgical complications (%)	37.20	61.10	<0.0001	26.30	50.00	<0.0001	16.40	37.20	<0.0001	10.30	25.30	<0.0001
Mortality (%)	2.30	8.30	<0.0001	0.90	4.00	<0.0001	0.30	1.60	<0.0001	0.10	0.50	<0.0001
LOS (mean days)	6.77 (SD 6.46)	11.91 (SD 10.07)	<0.0001	5.01 (SD 5.72)	10.29 (SD 10.34)	<0.0001	3.8 (SD 4.8)	8.1 (SD 9.6)	<0.0001	3.1 (SD 3.4)	6.2 (SD 7.9)	<0.0001
Cost (mean in 2005$)	15,030 (SD 15,100)	26,342 (SD 27,611)	<0.0001	12,451 (SD 13,723)	24,060 (SD 30,200)	<0.0001	10,425 (SD 11,369)	19,651 (SD 27,588)	<0.0001	8,858 (SD 8,051)	15,723 (SD 21,811)	<0.0001
Discharge disposition (%)			<0.0001			<0.0001			<0.0001			<0.0001
Routine home	63.20	37.00		86.60	66.00		95.80	85.30		98.40	92.70	
Short-term hospital	1.10	1.20		0.70	1.10		0.50	0.80		0.40	0.70	
Intermediate care	21.80	37.30		6.20	14.60		1.50	4.30		0.50	1.70	
Home health	11.60	16.20		5.60	14.30		1.80	7.80		0.60	4.20	
Against medical advice	0.07	0.04		0.07	0.06		0.12	0.13		0.13	0.20	
Died	2.30	8.27		0.87	3.95		0.26	1.61		0.06	0.53	
Unknown	0.01	0.04		0.01	0.01		0.01	0.01		0.00	0.01	

a well-validated and rigorously maintained database with a low error rate. Operative details such as operative duration, findings of gangrenous or perforated cholecystitis, postdischarge followup including readmissions, and postdischarge mortality are not available in HCUP-NIS. A limitation of the NIS database, however, is that ASA class is not available. We were able to assess the comorbidities of the elderly and the nonelderly patients, but the focus of this study is on the discrepancy in the rates of performance of laparoscopy in the elderly compared with the nonelderly. While we could not match the elderly and the nonelderly by comorbidity or severity of biliary 12 disease, we did note in this epidemiological study that the performance of laparoscopic cholecystectomy in the elderly group was lagging compared to their younger counterparts. The comparative effectiveness of laparoscopic over open cholecystectomy is clear from previous data with the advantage of laparoscopy.

This epidemiological study delineates that the performance of a laparoscopic approach for cholecystectomy in the elderly lags behind their younger counterparts.

5. Conclusion

In this large nationwide cross-sectional study of patients undergoing cholecystectomy, we observed an improvement in clinical outcomes for all patients in the laparoscopic arm with a large benefit noted in elderly patients. This coincided with an increasing trend in the adoption of laparoscopic cholecystectomy. Though elderly patients experienced a significant benefit in laparoscopic surgery, with fewer postoperative complications and lower mortality rates, they still lag significantly behind younger patients in undergoing laparoscopic cholecystectomy. However, we recognise that more data is needed, including data of elderly patients managed as outpatients and the investigation of 1-year mortality rates. Laparoscopic cholecystectomy is a valid primary option for biliary disease and should be considered the procedure of choice in all age groups.

References

[1] Institute of Medicine, Committee on the Future Healthcare Workforce for Older Americans. Retooling for an aging America: building the health care work force. Washington, DC, USA, National Academies Press, 2008.

[2] Consensus conference NIH Consensus conference, "Gallstones and laparoscopic cholecystectomy," *Journal of the American Medical Association*, vol. 269, no. 8, pp. 1018–1024, 1993.

[3] "Gallstones and laparoscopic cholecystectomy. NIH Consensus Development Panel on Gallstones and Laparoscopic Cholecystectomy," *Surgical Endoscopy*, vol. 7, no. 3, pp. 271–279, 1993.

[4] S. Kuy, J. A. Sosa, S. A. Roman et al., "Age matters: a study of clinical and economic outcomes following cholecystectomy in elderly Americans," *The American Journal of Surgery*, vol. 201, no. 6, pp. 789–796, 2011.

[5] H. Quan, V. Sundararajan, P. Halfon et al., "Coding algorithms for defining comorbidities in ICD-9-CM and ICD-10 administrative data," *Medical Care*, vol. 43, no. 11, pp. 1130–1139, 2005.

[6] F. M. Tagle, J. Lavergne, J. S. Barkin, and S. W. Unger, "Laparoscopic cholecystectomy in the elderly," *Surgical Endoscopy*, vol. 11, no. 6, pp. 636–638, 1997.

[7] A. Polychronidis, S. Botaitis, A. Tsaroucha et al., "Laparoscopic cholecystectomy in elderly patients," *Journal of Gastrointestinal and Liver Diseases*, vol. 17, no. 3, pp. 309–313, 2008.

[8] R. K. Annamaneni, D. Moraitis, and C. G. Cayten, "Laparoscopic cholecystectomy in the elderly," *Journal of the Society of Laparoendoscopic Surgeons*, vol. 9, no. 4, pp. 408–410, 2005.

[9] V. J. Legner, N. N. Massarweh, R. G. Symons et al., "The significance of discharge to skilled care after abdominopelvic surgery in older adults," *Annals of Surgery*, vol. 249, no. 2, pp. 250–255, 2009.

[10] B. Kirshtein, M. Bayme, A. Bolotin et al., "Laparoscopic cholecystectomy for acute cholecystitis in the elderly: is it safe?" *Surgical Laparoscopy Endoscopy and Percutaneous Techniques*, vol. 18, no. 4, pp. 334–339, 2008.

[11] L. M. Brunt, M. A. Quasebarth, D. L. Dunnegan, and N. J. Soper, "Outcomes analysis of laparoscopic cholecystectomy in the extremely elderly," *Surgical Endoscopy*, vol. 15, no. 7, pp. 700–705, 2001.

[12] S. J. Margiotta Jr., J. R. Horwitz, I. H. Willis, and M. K. Wallack, "Cholecystectomy in the elderly," *The American Journal of Surgery*, vol. 156, no. 6, pp. 509–512, 1988.

[13] J. Uecker, M. Adams, K. Skipper, and E. Dunn, "Cholecystitis in the octogenarian: is laparoscopic cholecystectomy the best approach?" *The American Surgeon*, vol. 67, no. 7, pp. 637–640, 2001.

[14] D. S. Kauvar, B. D. Brown, A. W. Braswell, and M. Harnisch, "Laparoscopic cholecystectomy in the elderly: Increased operative complications and conversions to laparotomy," *Journal of Laparoendoscopic and Advanced Surgical Techniques A*, vol. 15, no. 4, pp. 379–382, 2005.

[15] D. Hazzan, N. Geron, D. Golijanin, P. Reissman, and E. Shiloni, "Laparoscopic cholecystectomy in octogenarians," *Surgical Endoscopy and Other Interventional Techniques*, vol. 17, no. 5, pp. 773–776, 2003.

[16] P. A. Clavien, J. R. Sanabria, and S. M. Strasberg, "Proposed classification of complications of surgery with examples of utility in cholecystectomy," *Surgery*, vol. 111, no. 5, pp. 518–526, 1992.

8

Neuroendoscopic Resection of Intraventricular Tumors and Cysts through a Working Channel with a Variable Aspiration Tissue Resector

Edjah Kweku-Ebura Nduom,[1] Eric A. Sribnick,[1] D. Ryan Ormond,[1] and Costas G. Hadjipanayis[1,2]

[1] *Department of Neurosurgery, Emory University School of Medicine, 1365B Clifton Road NE, Suite 6200, Atlanta, GA 30322, USA*
[2] *Winship Cancer Institute of Emory University, Atlanta, GA, USA*

Correspondence should be addressed to Costas G. Hadjipanayis; chadjip@emory.edu

Academic Editor: Peng Hui Wang

Pure neuroendoscopic resection of intraventricular lesions through a burr hole is limited by the instrumentation that can be used with a working channel endoscope. We describe a safety and feasibility study of a variable aspiration tissue resector, for the resection of a variety of intraventricular lesions. Our initial experience using the variable aspiration tissue resector involved 16 patients with a variety of intraventricular tumors or cysts. Nine patients (56%) presented with obstructive hydrocephalus. Patient ages ranged from 20 to 88 years (mean 44.2). All patients were operated on through a frontal burr hole, using a working channel endoscope. A total of 4 tumors were resected in a gross total fashion and the remaining intraventricular lesions were subtotally resected. Fifteen of 16 patients had relief of their preoperative symptoms. The 9 patients who presented with obstructive hydrocephalus had restoration of cerebrospinal fluid flow though one required a ventriculoperitoneal shunt. Three patients required repeat endoscopic resections. Use of a variable aspiration tissue resector provides the ability to resect a variety of intraventricular lesions in a safe, controlled manner through a working channel endoscope. Larger intraventricular tumors continue to pose a challenge for complete removal of intraventricular lesions.

1. Introduction

The resection of lesions within the ventricular system presents a challenge to neurosurgeons. The deep location of intraventricular tumors or cysts can lead to neurological sequelae before or after surgery. With the use of the operative microscope, most lesions of the lateral and third ventricles are accessed by a craniotomy and either a transcortical or interhemispheric transcallosal approach. These approaches are associated with brain retraction that can result in seizures, focal neurologic deficits, and cognitive impairment. A pure neuroendoscopic approach for the management of intraventricular lesions has been described and remains a minimally invasive approach that avoids brain retraction and provides direct lesion visualization [1, 2]. Access to the ventricular system through a burr hole and use of a working channel endoscope can permit endoscopic visualization of tumors and cysts that may be sampled or resected. Reestablishment of CSF communication pathways is also possible endoscopically when patients develop obstructive hydrocephalus due to their intraventricular pathology. The neuroendoscopic resection of intraventricular cysts and tumors is limited by the appropriate instrumentation that can be used with a working channel endoscope. Conventional instruments used through the working channel endoscope include cautery, grasping forceps, and aspiration devices. This has limited tumor and cyst resection through a working channel endoscope to piecemeal removal of intraventricular lesions [1]. Here we describe our initial experience with a 1.9 and 1.1 mm variable aspiration tissue resector used through the working channel

Table 1: Patient characteristics.

Patient number	Age	Sex	Disposition	Obstructive HCP	Diagnosis	Outcome
Patient 1	37	M	Home	No	Lateral ventricular arachnoid cyst	Improvement of headaches, discharged home
Patient 2	30	M	Rehab	Yes	3rd ventricular immature teratoma	Underwent suboccipital craniotomy for pineal region immature teratoma. VPS placed for communicating hydrocephalus. Patient died from complications resulting from diabetes insipidus (DI)
Patient 3	71	F	SNF	No	Third ventricular epidermoid	Headaches improved, discharged for rehabilitation
Patient 4	43	F	Home	No	Lateral ventricular arachnoid cyst	Resolution of headaches, discharged home
Patient 5	27	F	Home	Yes	Pineal region cyst	Resolution of headaches, discharged home
Patient 6	72	F	Home	No	Lateral ventricular mixed astroglial cyst	Improvement of headaches, discharged home
Patient 7	88	F	SNF	Yes	Ventricular astrocytoma	Resolution of gait difficulties, discharged for rehabilitation, now resides in assisted living facility
Patient 8	47	M	Rehab	Yes	Ventricular/suprasellar pituitary adenoma	Had endoscopic transsphenoidal approach for further resection of giant pituitary adenoma, discharged for rehabilitation, headaches improved
Patient 9	47	M	Home	Yes	Hypothalamic myxopapillary ependymoma	Resolution of headaches, discharged home
Patient 10	40	F	Rehab	Yes	Pineal parenchymal tumor of intermediate differentiation	Headaches, gait difficulties, and diplopia resolved, discharged for rehabilitation. Received postoperative IMRT
Patient 11	20	M	Home	No	Subependymal giant-cell astrocytoma	Patient required repeat resection and ETV, had resolution of headaches, nausea and vomiting, and then discharged home
Patient 12	32	M	Home	No	Dysembryoplastic neuroepithelial-like tumor	Resolution of seizures, discharged home, now off of antiepileptic medications
Patient 13	36	F	Home	Yes	Lateral ventricular arachnoid cyst	Headaches improved, discharged home
Patient 14	20	F	Home	Yes	Pilocytic astrocytoma	Headaches improved, discharged home
Patient 15	20	M	Home	Yes	Colloid Cyst	Resolution of headaches, discharged home
Patient 16	77	M	Home	No	Craniopharyngioma	Headaches improved, discharged home

ETV: endoscopic third ventriculostomy; VPS: ventriculoperitoneal shunt.

endoscope for the resection of a variety of intraventricular tumors and cysts. Feasibility and safety were assessed in this series of patients.

2. Materials and Methods

Our initial experience using the variable aspiration tissue resector (NICO Myriad, NICO, Corp., Indianapolis, IN, USA) involves 16 patients (Table 1) with a variety of intraventricular pathologic lesions in the lateral ($n = 8$) or third ventricles ($n = 8$). Tumors or cysts treated include a pineal cyst, lateral ventricle arachnoid cysts ($n = 3$), a large colloid cyst, a benign mixed astroglial cyst, low-grade gliomas ($n = 4$) (1 myxopapillary ependymoma, 1 WHO grade II astrocytoma, 1 pilocytic astrocytoma, and 1 subependymal giant cell astrocytoma (SEGA)), a dysembryoplastic neuroepithelial-like tumor (DNET), an epidermoid tumor, an immature teratoma, a craniopharyngioma, a giant pituitary macroadenoma with intraventricular extension, and a pineal parenchymal tumor (intermediate differentiation). Patient ages ranged from 20 to 88 (mean 44.2). Nine patients (56%) presented with ventriculomegaly and obstructive hydrocephalus due to their intraventricular lesion. Five patients presented with memory difficulties, and two presented with seizures as part of their initial presentation. Fourteen out of 16 patients presented with progressive headaches.

All patients underwent neuroendoscopic resection through a single frontal burr hole. Neuronavigation (Medtronic StealthStation TREON) was used in all cases and registration of the working channel endoscope was performed. The majority ($n = 14$) of patients underwent neuroendoscopic resection utilizing a 30-degree Aesculap MINOP working channel endoscope (Aesculap Co., Tuttlingen, Germany). Two patients underwent surgery with use of the smaller diameter 30-degree Oi Handypro working channel endoscope (Karl Storz Co., Tuttlingen, Germany). A 1.9 mm diameter variable aspiration tissue resector was used with the Aesculap MINOP working channel endoscope and a 1.1 mm device was used with the Oi Handypro endoscope. All surgeries were performed by the senior surgeon (CH). Patient information for this study was collected with approval from the Institutional Review Board at Emory University. Extent of resection was calculated using the Osirix Open Source Imaging Software.

2.1. Technique. Each patient in the supine position was placed in a 3-pin Mayfield fixation device allowing for neutral positioning of the head. Neuronavigation was used for each patient to aid in cannulating the ventricular system and also for determining the proper trajectory to the intraventricular lesion. Registration of the tip of the working channel endoscope was also performed in all cases for navigation in the ventricular system and for the tumor or cyst resections. The right lateral ventricle was cannulated in 13 cases, and the left lateral ventricle in 3 cases.

A 2 cm frontal vertical incision was made 3 cm lateral to midline in the region of the coronal suture. A single burr hole was placed with a high-speed drill measuring at least 7 mm. After opening the dura and cauterization, a 19 or 12 French peel-away sheath catheter was passed into the lateral ventricle at 5-6 cm with neuronavigation and secured in position. The Xomed Endo Scrub (Medtronic Inc.) irrigation system was attached to a port on the working channel of the endoscope in addition to suction. A high-definition (1080 p) camera head and light source were used for illumination and visualization.

After insertion of the neuroendoscope working channel and identification of the intraventricular lesion, cautery of the tumor or cyst capsule was performed through the working channel. The variable aspiration tissue resector was subsequently placed through the working channel of the endoscope and secured in place with a tightening screw (Figure 1). The depth of insertion and rotation of the aperture of the resector was controlled with use of thumb dials on the device. Tissue resection was performed with the foot pedal control, and the intensity of aspiration and resection could be set with the console.

Any bleeding encountered during each neuroendoscopic procedure was controlled with irrigation or bipolar cautery through the working channel of the endoscope.

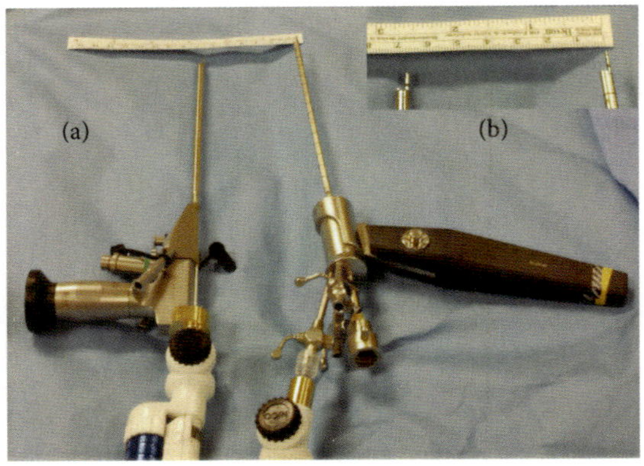

FIGURE 1: The NICO Myriad variable aspiration tissue resector. (a) On the left, the 1.9 mm device has been placed through the working channel of the Aesculap MINOP endoscopic system. On the right, the 1.1 mm device has been placed through the working channel of the Storz IO endoscopic system. (b) A closeup of the resecting tips extending beyond the endoscopes, showing the size of the complete system within the ventricle.

3. Results

3.1. Hospitalization, Follow-Up, and Symptom Resolution. The median length of hospitalization was 7 days. Eleven patients were discharged home, three to acute rehabilitation, and two patients to assisted living facilities. One patient died 135 days after surgery from complications related to diabetes insipidus. The median clinical followup was 4.35 months.

Fifteen patients (94%) had relief of their preoperative symptoms. Fourteen patients (88%) had preoperative headaches that improved after surgery. Eight of nine patients who presented with ventriculomegaly and obstructive hydrocephalus had ventricular decompression and restoration of cerebrospinal fluid flow without ventriculoperitoneal shunt (VPS) placement. One patient without hydrocephalus presented with simple partial seizures, which resolved after surgery.

3.2. Extent of Cyst or Tumor Resection. All three arachnoid cysts and the pineal cyst were partially resected. Of the intraventricular tumors, the large colloid cyst, epidermoid tumor including its capsule, immature teratoma, and the benign mixed astroglial cyst were resected in a gross total fashion. The remaining 8 intraventricular tumors were partially resected (Table 2). The pineal parenchymal tumor patient underwent fractionated intensity modulated radiotherapy (IMRT) for treatment of her residual tumor leading to complete resolution of her lesion ten months after treatment.

Three patients were taken back to the operating room for a repeat neuroendoscopic approach to further resect their residual intraventricular tumor (one with a SEGA; one with a DNET; and one with a teratoma) and reestablish cerebral spinal fluid flow communication to avoid placement of a VPS. In all three patients, during the initial procedure, neuroendoscopic resection with the variable aspiration tissue resector was stopped prematurely due to visualization problems after tumor bleeding. The intraventricular hemorrhage noted intraoperatively did not require conversion to an open craniotomy for hematoma evacuation in any of the patients. All three patients remained neurologically stable after their initial neuroendoscopic tumor resection. Placement of an EVD permitted clearing of blood from the ventricles prior to their second procedure. After discharge, no tumor or cyst has demonstrated recurrence or further needs for any surgical management.

3.3. Restoration of CSF Communication Pathways. All patients with intraventricular cysts had restoration of

Table 2: Extent of resection.

Patient no.	Diagnosis	Procedure	Extent of resection
Patient 1	Lateral ventricular arachnoid cyst	Cyst fenestration, ETV, SPF	Fenestration
Patient 2	3rd ventricular immature teratoma	Resection, ETV, SPF	Gross total resection
Patient 3	Third ventricular epidermoid	Resection, ETV, SPF	Gross total resection
Patient 4	Lateral ventricular arachnoid cyst	Cyst fenestration, ETV, SPF	Fenestration
Patient 5	Pineal region cyst	Resection, ETV, SPF	Gross total resection
Patient 6	Lateral ventricular mixed astroglial cyst	Resection, ETV, SPF	Gross total resection
Patient 7	Ventricular astrocytoma	Subtotal resection, ETV, SPF	22% resection
Patient 8	Ventricular/suprasellar pituitary adenoma	Subtotal resection, SPF	Postop MRI not available
Patient 9	Hypothalamic myxopapillary ependymoma	Resection, ETV, SPF	75% resection
Patient 10	Pineal parenchymal tumor of intermediate differentiation	Biopsy, ETV	22% resection
Patient 11	Subependymal giant-cell astrocytoma	Resection, SPF	92% resection
Patient 12	Dysembryoplastic neuroepithelial-like tumor	Subtotal resection, ETV, SPF	36% resection
Patient 13	Lateral ventricular arachnoid cyst	Cyst fenestration, SPF	Fenestration
Patient 14	Pilocytic astrocytoma	Subtotal resection, SPF	61% resection
Patient 15	2 cm colloid cyst	Subtotal resection, SPF	Gross total resection
Patient 16	Craniopharyngioma	Subtotal resection, ETV, SPF	53.6% resection

ETV: endoscopic third ventriculostomy; SPF: septum pellucidum fenestration.

CSF communication pathways with resolution of their obstructive hydrocephalus. No patients with intraventricular cysts required placement of a VPS. Restoration of CSF communication pathways was achieved in all tumor patients except for patient 2 who required placement of a VPS for persistent hydrocephalus and treatment of a pseudomeningocele. One patient was taken back to surgery for an endoscopic third ventriculostomy (ETV) and lysis of ventricular adhesions after inability to wean her EVD. Ten patients had an ETV performed at the time of their initial surgery, and two additional patients had an ETV performed in a subsequent case. Fourteen out of 16 patients had septum pellucidum fenestrations.

4. Illustrative Cases

4.1. Patient 13 (Arachnoid Cyst) (See Video 1 in the Supplementary Material Available Online at http://dx.doi.org/10.1155/2013/471805). A 35-year-old patient with no previous history of headaches presented with one month of progressive severe headaches. A CT scan, followed by an MRI of the brain, demonstrated a right lateral ventricle arachnoid cyst and associated ventriculomegaly of the right lateral ventricle. After three months of conservative medical management, the patient's headaches were persistent and associated with dizzy spells. A repeat MRI demonstrated unchanged findings of the right lateral ventricle arachnoid cyst and associated ventriculomegaly. The patient elected to proceed with a neuroendoscopic exploration and potential resection of her arachnoid cyst. With the variable aspiration tissue resector, the arachnoid cyst capsule was drawn into the side cutting aperture from the ependymal surface and partially resected, permitting reestablishment of CSF flow. The patient was discharged on postoperative day four without incident. Postoperative MRI demonstrated a reduction in ventricular size, and this remained stable at three-month follow-up (Figure 2). The patient had resolution of her severe presenting headaches.

4.2. Patient 14 (Pilocytic Astrocytoma) (Video 2). Patient 14 is a 20-year-old female who woke up the day of presentation with a severe headache. Both CT and MR images (Figure 3) were obtained revealing a left lateral ventricular lesion extending from the hypothalamic region. The patient was initially alert but became lethargic requiring EVD placement. The patient underwent a subtotal resection of her pilocytic astrocytoma with the variable aspiration tissue resector through the working channel endoscope (Figure 3). The patient's EVD was weaned successfully on post-operative day four, and she was discharged home on post-operative day seven, neurologically intact.

4.3. Patient 15 (Large Colloid Cyst) (Video 3). Patient 15 was a 20-year-old male presenting with progressive headache two days following an episode of transient confusion and word-finding difficulty. CT scan of the head demonstrated a 2.3 cm third ventricular cystic lesion. An MRI confirmed the suspected diagnosis of a colloid cyst (Figure 4), and a neuroendoscopic resection of the mass was performed. Initially, endoscopic cautery of the colloid cyst capsule was performed to shrink the colloid cyst permitting dissection off the roof of the third ventricle and the fornix. Due to the large size of the colloid cyst, en block resection was not possible. Evacuation of the contents of the colloid cyst was first performed followed by complete resection of cyst capsule with the variable aspiration tissue resector (Figure 4).

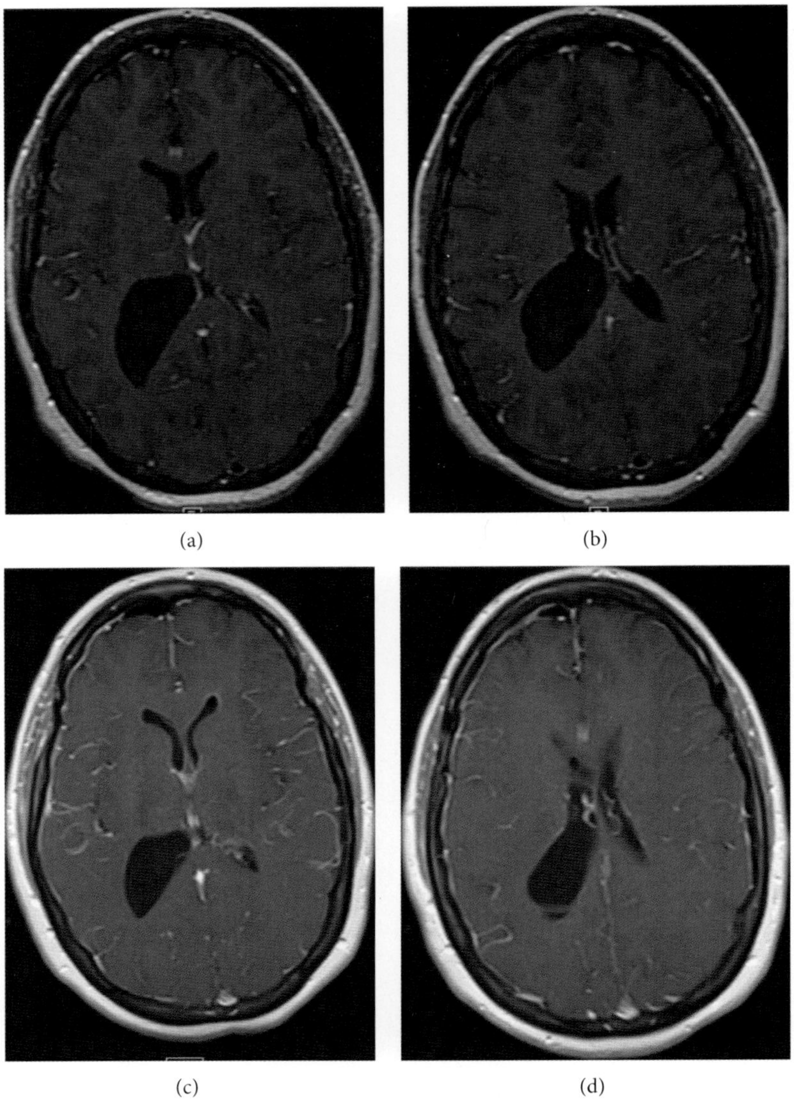

Figure 2: Patient 1, lateral ventricle arachnoid cyst. Preoperative ((a) and (c)) and postoperative ((b) and (d)) contrast enhanced axial T1-weighted magnetic resonance imaging, demonstrating decompression of the cyst and lateral ventricles.

5. Discussion

5.1. Microsurgical Approaches to Intraventricular Lesions. Use of a craniotomy and a transcallosal or transcortical microsurgical approach provides access to intraventricular pathology for resection purposes. These commonly used approaches have the advantage of allowing the surgeon to perform bimanual dissection with the microscope for tumor or cyst resection using a wide range of microscopic instruments and bipolar cautery. Microsurgical approaches to intraventricular lesions after a craniotomy can be associated with significant neurologic deficits due to brain retraction and possibly increased seizure risk postoperatively [3–6]. Others have described the use of tubular retractors in pediatric and adult patient populations for deep-seated lesions, but with limited experience with intraventricular lesions [7, 8].

5.2. Endoscopic Approaches to Intraventricular Lesions. There have been multiple reports of the resection of intraventricular lesions using a pure endoscopic approach with conventional working channel instruments, including suction, grasping forceps, and cutting instruments [1]. Souweidane and Luther reported the resection of 7 solid intraventricular brain tumors and outlined the difficulties associated with resecting these lesions given the restrictive instruments available to them at that time [2]. Their experience was also similar to that of Gaab and Schroeder who reported the purely endoscopic resection of intraventricular lesions [9]. In both series, the attempted resection of solid lesions with diameters greater than 20 mm was extremely difficult due to the small working channels of the endoscopes used and the length of surgery required in these cases.

The endoscope has also been used for assistance and visualization of deep structures while using a bimanual conventional open surgical technique. Interhemispheric endoscopic-assisted approaches have been reported, but this requires a large craniotomy and access near the superior sagittal sinus [10]. Mclaughlin et al. recently evaluated the use

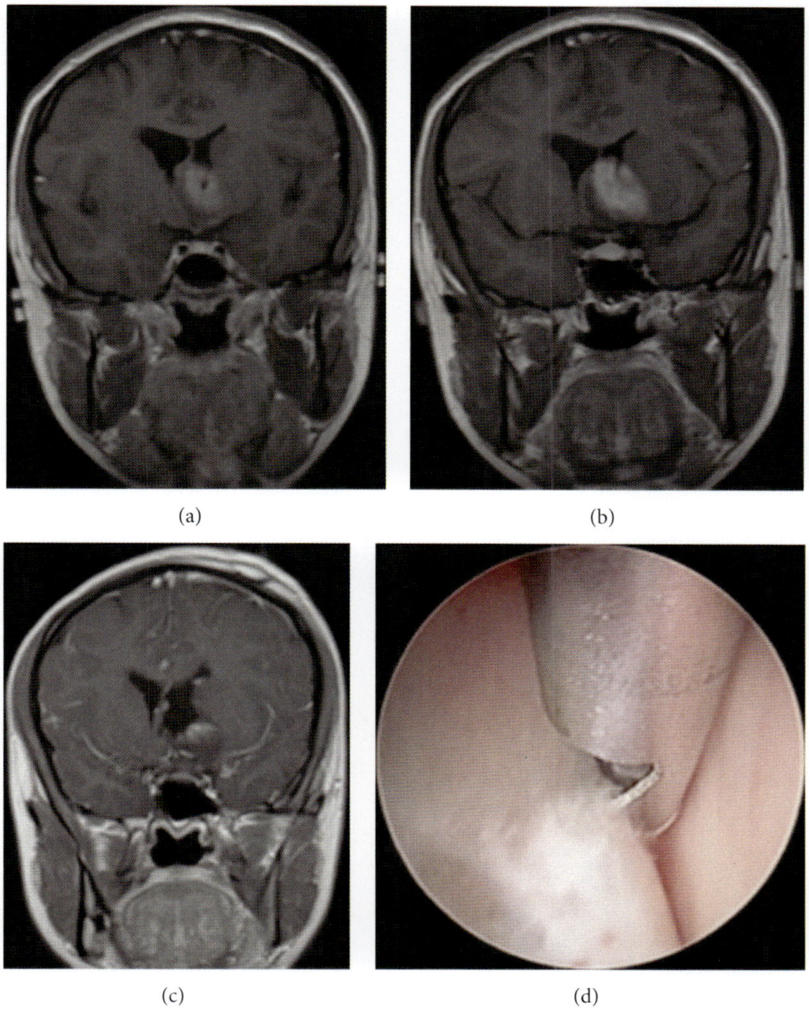

Figure 3: Patient 14, pilocytic astrocytoma. ((a) and (b)) Preoperative coronal T1-weighted contrast-enhanced magnetic resonance imaging showing enhancing lesion and obstructive hydrocephalus. (c) Decrease in ventricular size with interval debulking of lesion. (d) Intraoperative endoscopic view of the tissue aspirator resecting tumor.

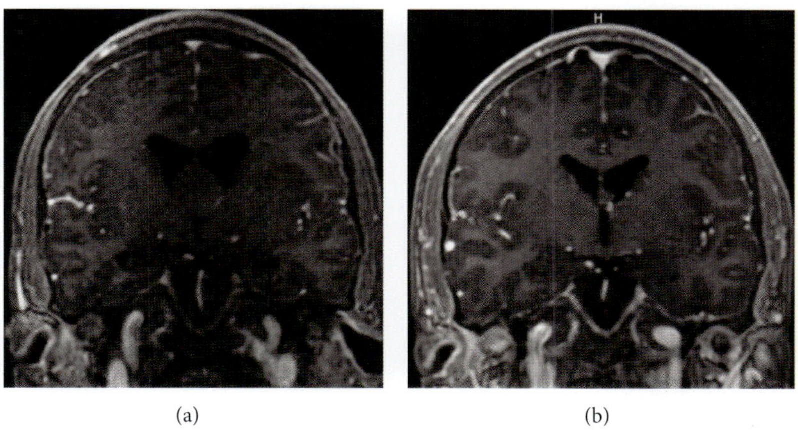

Figure 4: Patient 15, large colloid cyst. (a) Preoperative contrast enhanced coronal T1-weighted magnetic resonance imaging (MRI) showing a lesion with obstructive hydrocephalus. (b) 3-month follow-up MRI shows gross total resection of lesion and resolution of obstructive hydrocephalus.

of a port-assisted endoscopic technique for the resection of intraventricular lesions, allowing the use of bimanual technique [11]. This approach requires a craniotomy and placement of a 1.2 cm port through the brain to the tumor or cyst and use of a nonworking channel endoscope for visualization.

5.3. Previously Reported Use of Variable Aspiration Tissue Resectors. There have been limited reported case series on the use of variable-aspiration tissue resectors for the resection of intraventricular lesions. Lekovic et al. documented the use of a previous version to the current device in the resection of two hypothalamic hamartomas through a working channel endoscope [12]. Several studies have been performed on the use of the current variable aspiration tissue resector. Mohanty et al. described the sub- or near-total resection of large intraventricular tumors (two craniopharyngiomas and one subependymoma) [13]. Albright and Okechi described the resection of two pineal lesions without followup [14]. The two largest series to date were reported by Sood et al. and Dlouhy et al. [15, 16]. Sood et al. described their use of the device in resecting 23 lesions including brain and spinal lesions with good short-term follow-up results [15]. Dlouhy et al. describe their experience with the variable-aspiration tissue resector in fifteen patients [16]. These series, as with our series, all describe the benefits and limitations of the device, but our series is the largest to quantify extent of resection and how this relates to the use of the variable-aspiration tissue resector.

5.4. Strengths, Limitations, and Safety. The ability to rotate the aperture and lengthen or shorten the length of the variable aspiration tissue resector permitted safe resection of all lesions described in this series. Proper visualization of the aperture and placement away from neurovascular structures permitted controlled tissue resection with the foot pedal control. The console could be adjusted for greater or lesser aspiration and resection. In our limited experience, the variable aspiration tissue resector seemed to work best on soft tumors with minimal vascularity. One of the four tumors completely resected was a large colloid cyst, but, in our experience, colloid cysts can typically be resected without the use of the variable aspiration tissue resector. With larger cysts (>2 cm), rapid debulking of the cyst contents and complete resection of the capsule can be performed well with the variable aspiration tissue resector.

More vascular tumors, such as gliomas, were amenable to subtotal resection in our initial experience, which was often the goal of surgery. However, cautery is not provided by the variable aspiration tissue resector. Tumor resection was halted intermittently for hemostasis with irrigation and endoscopic cautery through the working channel. Use of multiple channels simultaneously has been reported with the working channel endoscope to optimize lesion resection [17]. We felt that the introduction of endoscopic cautery through a separate working channel with the variable aspiration tissue resector in place resulted in visual obstruction during tumor resection.

Due to inadequate hemostasis with the endoscopic cautery and poor endoscopic visualization from blood products in the ventricular system, three patients required repeat endoscopic operations for further tumor resection. We have found that adequate tumor capsule cautery prior to neuroendoscopic resection with the variable aspiration tissue resector may reduce bleeding from the residual tumor that may halt the surgery prematurely. While we did not have to convert to a craniotomy for evacuation of an intraventricular hematoma, aggressive resection with the variable aspiration tissue resector can result in intraoperative bleeding which may require an emergent craniotomy for definitive control. The development of newer bipolar cautery instruments that can be used through the working channel endoscope may provide the ability to better cauterize tumor capsules and intratumoral bleeding during resection with the variable aspiration tissue resector.

While we were able to completely resect one immature teratoma with a diameter of 29 mm, the remainder of lesions greater than 20 mm were subtotally resected. We did achieve our goal of significant debulking of these lesions with restoration of CSF flow in all but one of the cases, even when dealing with lesions with diameters up to 36 mm. A craniotomy and microsurgical technique may have precluded the need for neuroendoscopic reoperation in three cases, but the stated preoperative goal of subtotal resection was obtained in all cases without the need for conversion to an open craniotomy.

6. Conclusions

In summary, the variable aspiration tissue resector can be safely utilized for the resection of a variety of solid tumors or cysts involving the ventricular system through a working channel endoscope. This approach remains limited by difficulties in controlling bleeding encountered while resecting more vascularized lesions, and in maneuverability to visualize lesions greater than 2 cm.

References

[1] P. Cappabianca, G. Cinalli, M. Gangemi et al., "Application of neuroendoscopy to intraventricular lesions," *Neurosurgery*, vol. 62, supplement 2, pp. SHC575–SHC597, 2008.

[2] M. M. Souweidane and N. Luther, "Endoscopic resection of solid intraventricular brain tumors," *Journal of Neurosurgery*, vol. 105, no. 2, pp. 271–278, 2006.

[3] M. L. J. Apuzzo, O. K. Chikovani, and P. S. Gott, "Transcallosal, interfornical approaches for lesions affecting the third ventricle: surgical considerations and consequences," *Neurosurgery*, vol. 10, no. 5, pp. 547–554, 1982.

[4] W. A. Shucart and B. M. Stein, "Transcallosal approach to the anterior ventricular system," *Neurosurgery*, vol. 3, no. 3, pp. 339–343, 1978.

[5] A. Morita, P. J. Kelly, A. L. Rhoton, and B. M. Stein, "Resection of intraventricular tumors via a computer-assisted volumetric

stereotactic approach," *Neurosurgery*, vol. 32, no. 6, pp. 920–927, 1993.

[6] B. D. Milligan and F. B. Meyer, "Morbidity of transcallosal and transcortical approaches to lesions in and around the lateral and third ventricles: a single-institution experience," *Neurosurgery*, vol. 67, no. 6, pp. 1483–1496, 2010.

[7] P. F. Recinos, S. M. Raza, G. I. Jallo, and V. R. Recinos, "Use of a minimally invasive tubular retraction system for deep-seated tumors in pediatric patients: technical note," *Journal of Neurosurgery*, vol. 7, no. 5, pp. 516–521, 2011.

[8] S. M. Raza, P. F. Recinos, J. Avendano, H. Adams, G. I. Jallo, and A. Quinones-Hinojosa, "Minimally invasive trans-portal resection of deep intracranial lesions," *Minimally Invasive Neurosurgery*, vol. 54, no. 1, pp. 5–11, 2011.

[9] M. R. Gaab and H. W. Schroeder, "Neuroendoscopic approach to intraventricular lesions," *Neurosurgical Focus*, vol. 6, no. 4, article e5, 1999.

[10] S. Sood, N. Nundkumar, and S. D. Ham, "Interhemispheric endoscopic resection of large intraventricular and thalamic tumors: technical note," *Journal of Neurosurgery*, vol. 7, no. 6, pp. 596–599, 2011.

[11] N. McLaughlin, L. F. Ditzel Filho, D. M. Prevedello, D. F. Kelly, R. L. Carrau, and A. B. Kassam, "Side-cutting aspiration device for endoscopic and microscopic tumor removal," *Journal of Neurological Surgery B*, vol. 73, no. 1, pp. 11–20, 2012.

[12] G. P. Lekovic, L. F. Gonzalez, I. Feiz-Erfan, and H. L. Rekate, "Endoscopic resection of hypothalamic hamartoma using a novel variable aspiration tissue resector," *Neurosurgery*, vol. 58, no. 1, pp. S-166–S-168, 2006.

[13] A. Mohanty, B. J. Thompson, and J. Patterson, "Initial experience with endoscopic side cutting aspiration system in pure neuroendoscopic excision of large intraventricular tumors," *World Neurosurgy*, 2012.

[14] A. L. Albright and H. Okechi, "Use of the NICO Myriad device for tumor and cyst removals in a developing country," *Child's Nervous System*, vol. 28, no. 4, pp. 599–604, 2012.

[15] S. Sood, M. Hoeprich, and S. D. Ham, "Pure endoscopic removal of pineal region tumors," *Child's Nervous System*, vol. 27, no. 9, pp. 1489–1492, 2011.

[16] B. J. Dlouhy, N. S. Dahdaleh, and J. D. W. Greenlee, "Emerging technology in intracranial neuroendoscopy: application of the NICO Myriad Technical note," *Neurosurgical Focus*, vol. 30, no. 4, article E6, 2011.

[17] D. A. Wilson, D. J. Fusco, S. D. Wait, and P. Nakaji, "Endoscopic resection of colloid cysts: use of a dual-instrument technique and an anterolateral approach," *World Neurosurgery*, 2012.

9

Early Experience in Da Vinci Robot-Assisted Partial Nephrectomy

Francis Ting, Richard Savdie, Sam Chopra, Carlo Yuen, and Phillip Brenner

St Vincent's Hospital, Darlinghurst, Sydney, NSW 2010, Australia

Correspondence should be addressed to Phillip Brenner; pbrenner@stvincents.com.au

Academic Editor: Peng Hui Wang

Introduction and Objectives. To demonstrate the safety and efficacy of the robot-assisted partial nephrectomy (RAPN) technique in an Australian setting. *Methods.* Between November 2010 and July 2014, a total of 76 patients underwent 77 RAPN procedures using the Da Vinci Surgical System© at our institution. 58 of these procedures were performed primarily by the senior author (PB) and are described in this case series. *Results.* Median operative time was 4 hours (range 1.5–6) and median warm ischaemic time (WIT) was 8 minutes (range 0–30) including 11 cases with zero ischaemic time. All surgical margins were clear with the exception of one patient who had egress of intravascular microscopic tumour outside the capsule to the point of the resection margin. Complications were identified in 9 patients (15.8%). Major complications included conversion to open surgery due to significant venous bleeding ($n = 1$), reperfusion injury ($n = 1$), gluteal compartment syndrome ($n = 1$), DVT/PE ($n = 1$), and readmission for haematuria ($n = 1$). *Conclusion.* This series demonstrates the safety and efficacy of the RAPN technique in an Australian setting when performed by experienced laparoscopic surgeons in a dedicated high volume robotic centre.

1. Introduction

Partial nephrectomy (PN) is now the most commonly performed surgery for renal cell carcinoma (RCC) [1], with the AUA and EAU guidelines recommending PN as the standard of care for masses 4–7 cm [2, 3]. PN for RCC has been shown to have lower morbidity and equal oncological outcomes to radical nephrectomy as long as pathological/surgical margins are clear of tumour [4].

Furthermore, robotically assisted partial nephrectomy (RAPN) has surpassed laparoscopic partial nephrectomy (LPN) in the United States as the more frequently performed minimally invasive surgery for RCC [1].

Most surgeons continue to perform PN via an open approach as even those who are very skilled at laparoscopy find LPN technically challenging with long clamp times [4], potentially causing ischemic renal damage in the longer term. Additionally, the technical challenges presented by LPN have possibly led to the overuse of laparoscopic radical nephrectomy when PN may have been feasible [4].

There is increasing evidence that overall health is compromised in the presence of reduced renal function associated with a complete nephrectomy, with increased risk of cardiovascular events and hospitalisation being major contributors to long-term morbidity [5].

Da Vinci RAPN allows precise excision, greater dexterity, and ease of suturing to assist in renorrhaphy. This results in much shorter periods of ischaemia and potentially less renal ischaemic damage [4, 6]. It facilitates greater technical proficiency which expands the scope of minimally invasive partial nephrectomy to include more complex lesions, including lesions larger than T1a, hilar lesions, and those with venous tumour thrombosis [6, 7].

2. Methods

Between November 2010 and July 2014, a total of 76 patients underwent 77 RAPN procedures using the Da Vinci Surgical System© at St Vincent's Private Hospital by a selected team of surgeons, anaesthetists, and scrub staff dedicated to refining this procedure. The senior author performed the majority of the cases and these 58 cases have been highlighted in this case series.

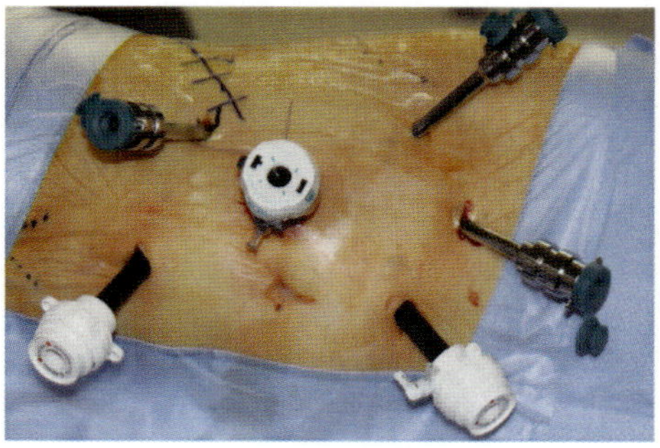

FIGURE 1: Port placement.

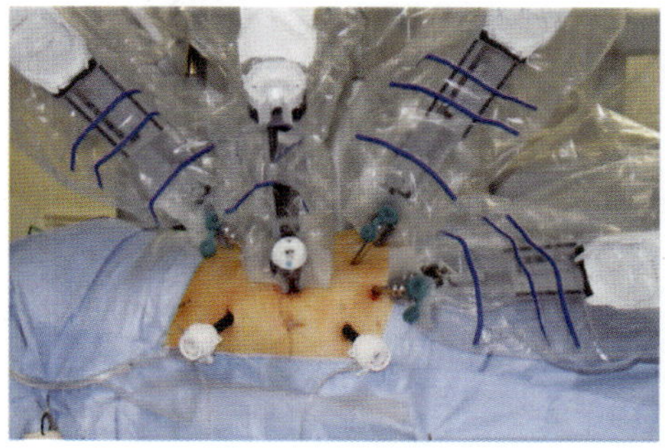

FIGURE 2: Port placement with Da Vinci robot.

Initially, the series consisted of patients with small renal tumours (T1A) in a favourable position but, as the series progressed, patients with solitary kidneys ($n = 5$) and multiple tumours ($n = 2$) and those with small (<4 cm) but unfavourably located tumours were also included ($n = 12$).

Preoperative work up included a serum creatinine and haemoglobin, a 24-hour creatinine clearance, DTPA with differential function, and calculated estimated glomerular filtration rate (eGFR).

Postoperatively, serum creatinine was assessed at one month, two months, three months, and six months, with a further DTPA scan at six months. DTPA scanning was discontinued after the first 12 patients as the literature indicated that a serum creatinine at this time would give similar information and this was consistent with our findings.

At the beginning of the series, standard renal imaging was accepted but, as the series progressed, a dedicated CT scan with arterial phase images at 3 mm cuts became mandatory for assessment of renal vasculature.

Complications from the procedure were recorded and graded according to the Clavien classification system.

2.1. Operative Technique. Patients were given routine intravenous hydration, but no Lasix or Mannitol was given intraoperatively.

Surgery was performed in standard flank position with usual attention to pressure areas. The anaesthetist placed an arterial line but not a central line as a routine. Ports were placed as shown in the diagram (Figures 1 and 2), with intermittent use of an extra port for the "Fourth Arm" when perceived to be of use. For right-sided tumours, it was occasionally necessary to place a 5 mm port for a liver retractor. Insufflation to achieve intraoperative laparoscopic pressures of between 6 and 8 cms H_2O was utilised to minimise compromise to renal function.

All renal arteries and renal veins were isolated and controlled with a Vesi-loop© using the preoperative CT as an adjunct in defining the arterial anatomy. If possible, the segmental vessel supplying the tumour alone was selectively isolated. Prior to clamping the renal artery, special care was taken to confirm that multiple preprepared sutures for the repair were available and that the robotic needle-drivers were available and functioning. Clamping of the renal vessel was done with laparoscopic bulldog clips, applied by the assistant.

Early in the series both renal artery and renal vein were clamped; currently only the artery is clamped. Intra-abdominal pressure was raised to between 15 and 20 cms of water for a few minutes if venous bleeding was apparent.

Ultrasound localisation of the tumour was performed intraoperatively to mark out the resection margins on the surface of the kidney. The area around the tumour was marked at a distance of 1 cm with cautery once the kidney was mobilised. The renal artery was then clamped and the tumour was excised with cold scissors to allow good visualisation. If the tumour was visualised, extra tissue was taken from the deep margin. No frozen sections were performed.

The defect was then repaired with a running 2.0 vicryl across the base of the defect and then interrupted one-vicryl sutures spaced one centimetre apart. We utilised the technique of sliding clip renorrhaphy [8] where large Hem-O-Lok are applied and fastened with the LapraTy© clip. The ability to tighten the Weck Haem-O-Lock clips© and then fasten with the LapraTy© was essential for haemostasis. Floseal was used for minor ooze but no bolsters were used.

Early unclamping of the renal artery was performed where possible after placing the running stitch at the base and the first one to two interrupted one-vicryl repair sutures before completing the renorrhaphy.

The perinephric fat was closed around the defect once haemostasis was ensured and a drain was placed in all patients.

3. Results

Demographic and tumour data is summarised in Table 1 and perioperative data is summarised in Table 2.

The mean operative time was 4.2 hours (range 1.5 to 6 hours), with a 98.3% procedural success rate due to one case requiring conversion to open. Intraoperative estimated blood loss (EBL) was between 50 and 100 mLs for 46 patients (79.3%). Seven patients (12.1%) had EBL of 200 mL, four patients (6.9%) had EBL of 400 to 500 mLs, and one patient (1.7%) had EBL of 1000 mL. Only two patients received a blood transfusion. Massive transfusion was given to one of these patients for significant venous bleeding which required conversion to open nephrectomy. The other patient received two units of packed red blood cells which were given post-operatively in intensive care for Haemoglobin (Hb) of 86 g/L

TABLE 1: Patient and tumour data.

Baseline data	
RAPN procedures (n)	77
Number of patients (n)	76
RAPN procedures, senior author	58
Mean age, y (range)	63 (36–83)
Sex (n)	
Male	41
Female	16
Tumour characteristics (procedures by senior author, $n = 58$)	
Side (n)	
Left	33
Right	25
Mean tumour size, mm (range, median)	30.5 (14–80, 28)
Pathology, n (percentage)	
Clear cell	36 (62.1%)
Papillary cell	8 (13.8%)
Oncocytoma	7 (12%)
Chromophobe	4 (7%)
Angiomyolipoma	2 (3.4%) (fat-poor)
Malakoplakia	1 (1.7%)
Negative margin status, n (%)	57 (98.3%)
Lymphovascular invasion at margin, n (%)	1 (1.7%)

TABLE 2: Perioperative data.

Perioperative data (procedures by senior author, $n = 58$)	
Median warm ischemia time, min (range)	8 (0–30)
Median operative time, hours (range)	4 (1.5–6)
Mean (hours)	4.2
Conversion to open, n (%)	1 (1.7%)
Intraoperative transfusion, n (%)	1 (1.7%)
Postoperative transfusion, n (%)	1 (1.7%)
Median length of stay, d (range)	6 (3–23)
Mean (d)	6.8

in the setting of known ischaemic heart disease (preoperative Hb of 113 g/L).

Overall, median warm ischaemic time (WIT) of eight minutes was achieved (range 0 to 30 minutes) by the senior author. It was noted that ischaemic times by the senior author dramatically improved as the series progressed. In the first ten patients, median WIT was 18 minutes. This improved to a median WIT of 4.5 minutes in the final 37 patients which included eleven patients with zero ischaemic time, that is, either no clamping or clamping of a third-order artery only (Table 3).

All surgical margins were clear with the exception of one who had egress of intravascular microscopic tumour outside

TABLE 3: Warm ischaemia times achieved by primary operator only (58 patients).

Patient number	Warm ischaemic time (range in minutes)	Warm ischaemic time (median in minutes)
1 to 10	10–30	18
11 to 21	6–20	9
22 to 58†	0–20	4.5†
Overall	0–30	8

†11 of these cases had zero ischaemic time.

the capsule to the point of the resection margin. The specimen was otherwise microscopically and macroscopically clear of the tumour bulk. All tumours were 80 mm or less, with a mean tumour size of 30.5 mm.

The pathology as expected from a group of mainly T1 patients was primarily clear cell renal cell carcinoma in 36 of the 58 (62.1%), papillary renal cell carcinoma in 8 (13.8%), renal oncocytoma in 7 (12%), chromophobe renal cell carcinoma in 4 (7%), two fat-poor angiomyolipoma (3.4%), and one malakoplakia (1.7%).

For the patients who did not fall into the solitary kidney group, at a minimum follow-up of three months all but three had creatinine within 20 micromol/L of preoperative levels. The first patient was early in the series and had a clamp time of thirty minutes. His postoperative DTPA showed loss of function in the left kidney. The second patient had a clamp time of only ten minutes but is presumed to have had reperfusion injury. Clinically, he developed pain and fever on day 1; angiogram showed normal vascularity and diagnostic laparoscopy was normal. The third had open conversion and nephrectomy.

In the five patients with solitary kidney, four of them maintained creatinine within 30 micromol/L of their preoperative level, including one who started with creatinine of 170 micromol/L.

Complications according to the Clavien classification system [9] are outlined in Table 4. Twelve postoperative complications were identified in nine patients (15.8%) with the remaining 48 patients (84.2%) being free of complications.

There were three Clavien Grade-3 complications. This included the previously mentioned reperfusion injury and also the patient who was discovered to have significant venous bleeding after completion of the partial nephrectomy, which required massive transfusion and conversion to open nephrectomy. The third patient was readmitted with haematuria two weeks postoperatively in the context of recommencing therapeutic Clexane for AF a few days before. Angiogram was unremarkable and the bleeding stopped spontaneously.

The commonest postoperative problem was atelectasis in three of the 57 patients (5.3%). One of these patients had pneumothorax (resolved without drain), and one patient required antibiotics for a pneumonia.

Gluteal compartment syndrome was diagnosed in one patient despite meticulous positioning. The patient was

TABLE 4: Complications by Clavien grade.

Grade I	(i) Atelectasis in 3 patients[†,‡] (ii) Pneumothorax, resolved without drain[†] (iii) Gluteal compartment syndrome[§]
Grade II	(i) Pneumonia (ii) Blood transfusion in 2 patients[‡,‖] (iii) DVT/PE
Grade IIIa	Haematuria requiring angiogram: negative study, haematuria spontaneously resolved
Grade IIIb	(i) Laparoscopy for investigation of acute abdomen, no abnormalities found, likely reperfusion injury (ii) Conversion to open nephrectomy for significant venous bleeding[‖]
Grade IV	None
Grade V	None

[†]One patient had both atelectasis and pneumothorax.
[‡]One patient had both blood transfusion and atelectasis.
[§]Conservative management only. Fasciotomy not required.
[‖]The patient who underwent conversion to open nephrectomy also received blood transfusion.

135 kgs and recovered completely without operative intervention.

One patient suffered a deep venous thrombosis with pulmonary embolus, but in retrospect this had likely been present prior to the surgery but was not detected or treated.

Most patients had a length of stay between 4 and 8 days, with a median stay of six days and a range between 3 and 23 days (patient with DVT and pulmonary embolus). This reflected an older age group of patients with comorbidities rather than surgical complications.

4. Discussion

This paper demonstrates the safety and efficacy of the RAPN technique in an Australian setting. RAPN has overtaken LPN in the US as the most commonly performed minimally invasive procedure for PN [1]. Much like the uptake of robot-assisted prostatectomy in our country, RAPN is sure to follow.

The earliest reported feasibility study on RAPN was in 2004 by Gettman et al. [10] in the Mayo Clinic. Since this initial study, there has been a multitude of reports on RAPN, with significant reported advancements in technique and technology, and RAPN is fast becoming the technique of choice for most T1a renal tumours, with the caveat being that the appropriate equipment and expertise are available [11].

Two recent meta-analyses comparing RAPN to LPN have been recently published which have shown that operating times, estimated blood loss, conversion rates, positive surgical margin rates, and complication rates are similar for both groups but with the advantage of significantly shorter WIT in RAPN compared to in LPN [4, 12]. The learning curve in LPN has been shown to be much steeper, with mastery of the procedure performed under warm ischaemia requiring completion of more than 500 cases [13], compared with much smaller numbers in RAPN of about 30 cases or fewer [11]. This has been complemented by the present series in which the median WIT of 12.5 minutes for the first 21 cases drastically dropped to almost a third of this to a median of 4.5 minutes for the last 37 cases for the senior author. However, it should be noted that many of these tumours were carefully selected and that the primary surgeons are experienced laparoscopic and robotic surgeons with a combined laparoscopic renal procedure history of over one thousand cases in a high volume tertiary referral centre, which would have had a considerable impact on the initial learning curve.

Selective segmental clamping was performed on nine of the patients in this series and no clamping of renal artery was performed in two patients with procedural success in all cases thus achieving avoidance of global renal ischaemia in 11 patients.

In our series, intraoperative ultrasound was critical in noting the deep extent of the tumour, particularly as the tumours always seemed to be deeper than estimated due to the magnified view at the surgeon console. Renal Doppler ultrasound would have been useful in the earlier stages to make sure that blood flow had stopped to the relevant area; particularly the micro probe would have been useful as it can be left on the kidney to monitor perfusion after renal clamping. To date, we have not used any intra-arterial fluorescence technology which has been used with some success at other centres [14].

For smaller tumours, clamping the artery alone was helpful as venous bleeding as a whole was not a problem and could be dealt with by increasing intra-abdominal pressure. In our experience, renal vein clamping is not necessary unless the tumour is centrally located and large venous branches are opened [15, 16].

Predictably, those patients with very short clamp times under ten minutes did not even have transient changes in serum creatinine, although it would be of value to follow renal function over a more extended period to see whether even a short period of renal ischaemia is damaging in the long term.

Long-term renal function outcomes and long-term oncological outcomes are obviously of the highest importance. While we are not able to report on these here, we will be monitoring them with interest. At the time of reporting none of the patients in the present series had any evidence of recurrence on routine follow-up imaging. A limited calculation based on 19 of our patients showed an average rise in total serum creatinine of 4.9% at an average follow-up of four months. In the literature, intermediate term data has been published with follow-up data at two to six years after RAPN in a group of 134 patients showing effective oncologic control and renal function preservation with an average drop of 8% in eGFR [17].

In terms of positive surgical margins (PSM), comparison between the gold standard of OPN and RAPN has been conducted with a multicentre comparison study of 198 OPN versus 105 RAPN showing no significant differences in PSM rates (5.6 versus 5.7%) [18]. For RAPN, the reported PSM rates vary widely. One series of 220 RAPN reported PSM of 8.2% [19], another series of 153 patients [20] reported PSM of 3.5%, and another series of 134 patients reported PSM of 0.7% [17]. Our series had no frankly positive margins; even if the one patient (1.7%) with lymphovascular invasion at the margin is counted our results are comparable to the literature.

Our overall complication rate of 15.8% is comparable to that achieved in the current standard of literature, with a US analysis of 886 patients undergoing RAPN at 5 US centres coming out with an overall complication rate of 15.6% [21]. However, it should be noted that over 66% of our complications were Clavien I and II and that progression to investigative intervention in two of our other patients did not reveal any complicating pathology. They reported a 4.6% perioperative transfusion rate, compared to our 3.4% transfusion rate, and the most common complication that they reported after RAPN was postoperative haemorrhage which can in most cases be managed conservatively [21].

In summary, the lessons we wish to impart include the following:

(i) The importance of dedicated CT arteriography to help in detecting a second or third renal artery, and in defining vascular anatomy to allow segmental clamping; as more complex tumour surgery is attempted, it is this segmental clamping that will allow us to avoid global ischaemia to the kidney.

(ii) The essential role of the sliding clip renorrhaphy technique with early unclamping.

(iii) The usefulness of intraoperative ultrasound.

(iv) The importance of having an experienced bedside assistant, preferably a second urologist with laparoscopic skills.

5. Conclusion

Use of the Da Vinci robot in assisting laparoscopic partial nephrectomy will allow experienced laparoscopic surgeons to perform the procedure with shorter ischaemic times to the kidney.

This series demonstrates that RAPN is feasible and can be performed safely with similar oncological outcomes to OPN in an Australian setting when performed by experienced laparoscopic surgeons in a dedicated high volume robotic centre.

References

[1] K. R. Ghani, S. Sukumar, J. D. Sammon, C. G. Rogers, Q.-D. Trinh, and M. Menon, "Practice patterns and outcomes of open and minimally invasive partial nephrectomy since the introduction of robotic partial nephrectomy: results from the nationwide inpatient sample," *Journal of Urology*, vol. 191, no. 4, pp. 907–913, 2014.

[2] B. Ljungberg, K. Bensalah, A. Bex et al., *Guidelines on Renal Cell Carcinoma*, European Association of Urology, 2013.

[3] S. C. Campbell, A. C. Novick, A. Belldegrun et al., "Guideline for management of the clinical T1 renal mass," *The Journal of Urology*, vol. 182, no. 4, pp. 1271–1279, 2009.

[4] X. Zhang, Z. Shen, S. Zhong, Z. Zhu, X. Wang, and T. Xu, "Comparison of peri-operative outcomes of robot-assisted vs laparoscopic partial nephrectomy: a meta-analysis," *BJU International*, vol. 112, no. 8, pp. 1133–1142, 2013.

[5] A. S. Go, G. M. Chertow, D. Fan, C. E. McCulloch, and C.-Y. Hsu, "Chronic kidney disease and the risks of death, cardiovascular events, and hospitalization," *The New England Journal of Medicine*, vol. 351, no. 13, pp. 1296–1305, 2004.

[6] R. Eyraud, J.-A. Long, D. Snow-Lisy et al., "Robot-assisted partial nephrectomy for hilar tumors: perioperative outcomes," *Urology*, vol. 81, no. 6, pp. 1246–1251, 2013.

[7] R. Abaza and J. Angell, "Robotic partial nephrectomy for renal cell carcinomas with venous tumor thrombus," *Urology*, vol. 81, no. 6, pp. 1362–1367, 2013.

[8] B. M. Benway, A. J. Wang, J. M. Cabello, and S. B. Bhayani, "Robotic partial nephrectomy with sliding-clip renorrhaphy: technique and outcomes," *European Urology*, vol. 55, no. 3, pp. 592–599, 2009.

[9] D. Dindo, N. Demartines, and P.-A. Clavien, "Classification of surgical complications: a new proposal with evaluation in a cohort of 6336 patients and results of a survey," *Annals of Surgery*, vol. 240, no. 2, pp. 205–213, 2004.

[10] M. T. Gettman, M. L. Blute, G. K. Chow, R. Neururer, G. Bartsch, and R. Peschel, "Robotic-assisted laparoscopic partial nephrectomy: technique and initial clinical experience with daVinci robotic system," *Urology*, vol. 64, no. 5, pp. 914–918, 2004.

[11] R. Gohil, K. Ahmed, G. Kooiman, M. S. Khan, P. Dasgupta, and B. Challacombe, "Current status of robot-assisted partial nephrectomy," *BJU International*, vol. 110, no. 11, pp. 1602–1606, 2012.

[12] O. M. Aboumarzouk, R. J. Stein, R. Eyraud et al., "Robotic versus laparoscopic partial nephrectomy: a systematic review and meta-analysis," *European Urology*, vol. 62, no. 6, pp. 1023–1033, 2012.

[13] I. S. Gill, K. Kamoi, M. Aron, and M. M. Desai, "Laparoscopic partial nephrectomies: a single surgeon series," *The Journal of Urology*, vol. 183, no. 1, pp. 34–42, 2010.

[14] L. S. Krane, T. B. Manny, and A. K. Hemal, "Is near infrared fluorescence imaging using indocyanine green dye useful in robotic partial nephrectomy: a prospective comparative study of 94 patients," *Urology*, vol. 80, no. 1, pp. 110–116, 2012.

[15] K. J. Kowalczyk, M. Alemozaffar, N. D. Hevelone et al., "Partial clamping of the renal artery during robot-assisted laparoscopic partial nephrectomy: technique and initial outcomes," *Journal of Endourology*, vol. 26, no. 5, pp. 469–473, 2012.

[16] L. S. Krane, P. W. Mufarrij, T. B. Manny, and A. K. Hemal, "Comparison of clamping technique in robotic partial nephrectomy: does unclamped partial nephrectomy improve perioperative outcomes and renal function?" *The Canadian Journal of Urology*, vol. 20, no. 1, pp. 6662–6667, 2013.

[17] A. Khalifeh, R. Autorino, R. Eyraud et al., "Three-year oncologic and renal functional outcomes after robot-assisted partial nephrectomy," *European Urology*, vol. 64, no. 5, pp. 744–750, 2013.

[18] G. Vittori, "Open versus robotic-assisted partial nephrectomy: a multicenter comparison study of perioperative results and complications," *World Journal of Urology*, vol. 32, no. 1, pp. 287–293, 2014.

[19] A. Masson-Lecomte, K. Bensalah, E. Seringe et al., "A prospective comparison of surgical and pathological outcomes obtained after robot-assisted or pure laparoscopic partial nephrectomy in moderate to complex renal tumours: results from a French multicentre collaborative study," *BJU International*, vol. 111, no. 2, pp. 256–263, 2013.

[20] L. Bi, C. Zhang, K. Li et al., "Robotic partial nephrectomy for renal tumors Larger than 4 cm: a systematic review and meta-analysis," *PLoS ONE*, vol. 8, no. 10, Article ID e75050, 2013.

[21] Y. S. Tanagho, J. H. Kaouk, M. E. Allaf et al., "Perioperative complications of robot-assisted partial nephrectomy: analysis of 886 patients at 5 United States centers," *Urology*, vol. 81, no. 3, pp. 573–579, 2013.

10

Converting Potential Abdominal Hysterectomy to Vaginal One: Laparoscopic Assisted Vaginal Hysterectomy

Jyothi Shetty,[1] Asha Shanbhag,[2] and Deeksha Pandey[1]

[1] *KMC, Manipal University, Manipal 576104, India*
[2] *KMC, Manipal University, Mangalore 575001, India*

Correspondence should be addressed to Deeksha Pandey; deekshiiiobg@gmail.com

Academic Editor: Peng Hui Wang

Background. The idea of laparoscopic assisted vaginal hysterectomy (LAVH) is to convert a potential abdominal hysterectomy to a vaginal one, thus decreasing associated morbidity and hastening recovery. We compared intraoperative and postoperative outcomes between LAVH and abdominal hysterectomy, to find out if LAVH achieves better clinical results compared with abdominal hysterectomy. *Material and methods.* A total of 48 women were enrolled in the study. Finally 17 patients underwent LAVH (cases) and 20 underwent abdominal hysterectomy (controls). All surgeries were performed by a set of gynecologists with more or less same level of surgical experience and expertise. *Results.*None of the patients in LAVH required conversion to laparotomy. Mean operating time was 30 minutes longer in LAVH group as compared to abdominal hysterectomy group (167.06 $\pm$ 31.97 min versus 135.25 $\pm$ 31.72 min; $P < 0.05$). However, the mean blood loss in LAVH was 100 mL lesser than that in abdominal hysterectomy and the difference was found to be statistically significant (248.24 $\pm$ 117.79 mL versus 340.00 $\pm$ 119.86 mL; $P < 0.05$). Another advantage of LAVH was significantly lower pain scores on second and third postoperative days. Overall complications and postoperative hospital stay were not significantly different between the two groups.

1. Background

Hysterectomy is the second most frequently performed major surgical procedure on women all over the world, next only to cesarean. The term "hysterectomy" though means removal of uterus; in practice it has a much wider classification depending upon the indication. At times, it is done without removal of the cervix (supracervical hysterectomy) or with removal of adnexa (hysterectomy with salpingooophorectomy). It can also be a part of staging laparotomy or radical hysterectomy. Hysterectomy can be performed abdominally, vaginally, or through abdominal ports with help of laparoscope. Approach depends on surgeon's preference, indication for surgery, nature of the disease, and patient characteristics. As any other surgery, hysterectomy is also associated with intraoperative and postoperative complications. Rates of various complications with hysterectomy have been reported in the range of 0.5% to 43% [1].

There is enough evidence from multiple randomized trials that vaginal hysterectomy is associated with fewer complications, a shorter hospital stay, more rapid recovery, and lower overall cost [2]. The idea of laparoscopic assisted vaginal hysterectomy (LAVH) is to convert a potential abdominal hysterectomy to a vaginal one, thus decreasing associated morbidity and hastening recovery. LAVH after being reported for the first time in 1989 gained wide popularity within a decade or two. Johnson et al. found that LAVH decreased pain, surgical site infections, and hospital stay and led to a quicker return to normal activities and fewer postoperative adhesions [3]. Quality of life studies also proved it to be better than abdominal hysterectomy at six weeks postoperatively [4]. However, Sculpher et al. could not demonstrate that LAVH was better than abdominal hysterectomy in their circumstances. The more we go through the literature and compare more variables among the two approaches, it is realized that the question of LAVH versus abdominal hysterectomy becomes more and more confusing [5].

Thus in this prospective study we aimed to compare the intraoperative and postoperative outcome between LAVH and abdominal hysterectomy, in order to find out if LAVH achieves better clinical results compared with abdominal hysterectomy.

2. Material and Methods

The present study was a prospective comparative study performed in a university teaching hospital from October 2007 to July 2009. The study was approved by the institutional ethical review board. Our study population was recruited from the set of women who were admitted in our hospital and required hysterectomy for the management of benign gynecological conditions. In order to convert a potential abdominal hysterectomy to a vaginal one with the help of LAVH we included those women who either had concomitant adnexal mass requiring adnexectomy, women who had undergone previous abdominopelvic surgery (like myomectomy, hysterotomy, surgeries on adnexa, and cesarean deliveries; and might require adhesiolysis), or women with history of pelvic inflammatory disease (PID) or endometriosis with suspected adhesions. Patients with one or more contraindications to LAVH were excluded from the study. This included cardiac or respiratory morbidity, frozen pelvis, broad ligament fibroid, and cervix flushed with vagina.

After recruiting the patients, they were informed about the study and written consent was obtained.

Women with benign gynecological conditions who required hysterectomy and where vaginal hysterectomy was not an option were recruited for the study. All these women were explained in detail about the advantages (abdominal hysterectomy: less operating time, regional anaesthesia, less cost; LAVH: less pain, cosmetic benefit) and disadvantages (abdominal hysterectomy: bigger incision, more postoperative pain; LAVH: chance of conversion to open method, only option of general anaesthesia, more time) of both the procedures with the help of a pre-prepared information leaflet which was based on the literature review. Patients were then allowed to choose from the two methods. A written consent was obtained from all the participants. All patients were given an oral gut lavage solution containing polyethylene glycol, sodium chloride, potassium chloride, and sodium bicarbonate, 1.5 liters ingested over 2-3 hours. Proctoclysis enema was administered the night before and also in the morning of the day of surgery. Patients were kept nil per oral for 12 hours before the surgery. Antiseptic vaginal douche was done preoperatively. All patients were subjected to prophylactic intravenous antibiotic half an hour before surgery and then eighth hourly in the postoperative period for 48 hours (amoxicillin 1000 mg + clavulanic acid 200 mg). Additional antibiotic was added if the same was deemed necessary due to any postoperative infection. General anesthesia was administered to all patients.

All surgeries were performed by a set of gynecologists with more or less same level of surgical experience and expertise. Abdominal hysterectomy was performed by the extrafascial technique and the vaginal cuff was sutured with interrupted sutures. LAVH was performed using video monitoring equipment. A 10 mm laparoscope with a Storz endovision camera was inserted in a subumbilical position. Three more 5 mm entry ports were created, one on each right and left spinoumbilical line and one on midline suprapubic region 3 cm above the symphysis pubis. Opening of bladder flap was done laparoscopically whereas bladder dissection was done during the vaginal phase of hysterectomy. Vaginal phase of hysterectomy was commenced with an anterior circumferential incision of the vagina. At the end after closing the vaginal cuff, a pneumoperitoneum was recreated to confirm hemostasis. A decision to convert a LAVH to an abdominal hysterectomy was readily made if difficulties were encountered. Following both, Foleys urinary catheter was left in situ and was removed after 24 hours or later depending upon the individual case. In LAVH, a vaginal pack was left in situ which was also removed 24 hours later. Postoperatively, all patients were prescribed an identical regimen of analgesia. A diclofenac rectal suppository was initially administered at the time of completion of the surgery. Following this, intramuscular tramadol and diclofenac rectal suppository were administered twice a day on the first postoperative day and then according to the patient's request.

2.1. Outcome Measures. The duration of surgery was calculated from the first surgical incision to the time when the last skin suture was applied. Blood loss during the laparoscopic phase was calculated as the difference between the volume of fluid aspirated and that of the fluid introduced into the pelvic cavity. Blood loss during the vaginal phase of LAVH or during abdominal hysterectomy was determined directly from the aspirated fluid collected in the calibrated container. Sponges used for mopping were also taken into consideration and one fully socked sponge was accounted for 50 mL of blood loss. All intraoperative complications—damage to ureter, urinary bladder, or major vessels and torrential hemorrhage requiring either transfusion or conversion of LAVH to open method—were noted. The specimen weight was obtained immediately after the surgery. Hemoglobin estimation was done for all patients 24 hours after surgery and blood transfusion was given if the hemoglobin was less than 8 gm/dL. Postoperative fever was considered as body temperature of more than 38.2°C for two consecutive measurements at least 6 hours apart, excluding the first 24 hours following the surgery. For comparing postoperative pain, we used visual analogue scale (VAS) in our study. Other postoperative complications like wound infection, secondary hemorrhage, or pulmonary embolism were also noted. For calculation of hospital stay, only days from surgery till discharge from the hospital were taken into account. The patients were discharged once they were able to tolerate oral diet, could void normally, were ambulatory, did not require parenteral medication, and had stable hematocrit.

2.2. Statistical Analysis. Statistical Package for the Social Sciences (SPSS 11.5 for Windows) was used for data compilation

Table 1: Demographic characteristics of the studied population.

Variables	LAVH $n = 17$	Abdominal hysterectomy $n = 20$	P value
Age (years)*			
Mean ± SD	43.2 ± 5.86	49.8 ± 8.59	0.010
Parity*			
Median (IQR)	2 (0–5)	2 (0–5)	0.619
Nulliparous	1	2	
Previous pelvic surgeries** (%)	9 (53)	9 (45)	0.193
BMI (kg/m^2)*			
Mean ± SD	24.8 ± 5.86	25.9 ± 5.86	0.473
Comorbidities			
Hypertension (%)	2 (11.7)	8 (40)	
Diabetes mellitus	1 (5.8)	3 (15)	
Thyroid disorder	3 (17.6)	3 (15)	
Bronchial asthma	0	2 (10)	

*Independent sample t-test; **Mann-Whitney test.

and statistical analysis. Independent sample t-test was used for discrete and continuous variables. Independent t-test was applied to test the difference between mean values of the variables in the two groups compared. Mann-Whitney test was used when variables had a nonparametric distribution (to compare number of previous surgeries, intraoperative blood loss, and weight of the retrieved specimen). Chi-square test was applied to those tests that evaluate the possible effect of one variable upon an outcome (postoperative complications). Fischer's exact test was used to compare the rate of postoperative wound infection, as the frequency was less than five.

3. Results

A total of 48 women were enrolled in the study. Out of these only 37 could be included as two were found to have frozen pelvis, one had broad ligament fibroid, and four menopausal women were found to have cervix flushed with vagina. In the remaining four women, their cardiorespiratory status contraindicated laparoscopy. Finally, 17 patients underwent LAVH (cases) and 20 underwent abdominal hysterectomy (controls). None of the patients in LAVH required conversion to laparotomy.

Demographic characteristics of both the groups have been tabulated in Table 1. Mean age of women in the LAVH group was 43.2 years as compared to 49.8 years in the abdominal hysterectomy group. Other characteristics like parity, cesarean deliveries, previous pelvic surgeries, and body mass index (BMI) were also comparable in both the groups. Even the comorbidities such as hypertension, diabetes mellitus, and thyroid disorders were also equally distributed between the two groups. Majority of women in both groups underwent hysterectomy for symptomatic fibroid uterus (58.8% in LAVH group and 45% in abdominal hysterectomy group), the next common indication being dysfunctional uterine bleeding (DUB) (23.5% in LAVH group and 25% in abdominal hysterectomy group).

It was observed that the mean operating time for LAVH was 30 minutes longer than that for abdominal hysterectomy and this was statistically significant (167.06±31.97 min versus 135.25 ± 31.72 min; $P < 0.05$). However the mean blood loss in LAVH was 100 mL lesser than that in abdominal hysterectomy and the difference was found to be statistically significant (248.24 ± 117.79 mL versus 340.00 ± 119.86 mL; $P < 0.05$). Four patients in the abdominal hysterectomy group required packed cell transfusion in the postoperative period while none of the patients required transfusion in the intraoperative or postoperative period. Weight of the uteri removed in both the groups was found to be comparable (223.82 ± 71.6 g in LAVH versus 252.00 ± 151.92 g in abdominal hysterectomy) (Table 2).

Six patients in the abdominal hysterectomy group required extra analgesia in the first postoperative day as compared to none in the LAVH group. The measurement of pain perception in the postoperative period was done with the help of VAS, where patients rated 10 for excruciating pain and 0 for no pain. It was seen that the level of pain (represented as mean ± standard deviation), perceived on the second and third postoperative days was significantly lower in the LAVH group. Difference of pain scores was not significant among the two procedures at Day 1 (Figure 1).

Table 3 shows the rate of postoperative complications in both the groups. In our study, the complications were more or less similar in both the groups. Even the postoperative hospital stay was also not significantly different in both the groups.

4. Discussion

In our study, it was found that the mean operating time was 30 minutes longer in LAVH group as compared to abdominal hysterectomy group. However the mean estimated blood loss was around 90 mL more in abdominal hysterectomy group. Another advantage of LAVH was significantly lower

TABLE 2: Intraoperative characteristics.

Characteristics	LAVH $n = 17$	Abdominal hysterectomy $n = 20$	P value
Operating time (min) Mean ± SD*	167.06 ± 31.97	135.25 ± 31.72	0.005
Estimated blood loss (mL) Mean ± SD**	248.24 ± 117.79	340.00 ± 119.86	0.003
Weight of specimen (g) Mean ± SD*	223.82 ± 71.6	252.00 ± 151.92	0.569

*Independent sample t-test; **Mann-Whitney test.

TABLE 3: Postoperative complications.

Complications	LAVH $n = 17$ (%)	Abdominal hysterectomy $n = 20$ (%)	P value
Febrile Morbidity*	3 (17.6)	1 (5)	0.482
Secondary hemorrhage*	3 (17.6)	1 (5)	0.482
Wound infection**	0	3 (15)	0.489

*Independent sample t-test; **Mann-Whitney test.

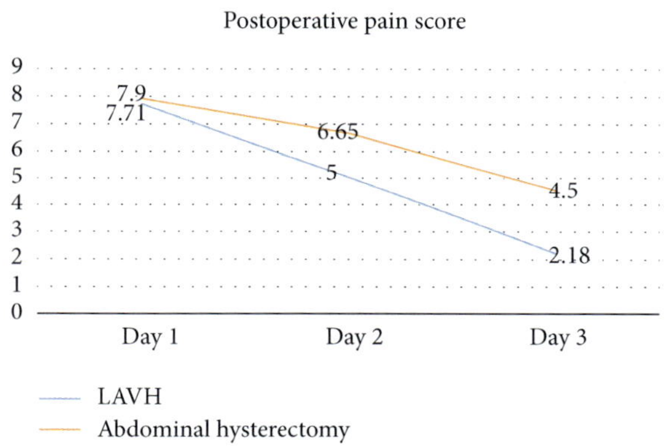

FIGURE 1: Pain scores among the two methods following surgery.

pain scores on second and third postoperative days. Overall complications were not significantly different between the two groups.

In a study conducted by Summitt et al. also the operative time averaged 30 minutes longer in LAVH and estimated blood loss averaged 100 mL greater in abdominal hysterectomy with no difference in the rate of overall complications [6]. While in another study by Marana et al. there was no difference between the operating time between the two groups. However, the estimated blood loss was around 89 mL higher in the abdominal hysterectomy group [7]. Similar to our observation, Marana et al. also found a significant reduced pain perception on second and third postoperative days in patients who underwent LAVH [7].

A recent meta-analysis which compared 23 randomized controlled trials concluded that LAVH has a significantly longer operation time than abdominal hysterectomy. This may be due to the learning curve for laparoscopy requiring a high level of skill and good hand-eye coordination. However, we also agree with the authors (Yi et al) that comprehensive training of surgeons and the development of surgical instruments may lead to a decrease in the operation time for LAVH in the future. Similar to our results in the meta-analysis also postoperative pain and hemoglobin drop were reduced significantly, and return to normal activities was significantly quicker following LAVH compared with abdominal hysterectomy [8]. It is supported by the observation that in the literature we found that the mean time taken to perform LAVH had a very wide range with a minimum of 77 minutes [9] to 179.8 minutes [6].

5. Conclusion

This study showed that LAVH had a disadvantage of longer operation time but had a definitive advantage of less blood loss and less postoperative pain. The skill of laparoscopy though has a learning curve but can be mastered over time, which will lead to combating the one and only negative issue of greater operative time.

Acknowledgment

The authors would like to acknowledge the help extended by Dr. Rajesh Bhakta during the surgical procedures.

References

[1] N. C. Lee, R. C. Dicker, G. L. Rubin, and H. W. Ory, "Confirmation of the preoperative diagnoses for hysterectomy," *American Journal of Obstetrics and Gynecology*, vol. 150, no. 3, pp. 283–287, 1984.

[2] D. Alan Johns, B. Carrera, J. Jones, F. DeLeon, R. Vincent, and C. Safely, "The medical and economic impact of laparoscopically assisted vaginal hysterectomy in a large, metropolitan, not-for-profit hospital," *American Journal of Obstetrics and Gynecology*, vol. 172, no. 6, pp. 1709–1719, 1995.

[3] N. Johnson, D. Barlow, A. Lethaby, E. Tavender, L. Curr, and R. Garry, "Methods of hysterectomy: systematic review and meta-analysis of randomised controlled trials," *British Medical Journal*, vol. 330, no. 7506, pp. 1478–1481, 2005.

[4] K. B. Kluivers, N. P. Johnson, P. Chien, M. E. Vierhout, M. Bongers, and B. W. J. Mol, "Comparison of laparoscopic and abdominal hysterectomy in terms of quality of life: a systematic review," *European Journal of Obstetrics Gynecology and Reproductive Biology*, vol. 136, no. 1, pp. 3–8, 2008.

[5] M. Sculpher, A. Manca, J. Abbott, J. Fountain, S. Mason, and R. Garry, "Cost effectiveness analysis of laparoscopic hysterectomy compared with standard hysterectomy: results from a randomised trial," *British Medical Journal*, vol. 328, no. 7432, pp. 134–137, 2004.

[6] R. L. Summitt Jr., T. G. Stovall, J. F. Steege, and G. H. Lipscomb, "A multicenter randomized comparison of laparoscopically assisted vaginal hysterectomy and abdominal hysterectomy in abdominal hysterectomy candidates," *Obstetrics and Gynecology*, vol. 92, no. 3, pp. 321–326, 1998.

[7] R. Marana, M. Busacca, E. Zupi, N. Garcea, P. Paparella, and G. F. Catalano, "Laparoscopically assisted vaginal hysterectomy versus total abdominal hysterectomy: a prospective, randomized, multicenter study," *American Journal of Obstetrics and Gynecology*, vol. 180, no. 2 I, pp. 270–275, 1999.

[8] Y.-X. Yi, W. Zhang, Q. Zhou, W.-R. Guo, and Y. Su, "Laparoscopic-assisted vaginal hysterectomy vs abdominal hysterectomy for benign disease: a meta-analysis of randomized controlled trials," *European Journal of Obstetrics Gynecology and Reproductive Biology*, vol. 159, no. 1, pp. 1–18, 2011.

[9] E.-M. Tsai, H.-S. Chen, C.-Y. Long et al., "Laparoscopically assisted vaginal hysterectomy versus total abdominal hysterectomy: a study of 100 cases on light-endorsed transvaginal section," *Gynecologic and Obstetric Investigation*, vol. 55, no. 2, pp. 105–109, 2003.

11

Minimally Invasive Mitral Valve Surgery

Fabiana Lucà,[1,2,3] Leen van Garsse,[1] Carmelo Massimiliano Rao,[2] Orlando Parise,[2] Mark La Meir,[1] Calogero Puntrello,[3] Gaspare Rubino,[3] Rocco Carella,[2] Roberto Lorusso,[2] Gian Franco Gensini,[2] Jos G. Maessen,[1] and Sandro Gelsomino[1,2]

[1] *Cardiothoracic and Cardiology Department, Maastricht University, The Netherlands*
[2] *Heart and Vessels Department, Careggi Hospital, Florence, Italy*
[3] *Cardiology Department, Paolo Borsellino Hospital, Marsala, Italy*

Correspondence should be addressed to Sandro Gelsomino; sandro.gelsomino@libero.it

Academic Editor: Gideon Uretzky

In the recent years minimally invasive mitral valve surgery (MIMVS) has become a well-established and increasingly used option for managing patients with a mitral valve pathology. Nonetheless, whether the purported benefits of MIMVS translate into clinically important outcomes remains controversial. Therefore, in this paper we provide an overview of MIMVS and discuss results, morbidity, mortality, and quality of life following mitral minimally invasive procedures. MIMVS has been proven to be a feasible alternative to the conventional full sternotomy approach with low perioperative morbidity and short-term mortality. Reported benefits of MIMVS include also decreased postoperative pain, improved postoperative respiratory function, reduced surgical trauma, and greater patient satisfaction. Finally, compared to standard surgery, MIMVS demonstrated comparable efficacy across a range of long-term efficacy measures such as freedom from reoperation and long-term survival.

1. Introduction

Minimally invasive mitral valve surgery (MIMVS) has been proven as a feasible alternative to conventional full sternotomy approach with low perioperative morbidity and short-term mortality [1, 2]. As a result, MIMVS is being employed increasingly as routine approach in many centers worldwide with excellent short-term and long-term results [3, 4].

During the past years, several studies on outcomes of MIMVS have been published in the literature [5–7]. Furthermore, since the first description of MIMVS by Cohn et al. [8] and Navia and Cosgrove [9] in the mid 1990s, various minimally invasive approaches have been reported including the parasternal, hemisternotomy, minithoracotomy, and totally endoscopic approaches [10–12]. However, despite the differences in surgical approaches, the shared goal of all these MIMVS procedures is to avoid median sternotomy-related complications such as infection, mediastinitis, and nerve injuries [8, 13–19] and, at the same time, to provide a safe and effective option for mitral valve surgery with the clinical benefits associated with a minimal access approach.

Nonetheless, whether the supposed benefits of MIMVS translate into clinical favorable outcomes still remains controversial, and there are conflicting opinions about whether minimally invasive surgery is ready for routine uptake in place of conventional open mitral valve surgery.

In this paper we provide an overview of MIMVS and discuss results, morbidity, mortality, and quality of life following mitral minimally invasive procedures.

2. Review Criteria

Papers selected for this review were identified on PUBMED using the search terms "minimally invasive mitral valve surgery."

All articles were reviewed and references were selected on the basis of historical contribution, number of patients, and new contributions to the field.

3. Surgical Procedure

MIMVS refers to a constellation of surgical techniques/technologies (Figure 1) that minimize surgical trauma through smaller incisions compared with a conventional sternotomy. The most common minimally invasive approach to the mitral valve includes a right minithoracotomy [8], a robotically assisted right thoracic approach [20], and a partial sternotomy [21].

In 1923 Elliot Carr Cutler, in conjunction with his cardiology colleague, Samuel Levine, performed a closed transventricular mitral commissurotomy on a 12-year-old patient with rheumatic mitral stenosis at the Peter Bent Brigham Hospital.

The patient survived surgery but died of pneumonia 4 years postoperatively. In the following years, Cutler performed seven more operations using his new cardiovalvulotome. Unfortunately, this concept did not promote long-term success and a moratorium for these operations was called in 1929. However, this pioneering effort in 1923 was the first successful operation to treat valvular heart disease by a surgical technique [22].

A transseptal approach to the mitral valve was described by Dubost and colleagues [23] using a biatrial incision and transecting the septum whereas Guiraudon and associates [24] described an approach via the right atrium.

By the mid 1990s, the success of laparoscopic operations in general surgery renewed an interest in minimally invasive approaches for cardiac surgery. During April and May 1996, minimally invasive mitral valve operations were performed on 25 patients by Navia and Cosgrove [8, 9]. All patients underwent mitral valve repair performed through a small right parasternal incision. Although the surgical field is smaller than a median sternotomy, the mitral valve is positioned in the center of the incision, and, if the atrium is small, extension of the incision over the dome of the left atrium provides a substantial improvement of exposure. There were no hospital deaths, reoperations for bleeding, embolic complications, wound infections, or valve repair failures. No sinus node dysfunction or atrioventricular dissociation resulted [9].

From 1996 to 1997, Cohn et al. [8] presented 84 minimally invasive cases (41 aortic, 43 mitral) using a right parasternal incision and excising the third and fourth costal cartilage. For mitral valve replacement or repair, all incisions were performed through a right parasternal incision, excising the third and fourth costal cartilage. The right atrium was exposed and opened after caval tapes were put down, isolating the right atrium. The aortic cross-clamp was applied before incising the right atrium. A transseptal incision then was made into the left atrium. Once the atrial septum was incised, the mitral valve was repaired or replaced by standard techniques [25, 26].

The operative mortality for mitral valve surgery was 0 (0%) of 43. There had been no perivalvular leaks in any of the valves implanted, and there has been excellent visualization of the mitral valves as to perform complicated repairs, including leaflet resection, chondroplasty, and commissuroplasty documented by intraoperative and postoperative transesophageal echo [8]. Smaller incisions lateral to the sternum have been introduced, with or without resection of the third or fourth costal cartilage. However, their disadvantages included femoral CPB cannulation, ligation of the right internal thoracic artery, occasional chest wall instability, and difficult conversion to full sternotomy [4].

In 1996, Carpentier et al. [27] performed the first video-assisted mitral valve repair through a minithoracotomy using ventricular fibrillation.

From 1996 to 1998 the Leipzig group [28] studied one hundred and twenty-nine patients with nonischemic mitral valve disease undergoing 3D video assisted mitral valve surgery via a 4 cm right lateral minithoracotomy using femorofemoral bypass and endoaortic clamping. After the initial series (group I, $n = 62$), a voice controlled robotic arm (AESOP 3000, Automated Endoscope System for Optimal Positioning; Computer Motion, Santa Barbara, CA) was employed to guide the video scope in the last series (group II, $n = 67$). Finally, intraoperative transesophageal echocardiography was introduced for real-time monitoring of cardiac distention, deairing, and cannula placement [29].

Felger et al. [30] evaluated a series of video-assisted minimally invasive mitral operations, showing safe progression toward totally endoscopic techniques. Consecutive patients with isolated mitral valve disease underwent either manually directed ($n = 55$) or voice-activated robotically directed ($n = 72$) video-assisted mitral operations. The consecutive series was evaluated in five cohorts comparing serial cross-clamp and perfusion times. Cold blood cardioplegia, a transthoracic aortic clamp, a 5 mm endoscope, and a 5 cm minithoracotomy were used. This video-assisted minimally invasive mitral operation cohort was compared with a previous sternotomy-based mitral operation cohort ($n = 100$). Repairs were performed in 61.8% manually directed (MD, $n = 34$), 75.0% robotically directed (RD, $n = 54$), and 54% sternotomy-based ($N = 54$) mitral operations. The robotically directed technique showed a significant decrease in blood loss, ventilator time, and hospitalization compared with the sternotomy-based technique. Manually directed mitral operations compared with robotically directed mitral operations had decreased arrest times (128.0 ± 4.5 minutes compared with 90.0 ± 4.6 minutes; $P < 0.001$) and decreased perfusion times (173.0 ± 5.7 minutes compared with 144.0 ± 4.6 minutes; $P < 0.001$). In the minimally invasive mitral operation cohort, complications included reexploration for bleeding (2.4%; $n = 3$) and one stroke (0.8%), whereas the 30-day mortality was 2.3% ($n = 3$). Operative times were significantly less with RD operations versus MD operations ($P < 0.002$) Table 1.

The next evolutionary bound in endoscopic mitral surgery was the development of three-dimensional (3D) vision and computer-assisted telemanipulation that could transpose surgical movements from outside the chest wall todeep within cardiac chambers; in that same year, Carpentier et al. [47] performed the first completely robotic MVR using the Da Vinci Surgical System (Intuitive Surgical,Inc., Sunnyvale, California, USA). Soon after, the East Carolina University group performed the first mitral valve replacement through a minithoracotomy, using video direction [8, 20].

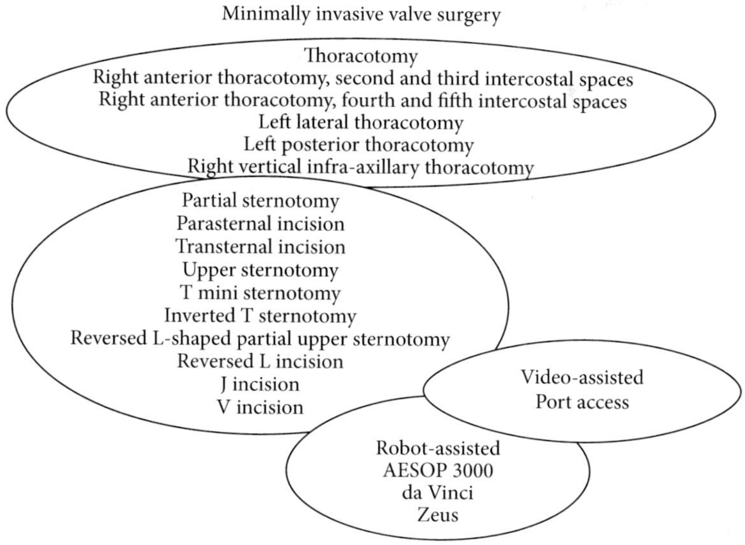

FIGURE 1: Minimally invasivemitral valve surgery: techniques overview.

TABLE 1: Most recent observational cohort studies of minimally invasive mitral valve surgery.

Authors	Year	Minimally invasive (number of patients)	Minithoracotomy (number of patients)	Approach	Valve	Differences
Cohn et al. [8]	1997	50	50	PS, UHS	MV, AV	Longer CBP/XT times in MI group
Navia and Cosgrove [9]	1996	31	100	MT	MV	Longer CBP/XT times, less transfusion, reduced CVA, shorter ICU/hospital stays in MI group
Glower et al. [31]	1998	21	20	MT	MV	Longer CBP/XT times, shorter return to normal activity time n MI group
Reichenspurner et al. [32]	1998	100	100	MT	MV	Reduced AF in MI group
Asher et al. [33]	1999	100	100	—	MV, AV	Longer CBP/XT times, shorter hospital stays in MI group
Grossi et al. [34]	1999	111	259	MT	MV, AV	Lower sepsis/wound complications, shorter hospital stays in MI group
Walther et al. [35]	1999	129	209	MT	MV, AV	Lower pain levels
Schneider et al. [36]	2000	21	13	MV	MT	Longer CPB time
Hamano et al. [37]	2001	21	27	PS, UHS, LHS	MV, AV	No differences
Grossi et al. [38]	2001	100	100	MT	MV	No differences
Grossi et al. [39]	2001	109	88	MT	MV, AV	Longer CBP/XT times, shorter hospital stays in MI group
Felger et al. [30]	2001	127	100	MT	MV	With AESOP shorter hospital stay time compared to ST group, shorter XC times compared to manually directed videoscope
Yamada et al. [40]	2003	66	50	LHS	MV, AV	Longer CBP/XT times in MI group
McCreath et al. [41]	2003	214	87	MT	MV	Reduced acute renal deseas in MI group
de Vaumas et al. [42]	2003	10	10	PS	MV	Longer CBP/XT times in PS group
Gaudiani et al. [43]	2004	205	616	UHS, LHS, MT	MV	Shorter hospital stay in MI repair group, less CVA in MI replacement group
Mihaljevic et al. [44]	2004	474	337	LHS, PS	MV	5-year survival better for MI group
Dogan et al. [45]	2005	20	20	MT	MV	Intraoperative complications in EABO group
Ryan et al. [46]	2005	117	117	MT	MV	Longer CBP/XT times in MI group

Another promising technique is the Port access for MIMVS [31, 48–50].

Stevens and colleagues at Stanford University introduced in Europe in March 1996 a surgical method for performing Port-access bypass grafting [51].

In 1998, Mohr reported the Leipzig University experience using the Port access technology, which was based on endoaortic balloon occlusion (EABO). The study recruited 51 consecutive patients with nonischemic mitral valve disease who undergone mitral repairment ($n = 28$) or replacement ($n = 23$) by means of a minimally invasive approach through a right lateral minithoracotomy and under videoscopic guidance. Acute retrograde aortic dissection occurred in two patients [50]. Both events were most likely caused by intimal dissection at the level of the iliac artery induced by the guide wire. Retrograde flow led to complete retrograde aortic dissection.

The Port access technology has some complicated aspects such as the introduction and the placement of the endoaortic balloon catheter and its intraoperative monitoring. Transesophageal echocardiography and fluoroscopy are used to verify proper positioning of the coronary sinus and pulmonary artery vent catheters and the venous drainage cannula and endoaortic balloon [52, 53]. During CPB, verification of proper positioning of the endoaortic balloon is vital because proximal migration can damage the aortic valve and distal migration can decrease cerebral perfusion by occluding the brachiocephalic artery [52]. Because distal migration may compromise cerebral blood flow, it is imperative to monitor endoaortic balloon position continuously. Multiple monitoring techniques are used to confirm proper positioning of the endoaortic balloon in the ascending aorta. Transesophageal echocardiography is useful in visualizing the ascending aorta and endoaortic balloon location [54], but it may become difficult to visualize the balloon position when the heart is fully arrested during CPB.

The implementation of continuous transcranial Doppler flow measurements of the middle cerebral arteries added an important safety measure, as right radial artery pressure measurements alone are not sensitive enough to immediately detect impairment of cerebral perfusion caused by balloon migration to the aortic arch [11].

However, the Port access technique still continues to be associated with significant risks such as peripheral CPB cannulation and a high rate of retrograde aortic dissection balloon catheter to occlude the aorta and provide cardioplegia.

An 8 cm anterolateral thoracotomy via the third intercostals space, direct aortic clamping, and cannulation has been described by Angouras and Michler [55].

Telemanipulators, robotics that allow a hand-like mechanism to be controlled by a human operator, were first used by Mohr et al. [28] and Falk et al. [11].

Chitwood et al. [56, 57] and Kypson et al. [58, 59] showed that this technique could be safely and effectively used. Recently, another group reported the results of 25 patients receiving successful telemanipulator-supported MIMVS [60]; however, long-term results are not available. Other centers had similar positive experiences using the telemanipulator-supported techniques in the late 1990s [61, 62]. However, they later abandoned this technique, given the lack of difference compared with their standard approaches. In 2009, Wang et al. [63] presented a new approach for MV replacement through a right vertical infra-axillary thoracotomy with excellent results (0.5% mortality).

4. Mortality

After reviewing all comparative miniVS studies evaluating mortality, no study showed a significant difference between minimally invasive and conventional approaches [32, 34, 38, 39, 42, 43, 46, 64].

Mihaljevic et al. compared 474 minimally invasive mitral operations (mostly lower sternotomy and right parasternal) with 337 median sternotomy procedures. The perioperative mortality was 0.2% for the minimally invasive group and this is compared favorably with 0.3% in the sternotomy patients. However, the MIMVS patients were found to be a lower risk group (better ejection fraction, more repairs, less symptomatic), and no attempt was made to adjust for these differences [44]; Furthermore, Grossi et al. matched 100 consecutive patients undergoing minimally invasive aortic and mitral valve surgery over a 2.5-year period (through either a 3rd or 4th interspace incision) to patients having the same valve surgery via a sternotomy [38]. They demonstrated no significant difference in hospital mortality (3.7% versus 3.4%, resp.) between groups, even though mean CPB times was 30 min longer in the minimally invasive group. Six studies met the inclusion criteria for our analysis and revealed no significant mortality difference between groups (1,641 patients, OR 0.46, 95% CI 0.15–1.42, $P = 0.18$) [38, 43, 44, 46].

5. Neurological Events

Due to the physical limitations of MIMVS, inadequate deairing leading theoretically to a higher incidence of neurological complications was a primary concern, making the use of transesophageal echocardiography mandatory. In his early series, Mohr [50] reported an 18% incidence of postoperative confusion; however, continuous Co_2 insufflation was not used, as in more recent series. One decade later, Seeburger et al. [3] observed postoperative neurological impairment in 41 of 1,339 patients (3.1%) who underwent mini MVS, with 28 (2.1%) minor and 13 (1.0%) major events. Ten studies reported no difference in the incidence of stroke [31, 39, 65, 66], while two showed a decreased incidence following a minimally invasive approach [43, 67]. In a systemic metaanalysis [3], there was no significant difference in neurological events in 6 eligible studies including a total of 1,801 patients.

Schneider et al. used transcranial Doppler to detect cerebral microemboli in 21 MIMVS patients undergoing endoaortic balloon occlusion with continuous Co_2 chest cavity insufflation. These were compared to 14 patients undergoing conventional mitral surgery [36]. They found no significant difference in the cerebral microembolic rate between either technique.

The Consensus Statement of the International Society of Minimally Invasive Coronary Surgery (ISMICS) 2010, based on a systematic review and meta-analysis of all available randomized and nonrandomized comparative trials of isolated mini versus conventional mitral valve surgery (two randomized trials and 33 nonrandomized studies for a total of 35 studies) [68], associated some adverse clinical outcomes with mini MVS compared with conv-MVS, including stroke, aortic dissection, and groin wound/vasculature complications. The absolute risk increase of stroke for mini MVS versus conv-MVS was 0.9% overall (2.1% versus 1.2%, RR 1.79, 95% CI 1.35–2.38; 13 studies, level B). Subanalysis of two propensity comparison studies also showed significant increase of stroke of 1% with mini MVS compared with conv-MVS (1.9% versus 0.9%, RR 2.02, 95% CI 1.40–2.94; two studies, level B) [69].

These findings are similar to those recently reported by a recent Society of Thoracic Surgeons-Adult Cardiac Surgical Database (STS-ACSD) publication made on 28,143 patients undergoing isolated mitral valve operations that examined the associations between operative strategy and the increased risk of stroke in the less-invasive group [70].

The markedly higher rate of permanent perioperative stroke in the less-invasive group compared with the conventional sternotomy group in unadjusted, adjusted, and propensity analyses was the most significant finding of this study. The adjusted OR for permanent stroke was 1.96 for less-invasive compared with conventional sternotomy operations in the multivariable analysis, and the likelihood of stroke was similarly increased in the propensity analysis. Among the 4,322 LIMV operations, there were 41 excess strokes compared with the propensity-matched group having conventional mitral valve operations. Additional analyses demonstrated a threefold higher risk of stroke for less-invasive operations performed without aortic occlusion (beating- or fibrillating-heart), which comprised 12% of the less invasive group. Femoral cannulation was not an independent predictor of stroke [70].

Grossi et al. [71] using an informal strategy of intraoperative echocardiographic analysis of the aortic arch and the descending aorta in 714 minimally invasive mitral valve procedures had excellent results from this approach avoiding the use of femoral perfusion when there was significant atherosclerotic burden [71]. In this cohort, where 30% of patients were >70 years of age, 15% were reoperations, and 12% were multivalve operations, femoral perfusion was used in nearly 80% of patients, with a 2.9% incidence of stroke. Afterwards they developed an aortic cannulation through a minithoracotomy incision that became the "go-to" approach for the majority of our minimally invasive mitral valve procedures, regardless of age.

The same group [72] reviewed a large minimally invasive valve experience using a robust data collection instrument. The study recruited 3,180 patients undergone to isolated, nonreoperative valve operations: 1,452 (45.7%) aortic valve replacements and 1,728 (54.3%) mitral valve procedures. The surgical approach was with standard sternotomy (n = 889; 28%) or by minimally invasive techniques (n = 2,291; 72%). Antegrade arterial perfusion was used in 2,646 (83.2%) cases and retrograde perfusion was used in 534 (16.8%) cases. Multivariable analysis revealed that age, atherosclerotic aorta, cerebrovascular disease, emergent procedure, ejection fraction less than 0.30, no use of aortic clamp, and retrograde perfusion were significantly associated with stroke. In patients 50 years old or younger (n = 662), retrograde perfusion had no significant impact on the incidence of stroke (1.6% versus 1.1%, $P = 0.57$). In this study, minimally invasive approaches for isolated aortic or mitral valve operations did not increase the perioperative risk of stroke when performed with antegrade perfusion. However, the risk of stroke did increase with the use of retrograde perfusion in older patients. Multivariable risk factors for stroke were retrograde perfusion (odds ratio 4.4; $P < 0.01$) and ejection fraction below 0.30 (odds ratio 2.1; $P = 0.09$). The authors concluded that the incidence of stroke in reoperative mitral operations was associated with perfusion strategies and not with the surgical approach [71]. The overall stroke rate was 2.2%, with increased stroke risk associated with an atherosclerotic aorta, cerebrovascular disease, emergent operation, ejection fraction <30% or retrograde perfusion ($P < 0.05$ for each), but not with incision location (P = 0.82). Additionally, the association of retrograde perfusion became insignificant when analyzing patients who were 50 years old or younger [72].

These results mirror those of a previous cohort of patients undergoing reoperative mitral valve procedures, which revealed that retrograde perfusion was the only independent risk factor for stroke (odds ratio 4.4; $P = 0.001$) [73].

Later, Grossi and colleagues presented a focused report on a more homogeneous subset of 1,282 first-time, isolated mitral valve operations performed through a right anterior minithoracotomy over a 12-year period [74]. This homogeneity allowed us greater discriminatory power to analyze the specific patient factors associated with an increased risk of stroke. The only significant risk factor interaction for neurologic complication identified was the use of retrograde perfusion in patients with high-risk comorbidities: peripheral vascular disease, cerebrovascular disease, atherosclerotic aortas, or dialysis dependence.

These data suggest that retrograde perfusion remains a viable option for younger patients without vascular comorbidities. In older patients or those with the risk factors discussed previously, performing a computed tomography angiography of the descending aorta with distal runoff in addition to an intraoperative transoesophageal echocardiographic assessment of the thoracic aorta [74, 75] is currently recommend. Such an approach has been shown to be effective by Murphy et al. [76], who demonstrated a 1.6% stroke rate using retrograde perfusion in similarly screened patients undergoing robotic cardiac procedures. Minimally invasive valve surgery with antegrade perfusion has a low risk of neurological complications and has excellent outcomes. Retrograde perfusion in older patients with significant vascular comorbidities is associated with an increased risk of stroke. The vast majority of patients currently undergo heart valve procedures through a right anterior minithoracotomy with antegrade perfusion via direct ascending aorta cannulation obviating the concerns associated with retrograde perfusion. For those procedures in which the direct access to the ascending aorta is extremely limited, in a recent editorials Yaffee et al. [75] recommend preoperative aortic screening to identify aortic pathology and to avoid retrograde perfusion in patients where high atheroembolic risk exists.

6. Bleeding, Transfusion, and Reexploration

A reduction in postoperative hemorrhage and transfusion requirements has been suggested as a potential advantage of minimally invasive valve surgery. This benefit is important given the significant morbidity and mortality associated with transfusions and reexploration for bleeding [77]. Smaller incisions should theoretically reduce postoperative bleeding and transfusion requirements, notably with the significant morbidity/mortality associated with transfusions and bleeding reexploration. Some studies report no difference in transfusion requirements [45]. Four comparative studies reported blood loss volume with three utilizing a minithoracotomy [28, 31, 66] and one selecting a parasternal approach [42].

Mohr et al. demonstrated no difference in blood loss or blood product transfusions in 31 videoscopic mitral procedures compared with a conventional sternotomy, despite fewer reexplorations for bleeding [28]. The robotically directed technique showed a significant decrease in blood loss as well as ventilator time and hospitalization compared with the sternotomy-based technique [30]. Felger et al. reported that there was no significant difference either in percentage of patients receiving transfusions or in the amount of packed red blood cells, fresh frozen plasma, or platelets transfused; however, postoperative chest tube drainage was significantly less in minimally invasive patients compared with sternotomy patients ($P = 0.006$). Because extreme values skewed the raw data for ventilator hours, a rank order analysis of variance was performed to provide homogeneity of the data. The ranked ventilator hours revealed a significant difference between conventional and minimally invasive patients ($P = 0.006$), but no difference was found between the RD and MD patients ($P = 0.984$). All three cohorts had similar intensive care unit lengths of stay (P = not significant). However, length of stay from operative procedure to discharge was significantly less in the RD and MD cohorts compared with conventional cohorts ($P = 0.001$). In all minimally invasive mitral valve operations the bleeding was controlled through the thoracotomy incision without the need for extension. However, there was no significant difference either in the percentage of patients receiving transfusions or the amount of blood products transfused [30] In addition, in a prospective, randomized trial, Dogan et al. [45] found a significant decrease in postoperative chest tube output in the miniVS group compared with the conventional group. In a consecutive series of 41 patients undergoing either Port access ($n = 21$) or sternotomy ($n = 20$) mitral surgery, Glower et al. demonstrated no significant difference in chest tube drainage or transfusion requirements despite longer CPB times in the former [31]. Grossi et al. [39] found that a right thoracotomy was associated with 51% fewer blood products than a conventional sternotomy.

In robotically assisted MVR, transfusion requirements are even lower (20% to 45% require transfusions) [11, 78]. Furthermore, 4 comparative studies found less blood loss: a minithoracotomy was used in 3 [26, 30, 31] and a parasternal approach was used in 1 [42]. Three of 10 studies found reduced transfusion requirements with a minimally invasive approach compared with conventional surgery [8, 34, 38] whereas the others showed no difference [31, 33, 42, 46, 65, 67, 77].

More convincing evidence came from a subsequent study by the same group that showed 13% fewer total transfusions with 1.8 fewer units of red blood cells using a minithoracotomy compared to a sternotomy [39].

Similar data from Cohn et al. confirm that patients undergoing minimally invasive valve surgery are transfused 1.8 units less compared to a conventional cohort [8]. Two of seven studies [56, 65] demonstrated a reduced need for reoperation for bleeding with a minimally invasive approach [38, 42, 44, 46]. Further, 5 studies showed a significant reduction in reoperations for bleeding with a minimally-invasive approach [32, 38, 42–44, 49, 64]. The recent data from the Leipzig group on postoperative course included reoperation for bleeding in 69 patients (5.1%) [3].

7. Atrial Fibrillation

It has been suggested that a less traumatic surgical approach would be a less potent trigger of postoperative AF. Nonetheless, 5 of 6 studies demonstrated that this is not the case [10, 30–33, 46], and on meta-analysis of four eligible studies, there was no significant difference between minimally invasive and sternotomy approaches (539 patients, OR 0.86, 95% CI 0.59–1.27, $P = 0.45$).

Asher et al. [33] addressed this question in a cohort of 100 patients having elective primary minimally invasive AV or MV surgery compared with a matched control group undergoing conventional sternotomy. They found a similar prevalence of post-operative AF using either method, even after stratifying for valve type. However, the PAIR registry reported a 10% incidence of new-onset AF with the port access technique, which is lower than that expected for sternotomy [33].

8. Septic Complications

The incidence of wound infections and septic complications is lower with a thoracotomy than with a median sternotomy. Of the three studies of minithoracotomy mitral valve surgery that reported wound complications compared to median sternotomy, Grossi et al. reported an incidence of 0.9% and 5.7% for minithoracotomy and sternotomy cases, respectively ($P = 0.05$) [34]. This increased to 1.8% and 7.7%, respectively, in elderly patients ($P = 0.03$) [34], whereas Felger et al. reported no significant difference [30].

9. Pain, Quality of Life and Speed of Recovery

Compared with a complete sternotomy, thoracotomy incisions are associated with less pain, discomfort, and postoperative analgesics [30]. Cohn's data show less pain in hospital and after discharge, less analgesic usage, greater patient satisfaction, and a return to normal activity 4.8 weeks ahead of sternotomy patients [8].

The most insightful evidence comes from 2 studies reporting that patients undergoing surgery via a minimally invasive approach as their second procedure all thought that their recovery was faster/less painful than their original sternotomy [30, 79].

10. Elderly Patients

Iribarne et al. demonstrated that MIMVS can be performed safely in patients at ≥75 years old [80]. Although the minimally invasive approach was associated with slightly longer CPB and cross clamp times than was the conventional sternotomy approach, there were no significant differences in postoperative morbidity and mortality. Importantly, patients undergoing MIMVS had approximate 3 days shorter mean and 1 day shorter median durations of hospitalization, a finding that has important implications for resource use. There were significant reductions in both mean and median costs of hospitalization associated with the minimally invasive approach, a finding that correlates with the observed difference in duration of hospitalization found between the groups. In addition, patients undergoing MIMVS had faster rates for both time to independent ambulation and time to independent sit-to-stand activity [80]. Grossi et al. analyzed 111 patients undergoing MIMVS who were at least 70 years old and compared these to 259 patients having a sternotomy and concluded that this approach can be used safely in operations on the elderly population with excellent result [34]. Felger et al. recently reported 123 cases of minimal invasive mitral valve repair in patients aged ≥70 years with 1.6% operative mortality as well as 5-year actuarial survival of 87% and 5-year freedom from reoperation of 93% [30, 79]. To date, no studies have assessed any difference in postoperative functional status by type of surgery.

11. Hospital Stay and Costs

Some of the reported benefits of MIMVS include decreased intensive care unit a and total hospital length of stay, faster physical rehabilitation, and decreased overall hospital resource use [35, 40, 81, 82]. MIMVS is a cost-effective and cost-saving strategy for mitral valve repair and replacement compared with the traditional approach with lower cost driven largely by a decreased length of stay [80].

12. Conclusions

MIMVS has been proven to be a feasible alternative to the conventional full sternotomy approach with low perioperative morbidity and short-term mortality.

Reported benefits of MIMVS include decreased postoperative pain, improved postoperative respiratory function, reduced surgical trauma, and greater patient satisfaction. Finally, compared to standard surgery, MIMVS demonstrated comparable efficacy across a range of long-term efficacy measures such as freedom from reoperation and long-term survival.

Acknowledgment

The authors gratefully thank MRS Judith Wilson for the English revision of the paper.

References

[1] A. M. Gilliov, M. K. Banbury, and D. M. Cosgrove, "Hemisternotomy approach for aortic and mitral valve surgery," *Journal of Cardiac Surgery*, vol. 15, no. 1, pp. 15–20, 2000.

[2] P. Modi, A. Hassan, and W. R. Chitwood Jr., "Minimally invasive mitral valve surgery: a systematic review and meta-analysis," *European Journal of Cardio-Thoracic Surgery*, vol. 34, no. 5, pp. 943–952, 2008.

[3] J. Seeburger, M. A. Borger, V. Falk et al., "Minimal invasive mitral valve repair for mitral regurgitation: results of 1339 consecutive patients," *European Journal of Cardio-Thoracic Surgery*, vol. 34, no. 4, pp. 760–765, 2008.

[4] J. D. Schmitto, S. A. Mokashi, and L. H. Cohn, "Minimally-invasive valve surgery," *Journal of the American College of Cardiology*, vol. 56, no. 6, pp. 455–462, 2010.

[5] R. S. McClure, L. H. Cohn, E. Wiegerinck et al., "Early and late outcomes in minimally invasive mitral valve repair: an eleven-year experience in 707 patients," *The Journal of Thoracic and Cardiovascular Surgery*, vol. 137, no. 1, pp. 70–75, 2009.

[6] J. S. Gammie, S. T. Bartlett, and B. P. Griffith, "Small-incision mitral valve repair: safe, durable, and approaching perfection," *Annals of Surgery*, vol. 250, no. 3, pp. 409–415, 2009.

[7] A. Iribarne, A. Karpenko, M. J. Russo et al., "Eight-year experience with minimally invasive cardiothoracic surgery," *World Journal of Surgery*, vol. 34, no. 4, pp. 611–615, 2010.

[8] L. H. Cohn, D. H. Adams, G. S. Couper et al., "Minimally invasive cardiac valve surgery improves patient satisfaction while reducing costs of cardiac valve replacement and repair," *Annals of Surgery*, vol. 226, no. 4, pp. 421–428, 1997.

[9] J. L. Navia and D. M. Cosgrove, "Minimally invasive mitral valve operations," *Annals of Thoracic Surgery*, vol. 62, no. 5, pp. 1542–1544, 1996.

[10] W. R. Chitwood Jr., C. L. Wixon, J. R. Elbeery, J. F. Moran, and W. H. Chapman, "Video-assisted minimally invasive mitral valve surgery," *The Journal of Thoracic and Cardiovascular Surgery*, vol. 114, no. 5, pp. 773–782, 1997.

[11] V. Falk, T. Walther, R. Autschbach, A. Diegeler, R. Battellini, and F. W. Mohr, "Robot-assisted minimally invasive solo mitral valve operation," *The Journal of Thoracic and Cardiovascular Surgery*, vol. 115, no. 2, pp. 470–471, 1998.

[12] N. Weinzweig and R. Yetman, "Transposition of the greater omentum for recalcitrant median sternotomy wound infections," *Annals of Plastic Surgery*, vol. 34, no. 5, pp. 471–477, 1995.

[13] A. Zacharias and R. H. Habib, "Factors predisposing to median sternotomy complications: deep versus superficial infection," *Chest*, vol. 110, no. 5, pp. 1173–1178, 1996.

[14] R. Moore, D. M. Follette, and H. A. Berkoff, "Poststernotomy fractures and pain management in open cardiac surgery," *Chest*, vol. 106, no. 5, pp. 1339–1342, 1994.

[15] C. D. Casscells, R. W. Lindsey, J. Ebersole, and B. Li, "Ulnar neuropathy after median sternotomy," *Clinical Orthopaedics and Related Research*, no. 291, pp. 259–265, 1993.

[16] A. J. Bryan, M. Lamarra, G. D. Angelini, R. R. West, and I. M. Breckenridge, "Median sternotomy wound dehiscence: a retrospective case control study of risk factors and outcome,"

Journal of the Royal College of Surgeons of Edinburgh, vol. 37, no. 5, pp. 305–308, 1992.

[17] A. P. Furnary, J. A. Magovern, K. A. Simpson, and G. J. Magovern, "Prolonged open sternotomy and delayed sternal closure after cardiac operations," *Annals of Thoracic Surgery*, vol. 54, no. 2, pp. 233–239, 1992.

[18] M. R. Hanson, A. C. Breuer, A. Furlan et al., "Mechanism and frequency of brachial plexus injury in open-heart surgery: a prospective analysis," *Annals of Thoracic Surgery*, vol. 36, no. 6, pp. 675–679, 1983.

[19] R. N. Merchant, W. F. Brown, and B. V. Watson, "Peripheral nerve injuries in cardiac anaesthesia," *Canadian Journal of Anaesthesia*, vol. 37, no. 4, part 2, p. S152, 1990.

[20] J. P. Greelish, L. H. Cohn, M. Leacche et al., "Minimally invasive mitral valve repair suggests earlier operations for mitral valve disease," *The Journal of Thoracic and Cardiovascular Surgery*, vol. 126, no. 2, pp. 365–373, 2003.

[21] D. S. Schwartz, G. H. Ribakove, E. A. Grossi et al., "Minimally invasive mitral valve replacement: port-access technique, feasibility, and myocardial functional preservation," *The Journal of Thoracic and Cardiovascular Surgery*, vol. 113, no. 6, pp. 1022–1031, 1997.

[22] E. C. Cutler and S. A. Levine, "Cardiotomy and valvulotomy for mitral stenosis," *The Boston Medical and Surgical Journal*, vol. 188, pp. 1023–1027, 1923.

[23] C. Dubost, D. Guilmet, B. Parades et al., "Nouvelle technique d'ouverture de l'oreillette gauche en chirurgie a coeur ouvert: l'abord bi-auriculair transseptal," *La Presse Médicale*, vol. 74, pp. 1607–1608, 1966.

[24] G. M. Guiraudon, J. G. Ofiesh, and R. Kaushik, "Extended vertical transatrial septal approach to the mitral valve," *Annals of Thoracic Surgery*, vol. 52, no. 5, pp. 1058–1062, 1991.

[25] L. H. Cohn, "Comparative morbidity of mitral valve repair versus replacement for mitral regurgitation with and without coronary artery disease: updated in 1995," *Annals of Thoracic Surgery*, vol. 60, no. 5, pp. 1452–1453, 1995.

[26] L. H. Cohn, D. P. Bichell, D. H. Adams et al., "Repair of mitral regurgitation from myxomatous degeneration in the patient with a severely calcified posterior annulus," *Journal of Cardiac Surgery*, vol. 10, pp. 281–284, 1995.

[27] A. Carpentier, D. Loulmet, A. Carpentier et al., "First open heart operation (mitral valvuloplasty) under videosurgery through a minithoracotomy," *Comptes Rendus de l'Academie des Sciences III*, vol. 319, no. 3, pp. 219–223, 1996.

[28] F. W. Mohr, J. F. Onnasch, V. Falk et al., "The evolution of minimally invasive mitral valve surgery—2 year experience," *European Journal of Cardio-Thoracic Surgery*, vol. 15, no. 3, pp. 233–239, 1999.

[29] I. Kronzon and T. G. Matros, "Intraoperative echocardiography in minimally invasive cardiac surgery and novel cardiovascular surgical techniques," *The American Heart Hospital Journal*, vol. 2, no. 4, pp. 198–204, 2004.

[30] J. E. Felger, W. R. Chitwood Jr., L. W. Nifong, and D. Holbert, "Evolution of mitral valve surgery: toward a totally endoscopic approach," *Annals of Thoracic Surgery*, vol. 72, no. 4, pp. 1203–1209, 2001.

[31] D. D. Glower, K. P. Landolfo, F. Clements et al., "Mitral valve operation via Port Access versus median sternotomy," *European Journal of Cardio-Thoracic Surgery*, vol. 14, supplement 1, pp. S143–S147, 1998.

[32] H. Reichenspurner, V. Gulielmos, J. Wunderlich et al., "Port-Access coronary artery bypass grafting with the use of cardiopulmonary bypass and cardioplegic arrest," *Annals of Thoracic Surgery*, vol. 65, no. 2, pp. 413–419, 1998.

[33] C. R. Asher, J. M. DiMengo, K. L. Arheart et al., "Atrial fibrillation early postoperatively following minimally invasive cardiac valvular surgery," *American Journal of Cardiology*, vol. 84, no. 6, pp. 744–747, 1999.

[34] E. A. Grossi, A. C. Galloway, G. H. Ribakove et al., "Minimally invasive port access surgery reduces operative morbidity for valve replacement in the elderly," *The Heart Surgery Forum*, vol. 2, no. 3, pp. 212–215, 1999.

[35] T. Walther, V. Falk, S. Metz et al., "Pain and quality of life after minimally invasive versus conventional cardiac surgery," *Annals of Thoracic Surgery*, vol. 67, no. 6, pp. 1643–1647, 1999.

[36] F. Schneider, J. F. Onnasch, V. Falk, T. Walther, R. Autschbach, and F. W. Mohr, "Cerebral microemboli during minimally invasive and conventional mitral valve operations," *Annals of Thoracic Surgery*, vol. 70, no. 3, pp. 1094–1097, 2000.

[37] K. Hamano, T. Kawamura, H. Gohra et al., "Stress caused by minimally invasive cardiac surgery versus conventional cardiac surgery: incidence of systemic inflammatory response syndrome," *World Journal of Surgery*, vol. 25, no. 2, pp. 117–121, 2001.

[38] E. A. Grossi, A. LaPietra, G. H. Ribakove et al., "Minimally invasive versus sternotomy approaches for mitral reconstruction: comparison of intermediate-term results," *The Journal of Thoracic and Cardiovascular Surgery*, vol. 121, no. 4, pp. 708–713, 2001.

[39] E. A. Grossi, A. C. Galloway, G. H. Ribakove et al., "Impact of minimally invasive valvular heart surgery: a case-control study," *Annals of Thoracic Surgery*, vol. 71, no. 3, pp. 807–810, 2001.

[40] T. Yamada, R. Ochiai, J. Takeda, H. Shin, and R. Yozu, "Comparison of early postoperative quality of life in minimally invasive versus conventional valve surgery," *Journal of Anesthesia*, vol. 17, no. 3, pp. 171–176, 2003.

[41] B. J. McCreath, M. Swaminathan, J. V. Booth et al., "Mitral valve surgery and acute renal injury: port access versus median sternotomy," *Annals of Thoracic Surgery*, vol. 75, no. 3, pp. 812–819, 2003.

[42] C. de Vaumas, I. Philip, G. Daccache et al., "Comparison of minithoracotomy and conventional sternotomy approaches for valve surgery," *Journal of Cardiothoracic and Vascular Anesthesia*, vol. 17, no. 3, pp. 325–328, 2003.

[43] V. A. Gaudiani, G. L. Grunkemeier, L. J. Castro, A. L. Fisher, and Y. Wu, "Mitral valve operations through standard and smaller incisions," *The Heart Surgery Forum*, vol. 7, no. 4, pp. E337–E342, 2004.

[44] T. Mihaljevic, L. H. Cohn, D. Unic et al., "One thousand minimally invasive valve operations: early and late results," *Annals of Surgery*, vol. 240, no. 3, pp. 529–534, 2004.

[45] S. Dogan, T. Aybek, P. S. Risteski et al., "Minimally invasive port access versus conventional mitral valve surgery: prospective randomized study," *Annals of Thoracic Surgery*, vol. 79, no. 2, pp. 492–498, 2005.

[46] W. H. Ryan, T. M. Dewey, M. J. Mack, M. A. Herbert, and S. L. Prince, "Mitral valve surgery using the classical 'heartport' technique," *The Journal of Heart Valve Disease*, vol. 14, no. 6, pp. 709–714, 2005.

[47] A. Carpentier, D. Loulmet, B. Aupècle et al., "Computer assisted open heart surgery. First case operated on with success,"

Comptes Rendus de l'Académie des Sciences, vol. 321, pp. 437–442, 1998.

[48] A. C. Galloway, R. J. Shemin, D. D. Glower et al., "First report of the port access international registry," *The Annals of Thoracic Surgery*, vol. 67, pp. 51–58, 1999.

[49] V. Gulielmos, J. Wunderlich, M. Dangel et al., "Minimally invasive mitral valve surgery, clinical experiences with port access system," *European Journal Cardio-Thoracic Surgery*, vol. 14, supplement 1, pp. S148–S153, 1998.

[50] F. W. Mohr, V. Falk, A. Diegeler et al., "Minimally invasive port-access mitral valve surgery," *The Journal of Thoracic and Cardiovascular Surgery*, vol. 115, no. 3, pp. 567–576, 1998.

[51] J. H. Stevens, T. A. Burdon, W. S. Peters et al., "Port-access coronary artery bypass grafting: a proposed surgical method," *The Journal of Thoracic and Cardiovascular Surgery*, vol. 111, pp. 567–573, 1996.

[52] L. C. Siegel, F. G. St Goar, J. H. Stevens et al., "Monitoring considerations for port-access cardiac surgery," *Circulation*, vol. 96, no. 2, pp. 562–568, 1997.

[53] F. Clements, S. J. Wright, and N. de Bruijn, "Coronary sinus catheterization made easy for Port-Access minimally invasive cardiac surgery," *Journal of Cardiothoracic and Vascular Anesthesia*, vol. 12, no. 1, pp. 96–101, 1998.

[54] M. A. Chaney, J. P. Sims, and B. Blakeman, "Port-access minimally invasive cardiac surgery in a patient without arms," *Journal of Cardiothoracic and Vascular Anesthesia*, vol. 13, no. 4, pp. 459–461, 1999.

[55] D. C. Angouras and R. E. Michler, "An alternative surgical approach to facilitate minimally invasive mitral valve surgery," *Annals of Thoracic Surgery*, vol. 73, no. 2, pp. 673–674, 2002.

[56] W. R. Chitwood Jr., J. R. Elbeery, W. H. H. Chapman et al., "Video-assisted minimally invasive mitral valve surgery: the 'micro- mitral' operation," *The Journal of Thoracic and Cardiovascular Surgery*, vol. 113, no. 2, pp. 413–414, 1997.

[57] W. R. Chitwood, "State of the art review: videoscopic minimally invasive mitral valve surgery. Trekking to a totally endoscopic operation," *The Heart Surgery Forum*, vol. 1, no. 1, pp. 13–16, 1998.

[58] A. P. Kypson, L. W. Nifong, and W. R. Chitwood Jr., "Robotic mitral valve surgery," *Surgical Clinics of North America*, vol. 83, no. 6, pp. 1387–1403, 2003.

[59] A. P. Kypson, J. E. Felger, L. W. Nifong, and W. R. Chitwood Jr., "Robotics in valvular surgery: 2003 and beyond," *Current Opinion in Cardiology*, vol. 19, no. 2, pp. 128–133, 2004.

[60] A. J. Tatooles, P. S. Pappas, P. J. Gordon, and M. S. Slaughter, "Minimally invasive mitral valve repair using the da Vinci robotic system," *Annals of Thoracic Surgery*, vol. 77, no. 6, pp. 1978–1984, 2004.

[61] T. Walther, C. Walther, V. Falk et al., "Early clinical results after stentless mitral valve implantation and comparison with conventional valve repair or replacement," *Circulation*, vol. 100, no. 19, pp. II78–II83, 1999.

[62] T. Walther, S. Lehmann, V. Falk et al., "Midterm results after stentless mitral valve replacement," *Circulation*, vol. 108, supplement 1, pp. II85–II89, 2003.

[63] D. Wang, Q. Wang, X. Yang, Q. Wu, and Q. Li, "Mitral valve replacement through a minimal right vertical infra-axillary thoracotomy versus standard median sternotomy," *Annals of Thoracic Surgery*, vol. 87, no. 3, pp. 704–708, 2009.

[64] J. F. Onnasch, F. Schneider, V. Falk, M. Mierzwa, J. Bucerius, and F. W. Mohr, "Five years of less invasive mitral valve surgery: from experimental to routine approach," *Heart Surgery Forum*, vol. 5, no. 2, pp. 132–135, 2002.

[65] J. E. Felger, L. W. Nifong, and W. R. Chitwood Jr., "The evolution of and early experience with robot-assisted mitral valve surgery," *Surgical Laparoscopy, Endoscopy and Percutaneous Techniques*, vol. 12, no. 1, pp. 58–63, 2002.

[66] J. E. Felger, L. W. Nifong, and W. R. Chitwood Jr., "The evolution and early experience with robot-assisted mitral valve surgery," *Current Surgery*, vol. 58, no. 6, pp. 570–575, 2001.

[67] W. R. Chitwood Jr., J. R. Elbeery, and J. F. Moran, "Minimally invasive mitral valve repair using transthoracic aortic occlusion," *Annals of Thoracic Surgery*, vol. 63, no. 5, pp. 1477–1479, 1997.

[68] J. Puskas, D. Cheng, J. Knight et al., "Off-pump versus conventional coronary artery bypass grafting: a meta-analysis and consensus statement from the 2004 ISMICS Consensus Conference," *Innovations*, vol. 1, no. 1, pp. 3–27, 2005.

[69] V. Falk, D. C. H. Cheng, J. Martin et al., "Minimally invasive versus open mitral valve surgery: a consensus statement of the international society of minimally invasive coronary surgery (ISMICS) 2010," *Innovations*, vol. 6, no. 2, pp. 66–76, 2011.

[70] J. S. Gammie, Y. Zhao, E. D. Peterson, S. M. O'Brien, J. S. Rankin, and B. P. Griffith, "Less-invasive mitral valve operations: trends and outcomes from the society of thoracic surgeons adult cardiac surgery database," *Annals of Thoracic Surgery*, vol. 90, no. 5, pp. 1401–1408, 2010.

[71] E. A. Grossi, A. C. Galloway, A. LaPietra et al., "Minimally invasive mitral valve surgery: a 6-year experience with 714 patients," *Annals of Thoracic Surgery*, vol. 74, no. 3, pp. 660–664, 2002.

[72] E. A. Grossi, D. F. Loulmet, C. F. Schwartz et al., "Minimally invasive valve surgery with antegrade perfusion strategy is not associated with increased neurologic complications," *The Annals of Thoracic Surgery*, vol. 92, no. 4, pp. 1346–1350, 2011.

[73] G. A. Crooke, C. F. Schwartz, G. H. Ribakove et al., "Retrograde arterial perfusion, not incision location, significantly increases the risk of stroke in reoperative mitral valve procedures," *Annals of Thoracic Surgery*, vol. 89, no. 3, pp. 723–730, 2010.

[74] E. A. Grossi, D. F. Loulmet, C. F. Schwartz et al., "Evolution of operative techniques and perfusion strategies for minimally invasive mitral valve repair," in *Proceedings of The American Association for Thoracic Surgery: Mitral Conclave*, New York, NY, USA, May 2011, http://www.aats.org/mitral/abstracts/2011/15.html.

[75] D. W. Yaffee, A. C. Galloway, and E. A. Grossi, "Editorial analysis: impact of perfusion strategy on stroke risk for minimally invasive cardiac surgery," *European Journal Cardio-Thoracic Surgery*, vol. 41, no. 6, pp. 1223–1224, 2012.

[76] D. A. Murphy, J. S. Miller, D. A. Langford, and A. B. Snyder, "Endoscopic robotic mitral valve surgery," *The Journal of Thoracic and Cardiovascular Surgery*, vol. 132, no. 4, pp. 776–781, 2006.

[77] G. J. Murphy, B. C. Reeves, C. A. Rogers, S. I. A. Rizvi, L. Culliford, and G. D. Angelini, "Increased mortality, postoperative morbidity, and cost after red blood cell transfusion in patients having cardiac surgery," *Circulation*, vol. 116, no. 22, pp. 2544–2552, 2007.

[78] L. W. Nifong, W. R. Chitwood, P. S. Pappas et al., "Robotic mitral valve surgery: a United States multicenter trial," *The Journal of Thoracic and Cardiovascular Surgery*, vol. 129, no. 6, pp. 1395–1404, 2005.

[79] A. A. Vlessis and S. F. Bolling, "Mini-reoperative mitral valve surgery," *Journal of Cardiac Surgery*, vol. 13, no. 6, pp. 468–470, 1998.

[80] A. Iribarne, R. Easterwood, M. J. Russo, E. Y. Chan, C. R. Smith, and M. Argenziano, "Comparative effectiveness of minimally invasive versus traditional sternotomy mitral valve surgery in elderly patients," *The Journal of Thoracic and Cardiovascular Surgery*, vol. 143, supplement 4, pp. S86–S90, 2012.

[81] M. Tabata and L. H. Cohn, "Minimally invasive mitral valve repair with and without robotic technology in the elderly," *The American Journal of Geriatric Cardiology*, vol. 15, no. 5, pp. 306–310, 2006.

[82] L. G. Svensson, F. A. Atik, D. M. Cosgrove et al., "Minimally invasive versus conventional mitral valve surgery: a propensity-matched comparison," *The Journal of Thoracic and Cardiovascular Surgery*, vol. 139, pp. 926–932, 2010.

12

Minimally Invasive Mitral Valve Procedures: The Current State

Bhuyan Ritwick, Krishanu Chaudhuri, Gareth Crouch, James R. M. Edwards, Michael Worthington, and Robert G. Stuklis

Darcy Sutherland Cardiothoracic Surgical Unit, Level 4, East Wing, Royal Adelaide Hospital, North Terrace, Adelaide, SA 5000, Australia

Correspondence should be addressed to Bhuyan Ritwick; drritwick72@gmail.com

Academic Editor: José PS Henriques

Since its early days, cardiac surgery has typically involved large incisions with complete access to the heart and the great vessels. After the popularization of the minimally invasive techniques in general surgery, cardiac surgeons began to experiment with minimal access techniques in the early 1990s. Although the goals of minimally invasive cardiac surgery (MICS) are fairly well established as decreased pain, shorter hospital stay, accelerated recuperation, improved cosmesis, and cost effectiveness, a strict definition of minimally invasive cardiac surgery has been more elusive. Minimally invasive cardiac surgery started with mitral valve procedures and then gradually expanded towards other valve procedures, coronary artery bypass grafting, and various types of simple congenital heart procedures. In this paper, the authors attempt to focus on the evolution, techniques, results, and the future perspective of minimally invasive mitral valve surgery (MIMVS).

1. Introduction

Minimally invasive mitral valve surgery (MIMVS) does not refer to a single approach but rather to a collection of new techniques and operation-specific technologies. These include enhanced visualization and instrumentation systems as well as modified perfusion methods, all directed toward minimizing surgical trauma by reducing the incision size [1].

2. History and Evolution of MIMVS

The first successful cardiac operation was performed on September 7, 1896, in Frankfurt, Germany, by Rehn [2]. The first successful cardiac valve operation was performed in 1912 by Tuffier [3] and the first successful mitral valve (MV) operation in 1923 by Cutler and Levine [4]. In 1956, Lillehei et al. repaired multiple valvular lesions through a right thoracotomy using cardiopulmonary bypass (CPB) [5]. The subsequent years have seen a glorious phase of mitral valve surgery with full sternotomy and use of conventional cardiopulmonary bypass techniques. This phase also witnessed the development of various valvular prostheses and mitral valve repair techniques. In the 1990s, the success of laparoscopic operations in general surgery renewed an interest in minimally invasive approaches for cardiac surgery. Navia and Cosgrove [6] and Cohn et al. [7] performed the first minimally invasive valve operations (via the right parasternal and transsternal approaches). These authors have shown that small incision mitral valve surgery can be conducted safely with equivalent outcomes.

Carpentier et al. [8] in February of 1996 performed the first video-assisted mitral valve repair (MVR) through a mini thoracotomy using ventricular fibrillation. Following this the East Carolina University group performed the first video-assisted mitral valve repair through a mini thoracotomy, using video-direction, a transthoracic aortic clamp, and retrograde cardioplegia [9]. In 1998, Mohr et al. reported the Leipzig University experience using port-access technology, which was based on endoaortic balloon occlusion (EABO) rather than direct aortic clamping [10]. The next major development was the introduction of a voice-controlled robotic camera arm (AESOP 3000, Computer Motion Inc., Santa Barbara, CA, USA) which allowed precise tremor-free camera movements with less lens cleaning. This technology translated into reduced cardiopulmonary bypass (CPB) and cross-clamp (XC) times [11, 12] and enabled even smaller

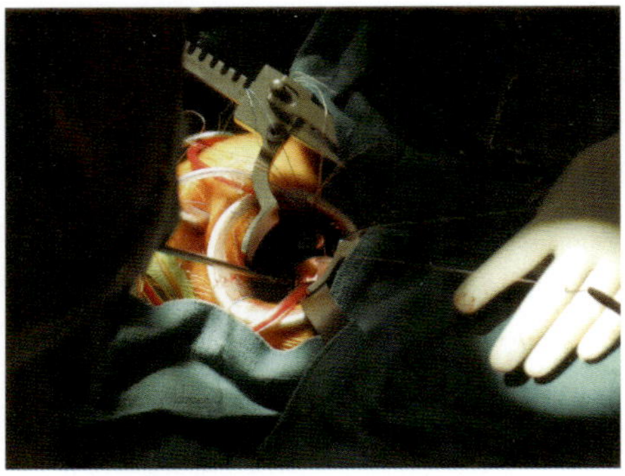

Figure 1: Level 2 minimally invasive approach (4–6 cm incision).

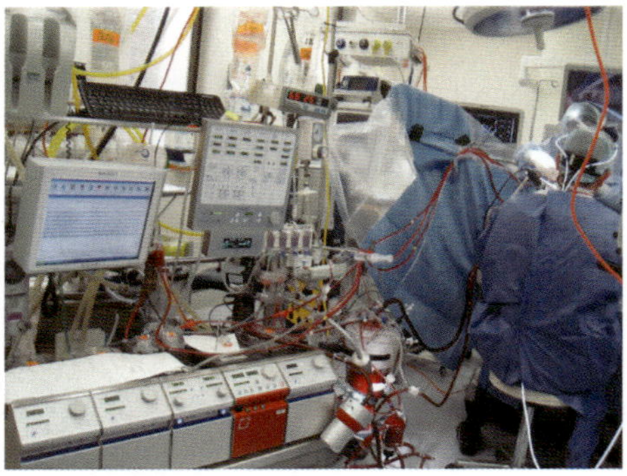

Figure 2: Heart Lung machine with peripheral cannulation via the femoral vessels.

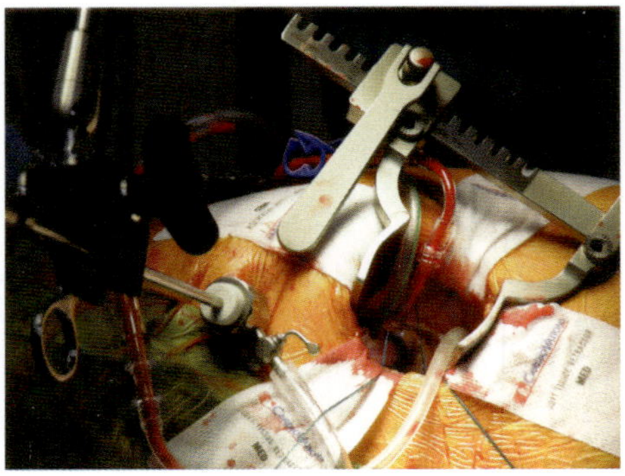

Figure 3: Direct transthoracic aortic clamping.

incisions with better valve and subvalvar visualization. The next major leap in the evolution of MIMVS was the development of robotic telemanipulation, and in 1998 Carpentier et al. [13] performed the first completely robotic mitral valve repair using the Da Vinci Surgical System (Intuitive Surgical, Inc., Sunnyvale, CA).

An important adjunct in the evolution of mini-valve surgery (mini-VS) is the parallel progress in perfusion technology [14]. First, smaller, nonkinking arterial and venous cannulae have been combined with vacuum-assisted venous drainage to allow maximal space use provided by the smaller incisions. Second, the implantation of transjugular coronary sinus catheters provides cardiac protection via retrograde cardioplegia. Third, the application of carbon dioxide (CO_2) into the operating field limits intracardiac air (to reduce air embolism), and finally intraoperative transesophageal echocardiography allows for real-time monitoring of cardiac distention, deairing, and cannula placement [15]. Thus, MIMVS has evolved into a routinely performed operation with excellent results in many specialized centers [14, 16–18].

Minimally invasive valve surgery evolved through graded levels of difficulty with less exposure and to a progressive reliance on video assistance. Loulmet and Carpentier classified these levels of minimally invasive cardiac surgery as shown in Box 1 (Figure 1). Current patient selection is shown in Box 2 [19].

The type of the musculoskeletal incision remains central to the discussion around minimally invasive cardiac surgery. A wide variety of modified small sternal, parasternal, and minithoracotomy incisions are used to access the cardiac valves. Although many surgeons prefer the hemisternotomy approach, a right minithoracotomy yields excellent exposure for both direct vision and videoscopic mitral valve access [19]. By the mid-1900s, parasternal and transsternal approaches were being described by Navia and Cosgrove [6] and Cohn et al. [7]. Smaller incisions lateral to the sternum were created, with or without resection of the third or fourth costal cartilage. However, their disadvantages included femoral CPB cannulation, ligation of the right internal thoracic artery, occasional chest wall instability, and difficult conversion to full sternotomy. In 1997, Cohn et al. [7] presented 84 minimally invasive cases (41 aortic and 43 mitral) using a right parasternal incision and excising the third and fourth costal cartilages. Interestingly, greater patient satisfaction, a decrease in postoperative atrial fibrillation (AF), and overall lower costs were found [7]. Later, Greelish et al. [20] primarily used a lower mini-sternotomy for mini-MVS with excellent results. Chitwood et al. [21] designed a new aortic clamp that allows transthoracic aortic occlusion. Video assistance has also been used for mini-MVS through small thoracotomies [9, 16, 17]. Although there are highly encouraging results using a right thoracotomy, several disadvantages exist, including peripheral CPB cannulation, the potential need for a double-lumen endotracheal tube, and occasional difficulty with MV exposure [16]. In contrast to this, the Leipzig Group has shown excellent results with their 5-6 cm right lateral minithoracotomy under video assistance with peripheral femoral cannulation (Figure 2), direct transthoracic aortic clamping and with single endotracheal tube (Figure 3), and use of cannulation of right internal jugular vein for concomitant tricuspid valve procedures [22, 23]. Several groups strongly advocate for intra-aortic balloon occlusion for minimally invasive and robotic mitral surgery [24–27]. Most commonly these devices are introduced as retrograde through the femoral artery. The occlusive balloon is usually positioned under echocardiographic guidance just above the sinotubular junction, and balloon has the potential hazard of migration either into the arch with neurological complications or to the left ventricle with resultant ventricular dysfunction. Balloon occlusion may be advantageous compared to the transthoracic clamp method when there is limited access to the

Level 1
Direct vision: Limited (10–12 cm) incisions
Level 2
Direct vision/video assisted: Mini (4–6 cm) incisions
Level 3
Video directed and robot assisted: Micro (1.2–4 cm) incisions
Level 4
Robotic (computer telemanipulation): Port (<1.2 cm) incisions

Box 1: Levels of ascent in minimally invasive cardiac surgery.

Suitable candidates:
- Patients with primary mitral valve disease
- Reoperative mitral valve patients
- Bileaflet and/or anterior leaflet prolapse
- Combined tricuspid and mitral operations
- Mild annular calcification
- Obese or large patients
- Elderly patients

Unsuitable candidates:
- Highly calcified mitral annulus
- Severe pulmonary hypertension, especially with a small right coronary artery
- Significant untreated coronary artery disease
- Severe peripheral atherosclerosis
- Prior right chest surgery
- Concomitant aortic or aortic valve pathology requiring surgical interventions

Box 2: Current patient selection: videoscopic or video-assisted mitral valve surgery.

aorta. Aortic dissection is a feared complication of using the endoballoon, but experience with this technique dramatically reduces the risk of this adverse event. However, some group demonstrated increased morbidity, cost, and operative/cross-clamp time when the endoballoon technique was used for mitral valve surgery [28]. Telemanipulators, robotics that allow a hand-like mechanism to be controlled by a human operator, were first used in Paris, France, by Carpentier et al. [8] and Falk et al. [12] in Leipzig, Germany. Telemanipulator-supported operations, which involve femoral cannulation and direct or endoluminal aortic clamping, have been used and propagated by Chitwood et al. [9, 18] and others [29, 30], who claim that this technique could be safely and effectively used [7]. Other centers (Leipzig) had similar positive experiences using the telemanipulator-supported techniques in the late 1990s [31, 32]. However, they later abandoned this technique, given the lack of difference compared with their "standard" approaches. Recently in 2012, Gao et al. reported successful robotically assisted mitral valve replacement with excellent results [33].

3. Results

During the past 16 years, cardiac surgeons worldwide have reported their MIMVS data with promising results. The majority of these results suggest that MIMVS provide excellent, safe, and familiar exposure of the mitral valve with results comparable to those with conventional approaches. Unfortunately we lack data from large prospective randomized control series comparing the results of minimally invasive versus the conventional sternotomy technique. We therefore have to rely on retrospective analysed registry data (mostly single centre).

4. Mortality

Reviewing all comparative MIMVS studies evaluating mortality, no study has shown a significant difference between minimally invasive and conventional approaches [34–40]. In 2003, Greelish et al. [20] reported the first long-term results (5-year followup) of mini-VS, indicating a freedom from mitral regurgitation and reoperation >90%. In their early port access cases, Mohr et al. [23] reported a high mortality rate (9.8%) for mini-MVS, partially procedure related, with 2 of 51 patients experiencing an aortic dissection [23]. After discontinuing the port access technique and modification and simplification of the surgical procedure, the mortality decreased to an in-hospital mortality rate of 3.9% [41]. The Leipzig long-term results revealed an actuarial survival rate of 83% at 6.8 years [42]. When excluding the initial 200 patients in whom an endoclamp was used, the overall results are even more impressive [42]. In 2002, Mohr's group (Onnasch et al. [36]) reported their 5-year experience performing mini-MVS in 449 patients, with a mean survival rate of 96.3% at 2-year followup. The East Carolina University group reported a combined series with Hargrove consisting of 1178 successful video-assisted mitral valve operations between 1996 and 2008 [43]. The operative mortality rates for mitral valve repair and replacement for this two center series were 2.1% and 4.6%, respectively, but only 0.2% for isolated primary mitral valve repair. A recent meta-analysis by Modi et al. [44] identified ten papers published between 1998 and 2005 which were suitable for analysis. This study included 1358 minimally invasive patients and 1469 sternotomy patients. Although cross-clamp and cardiopulmonary bypass time were longer in the minimally invasive group, there were no difference in mortality, stroke, reoperation for bleeding, new onset atrial fibrillation, or duration of ICU stay or hospital stay [44]. In a more recent study, Stevens et al. published the results of 2,255 patients who underwent MV operations, including 1,305 with isolated MV regurgitation operations (1,054 repairs and 251 replacements) [45]. The study period was between 1992 and 2009 and surgical approaches were sternotomy in 377, video-assisted right minithoracotomy in 481, or robot-assisted in 447. Mean followup was 6.4 ± 4.5 years (maximum, 19 years) [45]. The 30-day mortality for isolated MV repair was similar for all approaches ($P = 0.409$). Fewer neurological events were observed in the videoscopic and robotic groups ($P = 0.013$). Adjusted survival was similar for all approaches ($P = 0.357$) [45]. Galloway and associates at the New York University have reported the longest outcomes for minimally invasive mitral valve surgery to date [46]. Between 1996 and 2008, they performed 1071 minimally invasive mitral valve repairs and compared their results with a cohort of 1601 conventional procedures. Almost one third of the minimally invasive repairs included an anterior leaflet procedure and all patients received an annuloplasty device [46]. They reported a perioperative mortality of 1.3% in both groups with isolated mitral valve repair and no differences in major adverse events [46]. Long-term results were equivalent to sternotomy techniques. In isolated mitral valve repair, 8-year freedom from reoperation or severe recurrent insufficiency was 93% and freedom from all the valve related complications was 90%. At the same time, they had fewer transfusions, shorter lengths of hospital stay, and fewer septic complications [46].

5. Neurological Events

Due to the limited access to the operative field, there is the potential for inadequate deairing of the heart leading to an increased incidence of neurological events. Mohr et al. [23] in their early series reported an 18% incidence of confusion, but were not using the CO_2 insufflation—a technique they have since adopted. The same group after a decade observed postoperative neurological impairment in 41 of 1,339 patients (3.1%) who underwent mini-MVS, with 28 (2.1%) minor and 13 (1.0%) major events [22]. Grossi et al. [47] has recently published results of 1282 patients with an overall frequency of postoperative neurological event of 2.3% (30/1282). They also identified the high risk group for neurological event as those with peripheral vascular disease, cerebrovascular disease, dialysis, and atherosclerotic aortas [47] and also pointed out the use of retrograde arterial perfusion in diseased aortas as the most significant risk factor for the development of postoperative neurological event. In contrast to this, Gammie et al. maintained that neither retrograde arterial perfusion nor the use of end balloon were risk factors for development of postoperative neurological event [48]. This group studied 28,143 patients identified from the Society Of Thoracic Surgeons database and found a higher rate of permanent stroke, 1.87%, for the minimally invasive surgery group as opposed to 1.17% for the conventional sternotomy group) [48], and they observed a threefold higher rate of stroke in patients using fibrillatory arrest or beating heart technique without cross clamp. In their recent study, Stevens et al. have shown a reverse trend in their stroke rate (3.4%—sternotomy approach, 1.2%—videoscopic approach, and 0.7%—robotic mitral valve procedures) [49].

6. Bleeding Related Complications

Transfusion of allogenic red blood cells (RBCs) is recognized as a risk factor for adverse outcome after cardiac surgery [50]. Unnecessary transfusions are likely to be associated with unnecessary morbidity and additional indirect hospitalization costs.

Throughout the last decade, one of the major benefits of MIMVS has been claimed to be the less bleeding related complications and less usage of blood products [38, 51–54] as compared to the conventional sternotomy approach. Other authors have shown no difference in blood requirements in the two different groups [55]. In a recent study, Gammie et al. [48] could not show any difference in reexploration for bleeding in the MIMVS group when compared to the traditional sternotomy group but have shown a statistically significant higher use of perioperative red blood cell (52.6% for the open group and 41% for the MIMVS group) and platelet (25.3% for the open group and 15.8% for the MIMVS group) transfusion. However, when these outcomes were risk aadjusted there was no significant difference in the transfusion of either red blood cell or platelet [48]. Stevens et al. published their recent data with no difference in reexploration for bleeding in the three groups of conventional, videoscopic, and robotic mitral valve surgery (series of 2,255 patients) but with a significant difference in the requirement of blood transfusion (63%—conventional group, 43%—videoscopic, and 18%—robotic mitral valve procedures) [49].

7. Postoperative Atrial Fibrillation (AF)

There are conflicting data in the literature regarding the incidence of AF following MIMVS. It has been suggested that a less traumatic surgical approach would be a less potent trigger of postoperative AF. Five of six studies, however, demonstrated this not to be the case [11, 56–60], and on meta-analysis of four eligible studies, there was no significant difference between minimally invasive and sternotomy approaches (539 patients, OR 0.86, 95% CI 0.59–1.27, $P = 0.45$). More recently Gammie et al. [48], however, have shown a decreased incidence of postoperative AF (20.1% for the conventional sternotomy group and 15.9% for the less invasive group).

8. Septic Complications

The incidences of septic complications and wound infections are less in thoracotomy than with sternotomy. Of the three studies of mini-thoracotomy mitral valve surgery that reported wound complications compared to median sternotomy, Grossi et al. reported an incidence of 0.9% and 5.7% for mini-thoracotomy and sternotomy cases, respectively ($P = 0.05$) [61]. This increased to 1.8% and 7.7%, respectively, in elderly patients ($P = 0.03$) [37]. Santana et al. [62] recently showed a major difference of sternal wound infections and septic complications comparing minimally invasive versus sternotomy mitral valve procedures in obese patients. This group showed a 0% incidence of sternal wound infections for the minimally invasive group against a 4.1% in the sternotomy group and septic complications of 6.25% and 1.56% in the sternotomy and the minimally invasive group, respectively.

9. Pain and Speed of Recovery

Of all the potential benefits of MIMVS, a reduction in pain and faster return to normal activity is the most consistent finding. All four studies that measured postoperative pain levels reported less compared to sternotomy [55, 59, 62, 63], and both studies reporting time to return to normal activities noted a significant advantage for a minimally invasive approach [59, 62]. In a nonrandomized study, Cohn et al. reported equivalent pain for the first two postoperative days when a minithoracotomy approach was compared to sternotomy with a subsequent significant reduction of pain in the MI group from day 3 onwards, a difference which progressively widened with time [63]. Better stability of the bony thorax led to earlier mobilization and a faster return to activities of daily living. Glower reported that postoperative pain tended to resolve more quickly with a minimally invasive approach and that these patients returned to normal activity 5 weeks more rapidly than those having a median sternotomy (4 ± 2 weeks versus 9 ± 1 weeks, $P = 0.01$) [59]. Cohn's data is concordant with less pain in hospital and after discharge, less analgesic usage, greater patient satisfaction, and a return to normal activity 4.8 weeks ahead of sternotomy patients [62]. Walther et al. reported that 94% of his patients report no or mild postoperative pain, 99.3% feel they have an aesthetically pleasing scar, 93% would choose the same procedure again if they had to have redo surgery, and 46% are back at work within 3 weeks [64]. However, perhaps the most insightful piece of evidence for patient preference of MIMVS comes from two studies reporting that those who have had an MI approach as their second procedure all felt that their recovery was more rapid and less painful than their original sternotomy [11, 65].

10. Hospital Stay and Cost Savings

Vlessis and Bolling conducted a cost analysis between conventional mitral valve repair with sternotomy (ST) and MIMVS, and MIMVS was associated with a $9054 ± $3302 lower mean total hospital cost ($P = 0.006$), driven largely by a reduction in direct ($P = 0.003$) versus indirect costs ($P = 0.06$) [66]. Among the 13 billing categories, MIMVS was associated with a significant reduction in costs of cardiac imaging ($P = 0.004$), laboratory tests ($P = 0.005$), boarding and nursing ($P = 0.001$), and radiology ($P = 0.002$). More patients in the ST group required intubation for more than 72 hours ($P = 0.019$); however, there were no differences in morbidity or long-term survival ($P = 0.334$). A higher proportion of MI patients were discharged home with no nursing services ($P = 0.018$), and a higher proportion of ST patients required readmission within 1 year ($P = 0.023$). Eight of 14 studies reported a shorter hospital stay with a minimally invasive approach [7, 9, 34, 37–39, 63, 67, 68]. Only 5 studies were eligible for the meta-analysis of Modi et al. [44], and although the trend indicated this to be the case, the result was not statistically significant (350 patients, $P = 0.07$). Chitwood et al. [9], Cohn et al. [7], and Navia and Cosgrove [6] equated this trend to a 34%, 20%, and 7% cost saving, respectively. Moreover, these patients had fewer requirements for rehabilitation, a significant advantage in health care savings; 91% were discharged home compared with 67% with conventional approach [7, 67].

11. Operative Time

Being one of the consistent findings from various case series from the last decade, it was evident that the operative time (cardiopulmonary bypass and cross clamp time) for MIMVS is more than that of conventional surgery. There was evidence suggesting that parity can be achieved with experience while certain high volume centres report shorter operative times with MIMVS [67]. Recent study by Gammie et al. [48] with a population of 28,143 patients from the STS database also showed that the median cardiopulmonary bypass and cross-clamp times were longer in the less-invasive group compared with the conventional group (cardiopulmonary bypass time 135 versus 108 minutes, respectively; $P < 0.0001$; cross-clamp time 100 versus 80 minutes, respectively; $P < 0.0001$). The median operative time was longer (4.2 versus 3.4 hours, $P < 0.0001$) in the less-invasive group.

12. Intermediate and Long-Term Results

Modi et al. [44], in his meta-analysis, considered recent data from 10 cohorts with 6479 patients and found that crude unadjusted mortality rates for the entire cohort are 1.1% for mitral valve repair and 4.9% for mitral valve replacement. Galloway et al. [46] have published the longest term of followup of their MIMVS and found hospital mortality to be 2.2% for all patients (36 of 1601), 1.3% for isolated minimally invasive (9 of 712), and 1.3% (3 of 223) for isolated sternotomy mitral valve repair, as well as 3.6% (24 of 666) for valve repair plus a concomitant cardiac procedure. For isolated valve repair, 8-year freedom from reoperation was 91% ± 2% for sternotomy and 95% ± 1% for minimally invasive ($P = 0.24$), and 8-year freedom from reoperation or severe recurrent insufficiency was 90% ± 2% for sternotomy and 93% ± 1% for minimally invasive ($P = 0.30$). Eight-year freedom from all valve-related complications was 86% ± 3% for sternotomy and 90% ± 2% for minimally invasive ($P = 0.14$) [46].

13. Limitations of MIMVS

Clearly, there is a learning curve for the surgeon as well as the anesthetists, perfusionists, and nursing teams. Mohr et al. reported a high mortality (9.8%) in his early port access cases, partially procedure related with two of 51 patients suffering an aortic dissection [10]. After simplification of the surgical procedure, the mortality decreased to 3%. Vanermen et al. demonstrated that ICU and hospital stays decrease with increasing experience [24]. There are potential vascular risks with femoral cannulation, especially with the larger port access femoral cannula. Groin seromas can be problematic but are kept to a minimum by dissection of only of the anterior surface of the vessels as well as clipping lymphatics. When the pericardium is opened too posteriorly, phrenic nerve palsy has been reported and can be avoided by placing the pericardiotomy at least 3 cm anterior to it. Excess tension by pericardial retraction sutures should be avoided.

14. Conclusion

Cardiac valve surgery operations have historically been performed via a standard median sternotomy and CPB. With the advent of minimally invasive surgery, several new observations regarding the treatment of patients with isolated valve disease have arisen. Over the last decade there has been transformation in the way cardiac surgeons, cardiologists, and patients decide the approach to cardiac therapies. Patients now demand less-invasive procedures with equivalent safety, efficacy, and durability. Any form of new technology must provide better outcome and have better efficiency in terms of safety and durability. If scientific evidence shows that mini-VS results in lower complication rates, surgeons must be trained in these newer techniques. However, with different training backgrounds, patient populations, and surgical approaches, surgeons should use the technique that they believe will result in the best outcome and with which they feel most comfortable. The recent STS data shows that 11.3% of isolated mitral valve repairs are performed with robotic assistance [19]. Up to 20% surgeons are using some minimally invasive methods for their repairs [19].

Critically appraising the results of MIMVS has several limitations, based on the paucity of randomised controlled trials and the reliance on single centre case series or few other review papers. Furthermore, the definition of "minimally invasive" is controversial. The STS [69] defines minimally invasive surgery as any procedure not performed with a full sternotomy and CPB; however, this definition does not really fit into valve surgery.

We have attempted to review the various aspects of MIMVS, and the studies reviewed do not show a significant difference in operative mortality between minimally invasive and conventional approaches. Moreover, the long-term outcomes of these procedures appear to be as durable as the conventional approaches (with followup of up to 8 years). There has been almost no doubt that these procedures reduce the length of hospital stay and blood transfusion while at the same time being cosmetically more attractive than the conventional approach.

One of the major areas for further research is in the field of neurological outcomes as there has been conflicting data with a wide variation in the reported incidence of stroke. Most of the published series continue to implicate MIMVS done on the beating heart as increasing the risk of perioperative stroke. Further disadvantages with MIMVS are related to the use of femoral cannulation and perfusion, with groin complications (e.g., infections and arterial dissections/haematoma) accounting for morbidity unseen with conventional sternotomy.

As for the future, minimally invasive cardiac surgery is likely to become more widely adopted as growth in this niche market and cardiac surgery as a whole is often patient-driven, much in the same way that percutaneous intervention for multivessel disease has been. In essence, patients do not want a sternotomy and it is important as a surgical community that we realize this. However, despite enthusiasm, caution cannot be overemphasized as traditional cardiac operations still enjoy proven long-term success and ever-decreasing morbidity and mortality and remain our benchmark measures for comparison. To pave the path towards totally endoscopic valve surgery, surgeons, cardiologists, and engineers must focus on improving the methods of computerization of the instruments. Patient requirements, technology development, and surgeon capabilities all must be aligned to drive these needed changes. Minimally invasive valve surgery is an evolutionary process, and there must be a well-balanced alignment between the surgeons and the cardiologists to derive the maximal benefit that this technology has to offer. Traditional valve operations enjoy proven long-term success with ever-decreasing morbidity and mortality and remain the gold standard. Minimally invasive surgeries are probably not going to replace the gold standard, but they should present themselves as an alternative for treatment of mitral valve diseases with equal long-term durability.

References

[1] E. G. Soltesz and L. H. Cohn, "Minimally invasive valve surgery," *Cardiology in Review*, vol. 15, no. 3, pp. 109–115, 2007.

[2] L. Rehn, "Zur Chirurgie des Herzens und des Herzbeutels," *Archiv Für Klinische Chirurgie*, vol. 55, pp. 315–329, 1897.

[3] T. Tuffier, "Etat actuel de la chirurgie intrathoracique," *Transactions International Congress Medicine*, vol. 7, p. 249, 1913.

[4] E. C. Cutler and S. A. Levine, "Cardiotomy and valvulotomy for mitral stenosis," *The Boston Medical and Surgical Journal*, vol. 188, p. 1023, 1923.

[5] C. W. Lillehei, V. L. Gott, R. A. Dewall et al., "The surgical treatment of stenotic and regurgitant lesions of the mitral and aortic valves by direct utilization of a pump oxygenator," *Journal of Thoracic Surgery*, vol. 35, no. 2, pp. 154–191, 1958.

[6] J. L. Navia and D. M. Cosgrove, "Minimally invasive mitral valve operations," *Annals of Thoracic Surgery*, vol. 62, no. 5, pp. 1542–1544, 1996.

[7] L. H. Cohn, D. H. Adams, G. S. Couper et al., "Minimally invasive cardiac valve surgery improves patient satisfaction

while reducing costs of cardiac valve replacement and repair," *Annals of Surgery*, vol. 226, no. 4, pp. 421–428, 1997.

[8] A. Carpentier, D. Loulmet, A. Carpentier et al., "First open heart operation (mitral valvuloplasty) under videosurgery through a minithoracotomy," *Comptes Rendus de l'Academie des Sciences III*, vol. 319, no. 3, pp. 219–223, 1996.

[9] W. R. Chitwood, J. R. Elbeery, W. H. Chapman et al., "Video-assisted minimally invasive mitral valve surgery: the "micro-mitral" operation," *Journal of Thoracic and Cardiovascular Surgery*, vol. 113, no. 2, pp. 413–414, 1997.

[10] F. W. Mohr, V. Falk, A. Diegeler et al., "Minimally invasive port-access mitral valve surgery," *Journal of Thoracic and Cardiovascular Surgery*, vol. 115, no. 3, pp. 567–576, 1998.

[11] J. E. Felger, W. R. Chitwood, L. W. Nifong, and D. Holbert, "Evolution of mitral valve surgery: toward a totally endoscopic approach," *Annals of Thoracic Surgery*, vol. 72, no. 4, pp. 1203–1209, 2001.

[12] V. Falk, T. Walther, R. Autschbach, A. Diegeler, R. Battellini, and F. W. Mohr, "Robot-assisted minimally invasive solo mitral valve operation," *Journal of Thoracic and Cardiovascular Surgery*, vol. 115, no. 2, pp. 470–471, 1998.

[13] A. Carpentier, D. Loulmet, B. Aupècle et al., "Computer assisted open heart surgery. First case operated on with success," *Comptes Rendus de L'Académie des Sciences III*, vol. 321, no. 5, pp. 437–442, 1998.

[14] J. D. Schmitto, S. A. Mokashi, and L. H. Cohn, "Minimally-invasive valve surgery," *Journal of the American College of Cardiology*, vol. 56, no. 6, pp. 455–462, 2010.

[15] I. Kronzon and T. G. Matros, "Intraoperative echocardiography in minimally invasive cardiac surgery and novel cardiovascular surgical techniques," *The American Heart Hospital Journal*, vol. 2, no. 4, pp. 198–204, 2004.

[16] F. J. Benetti, J. L. Rizzardi, L. Pire, and A. Polanco, "Mitral valve replacement under video assistance through a minithoracotomy," *Annals of Thoracic Surgery*, vol. 63, no. 4, pp. 1150–1152, 1997.

[17] D. F. Loulmet, A. Carpentier, P. W. Cho et al., "Less invasive techniques for mitral valve surgery," *Journal of Thoracic and Cardiovascular Surgery*, vol. 115, no. 4, pp. 772–779, 1998.

[18] W. R. Chitwood, "State of the art review: videoscopic minimally invasive mitral valve surgery. Trekking to a totally endoscopic operation," *The Heart Surgery Forum*, vol. 1, no. 1, pp. 13–16, 1998.

[19] W. R. Chitwood WR, E. Rodriguez, E. J. Lehr et al., "Minimally invasive and robotic mitral valve surgery," in *Cardiac Surgery in the Adult*, L. H. Cohn, Ed., pp. 887–910, McGraw-Hill, New York, NY, USA, 4th edition, 2012.

[20] J. P. Greelish, L. H. Cohn, M. Leacche et al., "Minimally invasive mitral valve repair suggests earlier operations for mitral valve disease," *Journal of Thoracic and Cardiovascular Surgery*, vol. 126, no. 2, pp. 365–371, 2003.

[21] W. R. Chitwood Jr., J. R. Elbeery, and J. F. Moran, "Minimally invasive mitral valve repair using transthoracic aortic occlusion," *Annals of Thoracic Surgery*, vol. 63, no. 5, pp. 1477–1479, 1997.

[22] J. Seeburger, M. A. Borger, V. Falk et al., "Minimal invasive mitral valve repair for mitral regurgitation: results of 1339 consecutive patients," *European Journal of Cardio-thoracic Surgery*, vol. 34, no. 4, pp. 760–765, 2008.

[23] F. W. Mohr, V. Falk, A. Diegeler et al., "Minimally invasive port-access mitral valve surgery," *Journal of Thoracic and Cardiovascular Surgery*, vol. 115, no. 3, pp. 567–576, 1998.

[24] H. Vanermen, F. Farhat, F. Wellens et al., "Minimally invasive video-assisted mitral valve surgery: from port-access towards a totally endoscopic procedure," *Journal of Cardiac Surgery*, vol. 15, no. 1, pp. 51–60, 2000.

[25] H. Vanermen, F. Wellens, R. de Geest, I. Degrieck, and F. van Praet, "Video-assisted Port-Access mitral valve surgery: from debut to routine surgery. Will Trocar-Port-Access cardiac surgery ultimately lead to robotic cardiac surgery?" *Seminars in thoracic and cardiovascular surgery*, vol. 11, no. 3, pp. 223–234, 1999.

[26] D. A. Murphy, J. S. Miller, D. A. Langford, and A. B. Snyder, "Endoscopic robotic mitral valve surgery," *Journal of Thoracic and Cardiovascular Surgery*, vol. 132, no. 4, pp. 776–781, 2006.

[27] S. B. Colvin, A. C. Galloway, G. Ribakove et al., "Port-access(TM) mitral valve surgery: summary of results," *Journal of Cardiac Surgery*, vol. 13, no. 4, pp. 286–289, 1998.

[28] H. Reichenspurner, C. Detter, T. Deuse, D. H. Boehm, H. Treede, and B. Reichart, "Video and robotic-assisted minimally invasive mitral valve surgery: a comparison of the port-access and transthoracic clamp techniques," *Annals of Thoracic Surgery*, vol. 79, no. 2, pp. 485–490, 2005.

[29] A. P. Kypson, L. W. Nifong, and W. R. Chitwood Jr., "Robotic mitral valve surgery," *Surgical Clinics of North America*, vol. 83, no. 6, pp. 1387–1403, 2003.

[30] A. P. Kypson, J. E. Felger, L. W. Nifong, and W. R. Chitwood, "Robotics in valvular surgery: 2003 and beyond," *Current Opinion in Cardiology*, vol. 19, no. 2, pp. 128–133, 2004.

[31] T. Walther, C. Walther, V. Falk et al., "Early clinical results after stentless mitral valve implantation and comparison with conventional valve repair or replacement," *Circulation*, vol. 100, no. 19, pp. II78–II83, 1999.

[32] T. Walther, S. Lehmann, V. Falk et al., "Midterm results after stentless mitral valve replacement," *Circulation*, vol. 108, no. 10, pp. II85–II89, 2003.

[33] C. Gao, M. Yang, C. Xiao et al., "Robotically assisted mitral valve replacement," *Journal of Thoracic and Cardiovascular Surgery*, vol. 143, no. 4, supplement, pp. S64–S67, 2012.

[34] W. H. Ryan, T. M. Dewey, M. J. Mack, M. A. Herbert, and S. L. Prince, "Mitral valve surgery using the classical "heartport" technique," *The Journal of Heart Valve Disease*, vol. 14, no. 6, pp. 709–714, 2005.

[35] E. A. Grossi, A. LaPietra, G. H. Ribakove et al., "Minimally invasive versus sternotomy approaches for mitral reconstruction: comparison of intermediate-term results," *Journal of Thoracic and Cardiovascular Surgery*, vol. 121, no. 4, pp. 708–713, 2001.

[36] J. F. Onnasch, F. Schneider, V. Falk, M. Mierzwa, J. Bucerius, and F. W. Mohr, "Five years of less invasive mitral valve surgery: from experimental to routine approach," *Heart Surgery Forum*, vol. 5, no. 2, pp. 132–135, 2002.

[37] E. A. Grossi, A. C. Galloway, G. H. Ribakove et al., "Minimally invasive port access surgery reduces operative morbidity for valve replacement in the elderly," *The Heart Surgery Forum*, vol. 2, no. 3, pp. 212–215, 1999.

[38] E. A. Grossi, A. C. Galloway, G. H. Ribakove et al., "Impact of minimally invasive valvular heart surgery: a case-control study," *Annals of Thoracic Surgery*, vol. 71, no. 3, pp. 807–810, 2001.

[39] C. de Vaumas, I. Philip, G. Daccache et al., "Comparison of minithoracotomy and conventional sternotomy approaches for valve surgery," *Journal of Cardiothoracic and Vascular Anesthesia*, vol. 17, no. 3, pp. 325–328, 2003.

[40] L. G. Svensson, F. A. Atik, D. M. Cosgrove et al., "Minimally invasive versus conventional mitral valve surgery: a propensity-matched comparison," *Journal of Thoracic and Cardiovascular Surgery*, vol. 139, no. 4, pp. 926.e1-2–932.e1-2, 2010.

[41] T. Walther, V. Falk, and F. W. Mohr, "Minimally invasive surgery for valve disease," *Current Problems in Cardiology*, vol. 31, no. 6, pp. 399–437, 2006.

[42] J. Seeburger, M. A. Borger, V. Falk et al., "Minimal invasive mitral valve repair for mitral regurgitation: results of 1339 consecutive patients," *European Journal of Cardio-thoracic Surgery*, vol. 34, no. 4, pp. 760–765, 2008.

[43] P. Modi, E. Rodriguez, W. C. Hargrove, A. Hassan, W. Y. Szeto, and W. R. Chitwood, "Minimally invasive video-assisted mitral valve surgery: a 12-year, 2-center experience in 1178 patients," *Journal of Thoracic and Cardiovascular Surgery*, vol. 137, no. 6, pp. 1481–1487, 2009.

[44] P. Modi, A. Hassan, and W. R. Chitwood Jr., "Minimally invasive mitral valve surgery: a systematic review and meta-analysis," *European Journal of Cardio-thoracic Surgery*, vol. 34, no. 5, pp. 943–952, 2008.

[45] L. M. Stevens, E. Rodriguez, E. J. Lehr et al., "Impact of timing and surgical approach on outcomes after mitral valve regurgitation operations," *Annals of Thoracic Surgery*, vol. 93, no. 5, pp. 1462–1468, 2012.

[46] A. C. Galloway, C. F. Schwartz, G. H. Ribakove et al., "A decade of minimally invasive mitral repair: long-term outcomes," *Annals of Thoracic Surgery*, vol. 88, no. 4, pp. 1180–1184, 2009.

[47] E. A. Grossi, D. F. Loulmet, C. F. Schwartz et al., "Evolution of operative techniques and perfusion strategies for minimally invasive mitral valve repair," *Journal of Thoracic and Cardiovascular Surgery*, vol. 143, no. 4, supplement, pp. S68–S70, 2012.

[48] J. S. Gammie, Y. Zhao, E. D. Peterson, S. M. O'Brien, J. S. Rankin, and B. P. Griffith, "Less-invasive mitral valve operations: trends and outcomes from the society of thoracic surgeons adult cardiac surgery database," *Annals of Thoracic Surgery*, vol. 90, no. 5, pp. 1401–1410, 2010.

[49] L. M. Stevens, E. Rodriguez, E. J. Lehr et al., "Impact of timing and surgical approach on outcomes after mitral valve regurgitation operations," *Annals of Thoracic Surgery*, vol. 93, no. 5, pp. 1462–1468, 2012.

[50] C. G. Koch, L. Li, A. I. Duncan et al., "Morbidity and mortality risk associated with red blood cell and blood-component transfusion in isolated coronary artery bypass grafting," *Critical Care Medicine*, vol. 34, no. 6, pp. 1608–1616, 2006.

[51] F. Schneider, J. F. Onnasch, V. Falk, T. Walther, R. Autschbach, and F. W. Mohr, "Cerebral microemboli during minimally invasive and conventional mitral valve operations," *Annals of Thoracic Surgery*, vol. 70, no. 3, pp. 1094–1097, 2000.

[52] D. Moher, D. J. Cook, S. Eastwood, I. Olkin, D. Rennie, and D. F. Stroup, "Improving the quality of reports of meta-analyses of randomised controlled trials: the QUOROM statement," *The Lancet*, vol. 354, no. 9193, pp. 1896–1900, 1999.

[53] S. Dogan, T. Aybek, P. S. Risteski et al., "Minimally invasive port access versus conventional mitral valve surgery: prospective randomized study," *Annals of Thoracic Surgery*, vol. 79, no. 2, pp. 492–498, 2005.

[54] L. W. Nifong, W. R. Chitwood, P. S. Pappas et al., "Robotic mitral valve surgery: a United States multicenter trial," *Journal of Thoracic and Cardiovascular Surgery*, vol. 129, no. 6, pp. 1395–1404, 2005.

[55] T. Yamada, R. Ochiai, J. Takeda, H. Shin, and R. Yozu, "Comparison of early postoperative quality of life in minimally invasive versus conventional valve surgery," *Journal of Anesthesia*, vol. 17, no. 3, pp. 171–176, 2003.

[56] W. R. Chitwood Jr, C. L. Wixon, J. R. Elbeery, J. F. Moran, W. H. Chapman, and R. M. Lust, "Video-assisted minimally invasive mitral valve surgery," *Journal of Thoracic and Cardiovascular Surgery*, vol. 114, no. 5, pp. 773–782, 1997.

[57] H. Reichenspurner, A. Welz, V. Gulielmos, D. Boehm, and B. Reichart, "Port-access(TM) cardiac surgery using endovascular cardiopulmonary bypass: theory, practice, and results," *Journal of Cardiac Surgery*, vol. 13, no. 4, pp. 275–280, 1998.

[58] W. H. Ryan, T. M. Dewey, M. J. Mack, M. A. Herbert, and S. L. Prince, "Mitral valve surgery using the classical "heartport" technique," *The Journal of Heart Valve Disease*, vol. 14, no. 6, pp. 709–714, 2005.

[59] D. D. Glower, K. P. Landolfo, F. Clements et al., "Mitral valve operation via Port Access versus median sternotomy," *European Journal of Cardio-thoracic Surgery*, vol. 14, supplement 1, pp. S143–S147, 1998.

[60] C. R. Asher, J. M. DiMengo, K. L. Arheart et al., "Atrial fibrillation early postoperatively following minimally invasive cardiac valvular surgery," *American Journal of Cardiology*, vol. 84, no. 6, pp. 744–747, 1999.

[61] E. A. Grossi, A. C. Galloway, G. H. Ribakove et al., "Impact of minimally invasive valvular heart surgery: a case-control study," *Annals of Thoracic Surgery*, vol. 71, no. 3, pp. 807–810, 2001.

[62] O. Santana, J. Reyna, R. Grana, M. Buendia, G. A. Lamas, and J. Lamelas, "Outcomes of minimally invasive valve surgery versus standard sternotomy in obese patients undergoing isolated valve surgery," *Annals of Thoracic Surgery*, vol. 91, no. 2, pp. 406–410, 2011.

[63] L. H. Cohn, D. H. Adams, G. S. Couper et al., "Minimally invasive cardiac valve surgery improves patient satisfaction while reducing costs of cardiac valve replacement and repair," *Annals of Surgery*, vol. 226, no. 4, pp. 421–428, 1997.

[64] T. Walther, V. Falk, S. Metz et al., "Pain and quality of life after minimally invasive versus conventional cardiac surgery," *Annals of Thoracic Surgery*, vol. 67, no. 6, pp. 1643–1647, 1999.

[65] F. P. Casselman, S. van Slycke, F. Wellens et al., "Mitral valve surgery can now routinely be performed endoscopically," *Circulation*, vol. 108, no. 10, pp. II48–II54, 2003.

[66] A. A. Vlessis and S. F. Bolling, "Mini-reoperative mitral valve surgery," *Journal of Cardiac Surgery*, vol. 13, no. 6, pp. 468–470, 1998.

[67] A. Iribarne, R. Easterwood, M. J. Russo et al., "A minimally invasive approach is more cost-effective than a traditional sternotomy approach for mitral valve surgery," *Journal of Thoracic and Cardiovascular Surgery*, vol. 142, no. 6, pp. 1507–1514, 2011.

[68] J. E. Felger, L. W. Nifong, and W. R. Chitwood Jr., "The evolution of and early experience with robot-assisted mitral valve surgery," *Surgical Laparoscopy, Endoscopy and Percutaneous Techniques*, vol. 12, no. 1, pp. 58–63, 2002.

[69] V. A. Gaudiani, G. L. Grunkemeier, L. J. Castro, A. L. Fisher, and Y. Wu, "Mitral valve operations through standard and smaller incisions," *The Heart Surgery Forum*, vol. 7, no. 4, pp. E337–E342, 2004.

13

Transvaginal Appendectomy: A Systematic Review

Mehmet Ali Yagci and Cuneyt Kayaalp

Department of Surgery, Turgut Ozal Medical Center, Inonu University, 44315 Malatya, Turkey

Correspondence should be addressed to Cuneyt Kayaalp; cuneytkayaalp@hotmail.com

Academic Editor: Peng Hui Wang

Background. Natural orifice transluminal endoscopic surgery (NOTES) is a new approach that allows minimal invasive surgery through the mouth, anus, or vagina. *Objective.* To summarize the recent clinical appraisal, feasibility, complications, and limitations of transvaginal appendectomy for humans and outline the techniques. *Data Sources.* PubMed/MEDLINE, Cochrane, Google-Scholar, EBSCO, clinicaltrials.gov and congress abstracts, were searched. *Study Selection.* All related reports were included, irrespective of age, region, race, obesity, comorbidities or history of previous surgery. No restrictions were made in terms of language, country or journal. *Main Outcome Measures.* Patient selection criteria, surgical techniques, and results. *Results.* There were total 112 transvaginal appendectomies. All the selected patients had uncomplicated appendicitis and there were no morbidly obese patients. There was no standard surgical technique for transvaginal appendectomy. Mean operating time was 53.3 minutes (25–130 minutes). Conversion and complication rates were 3.6% and 8.2%, respectively. Mean length of hospital stay was 1.9 days. *Limitations.* There are a limited number of comparative studies and an absence of randomized studies. *Conclusions.* For now, nonmorbidly obese females with noncomplicated appendicitis can be a candidate for transvaginal appendectomy. It may decrease postoperative pain and enable the return to normal life and work off time. More comparative studies including subgroups are necessary.

1. Introduction

Since its original description by Mc Burney in 1894, appendectomy has been one of the most common surgical procedures performed by surgeons. In the last decades, laparoscopic appendectomy was an increasingly accepted treatment method for acute appendicitis, particularly for obese or female patients [1]. Natural orifice transluminal endoscopic surgery (NOTES) is a new approach that allows for minimal invasive surgery through the natural orifices such as mouth, anus, or vagina. This technique aims to avoid any visible scars on the body surface. Less incision on the abdomen helps to reduce surgical pain, analgesic requirement, recovery time, hernia formation, intra-abdominal adhesion, and surgical site infection. However, NOTES has several disadvantages and limitations with the currently available instruments, including limited access and less familiar working angles and operative views. In the past few years, many centers have published their experiences with NOTES appendectomies in humans. This study aimed to summarize the recent clini-
transvaginal appendectomy for humans and to outline techniques.

2. Material and Methods

Electronic searches in December 2013 of the PubMed/MEDLINE, Cochrane, Google Scholar, and EBSCOhost-Academic Search Complete, including CINAHL, used the key words [(vaginal OR transvaginal) AND (appendectomy OR appendectomies OR appendicectomy OR appendicectomies)]. All the studies including congress proceedings and abstracts that describe the clinical course of patients were accepted for the analysis. Two reviewers (Mehmet Ali Yagci and Cuneyt Kayaalp) assessed the list of titles and/or abstracts of the scanned articles at PubMed/MEDLINE and Cochrane using the key words in a function of [all fields]. If the articles met our inclusion criteria, full-text versions were obtained for assessment. If the articles were obviously irrelevant to the aim of this systematic review, they were excluded. Additional studies were also excluded due to their content (editorial letters, reviews, experimental studies, duplicated studies, technical notes not including patient data, and survey studies including questionnaires). After PubMed and Cochrane searches, we scanned the EBSCOhost-Academic Search Complete and Google Scholar databases with the same key words but using the [title] function. If any additional studies were found, they were added to the first search results. The unpublished, potentially relevant, trials at the registered trials database at https://www.clinicaltrials.gov/ were searched as well. The references of the selected relevant articles were cross checked to decrease the possibility of missing publications.

Transvaginal appendectomy was defined as a way of natural orifice translumenal endoscopic surgery for the appendix. Studies describing concomitant appendectomies during transvaginal hysterectomy were not considered for this systematic review. All the patients were included, irrespective of age, region, race, obesity, comorbidities, or history of previous surgery. No restrictions were made on language, country, or journal. In cases of disagreement during the study selection and analysis, the reviewers discussed the disagreement and a consensus was reached. Data for affiliation, number of the patients, age, clinical findings, inclusion and exclusion criteria, body mass index, history of previous abdominal surgery, trocar sites (pure or hybrid) and types, scope site and types (flexible or rigid), vaginal access and colpotomy closure techniques, intraoperative and postoperative complications, operating time, conversion to conventional laparoscopy or open surgery, postoperative pain, length of hospital stay, time off work, long term sexual function, and cosmetic satisfaction were recorded. A computer program including spreadsheet was used for records (Excel 2013, Microsoft Windows). If there were any missing data, we tried to contact the authors via e-mail.

Data were tabulated in tables, and column sums were created with the numbers or the means ± standard deviations, or the ranges of relevant parameters. When studies reported the median and range, we estimated the mean and standard deviation using the method described by Hozo et al. [2]. Basic calculations were used for the total numbers of the dichotomous outcomes and weighted means with ranges for the continuous outcomes. Chi-square test or the Fisher exact test (if expected values were less than 5) and Student's t-test were used for statistical analysis of both dichotomous and continuous variables (SPSS 13.0). A P value <.05 was considered significant.

3. Results

A total of 154 articles were retrieved from the PubMed/MEDLINE database and no additional study was available in the Cochrane library. After the elimination of the 96 irrelevant studies, the remaining 58 were selected for full-text examination. Google Scholar, EBSCOhost-Academic Search Complete, https://www.clinicaltrials.gov/, and reference cross-checking defined 26, 17, 6, and 2 studies, respectively (Figure 1). After the elimination of repetitive studies in several databases or sources, seven studies were added to the previously selected 58 articles. Studies including inadequate patient data, concomitant hysterectomy, experimental studies, and duplicated data were eliminated and finally 13 articles [3–15] were selected for the analysis (Figure 1). Two studies [10, 11] belonged to the same clinical series and their data were complementary (early and late results). As a result, we analyzed 12 clinical studies contained in 13 articles. Some studies had duplicated results [16–22] and their latest or the most comprehensive versions were accepted for the analysis [6, 10–13].

There were a total of 112 transvaginal appendectomies. Studies originated in Europe, North/South America, and Asia, and two of them included international multicenter data [6, 13]. Publications were generally (11/13) in English but one was in German [9], and one was in Japanese [14]. The patients' ages were generally in the mid-twenties or mid-thirties; however, there was a large age range (18–74 years). Inclusion criteria of the studies for transvaginal appendectomy are summarized in Table 1. All the patients were in the American Society of Anesthesia (ASA) I-II scores. A diagnosis of complicated appendicitis (perforation, abscess, and mass) was usually an exclusion criterion. Morbidly obese patients (body mass index more than 35 kg/m^2) were also excluded, and the mean body mass index of the patients in this systematic review was 23.2 kg/m^2 (Table 2) [4, 7–9, 13, 14]. Previous abdominal or pelvic surgery was not an exclusion criterion in all studies and 11% of the patients had a history of abdominal or pelvic surgery [9, 15]. Most of the cases (96%) were of acute appendicitis, while others (4%) were chronic appendicitis or incidental appendectomies.

Mean operating time was 53.3 minutes and ranged from 25 to 130 minutes. There were nine complications reported in 109 cases (8.2%). Four of them were intraoperative complications: appendicular artery hemorrhage (n: 3) and inability to sustain the pneumoperitoneum (n: 1). Those cases required additional abdominal trocar access and were accepted as a conversion to conventional laparoscopy (3.6%), but no case required conversion to open surgery. Postoperative complications occurred in five patients and all were treated by nonsurgical methods (Table 3). Intra-abdominal abscess, urinary retention, urinary infection, and dyspareunia were treated by percutaneous drainage plus antibiotics, Foley catheter placement, antibiotics, and just waiting, respectively. Mean length of hospital stay was 1.9 days for all studies. The mean length of hospital stay was longer in the German series (3.4 days) because of their national health system, [3, 9], and the mean length of hospital stay was 1.25 days for the rest of the studies.

There was no standard surgical technique for transvaginal appendectomy (Figure 2). Some studies used only the transvaginal access, called a pure or totally transvaginal appendectomy. Others used an abdominal assistance (usually a 5 mm umbilical trocar) to the transvaginal access and are called a hybrid technique (Table 4). Pure transvaginal appendectomy was performed on only 22% of the cases and the remaining were hybrid procedures (78%). When we compared the operating time and the complications for both techniques, there were no differences. The operating times

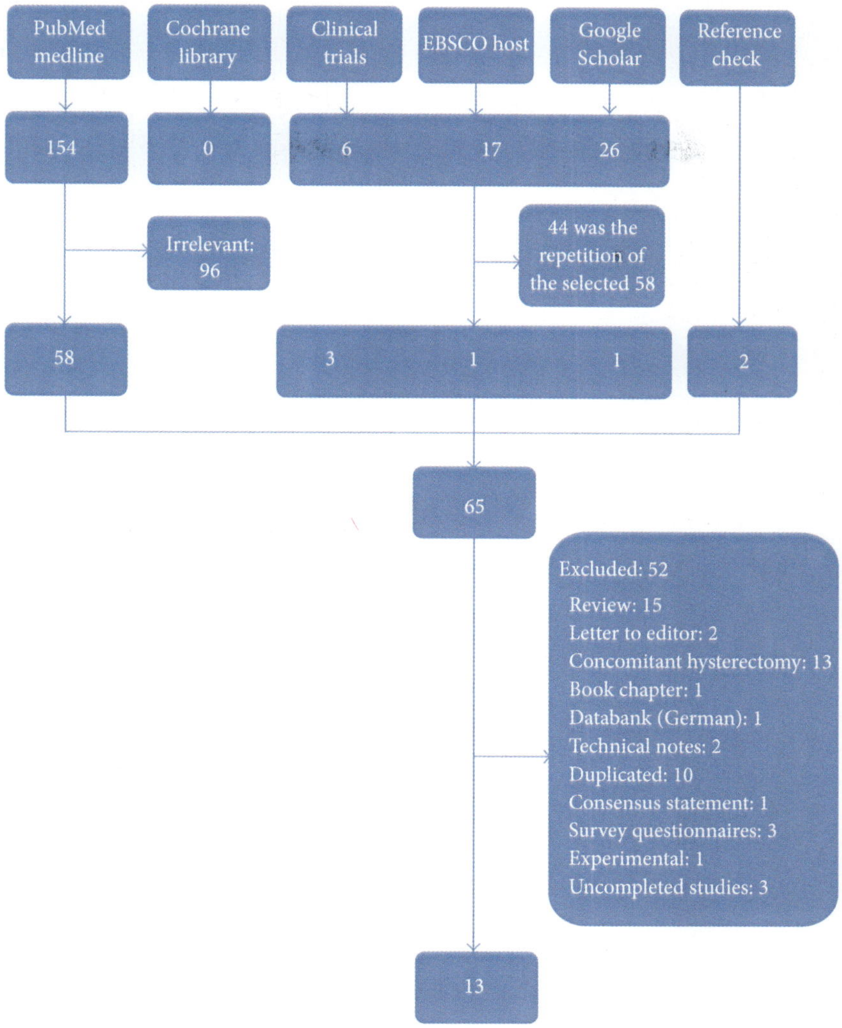

FIGURE 1: Flowchart of the systematic review.

for pure [4, 10] and hybrid [5, 9, 12–15] techniques were 48.3 ± 11.8 minutes and 49.6 ± 25.5 minutes, respectively (P = 0.83). Complication rates for pure [3, 4, 10] and hybrid [5, 7–9, 12–15] techniques were 19.0% and 5.5%, respectively (P = 0.09). Another technical difference was related to the type of scope. Some authors used flexible endoscopes (20%) and others preferred rigid laparoscopes (80%). Operating times with flexible endoscopes [4, 5, 12, 13] and rigid laparoscopes [9, 10, 13–15] were 71.9 ± 13.3 minutes and 45.2 ± 21.6 minutes, respectively (P = 0.0007). Complication rates for using flexible [3–5, 8, 12, 13] and rigid [7, 9, 10, 13–15] scopes were 0% and 11.4%, respectively (P = 0.33).

4. Discussion

Transvaginal appendectomy during vaginal hysterectomy was first described in 1949 [23] and, at the time, was performed by the gynecologists with the aim of incidental appendectomy [6, 23]. Those studies did not include the acute appendicitis cases and their primary objectives were the treatment of gynecological pathologies, not the appendix. In 2008, the first transvaginal appendectomy without vaginal hysterectomy was reported by Palanivelu and coworkers from India [22] and after a short period of time three more cases were reported one from Germany [3] and two from Georgia [4]. Interestingly, these first three separate reports of transvaginal appendectomies all described the totally transvaginal (pure) technique using only an endoscope [3, 4, 22]. In those cases, there was no abdominal trocar for assistance, nor was there any other transvaginal equipment except endoscopes. All the procedures were performed through the working channels of the endoscopes. Mesoappendixes were transected and the bases of the appendixes were secured with endoloops. Transection of the appendixes was done with scissors [3, 4] or snares [22] through the endoscopic channels. All the specimens were removed with the help of the endoscope and no extraction bags were used. Mean operating time was 95 minutes and ranged between 72 and 135 minutes. Palanivelu et al. reported that, before the first successful case, they experienced three prior conversions to conventional laparoscopic appendectomy due to technical difficulties with this pure endoscopic technique [22]. Bernhardt et al. used the same

Table 1: Inclusion criteria for transvaginal appendectomies.

Parameters	Zorron et al. [6]	Pérez et al. [7]	Roberts et al. [10]	Jacobsen et al. [12]	Noguera et al. [8]	Albrecht et al. [9]	Mofid et al. [15]
Age	NA	18–65	18–65	18–75	18–65	18–78	NA
ASA score	I-II	I-II	I-II	I-II	I-II	NA	NA
Disease severity	Mild symptoms and short duration of disease	No palpable mass No appendicular abscess	Not perforated at clinical and radiological evaluation	<48 hours of the onset No abdominal abscess No abdominal mass No sepsis No diffuse peritonitis	NA	Unclear abdominal discomfort in the sense of appendicitis	NA
Previous surgery	No history of hysterectomy Some centers avoided prior other abdominal surgeries	NA	No abdominal or pelvic surgery	NA	NA	Previous abdominal or pelvic surgery was not a contraindication	Previous abdominal or pelvic surgery was not a contraindication
Virginity or pregnancy	Not virgin Not pregnant	Not virgin Not pregnant	Not pregnant	Not pregnant	NA	NA	NA
BMI	NA	<35	<35	<35	NA	NA	<35
Gynecological pathologies	No vaginal infection No endometriosis No obliterating adhesions in the pouch of Douglas	No gynecological infection	NA	No history of ectopic pregnancy, PID, severe endometriosis, or perineal trauma	NA	NA	No known adhesions in the pelvis
Others	NA	NA	Not retrocecal at preoperative radiological evaluation	No immunosuppressive drug Not immunocompromised No blood thinner medication No platelet inhibitor drugs Normal coagulation tests	Previous delivery of at least one child	NA	No malignancy No previous pelvic radiotherapy

NA: not available, BMI: body mass index, ASA: American Society of Anesthesiology, and PID: pelvic inflammatory disease.

TABLE 2: Patient and article details.

Author	Year	Country	Number	Age (mean)	Appendectomy indication	BMI	Prior surgery
Bernhardt et al. [3]	2008	Germany	1	28	Subacute	NA	No
Tabutsadze and Kipshidze [4]	2009	Georgia	2	22, 28	Acute	22.2 & 23.5	No
Shin et al. [5]	2010	Korea	1	74	Acute	Not obese	No
Zorron et al. [6]	2010	International	37	NA	Acute	NA	Some
Pérez et al. [7]	2011	Cuba	8	29.6 (18–42)	Acute	<35	NA
Noguera et al. [8]	2011	Spain	4	NA	Acute (2), incidental (2)	NA	NA
Roberts et al. [10]	2012	USA	18	31.3	Acute	23.7	No
Albrecht et al. [9]	2013	Germany	30	33.9	Acute	23.7	Yes (5)
Jacobsen et al. [12]	2014	USA	3	NA	Acute	NA	NA
Arezzo et al. [13]	2013	International	5	31.2 (23–42)	Acute	18.9 (18-19)	NA
Wada et al. [14]	2013	Japan	1	50	Acute	24.2	No
Mofid et al. [15]	2013	Germany	2	NA	Chronic	NA	Yes (1)

BMI: body mass index.

TABLE 3: Results of transvaginal appendectomies.

Author	Number	Operating time (min) mean (range)	Complications (number)	Conversion to laparoscopy (number)	Length of stay (mean and range)
Bernhardt et al. [3]	1	NA	No	No	3
Tabutsadze and Kipshidze [4]	2	76 & 88	No	No	1.25 & 1.5
Shin et al. [5]	1	60	No	No	3
Zorron et al. [6]	37	60.5 (90 for flexible)	Appendicular artery hemorrhage (3)	Appendicular artery hemorrhage (3)	1.3
Pérez et al. [7]	8	48.3 (37–75)	No	No	1.1 (<1-2)
Noguera et al. [8]	4	61	No	No	NA
Roberts et al. [10]	18	44.4	Intra-abdominal abscess (1) Urinary retention (1) Unable to sustain pneumoperitoneum (1)	Unable to sustain pneumoperitoneum (1)	1.1
Albrecht et al. [9]	30	44.3	Urinary infection (1) Dyspareunia (2)	No	3.4
Jacobsen et al. [12]	3	71 (55–80)	NA	No	NA
Arezzo et al. [13]	5	Rigid: 42.5 (40–45) Flexible: 70 (60–90)	No	No	Rigid: 1.5 (1-2) Flexible: 1.3 (1-2)
Wada et al. [14]	1	130	No	No	1
Mofid et al. [15]	2	25 & 32	No	No	NA

technique and reported that their case was not an acute appendicitis, but a recurring subacute appendicitis [3]. We can conclude that, despite its minimal invasiveness, technical difficulties limit the application of the pure transvaginal technique to highly selected cases. Technological improvements may make its use more liberal in the future. But for now, this analysis revealed that this earliest described transvaginal appendectomy technique was the least commonly preferred one relative to others subsequently described.

Another technique for pure transvaginal appendectomy was reported using the placement of a single incision laparoscopic surgery (SILS) port into the incised posterior vaginal fornix [10]. There was no abdominal trocar assistance. The authors preferred a 5 mm 30° rigid telescope and two working ports (5 mm and 12 mm) on the SILS port [10]. They divided the mesoappendix with a stapler or an energy device and the appendix was likewise divided with an endoscopic stapler. The specimens were extracted with the endoscopic bags. They reported almost half the operating time (mean 44.4 minutes) of the previously described endoscope-only pure transvaginal appendectomy. Although this new technique seemed more adaptable to daily surgical practice, the authors warned that the SILS port was inadequate as it was too short, which made placement difficult. They concluded that there was still room for innovation in the development of the technique [10].

This analysis pointed out that hybrid procedures with umbilical port assistances were more common (72%) than the pure transvaginal techniques. Hybrid techniques had some

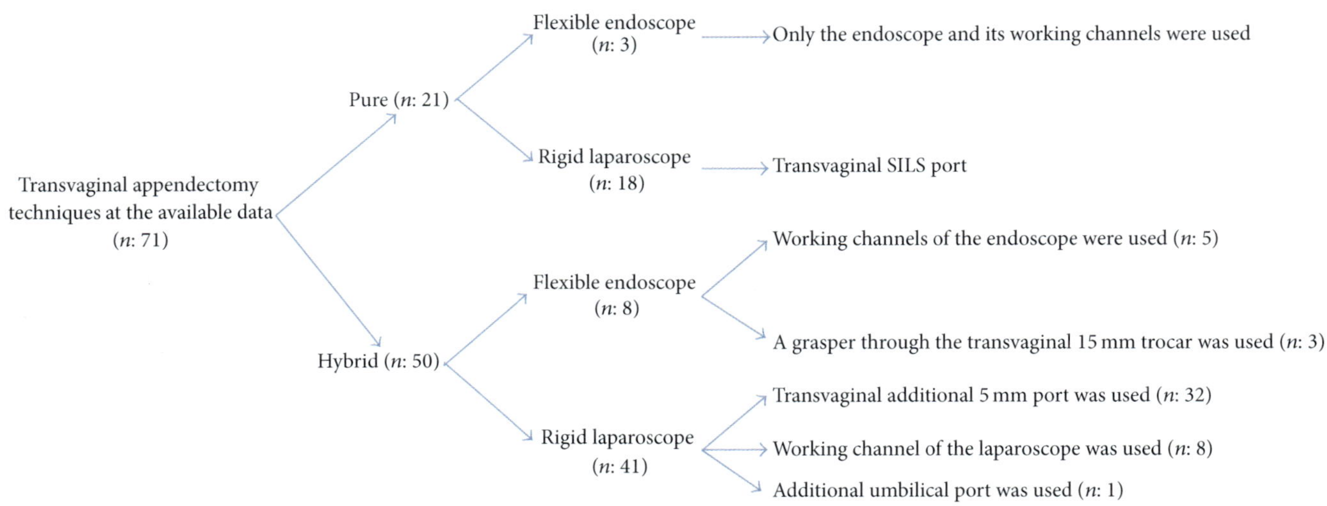

FIGURE 2: Technical details of the available transvaginal appendectomies.

TABLE 4: Technical details of transvaginal appendectomies.

Author	Number	Vaginal trocar	Umbilical assistance	Working access	Flexible or rigid scope
Bernhardt et al. [3]	1	No	No (pure)	Endoscope channel	Flexible
Tabutsadze and Kipshidze [4]	2	NA	No (pure)	Endoscope channel	Flexible
Shin et al. [5]	1	15 mm	5 mm (hybrid)	Endoscope channel	Flexible
Zorron et al. [6]	37	10 or 12 mm	No (pure) or 5 mm (hybrid)	NA	Both
Pérez et al. [7]	8	11 mm	5 mm (hybrid)	Laparoscope channel	Rigid
Noguera et al. [8]	4	15 mm	5 mm (hybrid)	Endoscope channel	Flexible
Roberts et al. [10]	18	SILS port	No (pure)	TV SILS port	Rigid
Albrecht et al. [9]	30	12 mm	5 mm (hybrid)	TV 5 mm port	Rigid
Jacobsen et al. [12]	3	15 mm	5 mm (hybrid)	Through TV 15 mm trocar	Flexible
Arezzo et al. [13]	5	12 mm	5 mm (hybrid)	NA	Flexible (3), rigid (2)
Wada et al. [14]	1	12 mm	5 mm (hybrid)	2.3 mm umbilical trocar	Rigid
Mofid et al. [15]	2	5 and 10 mm	5 mm (hybrid)	TV 5 mm trocar	Rigid

TV: transvaginal.

advantages over pure ones, such as safer transvaginal introduction under direct vision, transumbilical view when necessary, and two directional working in the abdominal cavity. A hybrid procedure was started with pneumoperitoneum via a Veress needle at the umbilicus and a 5 mm trocar was inserted via the umbilicus to inspect the abdominal cavity. After that a vaginal trocar (10–15 mm) was placed at the posterior fornix of the vagina. An additional working port was created in three different ways in the studies: (i) the channel of the laparoscope was used [7]; (ii) a second 5 mm trocar was inserted from the posterior fornix [15]; or (iii) a second 2.3 mm trocar was placed through the umbilicus [14]. Using a flexible endoscope instead of rigid laparoscope prolonged the operating time. No clear benefits of flexible endoscopes over the rigid scopes were seen in this systematic analysis.

Transferring the surgeons from open surgery to laparoscopic surgery provided the patients with a more comfortable postoperative course and a more rapid recovery. Another promising improvement was the single incision laparoscopic surgery. However, its benefits on postoperative pain and patient recovery were not as amazing as in the previous transfer from open to laparoscopy. A recent meta-analysis found no difference on postoperative pain and length of hospital stay between the single port and the multiport laparoscopic appendectomies [24]. Natural orifice surgery is a novel technique that can have a positive influence on postoperative pain and recovery. An important drawback of this technique may be the unfamiliarity of the access to the abdomen for surgeons who are generally familiar with abdominal incisions or transanal surgeries. A second point that may keep surgeons away from this technique is the idea that complicated surgical equipment is required. This systematic review demonstrated that, from the technical point of view, the equipment required for transvaginal appendectomy was not too distinct from the well-known existing conventional laparoscopic appendectomy equipment. There was no need for special equipment such as long trocars or flexible endoscopes.

Only two studies compared the results of transvaginal and conventional laparoscopic appendectomies [9, 10]. Despite the limited number of the patients in those studies, there was

TABLE 5: Comparison of transvaginal and conventional laparoscopic appendectomies.

Parameters	Studies	Transvaginal	Conventional	P
Operating time (minutes)	Albrecht et al. [9] (n: 30 versus n: 30)	44.3 ± 22.1	33.5 ± 10.0	0.02
	Roberts et al. [10] (n: 18 versus n: 22)	44.4 ± 4.5	39.8 ± 2.6	<0.01
Hospital stay (days)	Albrecht et al. [9] (n: 30 versus n: 30)	3.4 ± 1.2	5.0 ± 2.7	<0.01
	Roberts et al. [10] (n: 18 versus n: 22)	1.1 ± 0.1	1.2 ± 0.1	<0.01
Complications	Albrecht et al. [9] (n: 30 versus n: 30)	Urinary tract infection (1)	No	1.00
	Roberts et al. [10] (n: 18 versus n: 22)	Intra-abdominal abscess (1) Urinary retention (1)	Intestinal obstruction (1) Urinary retention (1)	1.00
Opioid requirement (mg)	Albrecht et al. [9] (n: 9 versus n: 9)	12.8 ± 7.0	14.7 ± 5.2	0.52
	Roberts et al. [10] (n: 18 versus n: 22)	8.7 ± 2.1	23.0 ± 3.4	<0.01
Return to normal activity after 2 weeks	Albrecht et al. [9] (n: 30 versus n: 30)	70%	59%	0.58
Return to normal activity (days)	Roberts et al. [10] (n: 18 versus n: 22)	3.3 ± 0.4	9.7 ± 1.6	<0.01
Return to work (days)	Roberts et al. [10] (n: 18 versus n: 22)	5.4 ± 1.1	10.7 ± 1.5	<0.01
Cosmetic satisfaction	Albrecht et al. [9] (n: 30 versus n: 30)	100%	80%	0.02
	Roberts et al. [10] (n: 18 versus n: 22)	NA	NA	NA

NA: not available.

a trend towards shorter hospital stays [9, 10], quicker recovery [10], and less analgesic requirement [10] for the transvaginal groups (Table 5). On the other hand, operating time was longer at transvaginal groups. There was no difference in morbidity. As expected, cosmetic satisfaction was better for the transvaginal group [9]. Recent meta-analyses including thousands of conventional laparoscopic appendectomies demonstrated that the wound infection rate was 3.3–4% and the length of hospital stay was 1.9–2.9 days [24, 25]. When compared to those results, this systematic review demonstrated that transvaginal appendectomy can be a rational alternative to conventional laparoscopic appendectomy in selected patients. It has very low wound infection rates (zero in this study) and short hospital stays (mean 1.9 days).

Today, two matters can limit the widespread use of transvaginal appendectomy. First, there is not enough data of this technique for the morbidly obese patients. There is a considerable amount of obese people in the western countries and transvaginal appendectomy studies are necessary including morbid obese patients. We believe that minimal invasive surgeries like transvaginal appendectomy can have a place for the morbid obese patients in future. Secondly, the risk of delving into the cultural sensitivity of using the vagina as an access point, particularly in third world countries can be a limitation. This can be a problem even in the most promiscuous cultures where virginity still runs some amount of the population.

As a conclusion, appendectomy is one of the most common emergency visceral surgical procedures. The early results of transvaginal appendectomy in this systematic review show some promise for improved postoperative pain and patient recovery. Using hybrid techniques with rigid laparoscopes may provide an easier adaptation for surgeons to this novel appendectomy method. For now, transvaginal appendectomy looks suitable for nonmorbid obese patients (BMI < 35) and noncomplicated appendicitis. Of course, its potential advantages and disadvantages will become clearer in the future with comparative studies. More studies are also necessary on the role of transvaginal appendectomy in some subgroups like morbidly obese patients or perforated appendicitis.

References

[1] S. Sauerland, T. Jaschinski, and E. A. Neugebauer, "Laparoscopic versus open surgery for suspected appendicitis," *Cochrane Database of Systematic Reviews*, vol. 10, Article ID CD001546, 2010.

[2] S. P. Hozo, B. Djulbegovic, and I. Hozo, "Estimating the mean and variance from the median, range, and the size of a sample," *BMC Medical Research Methodology*, vol. 5, article 13, 2005.

[3] J. Bernhardt, B. Gerber, H.-C. Schober, G. Kähler, and K. Ludwig, "NOTES—case report of a unidirectional flexible appendectomy," *International Journal of Colorectal Disease*, vol. 23, no. 5, pp. 547–550, 2008.

[4] T. Tabutsadze and N. Kipshidze, "New trend in endoscopic surgery: transvaginal appendectomy NOTES (Natural Orifice Transluminal Endoscopic Surgery)," *Georgian Medical News*, no. 168, pp. 7–10, 2009.

[5] E. J. Shin, G. A. Jeong, J. C. Jung et al., "Transvaginal endoscopic appendectomy," *Journal of the Korean Society of Coloproctology*, vol. 26, no. 6, pp. 429–432, 2010.

[6] R. Zorron, C. Palanivelu, M. P. Galvão Neto et al., "International multicenter trial on clinical natural orifice surgery-Notes IMTN study: preliminary results of 362 patients," *Surgical Innovation*, vol. 17, no. 2, pp. 142–158, 2010.

[7] R. C. Pérez, L. R. A. González, E. D. Reyes, J. C. D. Fernández, L. E. R. Arias, and M. O. Estrada, "The transvaginal approach in acute appendicitis," *Cirugia Espanola*, vol. 89, no. 8, pp. 517–523, 2011.

[8] J. F. Noguera, A. Cuadrado, F. M. Sánchez-Margallo et al., "Emergency transvaginal hybrid natural orifice transluminal endoscopic surgery," *Endoscopy*, vol. 43, no. 5, pp. 442–444, 2011.

[9] R. Albrecht, C. Bochmann, A. Süße, L. Jablonski, and U. Settmacher, "Hybrid NOS appendectomy (NA): clinical assessment of a new surgical technique," *Zentralblatt fur Chirurgie—Zeitschrift fur Allgemeine, Viszeral- und Gefasschirurgie*, vol. 138, no. 4, pp. 449–455, 2013.

[10] K. E. Roberts, D. Solomon, T. Mirensky et al., "Pure transvaginal appendectomy versus traditional laparoscopic appendectomy for acute appendicitis: a prospective cohort study," *Annals of Surgery*, vol. 255, no. 2, pp. 266–269, 2012.

[11] D. Solomon, R. Lentz, A. J. Duffy, R. L. Bell, and K. E. Roberts, "Female sexual function after pure transvaginal appendectomy: a cohort study," *Journal of Gastrointestinal Surgery*, vol. 16, no. 1, pp. 183–187, 2012.

[12] G. R. Jacobsen, J. S. Barajas-Gamboa, A. M. Coker et al., "Transvaginal organ extraction: potential for broad clinical application," *Surgical Endoscopy*, vol. 28, no. 2, pp. 484–491, 2014.

[13] A. Arezzo, C. Zornig, H. Mofid et al., "The EURO-NOTES clinical registry for natural orifice transluminal endoscopic surgery: a 2-year activity report," *Surgical Endoscopy and Other Interventional Techniques*, vol. 27, no. 9, pp. 3073–3084, 2013.

[14] N. Wada, M. Tanabe, F. Kataoka, and Y. Kitagawa, "Transvaginal hybrid natural orifice translumenal endoscopic surgery appendectomy," *Nihon Geka Gakkai zasshi*, vol. 114, no. 6, pp. 308–311, 2013.

[15] H. Mofid, A. Emmermann, M. Alm, H.-A. Von Waldenfels, C. Felixmüller, and C. Zornig, "Is the transvaginal route appropriate for intra-abdominal NOTES procedures? Experience and follow-up of 222 cases," *Surgical Endoscopy and Other Interventional Techniques*, vol. 27, no. 8, pp. 2807–2812, 2013.

[16] S. G. Wood, L. Panait, A. J. Duffy, R. L. Bell, and K. E. Roberts, "Complications of transvaginal natural orifice transluminal endoscopic surgery: a series of 102 patients," *Annals of Surgery*, vol. 259, no. 4, pp. 744–749, 2014.

[17] S. Horgan, O. R. Meireles, G. R. Jacobsen et al., "Broad clinical utilization of NOTES: is it safe?" *Surgical Endoscopy and Other Interventional Techniques*, vol. 27, no. 6, pp. 1872–1880, 2013.

[18] L. Panait, S. G. Wood, R. L. Bell, A. J. Duffy, and K. E. Roberts, "Transvaginal natural orifice transluminal endoscopic surgery in the morbidly obese," *Surgical Endoscopy and Other Interventional Techniques*, vol. 27, no. 7, pp. 2625–2629, 2013.

[19] S. Horgan, K. Thompson, M. Talamini et al., "Clinical experience with a multifunctional, flexible surgery system for endolumenal, single-port, and NOTES procedures," *Surgical Endoscopy*, vol. 25, no. 2, pp. 586–592, 2011.

[20] K. S. Lehmann, J. P. Ritz, A. Wibmer et al., "The German registry for natural orifice translumenal endoscopic surgery: report of the first 551 patients," *Annals of Surgery*, vol. 252, no. 2, pp. 263–270, 2010.

[21] S. Horgan, J. P. Cullen, M. A. Talamini et al., "Natural orifice surgery: initial clinical experience," *Surgical Endoscopy and Other Interventional Techniques*, vol. 23, no. 7, pp. 1512–1518, 2009.

[22] C. Palanivelu, P. S. Rajan, M. Rangarajan, R. Parthasarathi, P. Senthilnathan, and M. Prasad, "Transvaginal endoscopic appendectomy in humans: a unique approach to NOTES—World's first report," *Surgical Endoscopy and Other Interventional Techniques*, vol. 22, no. 5, pp. 1343–1347, 2008.

[23] B. Bueno, "Primer caso de apendicectomia por via vaginal," *Toko-Ginecologia Practica*, vol. 8, pp. 152–154, 1949.

[24] S. R. Markar, A. Karthikesalingam, F. di Franco, and A. M. Harris, "Systematic review and meta-analysis of single-incision versus conventional multiport appendicectomy," *British Journal of Surgery*, vol. 100, no. 13, pp. 1709–1718, 2013.

[25] H. Ohtani, Y. Tamamori, Y. Arimoto, Y. Nishiguchi, K. Maeda, and K. Hirakawa, "Meta-analysis of the results of randomized controlled trials that compared laparoscopic and open surgery for acute appendicitis," *Journal of Gastrointestinal Surgery*, vol. 16, no. 10, pp. 1929–1939, 2012.

14

Single-Incision Single-Instrument Adnexal Surgery in Pediatric Patients

Tara Loux,[1] Gavin A. Falk,[1] Michaela Gaffley,[2] Stephanie Ortega,[3] Carmen Ramos,[1,2,4] Leopoldo Malvezzi,[1,2,4] Colin G. Knight,[1,2,4] and Cathy Burnweit[1,2,4]

[1]*Miami Children's Hospital, Miami, FL, USA*
[2]*Herbert Wertheim College of Medicine, Florida International University, Miami, FL, USA*
[3]*Florida International University, Miami, FL, USA*
[4]*Miami Associates in Pediatric Surgery, Miami, FL, USA*

Correspondence should be addressed to Colin G. Knight; colin.knight@mch.com

Academic Editor: Chih-Feng Yen

Introduction. Pediatric surgeons often practice pediatric gynecology. The single-incision single-instrument (SISI) technique used for appendectomy is applicable in gynecologic surgery. *Methods.* We retrospectively analyzed the records of patients undergoing pelvic surgery from 2008 to 2013. SISI utilized a 12 mm transumbilical trocar and an operating endoscope. The adnexa can be detorsed intracorporeally or extracorporealized via the umbilicus for lesion removal. *Results.* We performed 271 ovarian or paraovarian surgeries in 258 patients. In 147 (54%), the initial approach was SISI; 75 cases (51%) were completed in patients aged from 1 day to 19.9 years and weighing 4.7 to 117 kg. Conversion to standard laparoscopy was due to contralateral oophoropexy, solid mass, inability to mobilize the adnexa, large mass, bleeding, adhesions, or better visualization. When SISI surgery was converted to Pfannenstiel, the principal reason was a solid mass. SISI surgery was significantly shorter than standard laparoscopy. There were no major complications and the overall cohort had an 11% minor complication rate. *Conclusion.* SISI adnexal surgery is safe, quick, inexpensive, and effective in pediatric patients. SISI was successful in over half the patients in whom it was attempted and offers a scarless result. If unsuccessful, the majority of cases can be completed with standard multiport laparoscopy.

1. Introduction

Laparoscopic operations for benign adnexal pathology have been conducted for many years; minimally invasive surgery was, in fact, initially pioneered by gynecologists. In most centers without specialized pediatric gynecologists, pediatric surgeons perform the majority of adnexal operations. We have previously reported our "all-in-one" single-incision single-instrument (SISI) appendectomy as an essentially scarless operation with outcomes equivalent to multiport techniques at a lower cost [1]. Since 2008, we have extended the SISI approach to adnexal pathology and found it to be a useful approach for the treatment of pediatric and adolescent ovarian or paraovarian pathology, with easy conversion to standard two- or three-port laparoscopy or even open Pfannenstiel, if additional visualization were needed.

Several authors have described the use of expensive single-site laparoscopy systems for treatment of adnexal pathology in small series of children and adolescents [2–8], and others have described similar approaches in adults [9–14], although many of these reports are for single-incision multiple-instrument methods. A few authors have also described the use of transumbilical operations for cystic ovarian lesions in small series of infants, whether laparoscopic-assisted or via minilaparotomy [15–19]. Only one other author has utilized our same approach in 15 children and adolescents [20].

A survey conducted among members of the International Pediatric Endosurgery Group (IPEG) divulged that only 7% of this highly selected group's respondents had performed single-incision pediatric endoscopic surgery (SIPES) for gynecologic pathology [21]. A quarter of respondents to this

Table 1: Select demographic characteristics of patients with ovarian pathology undergoing operation.

	Operative technique (initial approach : final approach)					
Demographic variable	SISI : SISI	SISI : multiport	SISI : Pfannenstiel	Multiport : multiport	Multiport : Pfannenstiel	Open
Number of pt. (% of cohort)	75 (27.7)	53 (19.6)	19 (7.0)	97 (35.8)	5 (1.8)	22 (8.1)
Mean age, yrs (range)	14.6 (1 d–19.9 y)	14.2 (1 m–9.6 y)	14.9 (9.7–18.8 y)	14.5 (3 m–9.9 y)	12.7 (8.3–15.1 y)	13.3 (3.8–18.2 y)
Mean weight, kgs (range)	61.0 (4.7–117)	62.7 (4.6–110)	65.3 (30.5–117)	63.5 (5.6–140)	64.1 (28.6–106)	53.8 (19.2–93)

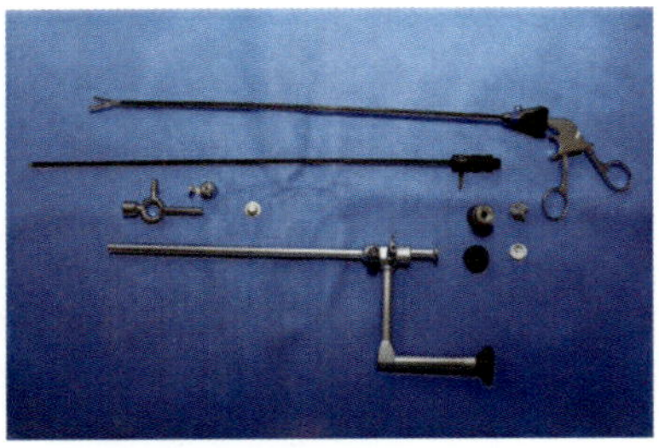

Figure 1: Picture of our 10 mm operating endoscope with periscope eyepiece and 5 mm instrument port.

survey who did not perform SIPES at all cited inadequate resources as the reason. The purpose of the current study was to describe our high-volume, extensive experience with SISI surgery applied to adnexal pathology as a low-cost, simple, efficient, and cosmetically appealing solution for pelvic surgery in children of all ages and sizes.

2. Methods

Our surgical billing database was queried for Current Procedural Technology (CPT) codes indicating partial or total oophorectomy (58661, 58662, 58720, 58900, 58925, 58940) from January 1, 2008, to November 30, 2013. Five attending surgeons performed or supervised all procedures, and all surgeons had been performing SISI appendectomy for at least 2 years. We extracted data retrospectively through review of hospital and clinic charts. Data extracted included patient age and weight at time of surgery, surgical start and end times, type of surgery performed (including surgical approach at beginning, intraoperative change of approach, and reason for conversion), final pathology and cytology results, total hospital length of stay, postoperative complications, and overall length of follow-up time. This study met criteria for exempt review, determined by the Western Institutional Review Board (Case number 1-814812-1).

Our SISI approach utilized a 12-millimeter standard laparoscopy trocar introduced transumbilically, after placement of an indwelling bladder catheter. We then inserted an operating endoscope (Karl Storz, product number 26036AA, Figure 1), which combines a 10-millimeter, 0-degree lens with an offset eyepiece and a 5-millimeter port through which a long instrument, such as a toothed grasper or suction, can be introduced. Ovarian torsions can almost always be reduced with this instrument. For large simple cystic lesions, aspiration of the cyst fluid was performed with a spinal needle introduced through the anterior abdominal wall under direct vision while stabilizing the lesion with the grasper or by cauterizing a hole in the cyst with the long suction and then inserting it inside the cyst. Such decompression afforded increased mobility of the adnexa. If the cystic lesion was so large that it extended out of the pelvis and could be directly visualized through the umbilical incision, it was grasped with an atraumatic clamp. A purse-string suture was then placed in the cyst wall, and a suction device was inserted for decompression of fluid. Once the adnexa was mobile, it was extruded through the umbilical incision, using a fascial extension if needed. Ovarian-sparing procedures were attempted when thought possible, with the cystic or solid lesions being dissected off the normal ovarian parenchyma, which was dropped back into the abdomen after achieving hemostasis. Total oophorectomy, sparing the fallopian tube, was utilized when normal-appearing ovarian parenchyma could not be distinguished from a solid mass of undetermined character. Rarely, full salpingooophorectomy was performed in cases of suspected malignancy. Conversion to standard laparoscopy was dependent upon the experience and comfort of the surgeon with each individual case. Alternatively, Pfannenstiel incision was performed if the surgeon deemed an open operation advisable.

Statistics utilized included the Student t-test, Chi-square test, and Fisher exact test where appropriate, with $p < 0.05$ considered statistically significant.

3. Results

We pulled 279 codes meeting the criteria from our surgical database. Eight operations had two procedure codes; five patients were excluded for nonovarian primary surgery. Four patients were found to have had a repeat operation that was not elicited in our code search. The end result was 271 evaluable operations in 258 patients, 13 of whom had recurrent adnexal pathology. The most common indications for surgical intervention were pain, cyst greater than 5 centimeters in diameter, suspected torsion, and/or solid mass. Demographic and clinical data by initial and final approach are delineated in Table 1. Over half of our initial operative attempts were via SISI (147 of 271, 54%); about half of these were converted to either standard laparoscopy or Pfannenstiel incision, resulting in 75 patients (28% of the total cohort, 51% of those started with SISI) completing treatment with

TABLE 2: Reason for change in approach, by initial approach.

Reasons for change	Number of patients SISI : multiport	SISI : Pfannenstiel	Multiport : Pfannenstiel
Oophoropexy	19		
Solid mass	7	16	4
Inability to mobilize adnexa	6		
Large size	4	2	1
Additional procedure	4		
Bleeding	3		
Adhesions	1	1	
Better visualization	3		
No reason given	6		
Total	**53**	**19**	**5**

TABLE 3: Surgical pathology and cytology results.

Pathology	Number of patients ($n = 255$)*	Percentage of cohort	Cytology	Number of patients ($n = 263$)**	Percent of cohort
Simple cyst or serous cystadenoma	84	32.9%	No specimen sent	188	71.5%
Mucinous cystadenoma	9	3.5%	Benign mesothelial, epithelial, mucin-producing, or ciliated tubal cells	41	15.6%
Hemorrhagic follicle	37	14.5%	Degenerated cells	6	2.3%
Ovarian torsion	17	6.7%	Various benign leukocytes	6	2.3%
Normal ovary	2	0.8%	Benign cystic teratoma	1	0.4%
Paratubal or paraovarian cyst	35	13.7%	Mesothelial cells and leukocytes	3	1.1%
Hydrosalpinx	4	1.6%	Red blood cells	10	3.8%
Mature teratoma	55	21.6%	Nondiagnostic (no cells)	7	2.7%
Malignant or premalignant lesion	12	4.7%	Atypical cells	1	0.4%

*For 1 patient no report was available and in 11 operations no specimen was sent.
**In 8 patients no report was available.

the technique. The SISI method was completed in patients ranging in age from 1 day to 19.9 years (median 15.3 years) and with weights from 4.7 to 117 kilograms (median 59.4 kilograms). Reasons for change in approach are delineated in Table 2 and were dominated by desire to perform contralateral oophoropexy or presentation of a solid mass.

Twenty-two patients underwent oophoropexy (8.1% of the total cohort) at the discretion of attending surgeon, usually in the case of residual solitary ovary such as with tumor resection or from contralateral torsion with probable gonadal compromise.

With progression of time, SISI use increased and standard multiport laparoscopy use decreased; successful SISI surgery comprised only 9.3% of all operations in 2008 compared with 34% in 2013, while multiport laparoscopy decreased from 42% to 24% over the same time period. The rate of converted SISI operations was stable at around 25% each year. Successful SISI surgery was significantly shorter than all other approaches (46 mins versus 59 mins for standard laparoscopy, t-test, $p < 0.001$). Length of stay (0.77 days) was shorter in the successful SISI surgery group when compared with standard laparoscopy (0.92 days), but this did not reach statistical significance.

Surgical pathology results are delineated in Table 3. Only 4.7% of the cohort was found to have a malignant or premalignant condition, and these 12 cases are broken down in detail in Table 4. No case of malignant or premalignant lesion was completed with the SISI technique.

Follow-up has ranged from 0 to 72 months (median 14.2 months). Thirty minor complications occurred in 28 patients (11% of operations). SISI converted to Pfannenstiel incision had a significantly higher rate of complications (42%, $p < 0.002$) than either successful SISI (6.7%), SISI converted to multiport laparoscopy (15%), initial multiport laparoscopy (8.2%), or initial Pfannenstiel approach (6.3%). There were no major complications of surgery, although there were five

Table 4: Breakdown of clinical and pathology characteristics of patients with malignant or premalignant lesions (4.7% of total patients).

Patient number	Age (yrs)	Weight (kg)	Timing of operation	Initial operative approach	Final operative approach	Reason for change	OR time (hr:min)	Side of pathology	Reason for operation	Final surgical pathology
3	17.8	105	Urgent	SISI	Multiport laparoscopy	Solid mass	1:51	Right	Hirsutism, solid mass	Sex cord stromal tumor
57	15.5	88.2	Elective	SISI	Multiport laparoscopy	Unable to mobilize	1:31	Right	Cyst > 5 cm	Low grade mucinous tumor of ovary
66	13.9	50	Urgent	Multiport laparoscopy	Multiport laparoscopy	No change	2:10	Left	Pain, solid mass	Yolk sac tumor
99	17.2	48	Urgent	Midline	Midline	No change	1:38	Right	Bowel obstruction, solid mass	Burkitt lymphoma
117	16.7	61	Urgent	Midline	Midline	No change	1:47	Right	Bowel obstruction, solid mass	Dysgerminoma
126	3.8	19.2	Urgent	Midline	Midline	No change	1:05	Right	Pain, solid mass	Sex cord stromal tumor
144	15.2	93	Elective	Midline	Midline	No change	2:15	Right	Ascites, pleural effusions, solid mass	Sex cord stromal tumor
163	14.2	38.7	Elective	Multiport laparoscopy	Multiport laparoscopy	No change	0:55	Bilateral	Turner syndrome, virilization	Dysgenetic gonads
198	11.9	33.5	Urgent	Pfannenstiel	Pfannenstiel	No change	0:33	Left	Cyst > 5 cm, solid mass	Immature teratoma
215	2.9	16.8	Elective	Multiport laparoscopy	Multiport laparoscopy	No change	1:03	Right	Precocious puberty, solid mass	Steroid-producing ovarian tumor
220	14.4	53.6	Urgent	Pfannenstiel	Pfannenstiel	No change	1:08	Left	Cyst > 5 cm	Borderline cystic mucinous tumor
270	8.6	32	Elective	Pfannenstiel	Pfannenstiel	No change	0:59	Left	Solid mass	Immature teratoma

recurrences of benign disease scattered across four of the different surgical techniques, which were all treated with repeat operation. Two deaths occurred in our cohort during long-term follow-up, one due to overwhelming oncologic disease (Burkitt lymphoma) and the second from peritonitis 7 months postoperatively. This was associated with a peritoneal dialysis catheter and unrelated to the ovarian pathology.

In regard to cytologic collection from peritoneal washings or cyst aspiration, 83 of 271 patients in the cohort (31%) had samples generated. In all but one case, the specimen yielded benign or nondiagnostic results. Cytology was sent in only 6 of 12 malignant or premalignant lesions, and a single specimen in a girl with a yolk sac tumor showed atypical cells.

4. Discussion

We report here our series of single-incision, single-instrument (SISI) operations for adnexal pathology in infants, children, and adolescent girls. Our series is the largest reported in the English-language literature to date. We feel our approach is useful as a cost-effective, simple, safe, and cosmetically appealing procedure for treating gynecologic pathology in children. We have gone on to utilize our SISI approach for other pathologies as well, including resection of Meckel diverticulum and duplications, reduction of intussusception, segmental colon resection, treatment of empyema, and extraction of multiple gastric or intestinal tract magnets. We feel this technique is broadly applicable and are continuously looking for new ways to safely limit expenses and improve outcomes with its employment.

One of the major decisions both prior to initiating a SISI approach and once inspecting the pelvic pathology is whether or not there is an immature or cancerous component to the pathology, for avoidance of rupture in these cases may be critical. We have found that the majority of cases can be approached with SISI, as long as the radiology is consistent with benign pathology (i.e., simple appearing cyst without solid component, hemorrhagic cyst, torsion, or solid mass consistent with teratoma based on appearance of fat or calcifications) and the hormonal markers are normal. Any indication of malignancy (peritoneal studding, retroperitoneal lymphadenopathy, noncalcified or highly vascularized solid mass, or elevated hormonal markers) should discourage use of the SISI technique. In these situations, multiport or multi-instrument single-incision laparoscopy (e.g., LESS) can be considered, although the standard is open surgery.

Intraoperatively, additional care must be taken as risk of spill in ovarian malignancy must be avoided with aspiration or attempts at mobilization. Intracorporeal needle decompression or periumbilical mobilization with purse-string evacuation is only undertaken in simple cystic lesions without solid component, unless the lesions are small and mobile enough to extrude easily through the umbilicus. In the present series, it is noteworthy that while malignancy was uncommon, no patient with malignancy was completed with the SISI technique. In cases of suspected malignancy or uncertain pathology, multiport laparoscopy with endobag extraction or Pfannenstiel incision is utilized. This latter option affords the opportunity to extracorporeally attempt the tedious dissection often required to perform an ovarian-sparing procedure while guarding against intra-abdominal rupture in benign but very large tumors such as teratomas. Occasionally, with a very large or clearly malignant tumor, we utilized a midline laparotomy.

Teratomas form an interesting group of neoplasms for which the SISI technique is particularly applicable. Usually mature but occasionally massive, they may be bilateral in 10% of cases [22], whether synchronously or metachronously. We follow these patients for a period of at least 5 years after diagnosis, which allows small, metachronous lesions to be identified early, making ovarian preservation easier. Small ovarian dermoids found during surveillance are easily treated using SISI instrumentation to exteriorize the ovary through the umbilicus for excision.

Based on the data gleaned from our sizable cohort, and contrary to the accepted practice in adult patients, peritoneal washing and/or cyst fluid collection for cytology may be unnecessary when benign disease is suspected. In no case did the results change either the diagnosis or the treatment, while adding a significant cost to the patient's care. Larger studies would be needed before recommending the abandonment of this diagnostic modality, but a prospective, multicenter investigation of cytology in pediatric adnexal pathology would be a fertile area for future investigation.

Limitations of our study include its retrospective and therefore descriptive nature. The conclusions herein are meant to encourage the application of this technique, while recognizing that surgeon judgment will always be principal when considering operative approach. Our report, the largest reported experience to date, reveals that a significant subset of girls with adnexal pathology can undergo successful treatment with the single-incision single-instrument technique, allowing for scarless surgery, minimal discomfort, and same-day discharge. We advocate further implementation of this safe, low-cost, and cosmetically appealing solution to the treatment of pediatric surgical illness.

References

[1] S. Stylianos, L. Nichols, N. Ventura, L. Malvezzi, C. Knight, and C. Burnweit, "The "all-in-one" appendectomy: quick, scarless, and less costly," *Journal of Pediatric Surgery*, vol. 46, no. 12, pp. 2336–2341, 2011.

[2] C. Litz, P. D. Danielson, and N. M. Chandler, "Single incision laparoscopic surgery for pediatric adnexal pathology," *Journal of Pediatric Surgery*, vol. 49, no. 7, pp. 1156–1158, 2014.

[3] M. Lacher, J. F. Kuebler, G. R. Yannam et al., "Single-incision pediatric endosurgery for ovarian pathology," *Journal of Laparoendoscopic and Advanced Surgical Techniques*, vol. 23, no. 3, pp. 291–296, 2013.

[4] O. Ergün, S. Tiryaki, and A. Çelik, "Single center experience in single-incision laparoscopic surgery in children in Turkey," *Journal of Pediatric Surgery*, vol. 46, no. 4, pp. 704–707, 2011.

[5] S. S. Rothenberg, K. Shipman, and S. Yoder, "Experience with modified single-port laparoscopic procedures in children," *Journal of Laparoendoscopic and Advanced Surgical Techniques*, vol. 19, no. 5, pp. 695–698, 2009.

[6] H. Till, R. Wachowiak, U. Waldschmidt, R. Metzger, W. Hirsch, and H. Christiansen, "Single incision laparoscopic surgery (SILS) for ovarian masses (including teratoma) in adolescent girls," *European Journal of Pediatric Surgery*, vol. 20, no. 6, pp. 425–426, 2010.

[7] A. Takeda, S. Imoto, and H. Nakamura, "Management of pediatric and adolescent adnexal masses by gasless laparoendoscopic single-site surgery," *European Journal of Obstetrics Gynecology & Reproductive Biology*, vol. 181, pp. 66–71, 2014.

[8] S. Pérez-Bertólez, M. González, N. de los Reyes, and I. Fernández-Pineda, "Laparoendoscopic single-site ovarian cystectomy and concomitant appendectomy in an adolescent," *Journal of Pediatric and Adolescent Gynecology*, vol. 27, no. 1, pp. e13–e16, 2014.

[9] D. R. Scribner Jr., E. Lara-Torre, and P. M. Weiss, "Single-site laparoscopic management of a large," *Journal of the Society of Laparoendoscopic Surgeons*, vol. 17, no. 2, pp. 350–353, 2013.

[10] A. Fagotti, C. Bottoni, G. Vizzielli et al., "Laparoendoscopic single-site surgery (LESS) for treatment of benign adnexal disease: single-center experience over 3-years," *Journal of Minimally Invasive Gynecology*, vol. 19, no. 6, pp. 695–700, 2012.

[11] S. W. Yi, "Minimally invasive management of huge ovarian cysts by laparoscopic extracorporeal approach," *Minimally Invasive Therapy and Allied Technologies*, vol. 21, no. 6, pp. 429–434, 2012.

[12] W.-C. Kim, K.-S. Im, and Y.-S. Kwon, "Single-port transumbilical laparoscopic-assisted adnexal surgery," *Journal of the Society of Laparoendoscopic Surgeons*, vol. 15, no. 2, pp. 222–227, 2011.

[13] Y.-Y. Lee, T.-J. Kim, C.-J. Kim et al., "Single port access laparoscopic adnexal surgery versus conventional laparoscopic adnexal surgery: a comparison of peri-operative outcomes," *European Journal of Obstetrics Gynecology and Reproductive Biology*, vol. 151, no. 2, pp. 181–184, 2010.

[14] P. F. Escobar, M. A. Bedaiwy, A. N. Fader, and T. Falcone, "Laparoendoscopic single-site (LESS) surgery in patients with benign adnexal disease," *Fertility and Sterility*, vol. 93, no. 6, pp. 2074.e7–2074.e10, 2010.

[15] T. Tajiri, S. Ieiri, Y. Kinoshita, K. Masumoto, Y. Nishimoto, and T. Taguchi, "Transumbilical approach for neonatal surgical diseases: woundless operation," *Pediatric Surgery International*, vol. 24, no. 10, pp. 1123–1126, 2008.

[16] C. Colby, M. Brindle, and R. L. Moss, "Minimally invasive laparotomy for treatment of neonatal ovarian cysts," *Journal of Pediatric Surgery*, vol. 36, no. 6, pp. 868–869, 2001.

[17] L. Schenkman, T. M. Weiner, and J. D. Phillips, "Evolution of the surgical management of neonatal ovarian cysts: laparoscopic-assisted transumbilical extracorporeal ovarian cystectomy (LATEC)," *Journal of Laparoendoscopic and Advanced Surgical Techniques*, vol. 18, no. 4, pp. 635–640, 2008.

[18] J.-Y. Lin, Z.-F. Lee, and Y.-T. Chang, "Transumbilical management for neonatal ovarian cysts," *Journal of Pediatric Surgery*, vol. 42, no. 12, pp. 2136–2139, 2007.

[19] T. Kosumi, A. Kubota, N. Usui, K. Yamauchi, M. Yamasaki, and H. Oyanagi, "Laparoscopic ovarian cystectomy using a single umbilical puncture method," *Surgical Laparoscopy, Endoscopy and Percutaneous Techniques*, vol. 11, no. 1, pp. 63–65, 2001.

[20] S.-Y. Lee, H.-M. Lee, C.-Y. Kao, and J.-H. Chuang, "Transumbilical 1-port laparoscopic resection of benign ovarian tumor," *Journal of Pediatric Surgery*, vol. 47, no. 7, pp. 1340–1344, 2012.

[21] B. S. Rich, J. Creasy, C. Afaneh, and O. J. Muensterer, "The international experience of single-incision pediatric endosurgery: current state of the art," *Journal of Laparoendoscopic and Advanced Surgical Techniques*, vol. 24, no. 1, pp. 43–49, 2014.

[22] I. M. Ehren, G. H. Mahour, and H. Isaacs Jr., "Benign and malignant ovarian tumors in children and adolescents. A review of 63 cases," *The American Journal of Surgery*, vol. 147, no. 3, pp. 339–344, 1984.

15

How to Evaluate Adenomyosis in Patients Affected by Endometriosis?

Nadine Di Donato and Renato Seracchioli

Minimally Invasive Gynaecological Surgery Unit, S. Orsola-Malpighi Hospital, University of Bologna, Via Massarenti 13, 40138 Bologna, Italy

Correspondence should be addressed to Nadine Di Donato; nadine.didonato@gmail.com

Academic Editor: Peng Hui Wang

Objective. The aim of the study is to evaluate adenomyosis in patients undergoing surgery for different type of endometriosis. It is an observational study including women with preoperative ultrasound diagnosis of adenomyosis. Demographic data and symptoms were recorded (age, body mass index, parity, history of previous surgery, dysmenorrhea, dyspareunia, dyschezia, dysuria, and abnormal uterine bleeding). Moreover a particular endometrial shape "question mark sign" linked to the presence of adenomyosis was assessed. *Results.* From 217 patients with ultrasound diagnosis of adenomyosis, we found 73 with ovarian histological confirmation of endometriosis, 92 with deep infiltrating endometriosis, and 52 patients who underwent surgery for infertility. Women with adenomyosis alone represented the oldest group of patients (37.8 ± 5.18 years, $P = 0.02$). Deep endometriosis patients were nulliparous more frequently ($P < 0.0001$), had history of previous surgery ($P = 0.004$), and complained of more intense pain symptoms than other groups. Adenomyosis alone was significantly associated with abnormal uterine bleeding ($P < 0.0001$). The question mark sign was found to be strongly related to posterior deep infiltrating endometriosis ($P = 0.01$). *Conclusion.* Our study confirmed the strong relationship between adenomyosis and endometriosis and evaluated demographic aspects and symptoms in patients affected by different type of endometriosis.

1. Introduction

Adenomyosis is a benign condition of the uterus, defined by the presence of endometrial glands and stroma within the myometrium. It is known as a histological diagnosis but it has a clinical dignity showing symptoms (dysmenorrhea, dyspareunia, abnormal uterine bleeding, and infertility) and sharing some pathogenic mechanisms with endometriosis [1]. Most of the major authors of the first half of the past century dealing with the disease considered pelvic endometriosis and uterine adenomyosis as variants of the same disease process [2, 3]. Also, Sampson (1927), although focusing mainly on the aetiology of the pelvic dissemination of the disease, mentioned uterine adenomyosis and referred to it as "primary endometriosis" [4]. Bazot and colleagues reported that 27% of women with endometriosis had concomitant adenomyosis [5]. Moreover, a 42.76% prevalence of adenomyosis in patients with endometriosis has been recently identified in patients reporting severe or incapacitating dysmenorrhea and deep dyspareunia and in patients with endometriosis of the rectosigmoid [6]. A common pathogenesis for adenomyosis and endometriosis has been hypothesized [7–9] and it was argued that endometrial stroma being in direct contact with the underlying myometrium allows communication and interaction, thus facilitating endometrial invagination or invasion of a structurally weakened myometrium during periods of regeneration, healing, and reepithelization [10]. Mechanical damage [11] to and/or physical disruption of the endometrial-myometrial interface may be due to dysfunctional uterine hyperperistalsis and/or dysfunctional contractility of the subendometrial myometrium.

Finally, considering adenomyosis as consequence of infiltration of basal endometrium into the underlying myometrium [8, 12], a correlation between the stage of endometriosis and the depth of adenomyotic infiltration has been reported [13]. Up to the present, in literature there is a lack of studies evaluating specifically demographic characteristics and symptoms in patients with adenomyosis and different type of endometriosis. In this view, we considered in our paper women with diagnosis of adenomyosis and endometriosis undergoing surgery and we recorded their demographic and clinical characteristics.

2. Materials and Methods

2.1. Design and Patients. For this observational study, ethical approval was obtained from the local ethics committee (198/2013/O/OssN). From January 2010 to December 2012, in the Minimally Invasive Gynecological Surgery Unit of the Department of Gynecology, S. Orsola-Malpighi Hospital, University of Bologna, women with ultrasound diagnosis of adenomyosis and endometriosis undergoing surgery for endometriosis and patients with ultrasound diagnosis of adenomyosis undergoing surgery for infertility were enrolled. Patients were divided according to the type of endometriosis (superficial, ovarian, and deep infiltrating endometriosis). This anatomic classification based on depth of infiltration of endometriotic nodules has been largely accepted by many authors [14, 15]. Deep infiltrating endometriosis was considered as a particular form of endometriosis that penetrates >5 mm under the peritoneal surface [15]. In case more than one condition was found, we considered the more advanced disease to classify women in the three different types of endometriosis. In endometriosis groups, histological confirmation of endometriosis was considered as an inclusion criterion. We excluded women who had previously undergone a hysterectomy, those who were pregnant women, those with malignant gynaecological disease, and those who received hormonal therapy (gonadotropin-releasing hormone agonist, levonorgestrel intrauterine system) in the preceding 3 months before surgery.

The following demographic data and symptoms were recorded: age, body mass index (BMI), history of previous surgery, dysmenorrhea, dyspareunia, dyschezia, dysuria, and abnormal uterine bleeding. The level of patient's discomfort and pain was evaluated by the visual analog scale (VAS) system, utilizing a 10 cm line with the extreme points 0 and 10 corresponding to "no pain" and "maximum pain," respectively. Menstrual bleeding was assessed with the use of the pictorial blood loss assessment chart (PBAC), [16] a validated method used to objectively estimate blood loss; monthly scores range from 0 to more than 500, with higher numbers indicating more bleeding, and menorrhagia was defined as a PBAC > 100 during 1 menstrual period, which corresponds to a blood loss of more than 80 mL.

A transvaginal ultrasound scan was then done before surgery by a single operator (G.M.) and other diagnostic tests, such as magnetic resonance imaging (MRI) and computed tomography (CT), were performed when indicated to evaluate the presence, the localization, and the extension of endometriosis lesions. Sonographic examinations were performed in a systematic manner by a single sonographer, using high-quality ultrasound machine (Voluson S8, GE Milwaukee, WI, USA) equipped with a transvaginal wideband 5.0–9.0 MHz transducer, which ensured a consistent approach to data collection and ultrasound examination. First, the uterus was examined in the longitudinal plane to identify the endometrium. The probe was then rotated 90° anticlockwise and cervical canal and the uterine cavity were visualized in the transverse plane. The myometrium was systematically examined for the sonographic features associated with adenomyosis. Diagnosis of adenomyosis was made when 3 or more of the following sonographic features were present: heterogeneous myometrial echotexture (presence of an indistinctly myometrial area with decreased or increased echogenicity), globular-appearing uterus (regular enlarged uterus), asymmetrical thickness of anteroposterior wall of the myometrium, subendometrial myometrial cysts (round anechoic areas of 1–7 mm diameter), subendometrial echogenic linear striations (radiate pattern of thin acoustic shadowing not arising from echogenic foci), or poor definition of the endometrial-myometrial junction, according to previous studies [17–19].

Moreover, ultrasound diagnosis of endometriosis was made when ovarian endometriomas or endometriotic nodules were visualized. Ovarian cysts were classified as endometriomas when they appeared as well-circumscribed thick-walled cysts that contained homogeneous low-level internal echoes ("ground glass"). Endometriotic nodules were typically visualized as stellate hypoechoic or isoechogenic solid masses with irregular outer margins which were tender on palpation and fixed to the surrounding pelvic structures, as previously described [20–23]. The diagnosis of DIE was made if at least 1 structure in the anterior or posterior compartment showed the presence of retroperitoneal abnormal hypoechoic linear or nodular thickening with irregular contours and no vascular Doppler signals, as described previously and validated ultrasonographic criteria [24, 25]. Locations for DIE in the anterior (bladder) or posterolateral compartment (vagina, rectovaginal septum, torus and uterosacral ligaments, parametria and ureteral involvement, rectum, and rectosigmoid junction) were examined. Concerning ultrasound adenomyosis evaluation, we described and recorded an additional finding which has been observed in our clinical practice. In adenomyosis cases, we identified a particular endometrial shape named *question mark sign ("?")*. The *"?" sign* was considered positive when the endometrium of the uterine fundus was deviated versus the pelvis posterior compartment (Figures 1 and 2).

2.2. Statistical Analysis. We reported means, standard deviations and medians for continuous variables, and frequency counts and percentages for nominal or categorical variables. To assess differences between groups of women, Fisher's exact test generalized for more than two groups was performed for nominal and categorical variables. Continuous data were analyzed with one-way ANOVA and Tukey's post hoc pair wise comparisons for continuous variables. An effect was deemed statistically significant at 0.05. All the analysis was performed with the software SPSS 11.0 software (SPSS Inc., Chicago, IL, USA).

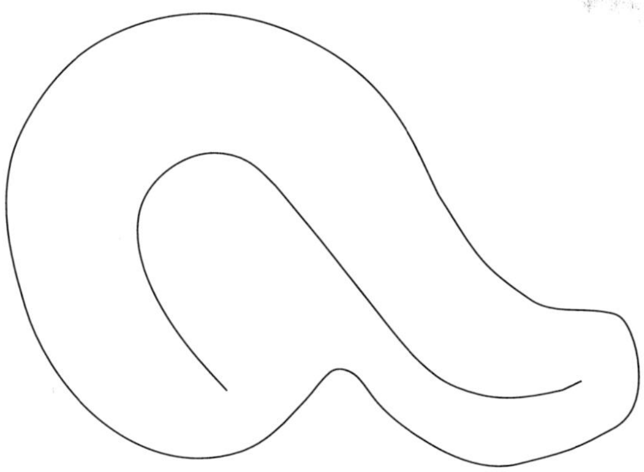

FIGURE 1: Question mark sign.

3. Results

Demographic and clinical characteristics of women included in the study are summarized in Table 1.

A total of 268 women were enrolled. Of the 268 women, 51 were excluded from the data analysis as 21 patients had no histological diagnosis of endometriosis, 26 had intolerance to transvaginal ultrasound examination, and 4 had previously undergone a hysterectomy.

From 217 patients included in the study with ultrasound diagnosis of adenomyosis, we found 66 with ovarian histological confirmation of endometriosis, 92 with DIE, and 52 patients who underwent surgery for infertility. Only seven women were found with superficial endometriosis alone. For the analysis of data, we considered them together with the ovarian group. Nine women during laparoscopic surgery for endometriosis underwent hysterectomy. For all of them adenomyosis diagnosis was histologically confirmed.

Women with adenomyosis alone represented the oldest group of patients (37.8 ± 5.18 years, $P = 0.02$); instead, BMI did not differ between groups. Concerning the characteristics recorded, we found that patients with DIE were nulliparous more frequently than other groups ($P < 0.0001$) and comparing to endometriosis patients (87/92, 94.6% DIE; 54/73, 73.9% ovarian endometriosis), only 27 (27/52 51.9%) women with adenomyosis alone were nulliparous. Moreover, in women with one or more births adenomyosis alone was significantly more frequent than in the others ($P < 0.0001$).

We evaluated the history of previous surgical procedures and we found that women with adenomyosis and DIE had more frequently a history of previous surgery ($P = 0.004$). Regarding symptoms, DIE group complained of more intense pain symptoms (dysmenorrhea, chronic pelvic pain, dyspareunia, dysuria, and dyschezia) than other groups. Moreover, patients with only adenomyosis were more likely to have abnormal uterine bleeding ($P < 0.0001$) (Table 2).

Describing the particular endometrial shape mentioned above, we found a strong relationship between this sonographic sign and adenomyosis associated deep infiltrating endometriosis. It was significantly ($P < 0.0001$) more present in DIE group (34/92 [37%]) than in the others (ovarian 7/73 [9.6%] and adenomyosis alone 4/52 [7.7%]). Specifically, evaluating the different localizations of DIE (anterior and posterior), we reported that it was significantly ($P = 0.01$) associated with posterior deep nodule (23/46 [50%] posterior DIE versus 11/46 [23.9%] anterior DIE).

TABLE 1: Demographic and clinical characteristics of all women included.

Variables	$n = 217$
Age (y) (mean ± SD)	35.3 ± 5.88
BMI (body mass index kg/m^2) (mean ± SD)	22.9 ± 3.57
Parity (N [%])	
0	168 (77.4%)
≥1	49 (22.6%)
Endometriosis (N [%])	
Adenomyosis alone	52 (24%)
Ovarian	73 (33.6%)
DIE	92 (42.4%)
Symptoms	
Dysmenorrhea (mean ± SD)	6.49 ± 3.26
Chronic pelvic pain (mean ± SD)	2.94 ± 3.45
Dyspareunia (mean ± SD)	3.03 ± 3.36
Dysuria (mean ± SD)	0.67 ± 2.05
Dyschezia (mean ± SD)	2.02 ± 3.31
Abnormal uterine bleeding (N [%])	49 (22.6%)

4. Discussion

Today, several authors have described the association between adenomyosis and endometriosis, particularly DIE [26–28]. In a prospective study Kissler et al. found that severe dysmenorrhea of long duration in patients with endometriosis is significantly related to uterine adenomyosis [27]. Moreover, Larsen et al. found a correlation between the severity of endometriosis and the degree of uterine adenomyosis and Gonzalez et al. found again a correlation between uterine adenomyosis and deep endometriosis with poor prognosis, particularly endometriosis of the recto-sigmoid [6]. In our study, we evaluated clinical and demographic characteristics related to adenomyosis in patients undergoing surgery for different type of endometriosis. We identified a particular endometrial shape associated with adenomyosis and we named this specific endometrial finding "*question mark sign*." The endometrium was deviated versus the pelvis posterior compartment from the fundus to the cervix. Moreover, we reported that the question mark sign was strongly related to the presence of posterior deep infiltrating endometriosis.

Therefore, it is interesting to look for this endometrial sign during the preoperative ultrasound evaluation in the way to facilitate the diagnosis of both posterior deep infiltrating endometriosis and adenomyosis. Probably, the uterus is deviated by the nodule in the posterior compartment of the pelvis changing the normal endometrial shape. Commonly, endometriosis nodules have the capacity to attract structures around the pelvis. Moreover, from literature, the posterior

TABLE 2: Demographic and clinical characteristics in the different patient groups.

Variables	DIE + adenomyosis (92)	Ovarian + adenomyosis (73)	Adenomyosis alone (52)	*P* value
Age (y) (mean ± SD)	34.4 ± 5.34	34.7 ± 6.36	37.8 ± 5.18	$P = 0.021$
BMI	22.6 ± 3.87	23.2 ± 3.81	23.0 ± 2.54	$P = 0.541$
Parity (*N* [%])				
0	87 (94.6%)	54 (73.9%)	27 (51.9%)	$P < 0.0001$
≥1	5 (5.4%)	19 (26.1%)	25 (48.1%)	$P < 0.0001$
History of previous surgery (≥1)	26 (28.3%)	26 (35.6%)	5 (9.6%)	$P = 0.004$
Symptoms				
Dysmenorrhea (mean ± SD)	7.04 ± 3.47	6.00 ± 3.46	6.21 ± 2.39	$P = 0.096$
Chronic pelvic pain (mean ± SD)	3.79 ± 3.58	2.83 ± 3.55	1.59 ± 2.54	$P = 0.001$
Dyspareunia (mean ± SD)	3.47 ± 3.54	3.35 ± 3.64	1.84 ± 2.15	$P = 0.013$
Dysuria (mean ± SD)	1.84 ± 2.15	0.50 ± 1.70	1.18 ± 2.68	$P = 0.002$
Dyschezia (mean ± SD)	3.32 ± 3.86	1.83 ± 2.98	0.01 ± 0.01	$P < 0.0001$
Abnormal uterine bleeding (*N* [%])	5 (5.4%)	23 (31.5%)	21 (40.4%)	$P < 0.0001$

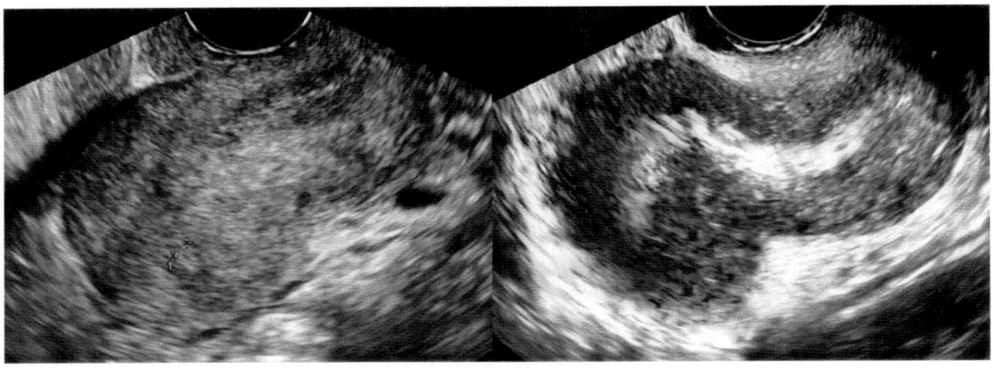

FIGURE 2: Ultrasound image of question mark sign.

wall of the uterus was predominantly affected by adenomyosis [29, 30]. However, no data are available that show an increased mechanical stress of the posterior uterine wall due to chronic uterine peristalsis and hyperperistalsis and a relationship of the site of predilection of adenomyosis with ante- or retroflection of the uterus [29, 30]. There is indirect evidence of an archimetral hyperestrogenism in women with endometriosis that interferes with the ovarian control of uterine peristaltic activity resulting in uterine hyperperistalsis [31, 32]. Moreover, it was argued that endometrial stroma being in direct contact with the underlying myometrium allows communication and interaction, thus facilitating endometrial invagination or invasion of a structurally weakened myometrium during periods of regeneration, healing, and reepithelization [10, 11].

From our results, we found that patients with DIE and adenomyosis were nulliparous more frequently and complained of more intense pain symptoms (dysmenorrhea, chronic pelvic pain, dyspareunia, dysuria, and dyschezia) than other groups with the exception of abnormal uterine bleeding which was complained by the majority of women with only adenomyosis. Heavy bleeding may be positively related to the depth of penetration of individual adenomyotic glands into the myometrium and to the density of deep endometrial glands within the myometrium [33].

In concordance with previous clinical evidence, we found that a high percentage of women with adenomyosis were multiparous [11, 18, 34, 35]. Instead, patients affected by endometriosis are frequently associated with infertility because of anatomical and immunological alterations caused by endometriosis. Generally, endometriosis is common in women with subfertility and can affect fertility at different level, from the induction of a local inflammation and decrease in endometrial receptivity to mechanical obstruction and altered sexual function [36].

There are some potential mechanisms associated with parity and adenomyosis pathology. First, pregnancy might facilitate formation of adenomyosis by allowing adenomyotic foci to be included in the myometrium due to the invasive nature of the trophoblast on the extension of myometrial fibers. Second, the possibility of Cesarean section may lead to iatrogenic adenomyosis [11, 37]. Third, the hormonal milieu of pregnancy may favour the development of islands of ectopic endometrium [38]. A recent review in 2013 defined a number of factors that encourage the development of adenomyosis (spontaneous miscarriage, curettage, hysteroscopic resection of the endometrium, uterine myomectomy, caesarean section, and taking Tamoxifen) and underlined that the main factor is having had more than one pregnancy [39]. In agreement with our data, Shrestha found that the frequency of adenomyosis was higher in parous women in comparison with nulliparous [40]. Moreover, Vercellini and colleagues suggested that parity may be associated with an increased frequency of adenomyosis [38]. Other studies reported the same relationship between parity and adenomyosis [34, 41].

Concerning symptoms, DIE is the most severe form of endometriosis, associated with infertility or pain symptoms, including chronic pelvic pain, dysmenorrhea, dyspareunia, dysuria, and dyschezia [42]. Nowadays, it is clarified that there is an overlap in the symptom complexes of both endometriosis and adenomyosis. In endometriosis, the presence of adenomyosis is found to be a risk factor for dysmenorrhea severity [6]. As described before, dysmenorrhea increases with greater depth of penetration of the adenomyotic process and to the density of deep endometrial glands into myometrium [43]; instead dyspareunia and chronic pain are not considered constant symptoms in patients with adenomyosis [5, 44]. Lazzeri and colleagues showed a persistence of dyspareunia in women after surgery for DIE when adenomyosis was present [45]. Another study reported pain recurrence in DIE, despite the radicality of the surgery [46]. Consequently, a correct counselling about pain recurrence is required in case of coexistence of both pathological entities. Surgery for posterior DIE with coexistence of adenomyosis could be not resolved for postoperative pain relief because of adenomyosis persistence. This information allows the chance of a correct counselling before surgery and should help to develop more effective treatment strategies in women affected by DIE and adenomyosis.

The strength of our study is the large number of women with endometriosis histologically confirmed and that it was conducted in a tertiary care university hospital, by clinicians highly skilled in endometriosis management. Moreover, sonographic examinations were performed in a systematic manner by a single sonographer, using high-quality ultrasound machine. The present study has also major limitations. First, the lack of histological confirmation of adenomyosis for the majority of patients included. However, recently transvaginal ultrasound has reached a high level of accuracy and many authors have reported the high agreement between ultrasound diagnosis of adenomyosis and histological findings [17, 47]. A recent review [48] reported that transvaginal ultrasound should be the primary tool for the diagnosis of adenomyosis, with MRI being used when transvaginal ultrasound is inconclusive or when large fibroids are present. Secondly, being patients included in the study with a mean age of 35 years old, it can be a possible bias for evaluation of the natural history of adenomyosis pathology. Since the adenomyotic nodules communicate with the uterine cavity, pathophysiologically a continuous process from initial to deep infiltration must exist. Authors reported that endometriosis-associated adenomyosis progresses with age [13, 49].

In conclusion, our data confirmed the strong relationship between adenomyosis and endometriosis and evaluated demographic aspects and symptoms in patients affected by different type of endometriosis. Our findings suggest that adenomyosis and endometriosis share same symptoms with important difference linked to the type of endometriosis and help to better understand the endometriosis-adenomyosis relationship and their associated factors.

References

[1] G. Leyendecker, L. Wildt, and G. Mall, "The pathophysiology of endometriosis and adenomyosis: tissue injury and repair," *Archives of Gynecology and Obstetrics*, vol. 280, no. 4, pp. 529–538, 2009.

[2] R. Meyer, "Über den stand der frage der adenomyositis und adenomyome im allgemeinen und insbesondere über adenomyositis seroepithelialis und adenomyometritis sarcomatosa," *Zentralbl Gynäkol*, vol. 36, pp. 745–750, 1919.

[3] T. S. Cullen, "The distribution of adenomyoma containing uterine mucosa," *Archives of Surgery*, vol. 1, pp. 215–283, 1920.

[4] J. A. Sampson, "Peritoneal endometriosis due to the menstrual dissemination of endometrial tissue into the peritoneal cavity," *American Journal of Obstetrics & Gynecology*, vol. 14, pp. 422–429, 1927.

[5] M. Bazot, O. Fiori, and E. Darai, "Adenomyosis in endometriosis—prevalence and impact on fertility. Evidence from magnetic resonance imaging," *Human Reproduction*, vol. 21, no. 4, pp. 1101–1102, 2006.

[6] M. Gonzales, L. A. de Matos, M. O. D. C. Gonçalves et al., "Patients with adenomyosis are more likely to have deep endometriosis," *Gynecological Surgery*, vol. 9, no. 3, pp. 259–264, 2012.

[7] G. Leyendecker, M. Herbertz, G. Kunz, and G. Mall, "Endometriosis results from the dislocation of basal endometrium," *Human Reproduction*, vol. 17, no. 10, pp. 2725–2736, 2002.

[8] G. Leyendecker, G. Kunz, M. Noe, M. Herbertz, and G. Mall, "Endometriosis: a dysfunction and disease of the archimetra," *Human Reproduction Update*, vol. 4, no. 5, pp. 752–762, 1998.

[9] G. Leyendecker, G. Kunz, L. Wildt, D. Beil, and H. Deininger, "Uterine hyperperistalsis and dysperistalsis as dysfunctions of the mechanism of rapid sperm transport in patients with endometriosis and infertility," *Human Reproduction*, vol. 11, no. 7, pp. 1542–1551, 1996.

[10] A. Ferenczy, "Pathophysiology of adenomyosis," *Human Reproduction Update*, vol. 4, no. 4, pp. 312–322, 1998.

[11] M. Levgur, M. A. Abadi, and A. Tucker, "Adenomyosis: symptoms, histology, and pregnancy terminations," *Obstetrics & Gynecology*, vol. 95, no. 5, pp. 688–691, 2000.

[12] M. Noe, G. Kunz, M. Herbertz, G. Mall, and G. Leyendecker, "The cyclic pattern of the immunocytochemical expression of oestrogen and progesterone receptors in human myometrial and endometrial layers: characterisation of the endometrial-subendometrial unit," *Human Reproduction*, vol. 14, no. 1, pp. 190–197, 1999.

[13] G. Kunz, D. Beil, P. Huppert, M. Noe, S. Kissler, and G. Leyendecker, "Adenomyosis in endometriosis—prevalence and impact on fertility: evidence from magnetic resonance imaging," *Human Reproduction*, vol. 20, no. 8, pp. 2309–2316, 2005.

[14] RCOG, "The investigation and management of endometriosis guideline," no. 24, 2006.

[15] P. Vercellini, L. Fedele, G. Aimi, G. Pietropaolo, D. Consonni, and P. G. Crosignani, "Association between endometriosis stage, lesion type, patient characteristics and severity of pelvic pain symptoms: a multivariate analysis of over 1000 patients," *Human Reproduction*, vol. 22, no. 1, pp. 266–271, 2007.

[16] J. M. Higham, P. M. S. O'Brien, and R. W. Shaw, "Assessment of menstrual blood loss using a pictorial chart," *British Journal of Obstetrics and Gynaecology*, vol. 97, no. 8, pp. 734–739, 1990.

[17] J. Naftalin, W. Hoo, K. Pateman, D. Mavrelos, T. Holland, and D. Jurkovic, "How common is adenomyosis? A prospective study of prevalence using transvaginal ultrasound in a gynaecology clinic," *Human Reproduction*, vol. 27, no. 12, pp. 3432–3439, 2012.

[18] T. Bergholt, L. Eriksen, N. Berendt, M. Jacobsen, and J. B. Hertz, "Prevalence and risk factors of adenomyosis at hysterectomy," *Human Reproduction*, vol. 16, no. 11, pp. 2418–2421, 2001.

[19] C. Reinhold, S. McCarthy, P. M. Bret et al., "Diffuse adenomyosis: comparison of endovaginal US and MR imaging with histopathologic correlation," *Radiology*, vol. 199, no. 1, pp. 151–158, 1996.

[20] L. Savelli, "Transvaginal sonography for the assessment of ovarian and pelvic endometriosis: how deep is our understanding?" *Ultrasound in Obstetrics and Gynecology*, vol. 33, no. 5, pp. 497–501, 2009.

[21] C. Exacoustos, E. Zupi, C. Carusotti et al., "Staging of pelvic endometriosis: role of sonographic appearance in determining extension of disease and modulating surgical approach," *The Journal of the American Association of Gynecologic Laparoscopists*, vol. 10, no. 3, pp. 378–382, 2003.

[22] L. Savelli, L. Manuzzi, P. Pollastri, M. Mabrouk, R. Seracchioli, and S. Venturoli, "Diagnostic accuracy and potential limitations of transvaginal sonography for bladder endometriosis," *Ultrasound in Obstetrics and Gynecology*, vol. 34, no. 5, pp. 595–600, 2009.

[23] L. Savelli, L. Manuzzi, M. Coe et al., "Comparison of transvaginal sonography and double-contrast barium enema for diagnosing deep infiltrating endometriosis of the posterior compartment," *Ultrasound in Obstetrics and Gynecology*, vol. 38, no. 4, pp. 466–471, 2011.

[24] O. Yeniel, T. Cirpan, M. Ulukus et al., "Adenomyosis: Prevalence, risk factors, symptoms and clinical findings," *Clinical and Experimental Obstetrics and Gynecology*, vol. 34, no. 3, pp. 163–167, 2007.

[25] F. Parazzini, V. Mais, S. Cipriani, M. Busacca, and P. Venturini, "Determinants of adenomyosis in women who underwent hysterectomy for benign gynecological conditions: results from a prospective multicentric study in Italy," *European Journal of Obstetrics Gynecology and Reproductive Biology*, vol. 143, no. 2, pp. 103–106, 2009.

[26] I. Brosens, G. Kunz, and G. Benagiano, "Is adenomyosis the neglected phenotype of an endomyometrial dysfunction syndrome?" *Gynecological Surgery*, vol. 9, no. 2, pp. 131–137, 2012.

[27] S. Kissler, S. Zangos, J. Kohl et al., "Duration of dysmenorrhoea and extent of adenomyosis visualised by magnetic resonance imaging," *European Journal of Obstetrics Gynecology and Reproductive Biology*, vol. 137, no. 2, pp. 204–209, 2008.

[28] S. B. Larsen, E. Lundorf, A. Forman, and M. Dueholm, "Adenomyosis and junctional zone changes in patients with endometriosis," *European Journal of Obstetrics Gynecology and Reproductive Biology*, vol. 157, no. 2, pp. 206–211, 2011.

[29] O. Käser, V. O. Friedberg, K. Ober, K. Thomsen, and E. Plotz, "Endometriose," in *Gynäkologie und Geburtshilfe Band III*, Thieme, Stuttgart, Germany, 1972.

[30] E. R. Novak and J. D. Woodruff, *Gynecologic and Obstetric Pathology*, W.B. Saunders Company, Philadelphia, Pa, USA, 8th edition, 1979.

[31] K. Takahashi, H. Nagata, and M. Kitao, "Clinical usefulness of determination of estradiol level in the menstrual blood for patients with endometriosis," *Acta Obstetrica et Gynaecologica Japonica*, vol. 41, no. 11, pp. 1849–1850, 1989.

[32] Y. Absenger, H. Hess-Stumpp, B. Kreft et al., "Cyr61, a deregulated gene in endometriosis," *Molecular Human Reproduction*, vol. 10, no. 6, pp. 399–407, 2004.

[33] M. G. Munro, H. O. Critchley, I. S. Fraser, and FIGO Menstrual Disorders Working Group, "The FIGO classification of causes of abnormal uterine bleeding in the reproductive years," *Fertility and Sterility*, vol. 95, no. 7, pp. 2204.e3–2208.e3, 2011.

[34] F. Parazzini, P. Vercellini, S. Panazza, L. Chatenoud, S. Oldani, and P. G. Crosignani, "Risk factors for adenomyosis," *Human Reproduction*, vol. 12, no. 6, pp. 1275–1279, 1997.

[35] C. Templeman, S. F. Marshall, G. Ursin et al., "Adenomyosis and endometriosis in the California Teachers Study," *Fertility and Sterility*, vol. 90, no. 2, pp. 415–424, 2008.

[36] C. Zeng, J. N. Xu, Y. Zhou, Y. F. Zhou, S. N. Zhu, and Q. Xue, "Reproductive performance after surgery for endometriosis: predictive value of the revised American Fertility Society classification and the endometriosis fertility index," *Gynecologic and Obstetric Investigation*, vol. 77, no. 3, pp. 180–185, 2014.

[37] U. R. Panganamamula, O. H. Harmanli, E. F. Isik-Akbay, C. A. Grotegut, V. Dandolu, and J. P. Gaughan, "Is prior uterine surgery a risk factor for adenomyosis?" *Obstetrics & Gynecology*, vol. 104, no. 5 I, pp. 1034–1038, 2004.

[38] P. Vercellini, P. Viganò, E. Somigliana, R. Daguati, A. Abbiati, and L. Fedele, "Adenomyosis: epidemiological factors," *Best Practice and Research: Clinical Obstetrics and Gynaecology*, vol. 20, no. 4, pp. 465–477, 2006.

[39] C. Tomassetti, C. Meuleman, D. Timmerman, and T. D'Hooghe, "Adenomyosis and subfertility: evidence of association and causation," *Seminars in Reproductive Medicine*, vol. 31, no. 2, pp. 101–108, 2013.

[40] A. Shrestha, "Risk factors for adenomyosis," *Journal of Nepal Health Research Council*, vol. 10, no. 22, pp. 229–233, 2012.

[41] D. Vavilis, T. Agorastos, J. Tzafetas et al., "Adenomyosis at hysterectomy: prevalence and relationship to operative findings and reproductive and menstrual factors," *Clinical and Experimental Obstetrics and Gynecology*, vol. 24, no. 1, pp. 36–38, 1997.

[42] P. R. Koninckx, A. Ussia, L. Adamyan, A. Wattiez, and J. Donnez, "Deep endometriosis: definition, diagnosis, and treatment," *Fertility and Sterility*, vol. 98, no. 3, pp. 564–571, 2012.

[43] C. C. Bird, T. W. McElin, and P. Manalo-Estrella, "The elusive adenomyosis of the uterus-revisited," *American Journal of Obstetrics and Gynecology*, vol. 112, no. 5, pp. 583–593, 1972.

[44] H. Peric and I. S. Fraser, "The symptomatology of adenomyosis," *Best Practice and Research: Clinical Obstetrics and Gynaecology*, vol. 20, no. 4, pp. 547–555, 2006.

[45] L. Lazzeri, A. Di Giovanni, C. Exacoustos et al., "Preoperative and postoperative clinical and transvaginal ultrasound findings of adenomyosis in patients with deep infiltrating endometriosis," vol. 21, no. 8, pp. 1027–1033, 2014.

[46] S. Ferrero, G. Camerini, M. V. Menada, E. Biscaldi, N. Ragni, and V. Remorgida, "Uterine adenomyosis in persistence of dysmenorrhea after surgical excision of pelvic endometriosis and colorectal resection," *Journal of Reproductive Medicine for the Obstetrician and Gynecologist*, vol. 54, no. 6, pp. 366–372, 2009.

[47] M. Dueholm, E. Lundorf, E. S. Hansen, J. S. Sorensen, S. Ledertoug, and F. Olesen, "Magnetic resonance imaging and transvaginal ultrasonography for the diagnosis of adenomyosis," *Fertility and Sterility*, vol. 76, no. 3, pp. 588–594, 2001.

[48] M. Dueholm, "Transvaginal ultrasound for diagnosis of adenomyosis: a review," *Best Practice and Research: Clinical Obstetrics and Gynaecology*, vol. 20, no. 4, pp. 569–582, 2006.

[49] B. Kunz, D. Beil, P. Huppert, and G. Leyendecker, "Structural abnormalities of the uterine wall in women with endometriosis and infertility visualized by vaginal sonography and magnetic resonance imaging," *Human Reproduction*, vol. 15, no. 1, pp. 76–82, 2000.

16

Short Hospital Stay after Laparoscopic Colorectal Surgery without Fast Track

Stefan K. Burgdorf and Jacob Rosenberg

Department of Surgical Gastroenterology, Herlev Hospital, University of Copenhagen, Herlev Ringvej 75, 2730 Herlev, Denmark

Correspondence should be addressed to Stefan K. Burgdorf, stefan@stefanburgdorf.dk

Academic Editor: Peng Hui Wang

Purpose. Short hospital stay and equal or reduced complication rates have been demonstrated after fast track open colonic surgery. However, fast track principles of perioperative care can be difficult to implement and often require increased nursing staff because of more concentrated nursing tasks during the shorter hospital stay. Specific data on nursing requirements after laparoscopic surgery are lacking. The purpose of the study was to evaluate the effect of operative technique (open versus laparoscopic operation), but without changing nurse staffing or principles for peri- or postoperative care, that is, without implementing fast track principles, on length of stay after colorectal resection for cancer. *Methods.* Records of all patients operated for colorectal cancer from November 2004 to December 2008 in our department were reviewed. No specific patients were selected for laparoscopic repair, which was solely dependent on the presence of two specific surgeons at the same time. Thus, the patients were not selected for laparoscopic repair based on patient-related factors, but only on the simultaneous presence of two specific surgeons on the day of the operation. *Results.* Of a total of 540 included patients, 213 (39%) were operated by a laparoscopic approach. The median hospital stay for patients with a primary anastomosis was significantly shorter after laparoscopic than after conventional open surgery (5 versus 8 days, $P < 0.001$) while there was no difference in patients receiving a stoma (10 versus 10 days, ns), with no changes in the perioperative care regimens. Furthermore there were significant lower blood loss (50 versus 200 mL, $P < 0.001$) and lower complication rate (21% versus 32%, $P = 0.006$) in the laparoscopic group. *Conclusion.* Implementing laparoscopic colorectal surgery in our department resulted in shorter hospital stay without using fast track principles for peri- and postoperative care in patients not receiving a stoma during the operation. Consequently, we aimed to reduce hospitalisation without increasing cost in nursing staff per hospital bed. Length of stay was not reduced in patients receiving a stoma pointing at this group for specific intervention in the future. Furthermore, the complication rate was reduced in the laparoscopic group.

1. Introduction

Colorectal cancer (CRC) is a common disease in the western world. Even though therapies like radio-, chemo- and newer immune-therapies have evolved and improved during the last decades, the prognosis for end-stage disease is still poor and surgery remains the only curative therapy [1]. Prognosis associated with CRC have improved due to earlier detection of malignancy, better and more radical surgical techniques and more effective adjuvant therapies, but there is still room for improvement.

Short hospital stay and equal or reduced complication rates have been demonstrated after fast track open colonic surgery [2]. Fast track principles of peri- and postoperative care, however, often require some changes in the surgical departments. As a consequence of more concentrated nursing tasks during the shorter hospital stay, increased nursing requirements per bed is required [3]. Implementation of these major changes has in many cases been problematic and unsuccessful [4]. However, in a gynaecological department enhanced recovery has been introduced without compromising the workload of the nurse staffing [5].

Laparoscopic colectomy was first reported by Jacobs et al. in 1991 [6] and since then minimally invasive gastrointestinal surgery has become more popular. The surgical trauma from laparoscopic surgery is significantly reduced compared with conventional open surgery. In spite of obvious advantages in laparoscopic surgery there is still an ongoing debate on complication rates, hospitalisation, nurse staff requirements, blood loss, radicality, conversion rate, learning curve and implementation difficulties, mortality, and overall survival in minimally invasive techniques compared with conventional open techniques [7]. Most studies have shown shorter hospitalisation for patients undergoing laparoscopic colonic surgery compared with open colonic surgery, but most of the available studies have either not been formally controlled randomised studies or not controlling perioperative care regimens. However, a recent randomised controlled 9-center trial concludes that the optimal perioperative treatment after segmental colectomy is laparoscopic approach in a fast track setting [7]. Data on nursing requirements after laparoscopic surgery are lacking. Therefore, possibly by only changing the operative procedure, a shorter hospitalisation may be obtained after laparoscopic surgery, without changing nurse staffing or principles for perioperative care, that is, without implementing fast track surgery principles.

The aim of this paper was to show the effect of laparoscopic surgery per se on hospital stay and complication rates after colonic and rectal resections in a retrospective controlled study in a setting where nurse staffing was not changed, but only changing the surgical procedures to a minimally invasive approach.

2. Methods

2.1. Patients. From the first laparoscopic operation in November 2004 through December 2008, 213 patients underwent laparoscopic and 327 patients underwent open surgery for CRC in the Department of Surgical Gastroenterology, Gentofte University Hospital, Copenhagen, Denmark. No specific patients were selected for laparoscopic repair, which was only dependent on the presence of two specific surgeons that both had to be working on the same day. If these two surgeons were available then the operation was laparoscopic and if not it was open. Thus, the selection procedure was based on logistics and not on patient factors. If possible for logistic reasons the patients were offered laparoscopic approach. Records of all patients going through colonic and/or rectal resections in the study period were reviewed. Only patients with verified colonic or rectal carcinomas who underwent elective surgery were included in this study.

The patients were all admitted to the same surgical department. Regardless of surgical approach they all received the same peri- and postoperative care by the same nurse staffing and the same doctors were doing the ward rounds. Fast track principles of peri- and postoperative care had not been implemented in the department. No certain criteria were used for discharge but was solely based on the doctors doing the ward rounds and was not dependent on the surgical approach.

2.2. Data Collection. All patient records were reviewed and all data extracted independently by two researchers and if inconsistencies consensus were made. The data retained from the patient records were demographics: sex, age, height, weight, and the American Society of Anaesthesiology (ASA) class; and parameters related to the operation: diagnosis, date of operation, primary anastomosis or stoma, blood loss, number of resected lymph nodes, and eventually conversion to open technique; and postoperative parameters: complications and duration of postoperative hospitalisation.

Since the study is a descriptive retrospective study neither consent nor ethical approval was obtained. This is in accordance with Danish law.

2.3. Implementation Setup. The surgeons in our department had experience with laparoscopic appendectomy, cholecystectomy, and hernia repair but most of these surgeons had little or no experience with surgery of the colon and rectum. The colorectal surgeons in our department had limited knowledge about it and very little experience in minimally invasive procedures. One colorectal surgeon (limited laparoscopic experience) was introduced to laparoscopic techniques and performed the operations with the experienced laparoscopist (limited experience in colorectal surgery) as an assistant. The only selection of patients for laparoscopic procedure was that these two surgeons had to be working on the day of the operation. If these two surgeons were present, the patient scheduled for operation that day underwent laparoscopic repair.

2.4. Statistical Analysis. A database with all relevant data was created in Microsoft Excel 2002 (Microsoft corp., USA). Statistical analyses were run on SPSS software version 15.0 (SPSS Inc., Chicago, USA). Differences between subgroups were analysed with the Mann-Witney or Fisher's Exact test where appropriate and $P \leq 0.05$ was considered statistically significant.

3. Results

A total of 540 patients were included in the study. The proportion of patients undergoing laparoscopic surgery was 39% (213/540). A comparison of the 213 laparoscopically treated patients with the 327 patients treated with conventional open surgery is shown in Table 1. Length of hospital stay was significantly shorter for patients going through laparoscopic surgery compared to open surgery (5 versus 8 days, $P < 0.001$). Numbers of the different surgical procedures are shown in Table 2. When comparing the open and laparoscopic groups there was no significant difference in sex, ASA class, and number of harvested lymph nodes.

Overall, the patients were equally distributed between men and women with a median age of 72 years (range 36–94 years) and a mean BMI of 23.7 kg/m^2 (range 13.9–42.3 kg/m^2). Most of the patients (78%) were given a primary anastomosis, while the rest received a temporary or permanent stoma. No 30-day mortality occurred in the laparoscopic cohort, but one patient died before discharge, 38 days after the primary operation after anastomosis leakage, open reoperation, abscesses, and finally lung edema. The patients in the laparoscopic group were significantly younger (70 versus 72 years, $P = 0.02$) and had a higher BMI (23.9 versus 23.4 kg/m^2, $P = 0.02$).

Table 1: Comparison of the 213 laparoscopic-treated patients with 327 patients treated with conventional open procedure in the same period (November 2004–December 2008) in our department.

Parameter	Laparoscopic procedure $n = 213$	Conventional open procedure $n = 327$	P value
Sex (male/female)	114/99	158/169	ns
Age (years, median (range))	70 (36–94)	72 (36–92)	0.002
BMI (kg/m^2, median (range))	23.9 (16.4–42.3)	23.4 (13.9–36.0)	0.023
ASA class (%)			
I	32 (16)	34 (11)	
II	145 (70)	218 (69)	ns
III	30 (15)	62 (20)	
IV	0 (0)	3 (1)	
Blood loss (mL, median (range))	50 (0–1600)	200 (0–2700)	<0.001
Number of patients with a primary anastomosis (%)	184 (86)	237 (72)	ns
Number of lymph nodes in resection (median (range))	15 (2–50)	15 (1–75)	ns
Hospital stay (days, median (range))			
With stoma	10 (5–24)	10 (5–14)	ns
With primary anastomosis	4 (1–55)	8 (2–109)	<0.001
Total	5 (1–55)	8 (2–109)	<0.001
Clavien-Dindo Classification of Surgical complications (%)			
No complications	168 (79)	223 (68)	0.006
Grade I	7 (3)	14 (4)	
Grade II	9 (4)	32 (10)	
Grade III-a	2 (1)	3 (1)	
Grade III-b	24 (11)	35 (11)	
Grade IV-a	2 (1)	3 (1)	
Grade IV-b	0 (0)	0 (0)	
Grade V	1 (0)	17 (5)	
Dukes classification (%)			
Dukes A	14 (7)	24 (7)	
Dukes B	106 (50)	148 (45)	
Dukes C	59 (28)	93 (28)	
Dukes D	28 (13)	47 (14)	
Not classified	6 (3)	15 (5)	

BMI: body mass index, ASA: American Society of Anaesthesiology, ns: nonsignificant ($P > 0.05$).

With regard to perioperative differences, the laparoscopic group had significantly lower blood loss (50 versus 200 mL, $P < 0.001$) and equal proportion of primary anastomoses (86% versus 72%, ns). Postoperative comparison showed significantly lower complication rates (Table 1, $P = 0.006$) in the laparoscopic group. Complications were graded according to the Clavien-Dindo Classification of Surgical Complications [8]. Finally, the analyses of postoperative hospitalisation showed no difference between the two groups for the patients who received a stoma (10 versus 10 days, ns), but a significant difference in the larger subgroup of patients with primary anastomoses (4 versus 8 days, $P < 0.001$). These differences are also shown graphically in Figure 1.

When comparing the laparoscopically treated patients who were given a stoma with those who received a primary anastomosis there was no significant difference in age (71 versus 69 years, $P = 0.74$), BMI (25.9 versus 23.6 kg/m^2, $P = 0.17$), blood loss (175 versus 100 mL, $P = 0.54$), or number of resected lymph nodes (14 versus 15, $P = 0.08$), but the patients with a stoma had significantly longer postoperative hospital stay compared with the patients not receiving a stoma (10 versus 4 days, $P = 0.001$). There were no significant differences in age ($P = 0.47$), blood loss ($P = 0.28$), number of resected lymph nodes ($P = 0.58$), and postoperative hospital stay ($P = 0.91$) between the male and female patients in the laparoscopic group.

4. Discussion

This retrospective controlled study showed shorter hospital stay and lower complication rates after laparoscopic CRC surgery compared with conventional open surgery. The reduction in postoperative hospital stay was achieved without implementing any changes in the surgical ward regarding fast track principles for perioperative care. Thus, we were

Table 2: Operative procedures.

Operative procedure	n (%)
Laparoscopic (n = 213)	
Sigmoid resection	72 (34)
Sigmoid resection with stoma	2 (1)
Left hemicolectomy	17 (8)
Right hemicolectomy	40 (19)
Transversum resection	2 (1)
Low anterior rectal resection	47 (22)
Low anterior resection with stoma	9 (4)
Hartmanns procedure	9 (4)
Abdominoperineal resection	6 (3)
Colectomy	3 (1)
Other	6 (3)
Open (n = 327)	
Sigmoid resection	27 (8)
Sigmoid resection with stoma	2 (1)
Left hemicolectomy	30 (9)
Left hemicolectomy with stoma	1 (0)
Right hemicolectomy	143 (44)
Transversum resection	4 (1)
Colectomy	7 (2)
Low anterior rectal resection	25 (8)
Low anterior resection with stoma	13 (4)
Hartmanns procedure	53 (16)
Abdominoperineal resection	14 (4)
Other	8 (2)

able to reduce hospitalisation without increasing nursing staff per hospital bed.

The setup with a colorectal surgeon without laparoscopic experience assisted by a laparoscopically experienced "upper" GI surgeon was simple and successful. With a median postoperative hospital stay of 5 days, median 15 lymph nodes in the specimens, and 79% of cases without complications, we were able to produce results comparable with, or even better than our nationwide data [9, 10] and large multicentre controlled trials [11–18].

Since the present results arise from a retrospective controlled study and not from a randomised controlled trial, and since the number of surgical procedures performed in the laparoscopic and open group is noncomparable, these results should be interpreted with caution. Nevertheless, they do indicate some of the advantages in laparoscopic CRC surgery and signify that laparoscopic CRC surgery may not be restricted to young and fit patients with low BMI and no comorbidities (low ASA class).

We reported a quite high mortality rate in the conventional open group. Some of the patients in the conventional open group died of reasons not directly related to the surgery, but the exact reasons were not reported and as a consequence the high incidence cannot be explained.

The large randomised controlled trials all confirm that laparoscopy has a positive impact on postoperative restitution with earlier recovery of bowel function, less need for postoperative analgesics, and shorter postoperative hospital stay compared with conventional open surgery [12–20]. A prospective database study by Abraham et al. [20] resulted in the same short-term conclusions and even suggested lower operative mortality rates and better 3-year survival for patients treated laparoscopically. The benefits for long-term outcomes have not been confirmed in large randomised controlled trials [11–14, 17–19] which have shown no significant differences in operative mortality and long-term survival between laparoscopic and open surgery. Though for patients with Dukes D cancer laparoscopy has resulted in better survival than open surgery [19]. The effect of laparoscopy on mortality and survival is therefore, in spite of solid evidence on short-term outcomes, still questionable. All of the studies have, like the present, shown equal, or even better, lymph node harvesting with laparoscopic technique [22]. A more complete lymph node resection would theoretically improve long-term outcomes, but this has not been documented yet. A recent study has shown that the postoperative immune function remains highest in patients undergoing laparoscopic surgery with fast track care [23].

Several studies have dealt with the aspect of learning difficulties in laparoscopic colonic and rectal resections [24–28]. The surgical procedures are technically difficult, but with previous laparoscopic experience from appendectomies, cholecystectomies, and hernia repair the learning curve is not differing from that of conventional open colorectal surgery [25]. A theory could be that older surgeons initially may have difficulties in seeing 3-dimensional structures on a 2-dimensional screen, while younger upcoming surgeons have grown up with this from for example, computer games [29]. Most studies defined learning curves from intraoperative complications, rate of conversion to open surgery, and eventually number of harvested lymph nodes and operating time. Adequate learning occurred after 5–80 interventions [24–28, 30]. The reasons for the wide spread in these results could be that the studies were based on a few surgeons and these results are of course very much dependent on the skills of the specific surgeon. In one study with three surgeons the time for adequate learning ranged from 5–17 interventions [24]. Based on these studies and our own experiences we believe that laparoscopic colonic and rectal resections can be learned as quickly, effectively, and safely as conventional open resections.

5. Conclusion

Implementing laparoscopic colonic and rectal resection for colorectal malignancies in our department resulted, for patients with primary anastomoses, in shorter hospital stay compared with conventional open surgical technique. The implementation of laparoscopic colorectal surgery was done without implementing fast track principles for perioperative care. This study confirms that laparoscopic CRC surgery can be implemented successfully. The short-term outcomes after laparoscopic CRC surgery are superior to conventional open surgery. The long-term effects have to be confirmed in large randomised controlled trials, but do not seem worse than

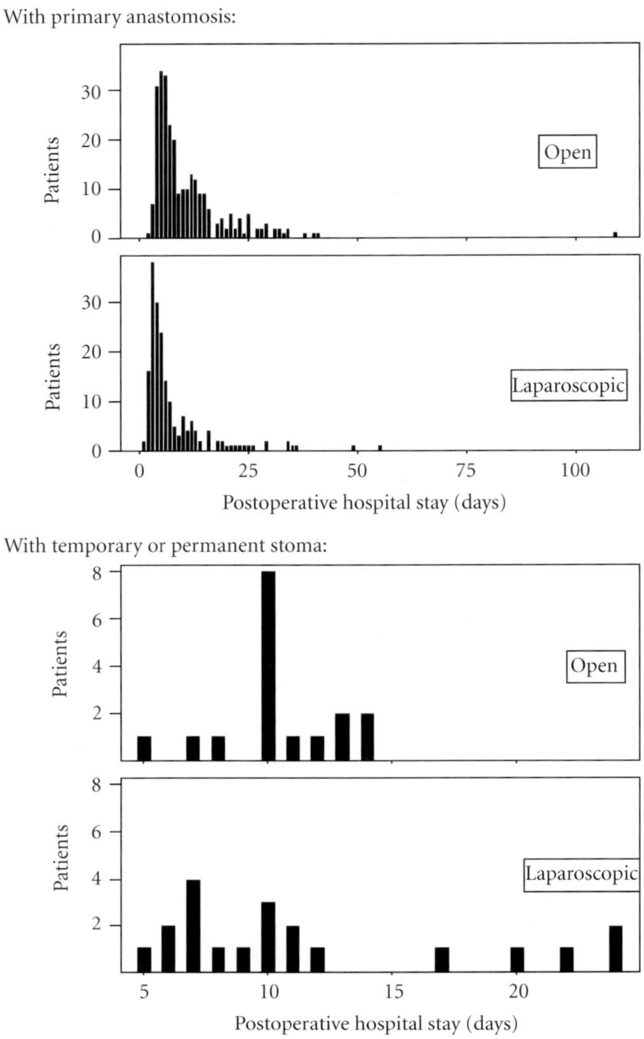

FIGURE 1: Histogram showing the frequencies of days of postoperative hospital stay after laparoscopic versus conventional open colonic and rectal resections for colorectal malignancies for patients with a stoma and for patients with primary anastomosis. For patients with a stoma there was no significant difference in postoperative hospital stay between laparoscopic and open surgery (median 10 versus 10 days, ns). For patients with primary anastomosis the median postoperative hospitalisation was significantly shorter (4 versus 8 days, $P < 0.001$) after laparoscopic repair.

after open repair. A part of our success with laparoscopic repair concerning length of hospital stay could theoretically be patient, surgeon, or nursing staff biased. Therefore, future studies should evaluate the effect of laparoscopic versus open surgery in a blinded trial and without implementing fast track principles for perioperative care.

Authors' Contribution

J. Rosenberg and S. K. Burgdorf carried out the data collection. J. Rosenberg and S. K. Burgdorf designed the study. S. K. Burgdorf performed the statistical analyses. S. K. Burgdorf drafted the manuscript. Both authors read and approved the final paper.

References

[1] S. K. Burgdorf, H. J. Nielsen, and J. Rosenberg, "Immunotherapy in colorectal cancer," *Scandinavian Journal of Gastroenterology*, vol. 44, no. 3, pp. 261–268, 2009.

[2] H. Kehlet, "Fast-track colorectal surgery," *The Lancet*, vol. 371, no. 9615, pp. 791–793, 2008.

[3] D. H. Jakobsen, E. Sonne, and H. Kehlet, "Nursing workload and fast track colonic surgery," *Journal of Advanced Perioperative Care*, vol. 2, no. 4, pp. 177–181, 2006.

[4] H. Kehlet, M. W. Büchler, R. W. Beart, R. P. Billingham, and R. Williamson, "Care after colonic operation—is it evidence-based? Results from a multinational survey in Europe and the United States," *Journal of the American College of Surgeons*, vol. 202, no. 1, pp. 45–54, 2006.

[5] I. S. Sjetne, U. Krogstad, S. Ødegård, and M. E. Engh, "Improving quality by introducing enhanced recovery after surgery in a gynaecological department: consequences for ward nursing practice," *Quality and Safety in Health Care*, vol. 18, no. 3, pp. 236–240, 2009.

[6] M. Jacobs, J. C. Verdeja, and H. S. Goldstein, "Minimally invasive colon resection (laparoscopic colectomy)," *Surgical Laparoscopy & Endoscopy*, vol. 1, no. 3, pp. 144–150, 1991.

[7] M. S. Vlug, J. Wind, M. W. Hollmann et al., "Laparoscopy in combination with fast track multimodal management is the best perioperative strategy in patients undergoing colonic surgery: a randomized clinical trial (LAFA-study)," *Annals of Surgery*, vol. 254, pp. 868–875, 2011.

[8] D. Dindo, N. Demartines, and P. A. Clavien, "Classification of surgical complications: a new proposal with evaluation in a cohort of 6336 patients and results of a survey," *Annals of Surgery*, vol. 240, no. 2, pp. 205–213, 2004.

[9] Annual report 2007-2008, "Nationwide database for colorectal cancer," DCCG 2009, http://www.dccg.dk/03_Publikation/02_arsraport_pdf/revideret_aarsrapport_2007_2009.pdf.

[10] S. Schulze, M. G. Iversen, A. Bendixen, T. S. Larsen, and H. Kehlet, "Laparoscopic colonic surgery in Denmark 2004–2007," *Colorectal Disease*, vol. 10, no. 9, pp. 869–872, 2008.

[11] E. Kuhry, W. Schwenk, R. Gaupset, U. Romild, and J. Bonjer, "Long-term outcome of laparoscopic surgery for colorectal cancer: a cochrane systematic review of randomised controlled trials," *Cancer Treatment Reviews*, vol. 34, no. 6, pp. 498–504, 2008.

[12] H. Nelson, D. J. Sargent, H. S. Wieand et al., "A comparison of laparoscopically assisted and open colectomy for colon cancer," *New England Journal of Medicine*, vol. 350, no. 20, pp. 2050–2059, 2004.

[13] P. J. Guillou, P. Quirke, H. Thorpe et al., "Short-term endpoints of conventional versus laparoscopic-assisted surgery in patients with colorectal cancer (MRC CLASICC trial): multicentre, randomised controlled trial," *The Lancet*, vol. 365, no. 9472, pp. 1718–1726, 2005.

[14] R. Veldkamp, E. Kuhry, A. van Buuren et al., "Laparoscopic surgery versus open surgery for colon cancer: short-term outcomes of a randomised trial," *Lancet Oncology*, vol. 6, no. 7, pp. 477–484, 2005.

[15] W. Schwenk, O. Haase, J. Neudecker, and J. M. Müller, "Short term benefits for laparoscopic colorectal resection," *Cochrane Database of Systematic Reviews*, no. 3, Article ID CD003145, 2005.

[16] M. S. Vlug, J. Wind, E. van der Zaag, D. T. Ubbink, H. A. Cense, and W. A. Bemelman, "Systematic review of laparoscopic vs open colonic surgery within an enhanced recovery programme," *Colorectal Disease*, vol. 11, no. 4, pp. 335–343, 2009.

[17] M. Buunen, R. Veldkamp, W. C. Hop et al., "Survival after laparoscopic surgery versus open surgery for colon cancer: long-term outcome of a randomised clinical trial," *The Lancet Oncology*, vol. 10, no. 1, pp. 44–52, 2009.

[18] G. D. McKay, M. J. Morgan, S.-K. C. Wong et al., "Improved short-term outcomes of laparoscopic versus open resection for colon and rectal cancer in an area health service: a multicenter study," *Diseases of the Colon and Rectum*, vol. 55, no. 1, pp. 42–50, 2012.

[19] A. M. Lacy, J. C. García-Valdecasas, S. Delgado et al., "Laparoscopy-assisted colectomy versus open colectomy for treatment of non-metastatic colon cancer: a randomised trial," *The Lancet*, vol. 359, no. 9325, pp. 2224–2229, 2002.

[20] N. S. Abraham, J. M. Young, and M. J. Solomon, "Meta-analysis of short-term outcomes after laparoscopic resection for colorectal cancer," *British Journal of Surgery*, vol. 91, no. 9, pp. 1111–1124, 2004.

[21] W. L. Law, Y. M. Lee, H. K. Choi, C. L. Seto, and J. W. C. Ho, "Impact of laparoscopic resection for colorectal cancer on operative outcomes and survival," *Annals of Surgery*, vol. 245, no. 1, pp. 1–7, 2007.

[22] R. C. Wright, C. A. Kim, I. Horner, and R. Wright, "Superior lymph node resection is achievable with laparoscopic colectomy: even in initial 30 cases," *American Surgeon*, vol. 74, no. 3, pp. 243–249, 2008.

[23] A. A. F. A. Veenhof, M. S. Vlug, M. H. G. M. Van Der Pas et al., "Surgical stress response and postoperative immune function after laparoscopy or open surgery with fast track or standard perioperative care: a randomized trial," *Annals of Surgery*, vol. 255, no. 2, pp. 216–221, 2012.

[24] D. H. Choi, W. K. Jeong, S. W. Lim et al., "Learning curves for laparoscopic sigmoidectomy used to manage curable sigmoid colon cancer: single-institute, three-surgeon experience," *Surgical Endoscopy and Other Interventional Techniques*, vol. 23, no. 3, pp. 622–628, 2009.

[25] L. Boni, M. Di Giuseppe, C. Bertoglio et al., "Preliminary results of laparoscopic colorectal resections: does surgeon's age influences outcomes?" *Surgical Oncology*, vol. 16, supplement 1, pp. 57–60, 2007.

[26] J. Kim, E. Edwards, W. Bowne et al., "Medial-to-lateral laparoscopic colon resection: a view beyond the learning curve," *Surgical Endoscopy and Other Interventional Techniques*, vol. 21, no. 9, pp. 1503–1507, 2007.

[27] D. J. Reichenbach, A. D. Tackett, J. Harris et al., "Laparoscopic colon resection early in the learning curve: what is the appropriate setting?" *Annals of Surgery*, vol. 243, no. 6, pp. 730–735, 2006.

[28] C. M. Schlachta, J. Mamazza, P. A. Seshadri, M. Cadeddu, R. Gregoire, and E. C. Poulin, "Defining a learning curve for laparoscopic colorectal resections," *Diseases of the Colon and Rectum*, vol. 44, no. 2, pp. 217–222, 2001.

[29] T. P. Grantcharov, L. Bardram, P. Funch-Jensen, and J. Rosenberg, "Impact of hand dominance, gender, and experience with computer games on performance in virtual reality laparoscopy," *Surgical Endoscopy and Other Interventional Techniques*, vol. 17, no. 7, pp. 1082–1085, 2003.

[30] S. Dinçler, M. T. Koller, J. Steurer et al., "Multidimensional analysis of learning curves in laparoscopic sigmoid resection: eight-year results," *Diseases of the Colon and Rectum*, vol. 46, no. 10, pp. 1371–1379, 2003.

17

How Predictable Is the Operative Time of Laparoscopic Surgery for Ovarian Endometrioma?

Pietro Gambadauro,[1,2] Vincenzo Campo,[2] and Sebastiano Campo[2]

[1]*Karolinska Institutet, LIME/NASP-C7, 17177 Stockholm, Sweden*
[2]*Department of Obstetrics and Gynaecology, Catholic University of the Sacred Heart, Largo A. Gemelli 8, 00168 Rome, Italy*

Correspondence should be addressed to Pietro Gambadauro; gambadauro@gmail.com

Academic Editor: Peng Hui Wang

Endometriosis is a tricky albeit common disease whose management largely relies on laparoscopy. We have studied the operative times of laparoscopic endometrioma surgery in order to assess their predictability and possible predictors. One hundred forty-eight laparoscopies were included, with a median operative time of 70 minutes (mean 75.14; 95% CI: 70.03–80.24). Half of the cases had a duration within 15–20 minutes above or below the median (IQR: 55–93.75), but the whole dataset ranged from 20 to 180 minutes, and the standard deviation was relatively large (31.4). Surgical times were significantly related to technical (number and size of the cysts) and nontechnical factors (age, parity, dysmenorrhea, and family history). At multiple logistic regression, after adjusting for number and size of the cysts, surgical times below the first quartile were associated with older age (>30 years old: aOR: 3.590; 95% CI: 1.417–9.091) and parity (≥1 delivery: aOR: 3.409; 95% CI: 1.343–8.651). Longer times, above the third quartile, were instead predicted by a familial anamnesis of endometriosis (aOR: 3.639; 95% CI: 1.246–10.627). Our findings indicate highly variable surgical times, which are predicted by unexpected nontechnical factors. This is consistent with the complexity of endometriosis and its treatment. Productivity and efficiency in endometriosis surgery should focus on the quality of healthcare outcomes rather than on the time spent in the operating theatres.

1. Introduction

Endometriosis is a tricky albeit common disease whose management still largely relies on laparoscopic surgery [1]. Surgical excision of ovarian endometrioma has positive effects on pain and on the chances of spontaneous conception in subfertile women [2]. However, endometrioma surgery is complicated by concerns about recurrence and ovarian reserve as well as by a relative lack of knowledge on the pathophysiology of the disease [3, 4].

Surgery also represents a major cost for public healthcare because of the valuable human, technical, and logistic resources needed to operate on any single patient. Frequently, the cost profile of surgery in public funded healthcare is also worsened by cascading factors such as delays, cancellations, and long waiting lists [5]. Therefore, the usage of the operating theatre (OT) is often under the spotlight of decision-makers [6]. In spite of evidence that a great proportion of the OT time is lost on nonsurgical activities [7, 8], most surgeons have probably felt the pressure to finish a procedure at the planned time, victims of the belief that operative times are predictable. Our need for certainty makes it difficult to question the often wrong but somehow necessary prediction of surgical procedures duration, which is the basis for OT daily planning [9].

Surgeons are naturally major determinants of surgical times, but no perfect predictive tool exists. In gynecological surgery, different operations require different times, but variability in the duration of the same intervention is also common [10]. Laparoscopic surgery for endometriosis, apart from being often advanced, is peculiar because of a double nature, diagnostic and operative. In fact, see-and-treat interventions can be considered the norm rather than an exception. Ovarian endometriomas, for instance, are typically diagnosed at ultrasound but they often coexist with adhesions and peritoneal implants which can only be seen at laparoscopy. Technical and anatomical factors are usually considered responsible for the duration of surgery, but it would clearly be interesting to know if and how the duration of endometriosis surgery is predictable.

In this study, we have analyzed the distribution of operative times from a series of laparoscopic removals of ovarian endometrioma, with a focus on possible predictive factors.

2. Materials and Methods

We performed an analysis of operative times from a database including 148 cases of laparoscopic removal of ovarian endometriomas at the Department of Obstetrics and Gynecology of the Catholic University of the Sacred Heart, Rome, Italy. Our database was created for a study on endometrioma recurrence published by our group in 2014 [11]. Only elective cases of laparoscopic excision of histologically confirmed endometriomas ≥2 cm in diameter were included, while cases with deep endometriosis were excluded. The cystectomy was always performed by means of laparoscopic stripping of the cystic capsule after careful identification of the cleavage plane. Laparoscopy was performed under the care of one experienced laparoscopic surgeon (SC) and in a standardized fashion, as elsewhere described by Campo et al. [11]. All patients gave their informed consent in written form preoperatively.

In order to identify factors affecting the length of surgery, skin-to-skin operative times were analysed statistically together with other anonymized data. The distribution of operative times was first analyzed by descriptive statistics. Operative times were then evaluated in bivariate analysis together with several anamnestic and clinicosurgical variables. Correlation between surgical time and continuous variables such as age, BMI, cysts number, and largest diameter (cm) was studied by Spearman's rho. Association between categorical variables and surgical time was assessed by Mann-Whitney *U* test or Kruskal-Wallis one-way analysis of variance. Variables of epidemiological and anamnestic interest included dysmenorrhea, parity (≥1 delivery), infertility, and family history of endometriosis. The following categorical variables of technical interest were also considered: cyst number (single/multiple); cyst size (largest diameter ≤5 cm/>5 cm); cyst location (right/left/bilateral); peritoneal implants and adhesions; and intraoperative spillage of cystic contents.

Furthermore, we aimed at identifying factors that could be associated with procedures which are either shorter or longer than the expected time according to measures of central tendency, such as the median. Hence, we divided the cases into three groups depending on surgical times. The reference group consisted of cases with a surgical time comprised within the first and the third quartiles (Q1–Q3), while the other two groups consisted of cases, respectively, below the first quartile (<Q1) and above the third quartile (>Q3). Separate comparisons between the reference group and the other two groups were carried out by Mann-Whitney *U* test for continuous variables and chi-square test or Fisher's exact test for categorical variables. Postoperative hospital stay and complications were compared among the groups in a similar fashion. Variables showing a significant association with surgical times in the previous analyses ($p < 0.05$) were considered for simple and multiple logistic regression analyses. Crude and adjusted odds ratios (OR and aOR), with 95% confidence intervals (CI), were calculated to express the strength of associations between selected variables and surgical times. A p value of less than 0.05 was considered statistically significant. The statistical analysis was performed with SPSS Statistics (IBM) for Mac OSX and manually.

3. Results

One hundred forty-eight laparoscopic surgeries for ovarian endometrioma were included in analysis. No conversion to laparotomy was recorded. The median operative time was 70 minutes (mean: 75.14; 95% CI: 70.03–80.24). However, analysis of the distribution showed a high dispersion of the data. While 50% of the cases had a surgical time within 15–20 minutes above or below the median (interquartile range, IQR: 55–93.75), the whole dataset ranged from 20 to 180 minutes, and the standard deviation was relatively large (31.4).

When analyzing the entire dataset (Table 1), no significant correlation was found between surgical times and age, BMI, and cystic diameter. Instead, the surgical time was significantly and positively correlated with the number of cysts ($r = 0.202$; $p = 0.014$). The median surgical time was significantly longer when multiple rather than single cysts were removed (77.50 versus 70 minutes; $p = 0.021$). Anamnestic factors such as dysmenorrhea and nulliparity were also significantly associated with longer operative times. The operative time was not significantly affected by cyst location, adhesions, peritoneal implants, spillage, or infertility.

The cases were divided into three groups as previously described (Table 2). The reference group, serving as control, included 78 cases with an operative time ranging from the first quartile to the third quartile of the series (median: 70 minutes; IQR: 60–80). A short time group (<Q1) included 33 cases with a median of 40 minutes, while the long time group (>Q3) consisted of 37 cases with a median of 115 minutes. Compared to the reference group, women in the short time group were significantly older (median age: 34 versus 30; $p = 0.018$), and their cysts were more frequently single (87.9% versus 69.2%; $p = 0.039$) and smaller than 5 cm (87.9% versus 62.8%; $p = 0.008$). Significantly less women in the short time group were nulliparous but the number of infertile patients was similar in both groups. No differences were found in adhesions and peritoneal implants rate, but the absence of spillage was associated with shorter times (69.7% versus 44.9%; $p = 0.017$).

No statistically significant differences were found between the reference group and the longer operative time group except for a positive family history of endometriosis. Twenty-seven percent of women in the long time group had a family history of endometriosis compared to 8.9% in the reference group (10/37 versus 7/78; $p = 0.011$).

Crude odds ratios, with 95% confidence intervals and p values, describing the strength of association between

Table 1: Factors affecting the operative time of laparoscopic surgery for ovarian endometrioma.

Variables		p value
Continuous variables	Spearman's rho	
Age	−0.113	0.172
BMI	0.066	0.425
Number of cysts	0.202	0.014
Largest diameter	0.084	0.309
Categorical variables	Operative time[a]	
Dysmenorrhea		
Yes (97)	75 (60–97.5)	0.038
No (51)	65 (40–90)	
Parity		
Yes (42)	60 (40–82.5)	0.020
No (106)	75 (60–95)	
Infertility		
Yes (35)	70 (60–90)	0.606
No (113)	70 (55–95)	
Positive family history		
Yes (20)	92.5 (56.25–110)	0.120
No (128)	70 (55–90)	
Cyst location		
Right (44)	60 (46.25–95)	0.258[b]
Left (73)	75 (50–90)	
Bilateral (31)	75 (60–100)	
Bilateral cysts[c]		
Yes (31)	75 (60–100)	0.570
No (13)	95 (57.5–115)	
Adhesions		
Yes (100)	72.5 (55–95)	0.093
No (48)	60 (45–90)	
Peritoneal implants		
Yes (62)	70 (55–91.25)	0.719
No (86)	70 (55–95)	
Spillage		
Yes (68)	72.5 (56.25–90)	0.564
No (80)	70 (45–95)	

[a]Operative times, in minutes, are presented as medians and interquartile range (IQR).
Comparisons for categorical variables were by Mann-Whitney U test.
[b]Calculated with Kruskal-Wallis test.
[c]Calculated only for cases with multiple cysts.

selected variables and operative times, respectively, shorter and longer than the reference group (Q1–Q3) are presented in Table 3.

A multiple logistic regression analysis, adjusting for the number and size of the removed cysts, identified older age and parity as independent predictors of shorter operative times (Table 4). Longer operations were instead significantly associated with a positive familial anamnesis (aOR: 3.639; 95% CI: 1.246–10.627; $p = 0.018$).

Finally, while shorter operative times did not appear to improve short-term postoperative outcomes, belonging to the long operative time group was associated with a significantly longer postoperative hospital stay (>1 day for 35.1% of patients versus 15.4% in the reference group; $p = 0.016$) and a nonsignificantly higher postoperative complication rate (5.4% versus 0% in the reference group).

4. Discussion and Conclusions

Surgery, as a tool to treat medical conditions and improve quality of life, is invaluable. At the same time, costly operating theatres are a natural target of efficiency improving efforts [12].

In our study, we analysed the operative times of laparoscopic surgery for endometrioma in order to evaluate to what extent they are predictable. Since historical data and the surgeon's expert judgement are, in combination, the most common predictive approach, we focused on their respective assumptions: a limited variation of operative times and adequate knowledge of predicting factors.

Various conclusions can be drawn from our results. The first one is the fact that the time needed to perform a laparoscopic removal of ovarian endometrioma is highly variable and, as such, difficult to predict by simply looking at historical data. This might sound familiar to endometriosis surgeons, but similar findings have rarely been described by dedicated scientific studies [10]. Although half of the cases will last something within 15 minutes above or below the median time, a large proportion of the patients will have surgical times which are 50% or more shorter or longer. Endometriosis is certainly a complex disease, and this may reflect on the variability of operative times. Nevertheless, the cases in our study were quite homogeneous, since we only included patients with ovarian endometriomas ≥2 cm but excluded cases with elsewhere located deep endometriosis. Moreover, all the cases were performed under the care of an experienced laparoscopic surgeon, with a standardized stripping technique, and at the same institution, which is a reference centre for the treatment of endometriosis. Those conditions reduce the risk of performance bias, which is not uncommon in surgical research [13, 14].

A peculiarity of our study lies in the attempt to identify predictors of surgical duration for laparoscopic endometrioma surgery. Operative times are correlated to some of the surgical factors that we have analyzed, such as number and size of the cysts. However, other factors that might be considered to increase the surgical difficulty and to require additional time, such as adhesions and peritoneal implants, were not associated with a longer duration of the procedures. On the contrary, nontechnical factors such as age, parity, and family history were significantly associated with operative times. This further confirms the peculiar nature of endometriosis whose clinical manifestations and behavior change from patient to patient depending on factors so far largely unknown. For instance, the association of shorter times with older age or parity could be linked to a milder disease. Similarly, a positive family history for endometriosis, which we found to be associated with higher endometrioma

TABLE 2: Comparison between groups of cases with shorter, average, and longer operative time.

	Short time group <Q1	Reference group Q1–Q3	Long time group >Q3
Number of cases	33	78	37
Operative time (min)	40 (30–45)	70 (60–80)	115 (100–132.50)
Continuous variables			
Age (years)	34 (28.50–43)[a]	30 (27–35)	30 (25–37.50)
Number of cysts	1 (1-1)[a]	1 (1-2)	1 (1-2)
Largest diameter (cm)	4.0 (3.0–5.0)[b]	5.0 (4.0–6.0)	5.0 (3.0–6.75)
Categorical variables			
Older age (>30)	23 (69.7)[c]	36 (46.2)	18 (48.6)
Single cyst	29 (87.9)[c]	54 (69.2)	21 (56.8)
Small cysts (≤5 cm)	29 (87.9)[c]	49 (62.8)	23 (62.2)
Dysmenorrhea	17 (51.5)	52 (66.7)	28 (75.7)
Parity (≥1)	15 (45.5)[c]	18 (23.1)	9 (24.3)
Infertility	7 (21.2)	20 (25.6)	8 (21.6)
Positive family history	3 (9.1)	7 (9)	10 (27)[c]
Cyst location			
Right	12 (36.4)	19 (24.3)	13 (35.1)
Left	19 (57.6)	39 (50)	15 (40.5)
Bilateral	2 (6.1)	20 (25.6)	9 (24.3)
Bilateral cysts[d]	2 (50)[d]	20 (83.3)[d]	9 (56.3)[d]
Adhesions	20 (60.6)	52 (66.7)	28 (75.7)
Peritoneal implants	13 (39.4)	34 (43.6)	15 (40.5)
Spillage	10 (30.3)[c]	43 (55.1)	15 (40.5)
Hospital stay > 1 day	6 (18.2)	12 (15.4)	13 (35.1)[c]
Complications	0 (0)	0 (0)	2 (5.4)

Values are given as medians (IQR) for continuous variables or n (%) for categorical variables.
Short time and long time groups have been, respectively, compared with the reference group. All differences are nonsignificant ($p \geq 0.05$) except for [a]$p < 0.05$ at Mann-Whitney U test, [b]$p < 0.01$ at Mann-Whitney U test, and [c]$p < 0.05$ at chi-square test.
[d]Calculated only for cases with multiple cysts.

TABLE 3: Factors associated with shorter or longer duration of laparoscopic surgery for ovarian endometrioma.

Variables	Shorter time <Q1			Longer time >Q3		
	OR	95% CI	p value	OR	95% CI	p value
Older age (>30)	2.683	1.129–6.377	0.025	1.105	0.505–2.419	0.802
Dysmenorrhea	0.531	0.232–1.217	0.531	1.556	0.641–3.774	0.329
Parity (≥1)	2.778	1.170–6.592	0.021	1.071	0.428–2.681	0.883
Positive family history	1.014	0.246–4.189	0.984	3.757	1.298–10.872	0.015
Single cyst (versus multiple)	3.222	1.020–10.183	0.046	0.583	0.260–1.310	0.192
Small cyst (≤5 cm)	4.291	1.370–13.440	0.012	0.972	0.434–2.180	0.946
Spillage	0.354	0.149–0.841	0.019	0.555	0.251–1.227	0.146

Crude odds ratios, with 95% confidence intervals and p values, describing the strength of association between selected variables and operative times, respectively, shorter and longer than the reference group (Q1–Q3).

recurrence rates [11], could be linked to a more severe disease and hence longer operative times.

Finally, shorter operative times do not seem to ensure short-term benefits in terms of postoperative stay or complications. This might depend on the fact that the overall operative times in this series were relatively low because of the team experience. On the other hand, patients whose surgical time was above the third quartile had a significantly longer postoperative stay, and the two postoperative complications of this series were found in this group. These findings cannot directly support a causal relationship and are limited by the sample size and a lack of controlling

Table 4: Nontechnical predictors of shorter and longer duration of laparoscopic surgery for ovarian endometrioma.

Variables	Shorter time <Q1			Longer time >Q3		
	aOR	95% CI	p value	aOR	95% CI	p value
Older age (>30)	3.590	1.417–9.091	0.007	1.009	0.453–2.249	0.983
Parity	3.409	1.343–8.651	0.010	1.031	0.408–2.605	0.948
Family history	1.304	0.298–5.707	0.724	3.639	1.246–10.627	0.018

Multinomial logistic regression analyses where the reference category of the dependent variable grouped laparoscopies with a surgical time between the first and third quartiles (Q1–Q3).
aOR: the odds ratios are adjusted for number of cysts (single/multiple) and largest diameter (≤5 versus >5 cm).

for possible confounders. However, they can be useful to formulate hypotheses on how to identify cases at risk at the time of surgery, allowing for tailored postoperative care planning.

Overall, our study highlights a new facet of the complexity of endometriosis and partially explains why it is difficult to predict operative times. The duration of laparoscopy is known to be less predictable than laparotomy [15], and this applies to different laparoscopic procedures [10]. Laparoscopy in endometriosis patients has a diagnostic value and often leads to see-and-treat management of unexpected findings [1]. Hence, strict time schedules are not convenient for endometriosis since they can lead to suboptimal surgery.

Besides, the heterogeneity of endometriosis seems to reflect also on the severity of the disease, for which we are still probably lacking important knowledge and a reliable staging system. Similar lesions, such as ovarian endometriomas, have variable pathological and clinical behaviors in different women [16], thus leading to surgical difficulty of unpredictable level or, as we have previously documented, different rates of recurrence [11].

Should we give up the efforts of making the operating theatre a more efficient place? Surely we should not do this, although proper targets should be identified.

To believe that surgical times, for any given operation, are standard and predictable according to historical measurements of central tendency such as the median, although tempting, is fallacious. The idea of standard procedures with standard times might satisfy our innate need for certainty and is also functional to other aspects of surgical planning, such as allocating instruments and staff [9]. However, because of the great dispersion of surgical times around the average values, scheduling according to historical averages is based on probability [9, 17]. The surgeons themselves, unfortunately, do not seem to be able to provide a more accurate estimate of operative times [18].

In this context, it would be reasonable to integrate predictive methods, based on historical data and the surgeon's estimate, with knowledge of the inevitable variability in operative time [19]. Measuring and adapting to the variability in surgical durations should be a key process of modern operating theatre management.

At the same time, efforts should be made in order to minimize the consequences to the patients and optimize resources' usage in other ways. On one hand, patient turnover could be improved by monitoring the time needed by standard perioperative procedures and activities [7, 8, 20]. On the other hand, we should maybe rethink our context where productivity is increasingly measured in number of procedures rather than in health outcomes, particularly in the case of such complex disease. Probably, the care of endometriosis patients should be provided by centres where the underlying production philosophy is mature enough to shift from a simplistic focus on quantity to a more refined demanding, but certainly patient-centered, interest for quality.

Acknowledgment

This study was based at the Institute of Obstetrics and Gynecology, Catholic University of the Sacred Heart, Rome, Italy.

References

[1] C. Farquhar, "Endometriosis," *British Medical Journal*, vol. 334, no. 7587, pp. 249–253, 2007.

[2] R. J. Hart, M. Hickey, P. Maouris, and W. Buckett, "Excisional surgery versus ablative surgery for ovarian endometriomata.," *Cochrane Database of Systematic Reviews*, no. 2, Article ID CD004992, 2008.

[3] T. A. Gelbaya and L. G. Nardo, "Evidence-based management of endometrioma," *Reproductive BioMedicine Online*, vol. 23, no. 1, pp. 15–24, 2011.

[4] I. Brosens, S. Gordts, P. Puttemans, and G. Benagiano, "Pathophysiology proposed as the basis for modern management of the ovarian endometrioma," *Reproductive BioMedicine Online*, vol. 28, no. 2, pp. 232–238, 2014.

[5] Audit Commission, *Operating Theatres: Review of National Findings*, HMSO, London, UK, 2003, http://webarchive.nationalarchives.gov.uk/20150220144004/http://archive.audit-commission.gov.uk/auditcommission/subwebs/publications/studies/studyPDF/3023.pdf.

[6] NHS Modernisation Agency, *Theatre Programme. Step Guide to Improving Operating Theatre Performance*, NHS Modernisation Agency, 2002.

[7] P. Saha, A. Pinjani, N. Al-Shabibi, S. Madari, J. Ruston, and A. Magos, "Why we are wasting time in the operating theatre?" *International Journal of Health Planning and Management*, vol. 24, no. 3, pp. 225–232, 2009.

[8] M. A. Lewis, R. D. Hall, S. Okolo, and W. Yoong, "How time flies: a prospective analysis of theatre efficiency during elective gynaecology lists," *Gynecological Surgery*, vol. 9, no. 2, pp. 213–217, 2012.

[9] A. Macario, "Truth in scheduling: is it possible to accurately predict how long a surgical case will last?" *Anesthesia & Analgesia*, vol. 108, no. 3, pp. 681–685, 2009.

[10] A. Shushan, H. Mohamed, and A. L. Magos, "How long does laparoscopic surgery really take? Lessons learned from 1000 operative laparoscopies," *Human Reproduction*, vol. 14, no. 1, pp. 39–43, 1999.

[11] S. Campo, V. Campo, and P. Gambadauro, "Is a positive family history of endometriosis a risk factor for endometrioma recurrence after laparoscopic surgery?" *Reproductive Sciences*, vol. 21, no. 4, pp. 526–531, 2014.

[12] J. J. Pandit, S. Westbury, and M. Pandit, "The concept of surgical operating list 'efficiency': a formula to describe the term," *Anaesthesia*, vol. 62, no. 9, pp. 895–903, 2007.

[13] D. P. Strum, A. R. Sampson, J. H. May, and L. G. Vargas, "Surgeon and type of anesthesia predict variability in surgical procedure times," *Anesthesiology*, vol. 92, no. 5, pp. 1454–1466, 2000.

[14] C. Paradis, "Bias in surgical research," *Annals of Surgery*, vol. 248, no. 2, pp. 180–188, 2008.

[15] A. Shushan, H. Mohamed, and A. L. Magos, "A case-control study to compare the variability of operating time in laparoscopic and open surgery," *Human Reproduction*, vol. 14, no. 6, pp. 1467–1469, 1999.

[16] P. Gambadauro, M. Olovsson, and P. Persson, "Unusually rapid growth of bilateral endometriomas and acute bilateral hydronephrosis," *Gynecological Endocrinology*, vol. 27, no. 11, pp. 948–950, 2011.

[17] J. Zhou, F. Dexter, A. Macario, and D. A. Lubarsky, "Relying solely on historical surgical times to estimate accurately future surgical times is unlikely to reduce the average length of time cases finish late," *Journal of Clinical Anesthesia*, vol. 11, no. 7, pp. 601–605, 1999.

[18] D. M. Laskin, A. O. Abubaker, and R. A. Strauss, "Accuracy of predicting the duration of a surgical operation," *Journal of Oral and Maxillofacial Surgery*, vol. 71, no. 2, pp. 446–447, 2013.

[19] F. Dexter, J. Ledolter, V. Tiwari, and R. H. Epstein, "Value of a scheduled duration quantified in terms of equivalent numbers of historical cases," *Anesthesia and Analgesia*, vol. 117, no. 1, pp. 205–210, 2013.

[20] F. Dexter and R. H. Epstein, "Increased mean time from end of surgery to operating room exit in a historical cohort of cases with prolonged time to extubation," *Anesthesia and Analgesia*, vol. 117, no. 6, pp. 1453–1459, 2013.

18

Teach and Playback Training Device for Minimally Invasive Surgery

Sriram Garudeswaran,[1] Sohyung Cho,[1] Ikechukwu Ohu,[2] and Ali K. Panahi[1]

[1]*Industrial Engineering, Southern Illinois University Edwardsville, Edwardsville, IL 62026, USA*
[2]*Industrial Engineering, Gannon University, Erie, PA 16541, USA*

Correspondence should be addressed to Sohyung Cho; scho@siue.edu

Academic Editor: Stephen Kavic

Recent technological progress offers the opportunity to significantly transform conventional open surgical procedures in ways that allow minimally invasive surgery (MIS) to be accomplished by specific operative instruments' entry into the body through key-sized holes rather than large incisions. Although MIS offers an opportunity for less trauma and quicker recovery, thereby reducing length of hospital stay and attendant costs, the complex nature of this procedure makes it difficult to master, not least because of the limited work area and constricted degree of freedom. Accordingly, this research seeks to design a Teach and Playback device that can aid surgical training by key-framing and then reproducing surgical motions. The result is an inexpensive and portable Teach and Playback laparoscopic training device that can record a trainer's surgical motions and then play them back for trainees. Indeed, such a device could provide a training platform for surgical residents generally and would also be susceptible of many other applications for other robot-assisted tasks that might require complex motion training and control.

1. Introduction

This past decade has seen an undeniable turn toward new approaches to minimally invasive surgery (MIS), fueled by modern enhancements to the designs of surgical instruments as well as to techniques for vision and image processing. MIS procedures are generally carried out through a half-inch incision (or multiple such incisions), offering patients benefits in comparison to traditional open surgery that include alleviated trauma level, brief hospital stay, and higher-quality care [1, 2]. Yet MIS is more challenging for the surgeon than open surgery is [3, 4]. Indeed in MIS, visual feedback from the operating area is available only by means of an endoscopic camera. Accordingly, rather than using direct observation, surgeons use a two-dimensional (2D) screen to monitor operations—an approach that deprives them of means for gauging depth. What is more, because of kinematic constraints at incision points, instruments' motions are restricted. Diminished visual and tactile perception and lack of scope for dexterity notwithstanding surgical approaches are trending toward minimally invasive techniques, seeking to offer patients additional benefits even if doing so increases stress on surgeons [5]. Accordingly, means of resolving these technical issues are in high demand, especially for complex tasks such as suturing. In particular, training in MIS procedures is required to ensure safe practice in a finite working space offering reduced tactile feedback. Thus recent studies have indicated a need for task-oriented tests that encompass the complexities of MIS as they relate to visual, spatial, cognitive, perceptual, and motor factors—which are also critical for investigating, classifying, and designing training programs for surgeons at all levels with a view to instituting preferred models for structured, quantitative, and objective education and assessment [6–9]. This research, then, seeks to meet these needs by developing a physical Teach and Playback training device.

Use of MIS improves surgical results while diminishing recovery time, but it has also complicated surgical tasks, increasing surgeons' stress levels as the intricacy of their work also increases. Surgical ergonomics research has naturally followed that has sought ways of reducing stress, improving skills, and assessing quantitative skills. This last object seeks to uncover vital information relating to a trainee surgeon's level of expertise as well as the effectiveness of the training process itself. Moreover, it can provide timely performance feedback to trainees at all levels, greatly assisting in competence reviews. Such an approach can drastically reduce training time—and researchers and expert surgeons, for their part, can use assessment information to aid their own research and analysis while improving the ergonomics of surgery.

Historically, assessment of surgical skills has been subjective, depending on direct observation, global assessments, and the use of checklists [10]. As part of this assessment, experienced surgeons observe trainees during MIS—a time-consuming approach that is also resource- and effort-intensive. Objective assessment, however, poses its own challenges, arising from differences in patients, surgical teams, and operational setup, among other factors [11]. In recognition of this, efforts at improving and formulating objective evaluation approaches have proliferated during the past few years [12]. As part of this effort, MI researchers, along with researchers in other areas, have collaborated to develop ways of objectively assessing surgical skills. Yet an extensive review of the literature reveals that a standalone solution to these challenges is not yet available—although use of virtual reality (VR) systems has shown some promise [11].

Patients increasingly prefer MIS, but the number of well-trained surgeons is falling short of the demand—partly owing to a lack of MIS equipment and partly because of the prohibitive cost of such equipment. As a result, little equipment is available, whether for the operating room (OR) or for training. What is more, no quantitative standard exists for real-time assessment of surgical skills. Accordingly, this research aims to provide a low-cost and portable Teach and Playback laparoscopic training device able to record a trainer's surgical motions and play them back for trainees. Using such a method would greatly speed learning time by providing ready access to expert practice, thereby avoiding subjective ("self-discovery") approaches to learning complex skills.

The Teach and Playback training device prototype offers a robot arm that enjoys 6 degrees of freedom (6DoF). Although, traditionally, DC servomotors comprise three terminals (positive, negative, and signal), a generally unused terminal within the servomotor's housing can be harnessed as a potentiometer, with the shaft of the servomotor itself acting as a variable rheostat. Accordingly, when key-framing motions use the Teach and Playback device, the 6DoF robot arm is able to encode angular information derived from the shafts of its six different servomotors, which also act as potentiometers, for processing and analysis. This simple design choice serves as the kernel of the idea of the Teach and Playback device and its construction: the device records a robot's end-effector motion path, physically key-framing it so as to reproduce precisely the same motions. Thus sensors eliminate complex inverse kinematic equations from the calculations.

2. System Structure

The system has a 6 DoF (degree of freedom) robotic construction that itself is built up out of six servomotors, mechanically connected to each other by aluminum links that form the robot's armature. Figure 1 shows the system structure. In its offline (nonexcited) mode, each servo also acts as a potentiometer so that, during physical key-framing, the armature with its six servomotors, all now acting as potentiometers, emits instantaneous angular information from the shaft of the servomotors for processing and analysis. Thus the sensors eliminate the need to solve complex inverse kinematic equations.

The signal and potentiometer terminals of each servo connect, respectively, to the "digital" output pins of a servo driver and the "analog" input pins of an Arduino microcontroller. These integrated circuits (ICs) exert control, route instructions, and allow receipt of data. The Arduino microcontroller is itself connected by universal serial bus (USB) to a PC or workstation, communicating serially in duplex (2-way) mode. Thus physically key-framed information is transmitted to a database hosted on the workstation for storage and processing—and can also be transmitted on demand to the Arduino microcontroller over the serial duplex channel. This is the whole of the system. The Adafruit® 16-channel 12-bit PWM/servo driver, built using the PCA9685, drives up to 16 servos over I^2C, making use of only two pins. The onboard PWM controller drives all 16 channels simultaneously, requiring no additional Arduino processing overhead. For purposes of expansion, up to 62 drivers can be chained to control up to 992 servos, all using the same two pins: the SDA (data) and SCL (clock) ports. Servo motors allowing for precise control of angular position, velocity, and acceleration are used, coupled to sensors for position feedback.

The Parallax Data Acquisition tool, commonly known as PLX-DAQ, is a software add-in for Microsoft Excel that acquires up to 26 channels of microcontroller data through serial communication, arranging the data into columns. The PLX-DAQ thus offers an easy means of conducting spreadsheet analysis of data collected in the field, along with laboratory analysis of sensors and real-time equipment monitoring.

2.1. Servo Modification. Traditionally, a servomotor accepting direct current (DC) input comprises three electrical terminals: positive, negative, and signal. In general, however, there is one more terminal for the IC to protect the servomotor from potential overcurrent faults and shocks. Tapping into this terminal allows the addition of a fourth and new connection, this one serving as a potentiometer, with the servo motor itself acting as a variable rheostat in its offline mode.

Accordingly, during physical key-framing of motions using the Teach and Playback device in its offline mode (i.e., when the servos are not driven), the armature and its six different servomotors, each now acting as a potentiometer, emits moment-by-moment angular information from the shaft of the servomotor for processing and analysis. This

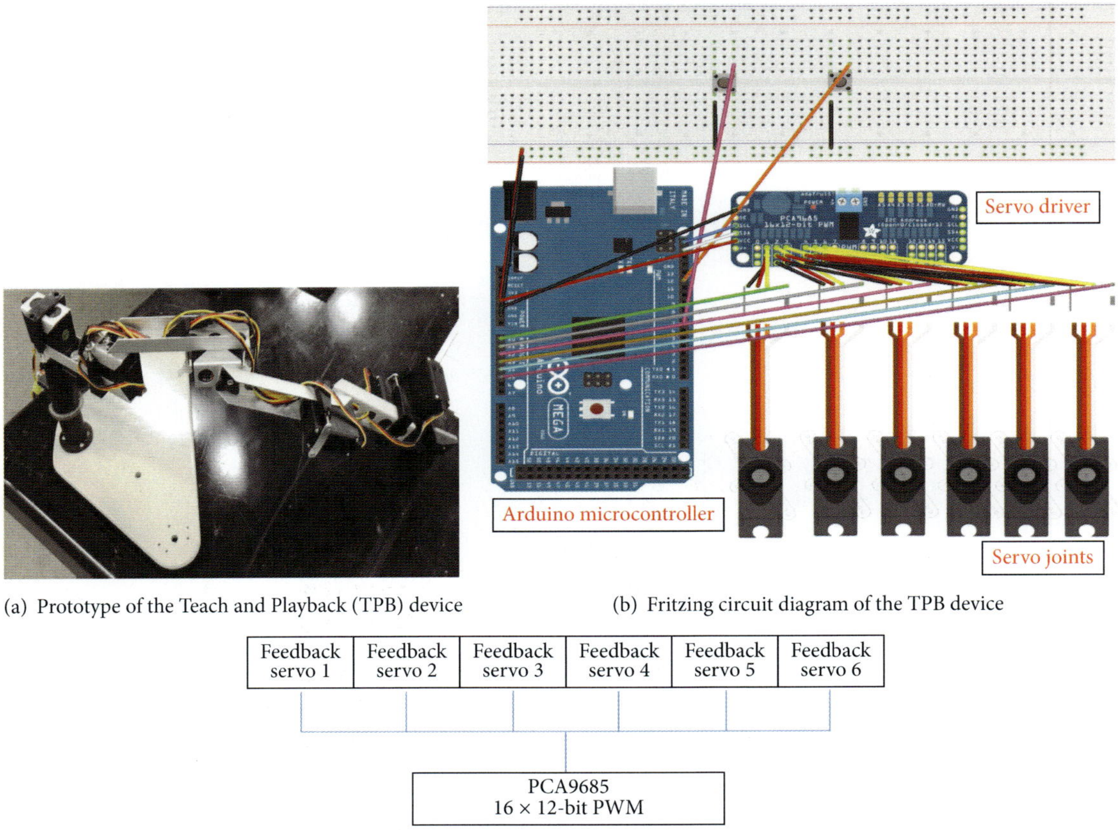

(a) Prototype of the Teach and Playback (TPB) device

(b) Fritzing circuit diagram of the TPB device

(c) Schematic diagram of the TPB device

FIGURE 1: The Teach and Playback device. (a) 6DoF Robot Arm. (b) Fritzing circuit diagram. (c) Fritzing block diagram.

simple concept, unique to this project, serves as the essential concept around which the Teach and Playback device is built.

2.2. Robot Kinematics. The kinematic equations for a robot's series chain are obtained using a rigid transformation Z to characterize the relative movement allowed at each joint and using a separate rigid transformation X to define the dimensions of each link. The resulting sequence is one of rigid transformations, alternating joint and link transformations from the base of the chain to its end link, the position of which is calculated as follows:

$$[T] = [Z_1][X_1][Z_2][X_2]\cdots[X_{n-1}][Z_n], \quad (1)$$

where T is the transformation locating the end link.

These equations represent the kinematics equations of the serial chain [13].

In 1955, Denavit and Hartenberg introduced a convention for defining joint matrices Z and link matrices X so as to standardize the coordinate frame for spatial linkages [14, 15]. This convention positions the joint frame such that it consists of a screw displacement along the Z-axis:

$$[Z_i] = \mathrm{Trans}_{Z i}(d_i)\,\mathrm{Rot}_{Z i}(\theta_i) \quad (2)$$

and positions the link frame such that it consists of a screw displacement along the X-axis:

$$[X_i] = \mathrm{Trans}_{X i}(a_{i,i+1})\,\mathrm{Rot}_{X i}(\alpha_{i,i+1}). \quad (3)$$

Using this notation, each transformation link going along a serial chain robot can be described by the coordinate transformation

$$\begin{aligned} {}^{i-1}T_i = [Z_i][X_i] &= \mathrm{Trans}_{Z i}(d_i)\,\mathrm{Rot}_{Z i}(\theta_i) \\ &\cdot \mathrm{Trans}_{X i}(a_{i,i+1})\,\mathrm{Rot}_{X i}(\alpha_{i,i+1}), \end{aligned} \quad (4)$$

where θ_i, d_i, $\alpha_{i,i+1}$, and $a_{i,i+1}$ are Denavit-Hartenberg parameters.

2.3. Kinematic Analysis. Through kinematic analysis, the designer can discover the position of each component of the mechanical system—data needed for subsequent dynamic analysis and control paths. Inverse kinematics exemplifies the analysis of a constrained system of rigid bodies, or a kinematic chain, such that a robot's kinematic equations can be used to define loop equations for a complex articulated system, which are nonlinear constraints on the configuration parameters of the system. The independent parameters in these equations are known as the system's degrees of freedom. Although analytical solutions to the inverse kinematics

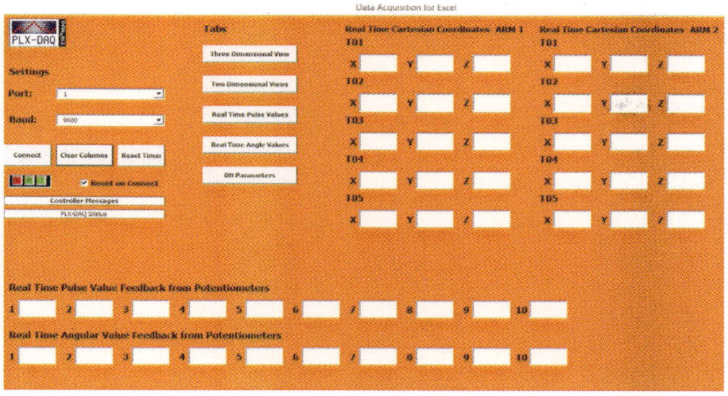

FIGURE 2: Graphical User Interface (GUI) for the "Teach and Playback" device system.

problem exist for a wide range of kinematic chains, computer modeling and animation tools often use Newton's method of solving nonlinear kinematics equations. Other applications of inverse kinematic algorithms include interactive manipulation, animation control, and collision avoidance.

3. System Programming

3.1. Communication Interface and Hardware Programming. Extensive programming was used to establish the communication interface and to program the microcontrollers to communicate among all interfaces in the control system, allowing for the sending, receiving, and routing of angular values as well as the use of a user interface. Communications to and from the Arduino microcontroller are conducted using the Arduino programming language, which resembles the C programming language and features C-style constructs. It is used to read and route, via the microcontroller, potentiometer values to a local computer database. Communication between potentiometers and Arduino microcontroller is established by means of the I^2C communication protocol, whereas communication between Arduino microcontroller and computer is by USB.

3.2. User Interface and Software Programming. The PLX-DAQ Microsoft Excel plugin is coded in the backend using Visual Basic for Applications (VBA), as is the custom-designed user interface, which can be tweaked to populate angular values and graphical illustrations in real time as shown in Figure 2. Figure 3 illustrates the sequence of *Teach* and *Playback* actions.

4. Data Validation

Rather than physically key-framing motions into the Teach and Playback device, the device is left energized, with values recorded by the servos during the "teach" and "playback" phases recorded and compared with one another. Table 1 and Figures 4 and 5 present observations from each servo, 1 through 6, during the Teach and Playback device as already discussed, when no motion is physically key-framed and when it is in its standstill state, with pulse values recorded at 40 Hz for 9 seconds. Angular values and percentage error were also computed for the pulse values, during the "teach" and "playback" phases. Table 1 lists average pulse values, percentage error, and standard deviation for servos 1–6 during the "teach" and "playback" phases.

The foregoing values show that the average error percentage calculated at the sixth joint or the sixth servo is far less than the average error percentage calculated at the first servo. Another interesting observation may also be made: the average error percentage increases from the sixth servo to the first. A similar pattern is also observed in the standard deviation calculated for each of the servos. As with the computed error percentages, the standard deviation possesses a higher value at the sixth servo than at the first servo, and the standard deviation value continually increases from the sixth servo joint to the first. Figure 4 shows the servo values at a fixed position during the "teach" and "playback" stages.

This behavior comports with existing knowledge: The load on the sixth servo is far less than that endured by the first, for the load on the sixth servo is directly applied to the fifth servo, taking weight off the sixth servo itself, and so on to the first. Thus the first servo, being in base position, bears the highest load of all. Accordingly, error and deviation of output from input are greatest at the first servo but decrease through to the sixth servo. In this manner, theoretical understanding is reinforced by calculated observations.

Figure 5 depicts the servo values in the "teach" and "playback" stages during a surgical exercise (peg transfer), during which the average error percentage calculated at the sixth joint or the sixth servo is noticeably less than that at the first servo. This echoes previous observations about the fixed position, which can be attributed to the difference in load endured by servos in various positions.

5. Conclusions

5.1. Design Contributions. In this study, a novel Teach and Playback training device was developed—essentially a 6 DoF robot that can be used to train novice surgeons to perform minimally invasive surgery by first recording the surgical motions of a trainer and then playing back those same motions for trainees. This device thus seeks to address the need for a quantitative standard for real-time surgical skills assessment.

In developing an interactive communication protocol for high-speed duplex communication, this study sought to seamlessly connect such a training device to a computer workstation or laptop by means of an open-source microcontroller, making use of the ubiquitous Microsoft Excel as a database for all physically key-framed angular information. Such a method combines visually pleasing access to raw data with the facility for instantaneous pattern recognition and identification, along with unlimited storage capacity and organized data storage.

This research also explains how a simple servo hack may accommodate a fourth terminal, enabling the servomotor

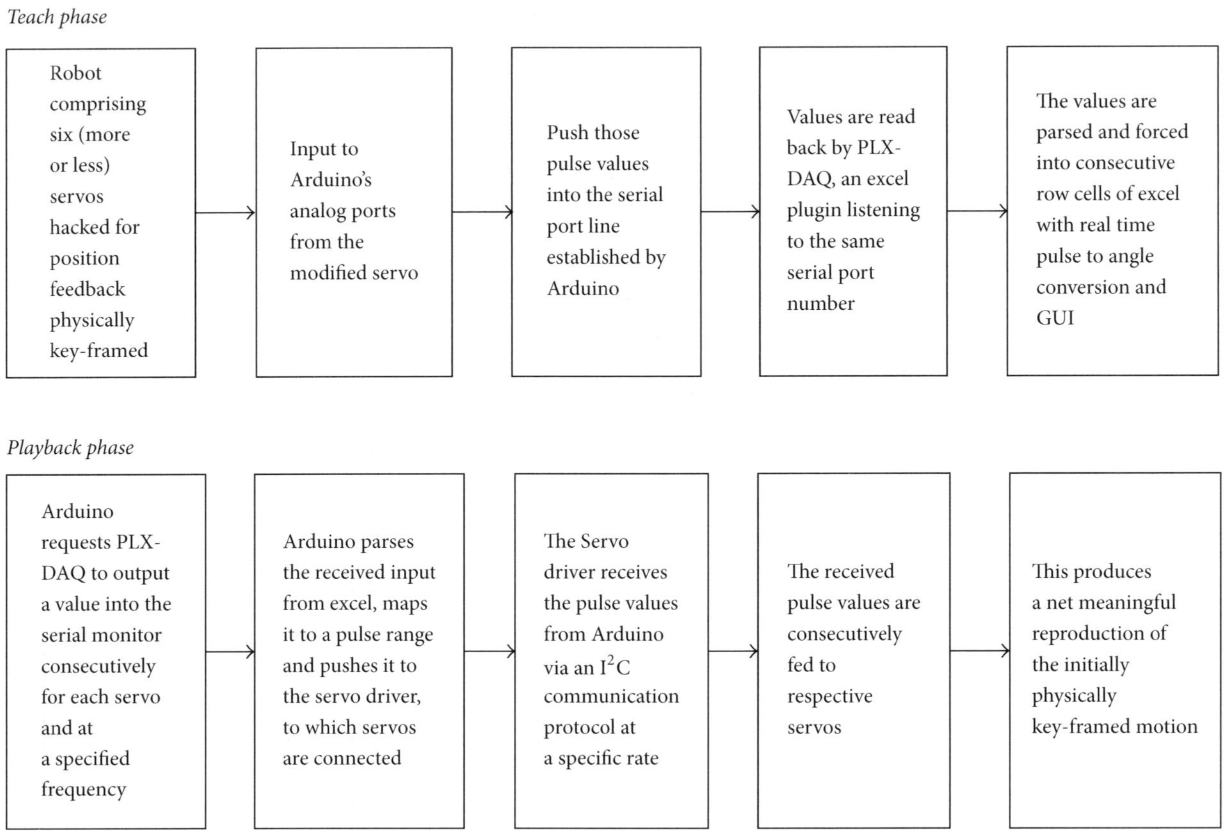

FIGURE 3: Logical activity flow during different phases of system operation.

TABLE 1: Mean pulse and standard deviation values in the "teach" and "playback" phases, and average percentage errors in the stationary and physically key-framed states.

	Teach phase (pulse value)		Playback phase (pulse value)		Average error (%)	
	Mean	St. dev.	Mean	St. dev.	Stationary	Key-framed
Servo 1	296.5	1.22	302.6	4.88	2.5	6.1
Servo 2	281.2	0.42	288.4	3.25	2.6	5.2
Servo 3	81.3	0.49	81.9	1.18	1.3	5.5
Servo 4	298.4	0.58	302.3	1.76	1.3	5.3
Servo 5	162.6	0.48	162.5	1.68	0.8	3.8
Servo 6	124.8	0.66	124.8	0.99	0.6	3.3

to act as a potentiometer in its standalone state and thereby form the entire basis for development of the low-cost Teach and Playback device in question. Notably, this research uses readily available and low-cost components and devices, together with open-source architecture and freeware, to facilitate construction.

During error analysis performed on the pulse and angular values recorded from the joints of the Teach and Playback device for each of the six servos in its standstill state, as well as when a practical action (peg transfer) was performed using the device, with motions physically key-framed into the device, observed percentage error values were within reasonable and permissible levels. Indeed, the average percentage error and standard deviation values recorded aligned with the system's theoretically expected behavior.

5.2. Recommendations for Future Research. The proposed design paradigm should thus be applied to an industrial-grade servo, allowing its performance to be gauged in a real-world situation. Also, the use of a more robust GUI-based middleware software package would enhance operation during the "playback" phase, making it smoother and more accurate. Blender [16] can be considered, a professional open-source 3D computer graphics software product was used to create animated films, visual effects, art, 3D-printed models,

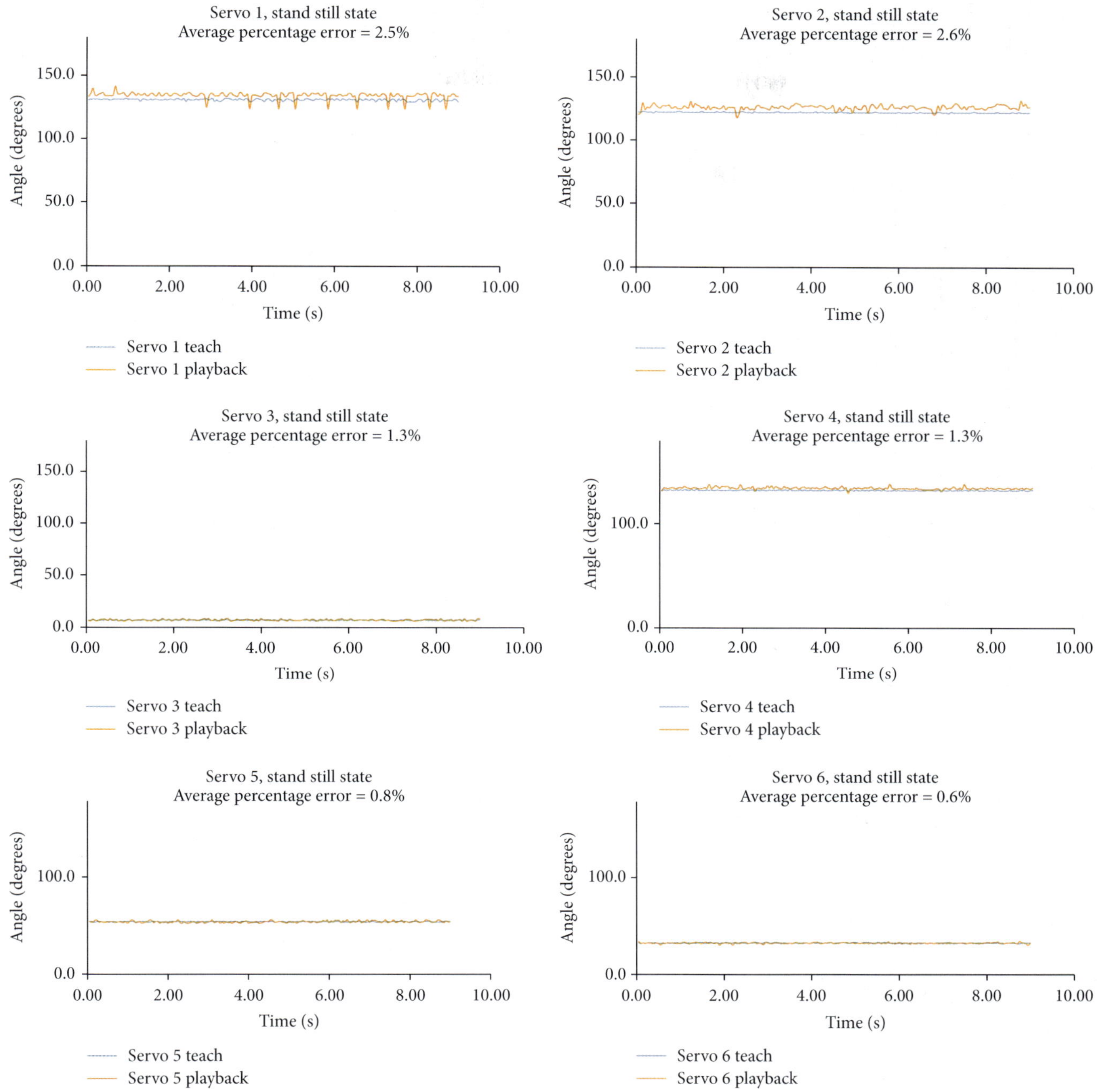

FIGURE 4: Fixed-position servo values during the "teach" and "playback" stages.

interactive 3D applications, and video game assets. Importantly, the game engine within this software application could be used to build a virtual model of the Teach and Playback device's entire armature. This same engine also flaunts an inverse kinematics system that could be used to compute joint positions and servo angles at a moment's notice and with far greater precision and accuracy. Accordingly, using this software would diminish the effects of rounding and would reduce the effects of other sources of potential noise arising during communication. Continuation of research in this vein could thus make use of the many features available in more sophisticated software packages to enhance precision, boost accuracy, and improve visualization.

Disclosure

The authors acknowledge that a part of the research work described in this paper was previously presented in 2016 Flexible Automation and Intelligent Manufacturing (FAIM) Conference.

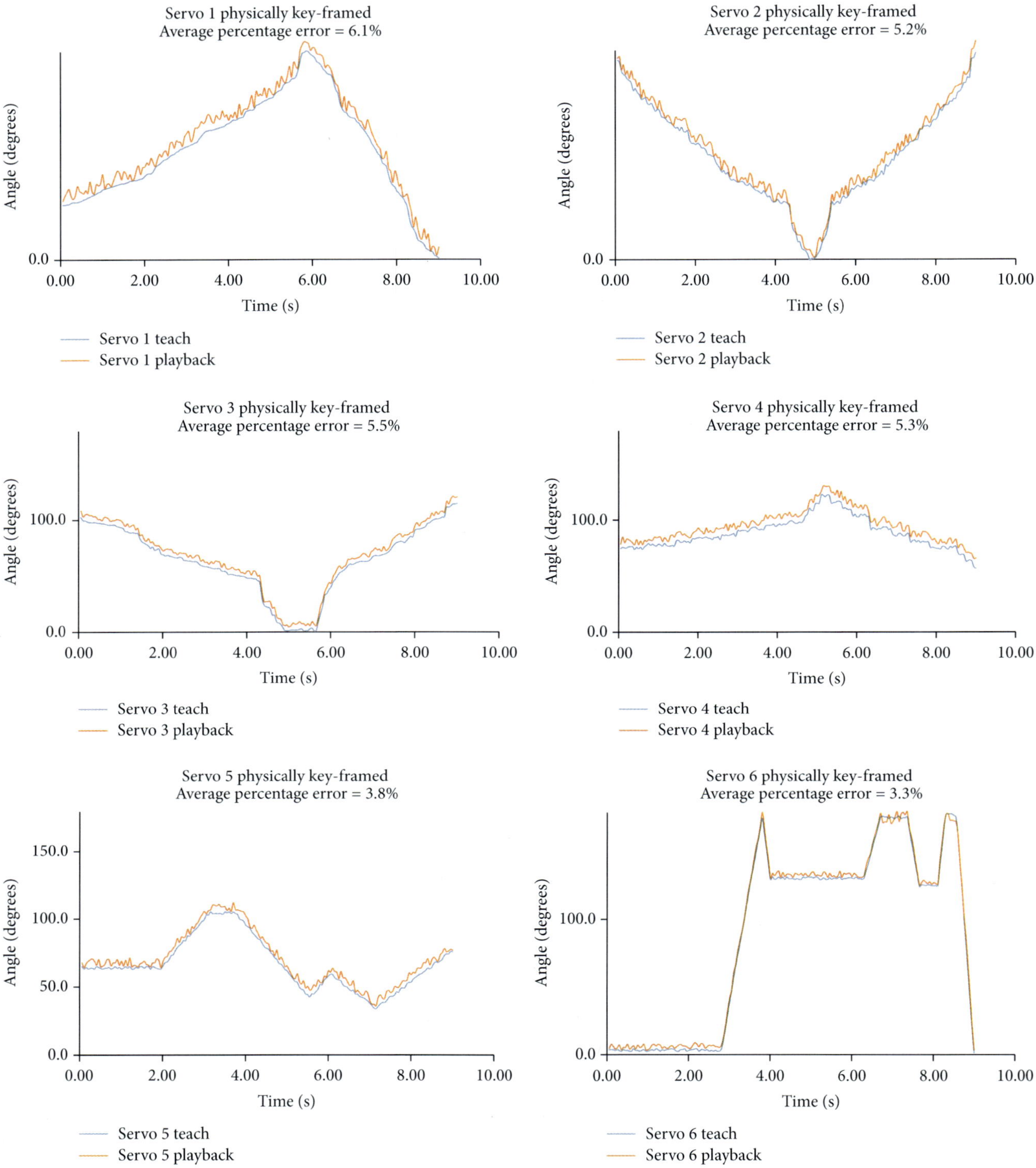

Figure 5: Servo values during the "teach" and "playback" stages of a surgical exercise (peg transfer).

References

[1] A. J. Karayiannakis, G. G. Makri, A. Mantzioka, D. Karousos, and G. Karatzas, "Postoperative pulmonary function after laparoscopic and open cholecystectomy," *British Journal of Anaesthesia*, vol. 77, no. 4, pp. 448–452, 1996.

[2] A. W. Majeed, G. Troy, J. P. Nicholl et al., "Randomised, prospective, single-blind comparison of laparoscopic versus small-incision cholecystectomy," *The Lancet*, vol. 347, no. 9007, pp. 989–994, 1996.

[3] M. K. Chen, K. P. Schropp, T. E. Lobe, and E. Wiener, "Complications of minimal-access surgery in children," *Journal of Pediatric Surgery*, vol. 31, no. 8, pp. 1161–1165, 1996.

[4] D. I. Watson, R. J. Baigrie, and G. G. Jamieson, "A learning curve for laparoscopic fundoplication: definable, avoidable, or a waste of time?" *Annals of Surgery*, vol. 224, no. 2, pp. 198–203, 1996.

[5] R. Berguer, W. D. Smith, and Y. H. Chung, "Performing laparoscopic surgery is significantly more stressful for the surgeon than open surgery," *Surgical Endoscopy*, vol. 15, no. 10, pp. 1204–1207, 2001.

[6] S. M. B. I. Botden, I. H. J. T. de Hingh, and J. J. Jakimowicz, "Meaningful assessment method for laparoscopic suturing training in augmented reality," *Surgical Endoscopy and Other Interventional Techniques*, vol. 23, no. 10, pp. 2221–2228, 2009.

[7] J. C. Rosser, L. E. Rosser, and R. S. Savalgi, "Objective evaluation of a laparoscopic surgical skill program for residents and senior surgeons," *Archives of Surgery*, vol. 133, no. 6, pp. 657–661, 1998.

[8] J. C. Rosser, L. E. Rosser, and R. S. Savalgi, "Skill acquisition and assessment for laparoscopic surgery," *Archives of Surgery*, vol. 132, no. 2, pp. 200–204, 1997.

[9] T. R. C. o. S. o. E. a. t. S. a. N. Foundation, Surgical Competence - Challenges of assessment in training and practice, 1999.

[10] K. Moorthy, Y. Munz, S. K. Sarker, and A. Darzi, "Objective assessment of technical skills in surgery," *British Medical Journal*, vol. 327, no. 7422, pp. 1032–1037, 2003.

[11] S. M. Cristancho, A. J. Hodgson, O. N. M. Panton, A. Meneghetti, G. Warnock, and K. Qayumi, "Intraoperative monitoring of laparoscopic skill development based on quantitative measures," *Surgical Endoscopy*, vol. 23, no. 10, pp. 2181–2190, 2009.

[12] K. Moorthy, Y. Munz, A. Dosis, F. Bello, and A. Darzi, "Motion analysis in the training and assessment of minimally invasive surgery," *Minimally Invasive Therapy and Allied Technologies*, vol. 12, pp. 137–142, 2003.

[13] J. M. McCarthy, *Introduction to Theoretical Kinematics*, MIT Press, Cambridge, UK, 1990.

[14] J. Denavit and R. S. Hartenberg, "A kinematic notation for lower-pair mechanisms based on matrices," *Journal of Applied Mechanics*, vol. 23, pp. 215–221, 1955.

[15] R. S. Hartenberg and J. Denavit, *Kinematic Synthesis of Linkages*, McGraw-Hill, New York, NY, USA, 1964.

[16] "Blender Software for 3D modeling," http://www.blender.org/.

19

The Application of Pediatric Ureteroscope for Seminal Vesiculoscopy

Shulin Guo,[1] Donghua Xie,[1] Xiangfei He,[2] Chuance Du,[1] Lunfeng Zhu,[1] Xiaolin Deng,[1] and Zhongsheng Yang[1]

[1]*Department of Urology, The Affiliated Ganzhou City People's Hospital of Nanchang University, Ganzhou, Jiangxi 341000, China*
[2]*Linyi City People's Hospital, Linyi, Shandong 276003, China*

Correspondence should be addressed to Shulin Guo; gshul2007@163.com

Academic Editor: Peng Hui Wang

To describe a novel technique of transurethral seminal vesiculoscopy using a pediatric ureteroscope in the diagnosis and management of persistent hematospermia, a retrospective study was carried out for 20 patients with recurrent hematospermia whom we evaluated and treated using a 6–7.5F (6F front end and 7.5F rear end) pediatric ureteroscope from August 2009 to September 2013. For the 20 patients, the age ranges from 25 to 48 years with a mean age of 36 years. The duration of the hematospermia ranges from 6 to 48 months with a mean duration of 18 months. Transurethral seminal vesiculoscopy was successfully performed in the 20 cases and the mean operative time was 35 min (ranges from 25 to 90 min). Among the 20 patients, 11 patients were found to have seminal vesiculitis, five were with seminal vesicle stone, one was with prostatic utricle stone, one was with prostate cyst, and one was with ejaculatory duct obstruction. The mean follow-up period was 7 months (ranged from 6 to 12 months). Hematospermia in 19 cases disappeared after the surgery and only in one patient the hematospermia recurred 6 months after the surgery. The cure rate was 95%. This study indicated that transurethral seminal vesiculoscopy could be performed easily using a semirigid pediatric ureteroscope with few complications and is an effective therapeutic approach for persistent hematospermia.

1. Introduction

Hematospermia is a common disease in andrology. The etiology is quite complex. However, the majority of hematospermia is related to infection in prostate and seminal vesicle. Symptom relief can be achieved for some of the patients after a course of anti-inflammatory therapy. However, symptoms in a small portion of the patients cannot be improved after medication and the hematospermia persists [1, 2]. From August 2009 to September 2013, we evaluated and treated 20 patients with recurrent hematospermia using the pediatric ureteroscopy with satisfactory outcome. We thus reported the results as below.

2. Methods

First of all, all the following work was conducted in accordance with the Declaration of Helsinki (1964). The study was conducted with the understanding and the consent of the patients as well as approval from the Ethical Committee of the Affiliated Ganzhou City People's Hospital of Nanchang University, China.

2.1. Patients. The study consists of 20 patients with age ranging from 25 to 48 years and a mean age of 36 years. The duration of the hematospermia ranges from 6 to 48 months with a mean duration of 18 months. All these patients presented with intermittent hematospermia. The color in patients with short interval of ejaculation was bright reddish or pinkish. The color in patients with longer interval of ejaculation was dark reddish or coffee colored. Routine and special tests were performed before the surgery. These include CBC, urinalysis, coagulation function index, and prostate fluid routine examination and culture. Per the prostate routine exam, there were 8 cases with elevated WBC count accompanied by decreased lecithin corpuscle. Per the prostate fluid culture, there were 2 cases infected with *E. coli*, 1 case with *Staphylococcus aureus*, and one case with Proteus syndrome. All the patients were found to have normal serum PSA level. Digital rectal exam revealed no abnormality on prostate. Transrectal color Doppler revealed one case with seminal vesicle cyst, 6 cases with inflamed prostate accompanied by calcification, and 5 cases with unilateral or bilateral seminal vesicle stones.

2.2. Surgical Procedure. All patients underwent the seminal vesiculoscopy using 6–7.5F pediatric ureteroscope under epidural anesthesia in lithotomy position. Pancystoscopy was performed initially to investigate prostate, bladder, and bilateral ureteral orifices before withdrawing the ureteroscope to the position of verumontanum. Under direct visualization, we initially located the opening of the verumontanum. With the guidance of an epidural catheter and mild flushing with saline, we then entered prostatic utricle for investigation. After careful examination of the prostate utricle, we withdrew the ureteroscope to the opening of the prostate utricle and looked for openings of bilateral ejaculatory ducts outside at 5 and 7 o'clock positions, under continuous saline flushing. Seminal vesicle was then entered under the guidance of the epidural catheter. For patients with unclear ejaculatory duct openings, we used transurethral plasmakinetic resectoscope to resect the verumontanum to expose the openings. Under the direct vision of ureteroscope, we examined carefully if there were congestion or edema on seminal vesicle mucosa, active bleeding or old blood clot, stone, anatomical abnormalities such as cyst, and new growth. We biopsied those lesions suspected to have pathological abnormality. For those small stones, sand-like stones, and old blood clots, we manually removed them using alligator forceps or flushed them out under pressure produced by bolus injection. For those larger stones inside the seminal vesicle, we cleared them by using Holmium laser (power of 2 joules, frequency 15 Hz) to powderize them followed by saline flushing. For seminal vesicle cysts, we also used the Holmium laser to unroof them. In the end, seminal vesicle cavities were irrigated with antibiotic. The same modalities were used for management of other sides of the seminal vesicle. Postoperatively, every patient was placed a Foley catheter and was treated with intravenous antibiotic for 3–5 days.

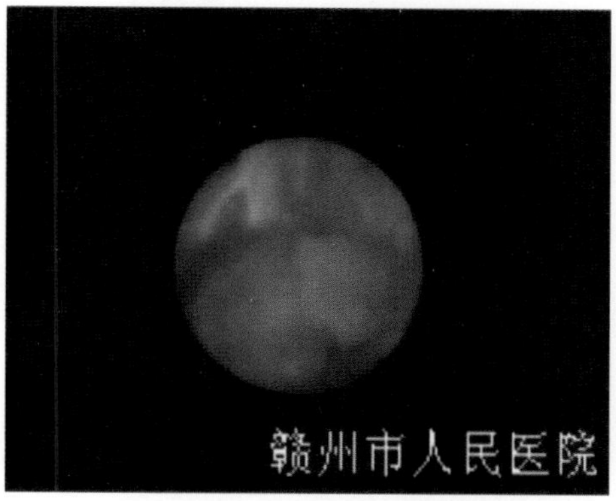

Figure 1: Stone in the cavity of seminal vesicle.

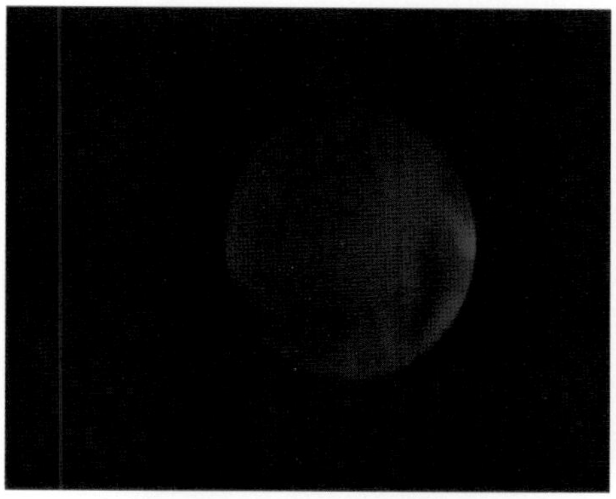

Figure 2: Stone in prostate utricle.

3. Results

All 20 cases were examined successfully for their seminal vesicles using the pediatric ureteroscopy. The operative time ranged from 25 to 90 minutes with a mean duration of 35 minutes. Eighteen of the 20 cases underwent exam, saline flushing, and antibiotic irrigation bilaterally while for the other 2 cases the exam and treatment were performed unilaterally. In 5 patients there were seminal vesicle stones (left side, 3 cases; right side, 2 cases, Figure 1) which were flushed out after being powderized by holmium laser. In two patients stones were found in prostate utricle (Figure 2), which were extracted manually using alligator forceps. One case of seminal vesicle cyst was unroofed using Holmium laser. One case of ejaculatory duct obstruction underwent transurethral plasmakinetic resection (Figure 3). Eleven cases were found to have edema and congestion in the inner wall of seminal vesicle cavities and a trace of old blood clots, consistent with seminal vesicle wall inflammatory hemorrhage (Figure 4). We followed the cases for 6 to 12 months and found that that there were rare complications. No postoperative epididymitis, retrograde ejaculation, urinary incontinence, and urethral stricture were found in this study. There was one case noticed to have recurrent hematospermia 6 months after surgery with transrectal color Doppler ultrasound revealing a 1.2 $*$ 0.8 cm left sided para-seminal vesicle cyst, which was improved after a course of anti-inflammatory and physical therapy. The recurrent rate of hematospermia in this series was 5%.

4. Discussion

The etiology of hematospermia is quite complex clinically. In general, the etiology can be divided into 3 types including organic, functional, and exigent. The most common circumstance for organic cause is seminal vesicle and prostate inflammation and infection. Other circumstances are ejaculatory duct obstruction, seminal vesicle and prostate stone or cyst, seminal vesicle tuberculosis, and ejaculatory duct injury including iatrogenic factors such as transrectal prostate biopsy [3–9]. In addition, some blood disorders and tumor invasion could also cause hematospermia. The common

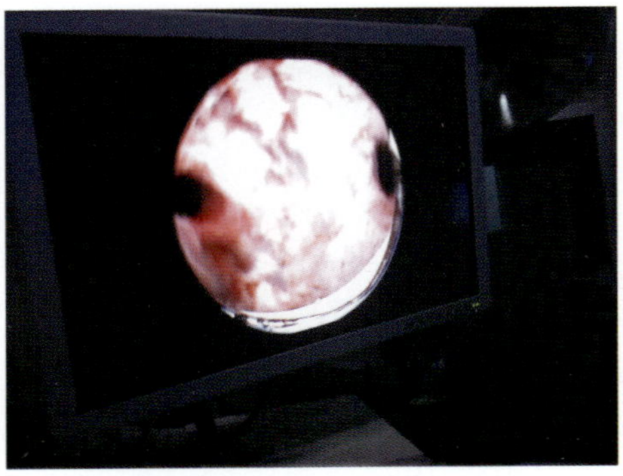

FIGURE 3: Opened ejaculatory ducts after transurethral plasmakinetic resection.

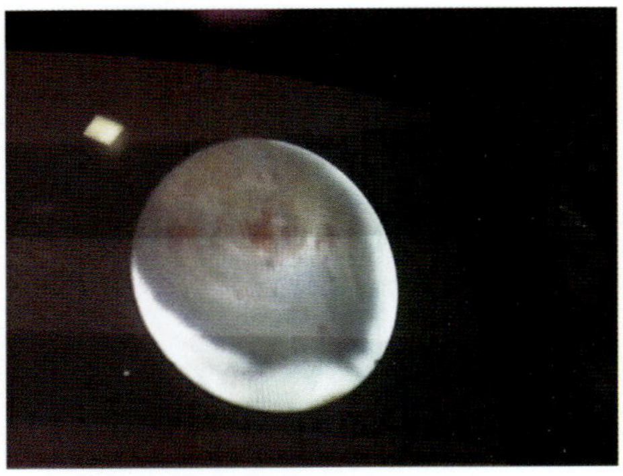

FIGURE 4: Seminal vesiculitis.

circumstances for the functional cause are excessive masturbation, excessive sexual intercourse, or too long abstinence time. The exigent cause of the hematospermia could result from minor damage to the ejaculatory duct. Seminal vesicle is the organ to store sperm with abundant vascular layer. When there is inflammatory reaction in the seminal vesicle, the mucosa became congested and edematous and the hematospermia occurs, which often leads to severe stress and fear to the patient [5]. In most patients, the hematospermia may resolve spontaneously in a few weeks or after a course of sensitive antibiotic. However, a small portion of the patients may have recurrent hematospermia resistant to routine therapy, which poses a big challenge for clinical diagnosis and treatment [3, 4].

According to the literature data retrieval, conventional treatment of hematospermia includes systemic administration and local treatment, the latter including prostate massage, hot water bath, physical therapy to improve local blood circulation and promote inflammation absorption and elimination. Due to the special anatomical and physiological characteristics of seminal vesicle and prostate, the treatment efficacy is often poor or not to work for the persistent hematospermia. Therefore, we used the 6–7.5F ureteroscope to investigate the seminal vesicle for those patients with persistent hematospermia, achieving good outcome in both finding out the etiology and delivering therapy.

There are different methods to enter a scope for vesiculoscopy for those patients with unclear ejaculatory duct openings. Some people performed blind insertion through prostate utricle using the scope body forcefully to create a hole, while others used transurethral plasmakinetic resection of verumontanum to expose the ejaculatory duct to enter the scope under direct visualization. We performed one of our 20 cases using the aforementioned blind insertion, which is the case in which recurrent hematospermia was found 6 months after the surgery with a color Doppler ultrasound revealing the left sided para-seminal vesicle cyst. We think this could be caused by seminal vasculitis resulting from blind insertion injury to the ejaculatory duct and incomplete absorption of the intraoperative saline extravasations. But because of the small number of cases and without the blind comparative study, the exact cause of the recurrence needs further investigation.

In our study, we found that the most important causes of hematospermia are inflammation, stenosis, and cyst. Ejaculatory duct stenosis further aggravates the inflammatory reaction. The infection, hemorrhage, and impeded drainage from narrowed ejaculatory duct opening may contribute to the formation of stones, posing a vicious cycle because the stone will further aggravate the stenosis leading to infection and stone formation. For those cases with ejaculatory ducts stenosis with bad exposure of ejaculatory duct opening, we used the transurethral plasmakinetic resection of verumontanum to expose spacious ejaculatory duct openings, not only removed the ejaculatory duct stenosis, but also dredged the ejaculatory duct. The drainage was thus improved, eliminating the root of hematospermia.

Our experiences using the pediatric ureteroscope for seminal vesiculoscopy include the following. (1) The ejaculatory duct openings are most commonly located at 5 and 7 o'clock positions outside the prostate utricle, which allow the 6–7.5F pediatric ureteroscopy to enter under direct visualization in most circumstances. However, it is very important to use epidural catheter as a guide instead of ureteral catheter to avoid edematous effect on the openings and bleeding which will make it difficult to find the openings afterwards. Compared to the ureteral catheter, the epidural catheter is smaller and smoother with better flexibility. Infusing saline through the epidural catheter can facilitate to extend ejaculatory duct openings by maintaining a pressure. (2) It is important to control flushing pressure and speed. We prefer a pressure at 200 mmHg and a speed at 0.2 L/min. (3) We used transurethral plasmakinetic resection of verumontanum instead of traditional vaporization resection for those patients with unclear ejaculatory duct openings, mainly because plasmakinetic resection does not produce coke attachments, reducing the likelihood of postoperative scar stenosis. (4) For patients with intractable hematospermia, we recommend prostate fluid culture and drug susceptibility before the vesiculoscopy and intraoperative irrigation of the seminal vesicle cavities using sensitive antibiotic plus saline.

In summary, we think seminal vesiculoscopy using a pediatric ureteroscope develops a new way to treat refractory hematospermia and plays an important role in promoting the understanding of the cause and treatment of hematospermia. Combining literature reports with our preliminary practical experience, the authors think that the pediatric ureteroscopic examination of seminal vesicle has the advantages of being simple operation, of less trauma, safe, and effective and can be widely used as one of effective methods of diagnosis and treatment of intractable hematospermia. But because of the small number of cases we carried out in the study and the lack of multicenter clinical study of large samples, especially the possible negative thermal effect of holmium laser lithotripsy on mucosa of seminal vesicle by using power of 2 joules and frequency of 15 Hz, the overall and long-term efficacy still needs further observation. Also, we understand that, in case of midline seminal vesicle cyst, we may be able to find the thin lining of mucosa to puncture and introduce the scope to seminal vesicle easily without a need of transurethral resection of verumontanum.

Authors' Contribution

Donghua Xie and Xiangfei He were involved in analysis and interpretation of data and drafting the report; Shulin Guo, Donghua Xie, Chuance Du, Lunfeng Zhu, and Zhongsheng Yang were involved in data acquisition; Shulin Guo and Donghua Xie were involved in conception and design; all the authors read and approved the final paper. Shulin Guo, Donghua Xie, and Xiangfei He contribute equally to the paper.

References

[1] R. Munkel witz, S. Krasnokutsky, J. Lie, S. M. Shah, J. Bayshtok, and S. A. Khan, "Current perspectives on hematospermia: a review," *Journal of Andrology*, vol. 18, no. 1, pp. 6–14, 1997.

[2] I. Ahmad and N. S. Krishna, "Hemospermia," *The Journal of Urology*, vol. 177, no. 5, pp. 1613–1618, 2007.

[3] B.-J. Li, C. Zhang, K. Li et al., "Clinical analysis of the characterization of magnetic resonance imaging in 102 cases of refractory haematospermia," *Andrology*, vol. 1, no. 6, pp. 948–956, 2013.

[4] Z.-Y. Liu, Y.-H. Sun, C.-L. Xu et al., "Transurethral seminal vesiculoscopy in the diagnosis and treatment of persistent or recurrent hemospermia: a single-institution experience," *Asian Journal of Andrology*, vol. 11, no. 5, pp. 566–570, 2009.

[5] B. Liu, J. Li, P. Li et al., "Transurethral seminal vesiculoscopy in the diagnosis and treatment of intractable seminal vesiculitis," *Journal of International Medical Research*, vol. 42, no. 1, pp. 236–242, 2014.

[6] S. C. Yang, K. H. Rha, S. K. Byon, and J. H. Kim, "Transutricular seminal vesiculoscopy," *Journal of Endourology*, vol. 16, no. 6, pp. 343–345, 2002.

[7] H. Wang, H. Ye, C. Xu et al., "Transurethral seminal vesiculoscopy using a 6F vesiculoscope for ejaculatory duct obstruction: initial experience," *Journal of Andrology*, vol. 33, no. 4, pp. 637–643, 2012.

[8] T. Song, X. Zhang, L. Zhang, F. Zhang, and W.-J. Fu, "Transurethral seminal vesiculoscopy in the diagnosis and treatment of seminal vesicle stones," *Chinese Medical Journal*, vol. 125, no. 8, pp. 1475–1478, 2012.

[9] C.-H. Han, Q. Liang, B.-Z. Dong et al., "The transurethral seminal vesiculoscopy in the diagnosis and treatment of the seminal vesicle disease," *Cell Biochemistry and Biophysics*, vol. 66, no. 3, pp. 851–853, 2013.

20

'True Day Case' Laparoscopic Cholecystectomy in a High-Volume Specialist Unit and Review of Factors Contributing to Unexpected Overnight Stay

A. Solodkyy, A. R. Hakeem, N. Oswald, F. Di Franco, S. Gergely, and A. M. Harris

Department of Upper Gastrointestinal Surgery, Hinchingbrooke Hospital, Hinchingbrooke Park, Huntingdon, Cambridgeshire PE29 6NT, UK

Correspondence should be addressed to A. M. Harris; adrianharris@nhs.net

Academic Editor: Peng Hui Wang

Introduction. Laparoscopic cholecystectomy (LC) is the gold standard treatment for gallstones. British Association of Day Case Surgery recommends at least 60% of LCs be performed as day cases. The aim of this study was to assess our rate of true day case LCs and review factors preventing same-day discharge. *Methods.* We prospectively collected data of all elective LCs performed in a district general hospital over 32 months. *Results.* 500 patients underwent LC during this period; 438 (88.2%) patients were planned day cases and 59 patients (11.8%) planned overnight stays. Of the planned day cases, 75.8% (n=332) were discharged on the same day and 106 (24.2%) had unexpected overnight stay (UOS). Most patients with BMI >35 and ASA3 planned day case patients were successfully discharged. Drain insertion, longer operations, and late recovery departure were the main reasons for UOS. There were more complications in this group compared to day cases. *Conclusions.* This unit has a high 'true day case' rate of 75.8%. High BMI and ASA3 should not be absolute contraindications to day case surgery. The majority of unexpected overnight stays are unavoidable but may be reduced by patient selection, stringent preoperative assessment, operation scheduling, and reduction in unnecessary drain insertion.

1. Introduction

Laparoscopic cholecystectomy (LC) is the gold standard of the treatment for gallstones [1]. Increasing the number of elective LCs performed as day case (at least 75%) is a key target in the National Health Service (NHS) plan issued by the UK Department of Health [2]. British Association of Day Surgery (BADS) recommends that at least 60% of LC operations should be performed as day cases both for optimal patient outcomes and cost-effectiveness [3]. Although a number of studies have reported that day case LC is feasible, effective, and safe, the national average for successful day case LC is reported to be only around 16% [3–6]. This may be in part due to use of so-called 'absolute criteria' guiding admission policies in many units.

There is still ambiguity in the way the day case LC data is presented in the literature, with considerable confusion between the so-called '23-hour' stay and true day cases where the patient is discharged on the same day of surgery [7, 8]. The definition of 'true day case' procedure as per BADS guidelines is as follows: a patient is admitted, has a procedure performed, requires recovery facilities, and is discharged on the same day and does not stay overnight in the hospital [3]. However, some units 'reinterpret' the definition and hence report those patients who stayed overnight and get discharged the following morning as 'day cases', based on the 23-hour stay guideline [7].

Unexpected admission following day case procedure is an unwanted outcome for the patient, the surgeon, and the trust [9, 10]. Overnight stay leads to inconvenience among the patients and carers and can lead to poor patient experience and satisfaction [11]. Admission of these patients increases the pressure on acute hospital beds and has significant economic implications. A high unexpected admission rate invariably reflects on the suboptimal efficiency of the trust and is considered as a failure of day care facilities [12, 13].

The aims of this study were to determine the rate of 'true day case' LCs in a high-volume setting and also to study the factors that lead to unexpected admissions following LC.

2. Methods

We prospectively collected data for all patients who underwent day case LC over a period of 32 months between March 2010 and October 2012. The Upper Gastrointestinal Unit at Hinchingbrooke Hospital performs around 300 LCs per year, of which 75-80% are elective planned admissions and the remainder done as emergencies. All patients for day case LC were listed following review in outpatient clinic or after emergency admission without requiring urgent surgery (when symptoms settled rapidly allowing discharge and a planned elective procedure). In every case gallstones were confirmed on ultrasound scan.

The patient inclusion and exclusion criteria for day case LC were based on agreed local trust guidelines on day case surgery and include three categories: social factors, medical factors, and surgical factors. The social factor includes their understanding of day case procedure, their social support for the first 24 hours, and domestic circumstances for postoperative care. The medical factors, such as their comorbidities and contraindications to day surgery, were reviewed by the consultant anaesthetists or specialist nurses, who had the final say on listing for day case or planned admission. The listing surgeon decides on the appropriateness of the laparoscopic procedure, including the risk of serious complications, recovery postprocedure, and mobility.

Our only absolute criterion for allocation to the overnight admission group is social, i.e., those patients who do not have a responsible adult at home to look after them for 24 hours postprocedure. The other criteria such as American Society of Anaesthesiology (ASA) class 3 and above, body mass index (BMI) above 35, previous severe pancreatitis, and previous extensive abdominal surgery are considered to be relative contraindications to being listed as day case procedure; while some of these patients inevitably require overnight stay, many are routinely planned as day cases. Patients with multiple comorbidities are all assessed and treated in this unit and not referred to a tertiary centre. Diabetic patients are routinely placed first on the morning list and usually discharged on the same day. Patients on anticoagulation present a range of clinical risk: those on prophylaxis for uncomplicated atrial fibrillation can often be successfully treated as day cases whereas those with higher risk disease (e.g., coronary stents or recurrent DVTs) are usually planned for overnight stay with advice sought where appropriate from cardiologist and/or anticoagulant nurse specialists. A diagnosis of common bile duct (CBD) stones elevates the complexity of the case; if preoperative endoscopic retrograde cholangiopancreatography (ERCP) successfully clears the duct, the patient may still be considered for day case surgery, but planned laparoscopic CBD exploration will inevitably require inpatient care.

Patients were admitted to the day case unit at 07:30 if their operation was scheduled for the morning list and 11:00 if scheduled for the afternoon. The patients wore thromboembolic deterrent (TED) stockings unless contraindicated. All patients had antibiotic prophylaxis at induction and intraoperative temperature was maintained by warming blanket. All patients underwent standard LC using four-port technique. Intra-abdominal CO_2 insufflation pressure was set at 10-12mmHg. The port sites were injected with 20ml of 0.25% bupivacaine. Drains were not placed routinely but used selectively where surgically indicated, e.g., after particularly difficult dissection with unexpected bleeding. This unit operates a selective policy for intraoperative cholangiography, depending on preoperative bloods and imaging; rarely it is required for difficult anatomy.

All patients were operated on by a consultant, or experienced registrar with consultant available for advice. Junior trainees not yet independent on this operation were supervised by the consultant scrubbed in theatre.

Postoperatively patients were transferred to recovery and then back to the day case ward, from where they could be discharged until 22:00 if they met day case unit criteria for discharge shown in the appendix. If there are any contraindications to discharge, they were admitted for overnight stay.

All patients were followed up by telephone at 4–6 weeks postoperatively by a surgical care practitioner who completed a follow-up questionnaire and collected outcome data prospectively including any postoperative complications such as wound infection, haematoma, and readmissions.

The data collected for this study included demographic details and operative details including timing of the procedure (AM or PM list), length of operation, use of on-table cholangiogram, insertion of drains, intraoperative complications, time of leaving theatre recovery, grade of operating surgeon, and any immediate postoperative complications. The reasons for overnight admission were categorised as pain control, nausea and vomiting, drain in situ, urinary retention, other anaesthetic and social issues, positive on-table cholangiogram (if there is a need for urgent postoperative ERCP), long operation, and late-evening completion of the procedure. Long operation was defined as 90 minutes or longer and late operation was defined as leaving recovery later than 18:30. Leaving recovery after this time would not allow 4 hours of recovery time before closure of the day case unit at 22:00.

2.1. Statistical Analysis. Categorical variables are expressed as the frequency and proportions (%), and continuous variables are presented as the mean ± standard deviation. Categorical variables were analysed by Fisher's exact or chi-square test and continuous variables by unpaired Student's *t*-test or one-way ANOVA (Analysis of Variance). P value <0.05 was considered significant.

The variables which showed statistical significance (p value <0.01) on univariate analysis were further subjected to multivariate analysis using logistic regression model, and odds ratio with 95% confidence interval was calculated. The variables significant on multivariate analysis (p value <0.05) were considered as independent prognosticators of unexpected overnight stay. All statistical analyses were carried out using SPSS for Windows version 20.0 (SPSS Inc., Chicago, IL, USA).

Table 1: Patient demographics: TDC versus UOS.

	Total (N=438)	TDC (n=332)	UOS (n=106)	P value
Age (years)	51.0±15.6	49.8±15.6	54.7±15.0	**0.005**
Female gender	347 (79.2%)	269 (81.0%)	78 (73.6%)	0.129
BMI (Kg/m^2)				
Mean ± SD	29.9±5.5	29.8±5.4	30.5±5.9	0.256
<18.5	2 (0.5%)	1 (0.3%)	1 (0.9%)	0.426
18.5-24.9	67 (15.3%)	56 (16.9%)	11 (10.4%)	0.122
25.0-29.9	164 (37.4%)	122 (36.7%)	42 (39.6%)	0.645
30.0-34.9	113 (25.8%)	83 (25.0%)	30 (28.3%)	0.525
≥35.0	92 (21.0%)	70 (21.1%)	22 (20.8%)	1.000
ASA				
1	184 (42.0%)	154 (46.4%)	30 (28.3%)	**0.001**
2	232 (53.0%)	163 (49.1%)	69 (65.1%)	**0.005**
3	22 (5.0%)	15 (4.5%)	7 (6.6%)	0.443

3. Results

During the study period, 500 patients underwent elective LC in our unit. Three patients were excluded from the study because they required CBD exploration; therefore 497 cases were analysed. Among those were 391 females and 106 males (ratio 4:1). The median age was 52 with a range of 16-85 years. The median body mass index (BMI) was 29 kg/m^2 with a range of 17-50 kg/m^2. The ASA status was ASA 1= 192 (38.6%), ASA 2= 266 (53.5%), and ASA 3= 39 (7.9%). Fifty-nine (11.8%) patients were planned for postoperative overnight stay due to either social or medical reasons. Therefore, overall 438 (88.2%) patients were planned for day case LCs, of which 332 (75.8%) were successfully completed as day case (true day case; TDC) and 106 (24.2%) patients stayed overnight due to various reasons (unexpected overnight stay; UOS).

4. Demographics: TDC versus UOS

Those patients who stayed overnight following day case LC were older (UOS; 54.7±15.0 years) when compared to TDC group (49.8±15.6 years; P=0.005). There was no difference between the two groups in terms of gender and BMI distribution; 76% patients with BMI >35 who were planned day cases were discharged on the day of surgery. There were significantly more ASA 2 patients in UOS group, when compared to TDC group (65.1% versus 49.1%; P=0.005). As expected, the TDC group had significantly more fit and healthy ASA 1 status patients (46.4%) when compared to UOS group (28.3%; P=0.001) (Table 1). Of the 22 ASA 3 patients who were planned day cases, 68% were successfully discharged on the day of surgery.

5. Reasons for Unexpected Overnight Admissions

The reasons for unexpected overnight admissions are listed in Table 2. Some of the patients stayed overnight due to multiple reasons. Twenty-six (24.6%) patients had drain inserted which was the main reason for UOS. The other common reasons for UOS was leaving theatre recovery after 18:30 (19.8%), anaesthetic/social issues such as prolonged postoperative nausea and vomiting or unanticipated lack of support at home (19.8%), and procedures lasting more than 90 minutes (17.9%).

Table 2: Reasons for unexpected overnight admissions (n=106).

Reason*	Number of Patients (%)
Long operation over 90 min	19 (17.9%)
Drain	26 (24.6%)
Left recovery after 18:30	21 (19.8%)
Post-operative pain	5 (4.7%)
Intra operative complications (small bowel injury)	1 (0.9%)
Retention of urine	7 (6.6%)
Other reasons (anaesthetic issues and social)	21 (19.8%)
Required ERCP post-op (positive OTC)	6 (5.7%)

*Main reason for unplanned overnight stay as per clinician decision listed in the table. Some patients stayed overnight due to multiple reasons.

6. Factors Contributing to UOS

There were significantly more patients aged more than 50 years in UOS group when compared with the TDC group

(64.1% versus 46.7%; P=0.001). The mean operating time was also longer in the UOS group, which explains why there was unexpected overnight admission in this group (82.5 versus 64.9 mins; P<0.001). The LC took more than 90 minutes in 35.8% of patients in the UOS group, whereas only 12.9% in the TDC group had procedure which was longer than this time (P<0.001). As expected, significantly more patients in the UOS group had OTCs performed (35.8% versus 25.3%; P=0.046) and these were more common when LC took more than 90 minutes (15.1% versus 4.5%; P<0.001). Similarly, 24.5% of patients in the UOS group had drain inserted, whereas no patients (0.0%) in the TDC group had drains (P<0.001).

The majority of patients in the UOS group were operated in the PM list (69.8%) when compared to the TDC group (49.7%; P<0.001). This also explains why significant proportion of UOS patients left recovery after 18:30 when compared to those who were discharged on the same day (22.6% versus 1.8%; P<0.001).

There was no difference in the intraoperative complications between the two groups; however, immediate postoperative complications such as bleeding from the port site and urinary retention were significantly higher in the UOS group (6.6% versus 0.0%; P<0.001). There was no difference in the number of LCs performed by the trainee registrar or staff grade between the TDC and UOS groups, respectively (18.1% versus 11.3%; P=0.131).

On multivariate analysis, age more than 50 years [OR 2.1 (95% CI 1.15-3.78); P=0.015], mean operating time [OR 1.0 (95% CI 1.00-1.04); P=0.017], leaving theatre recovery after 18:30 [OR 15.1 (95% CI 5.41-42.34); P<0.001)], and PM list [OR 2.4 (95% CI 1.30-4.61); P=0.005] were independent prognosticators contributing to unexpected overnight admissions following LC (Table 3).

There was no conversion to open procedure or reoperation during the study period in either group and there was also no bile leak or bile duct injury. There was no difference between the TDC and UOS groups in terms of number of readmissions following discharge [9 (2.7%) versus 2 (1.9%); P=1.000] (Table 4).

7. Discussion

It has long been established that LC can be performed safely and effectively as a day case procedure. However, this has usually applied to a selected group of patients using rigid exclusion criteria and thus results in an overall low rate of true day case surgery with implications for procedure cost and bed availability. Many units still routinely book high BMI patients, diabetic patients, and all those classified as ASA3 for an overnight stay.

In this study in a high-volume LC setting in a specialist DGH unit, three-quarters (75.8%) of our planned day case patients were discharged on the same day, which gives an excellent 'true day case' rate which is significantly higher than previous reports in the literature [5, 8, 9, 11, 13–19].

Day case LC has been shown to be safe, effective, and highly economical. The Cochrane review published in 2013 pooled data from six trials involving 492 patients undergoing LC, with 239 patients in the day case and 253 in the overnight stay group. The review reported no significant difference in postoperative pain scores on visual analogue scale, serious adverse events, hospital readmission rate, time to return to normal activity, return to work, and quality of life after LC. They concluded that day case LC is just as safe as overnight stay LC. However day case discharge did not seem to result in improvement in any patient-oriented outcomes such as return to normal activity or earlier return to work [19].

In a large sample size we have demonstrated that 75.8% patients can be discharged home safely on the day of LC. A number of small studies have demonstrated high rates of compliance with day case LC; however, most of them involve discharge within 23 hours of surgery, which actually means that the patient stays overnight and is discharged home the following morning. Jain et al. reported 269 patients over a 5-year period who underwent LC, of which 79% were discharged home within 8 hours of surgery, 95% were discharged on the same day, and 5% were admitted overnight. The patients in this study were highly selected with only 26% of all patients listed for day case LC, whereas we listed 88.2% of all patients for day case LC. Also the majority of patients in their study were ASA 1 (88%) and the remainder were ASA 2 (12%), there were no intraoperative cholangiograms, and 16% of the patients who stayed more than 8 hours were temporarily transferred to the main hospital surgical ward. Although the results from this study are commendable, any usage of general surgical non-day case bed following LC should be considered as failure of day case intention [20]. Similarly, a number of studies have demonstrated that LC can be performed as day case with careful patient selection. Metcalfe et al. reported no difference between the outcomes when comparison was made between day case LC patient selection with and without strict exclusion criteria such as thickness of gallbladder wall, patient age more than 55 years, and previous sphincterotomy [21], but this will inevitably result in higher rates of planned inpatient admission [7, 22, 23].

Many centres employ stringent or 'absolute' criteria for selection of patients for day case LC [21, 24, 25]. The common exclusion criteria are age more than 70 years, BMI > 35 kg/m^2, ASA grade 3 or more, complicated biliary disease (evidence of common bile duct stones or previous endoscopic retrograde cholangiogram, severe pancreatitis, and recurrent admissions with cholecystitis), previous extensive abdominal surgery, or a history of severe postoperative nausea and vomiting [8, 26]. Tescani et al. published a systematic review of 20 randomised controlled trials published on day case LCs between January 2000 and June 2008. Out of 20 trials, only one trial included patients of ASA grade III for day case LC, and only three trials included patients with high BMI (35 or more) for day case LC [24]. Our only absolute exclusion criterion was the absence of a responsible adult to stay with the patient following discharge. We suggest criteria other than social should be considered relative and selection should be done on a case by case basis. We have also demonstrated that the majority of patients with BMI > 35 kg/m^2 can be planned and successfully

Table 3: Univariate and multivariate analysis of factors contributing to UOS.

Parameter	TDC (N=332)	UOS (n=106)	Univariate Analysis	Multivariate Analysis		
				OR	95% CI	P value
Age (>50 years)	155 (46.7%)	68 (64.1%)	**0.001**	2.1	1.15-3.78	**0.015**
Age (>60 years)	97 (29.2%)	42 (39.6%)	0.055			
Age (> 70 years)	35 (10.5%)	18 (17.0%)	0.088			
Female gender	269 (81.0%)	78 (73.6%)	0.129			
BMI ≥ 30 Kg/m^2	153 (46.1%)	52 (49.0%)	0.655			
BMI ≥ 35 Kg/m^2	70 (21.1%)	22 (20.7%)	1.000			
BMI ≥ 40 Kg/m^2	19 (5.7%)	9 (8.5%)	0.361			
ASA 3	15 (4.5%)	7 (6.6%)	0.443			
Mean operation time (mins)	64.9±21.6	82.5±35.4	**<0.001**	1.0	1.00-1.04	**0.017**
Length of procedure (>90 minutes)	43 (12.9%)	38 (35.8%)	**<0.001**			
OTC performed	84 (25.3%)	38 (35.8%)	**0.046**			
OTCs in those who had > 90 minutes procedure	15 (4.5%)	16 (15.1%)	**<0.001**			
Drain insertion	0 (0.0%)	26 (24.5%)	**<0.001**			
Time leaving recovery (after 18:30 hrs)	6 (1.8%)	24 (22.6%)	**<0.001**	15.1	5.41-42.34	**<0.001**
Timing of procedure (PM list)	165 (49.7%)	74 (69.8%)	**<0.001**	2.4	1.30-4.61	**0.005**
Intra-operative complications (bowel injury, etc)	0 (0.0%)	1 (0.9%)	0.242			
Immediate post-operative complications (urine retention, bleeding)	0 (0.0%)	7 (6.6%)	**<0.001**			
Operations by trainee (Registrar)	60 (18.1%)	12 (11.3%)	0.131			

TABLE 4: Complications: TDC versus UOS.

Complications	TDC (n=332)	UOS (n=106)	P value
Readmissions	9 (2.7%)	2 (1.9%)	1.000
Retained stones	4	1	
Pain	3	1	
Wound infection	1	0	
Haematoma	1	0	
Total complications	6 (1.8%)	8 (7.5%)	**0.007**
	Wound infections (5), haematoma (1)	Small bowel injury (1), urine retention (7)	
Re-operation	0 (0.0%)	0 (0.0%)	1.000
Bile duct injury/bile leak	0 (0.0%)	0 (0.0%)	1.000
Conversion to open	0 (0.0%)	0 (0.0%)	1.000
30-day mortality	0 (0.0%)	0 (0.0%)	1.000

completed as day cases and the same applies to patients older than 50 years and ASA grade 3.

On multivariate analysis we identified patient's age more than 50 years, longer length of the procedure, PM operating list, and patient leaving theatre recovery after 18:30 as the independent prognosticators for unexpected admission following day case LC. Some of these factors such as age of the patient and length of the procedure cannot be altered. The prolonged procedure is mostly multifactorial, and in our cohort, it is possibly related to the time taken for OTC, difficult operation, intraoperative complication, and procedures requiring drain insertion. Hence, we recommend that procedures longer than 90 minutes should not be a contraindication for same-day discharge. Previous studies have reported longer operating durations when trainees were involved [27]. However, the longer operating times in our cohort were not related to inexperience of the surgeon, as only two of the 38 prolonged operations were operated by trainee surgeons.

Patients more than 50 years and those who are at risk of having prolonged surgery such as previous cholecystitis, ERCP procedure, and/or severe pancreatitis, high BMI (>35 kg/m^2), and previous abdominal surgery can be listed for AM rather than PM procedure. Appropriate list selection for these patients could make a substantial difference to the patient satisfaction and true day case rates, which in turn will have significant positive financial implications for the trust and also increase bed availability for emergency admissions at a time when this is sorely needed. Length of the operation and timing of the list have similarly contributed to overnight admission in other published series [6, 28]. Our readmission rate of 2.5% compares favourably with those reported by other centres, and there was no difference in readmission when patients were discharged home on the stay day or had overnight/further stay [28].

Drain insertion after LC is another aspect we have been auditing to see if the rates can be reduced. In this unit we do not insert drains routinely but only in difficult procedures, e.g., those with sepsis or significant intraoperative bleeding. Another option would be to send patients home with drain in situ, which can be monitored and removed by the community nurses. However, this is not without risk and involves utilisation of community resources. The other complications of drain insertion are localised pain (due to the presence of the tube) and poor patient mobility [29–31]. A recent meta-analysis of 12 randomised controlled trials involving 1939 patients randomised to drain (960) versus no drain (979) demonstrated lower morbidity in the no drain group (OR 1.97 (95% CI 1.26-3.10); P=0.003), lower wound infection (OR 2.35 (95% CI 1.22-4.51); P=0.010), and reduced pain 24 hours postsurgery (Standardised Mean Difference 2.30 (95% CI 1.27-3.34); P<0.0001). However they did not show any difference in the intra-abdominal collections and hospital stay [32].

8. Conclusion

The vast majority (88.2%) of our LCs were planned as day case, which is higher than those in most specialist units performing LCs. Three-quarters (75.8%) of our planned day case patients were discharged on the same day, which gives a high 'true day case' rate. The majority of unexpected overnight stays are unavoidable but this may potentially be reduced by a combination of patient selection, stringent preoperative assessment, operation scheduling, and reduction in unnecessary drain insertion. We recommend the reporting of day case surgery should be standardised in the literature to mean same-day discharge; patients who are predicted to have a long or difficult operation should be booked on a morning list to allow adequate recovery time and thus increase the chance of same-day discharge. Patients with BMI >35 or ASA 3 who are routinely scheduled for overnight stay in many units are in our experience often suitable for day case surgery. These measures may increase the overall rate of true day case surgery for LC and have a significant cost benefit by reducing the added bed pressures and financial costs of overnight or further hospital stay.

Appendix

Day Case Discharge Criteria

Discharge

OUTCOMES AND DISCHARGE CRITERIA	MET	If NO please give details
(i) Pain controlled with or without analgesia	□	
(ii) Patient made aware of care required post discharge	□	
(iii) Patient consent scanned and returned	□	

BP, pulse and blood loss stable and within normal range	YES	NO	N/A
Blood loss	□	□	
Tolerable nausea and no vomiting	□	□	
Passing urine normally if relevant	□	□	
Taken food and fluids	□	□	□
Mobile without feeling faint	□	□	□
IV cannula removed	□	□	□
Dressing clean and dry (please state types of dressing supplied)	□	□	□
Pressure areas checked	□	□	□
Patient safe on crutches	□	□	□
Post-op instructions and advise sheet given	□	□	□
Medication given and usage explained	□	□	□
Patient aware of re OPA_________/Details to be posted	□	□	□
Medical/Self certificate	□	□	□
Discharge letter: GP □ Practice nurse □ District nurse □	□	□	□
Day surgery only: Escort home and career to stay overnight	□	□	□
Social support (if yes, describe)	□	□	□
Telephone follow-up arranged for morning	□	□	□
Did Doctor see the patient before discharge?	□	□	□
Procedure specific protocol completed	□	□	□

DISCHARGE DATE: **TIME:**
NAME **SIGNATURE** **DESIGNATION**

I agree I am fit for discharge. Signature:..

I have been informed of my procedure and after care. Signature:..

Disclosure

Earlier version of this manuscript was orally presented in the 21st International Congress of the European Association for Endoscopic Surgery (EAES), Vienna, Austria, 19–22 June 2013.

Authors' Contributions

A. Solodkyy, A. R. Hakeem, and A. M. Harris conceptualised and designed the study. A. Solodkyy and N. Oswald collected the data. A. Solodkyy and A. R. Hakeem performed the statistical analysis and wrote the manuscript. A. R. Hakeem corrected the manuscript and prepared the final draft. F. Di Franco, S. Gergely, and A. M. Harris reviewed the manuscript and made the necessary corrections. A. M. Harris made the final corrections to the manuscript and is the corresponding author.

References

[1] F. Agresta, F. C. Campanile, N. Vettoretto et al., "Laparoscopic cholecystectomy: consensus conference-based guidelines," *Langenbeck's Archives of Surgery*, vol. 400, no. 4, article no. 1300, pp. 429–453, 2015.

[2] DOH, *The NHS Plan: a plan for investment, a plan for reform*, DoH, London, 2015.

[3] BADS, "Day Case Laparoscopic Cholecystectomy: NHS Institute Rapid Improvement Programme - British Association of Day Surgery," 2009, http://rcseng.ac.uk/policy/policy-seminars/day-surgery-and-enhanced-recovery/docs/ian_smith_2.pdf.

[4] G. van Boxel, M. Hart, A. Kiszely, and S. Appleton, "Elective day-case laparoscopic cholecystectomy: a formal assessment of the need for outpatient follow-up," *Annals of the Royal College of Surgeons of England*, vol. 95, no. 8, pp. 561–565, 2013.

[5] L. Graham, C. P. Neal, G. Garcea, D. M. Lloyd, G. S. Robertson, and C. D. Sutton, "Evaluation of nurse-led discharge following laparoscopic surgery," *Journal of Evaluation in Clinical Practice*, vol. 18, no. 1, pp. 19–24, 2012.

[6] J. A. Akoh, W. A. Watson, and T. P. Bourne, "Day case laparoscopic cholecystectomy: Reducing the admission rate," *International Journal of Surgery*, vol. 9, no. 1, pp. 63–67, 2011.

[7] J. Young and B. O'Connell, "Recovery following laparoscopic cholecystectomy in either a 23 hour or an 8 hour facility," *Journal of Quality in Clinical Practice*, vol. 21, no. 1-2, pp. 2–7, 2001.

[8] A. W. Chieh Kow, A. Tan, S. P. Chan et al., "An audit of ambulatory laparoscopic cholecystectomy in a Singapore institution: Are we ready for day-case laparoscopic cholecystectomy?" *HPB*, vol. 10, no. 6, pp. 433–438, 2008.

[9] J. M. Kiely, A. Brannigan, E. Foley, S. Cheema, W. O'Brien, and P. V. Delaney, "Day case laparoscopic cholecystectomy is feasible," *Irish Journal of Medical Science*, vol. 170, no. 2, pp. 98-99, 2001.

[10] M. A. Rathore, S. I. H. Andrabi, M. Mansha, and M. G. Brown, "Day case laparoscopic cholecystectomy is safe and feasible: A case controlled study," *International Journal of Surgery*, vol. 5, no. 4, pp. 255–259, 2007.

[11] K. S. Gurusamy, S. Junnarkar, M. Farouk, and B. R. Davidson, "Day-case versus overnight stay in laparoscopic cholecystectomy.," *Cochrane Database of Systematic Reviews (Online)*, no. 1, p. CD006798, 2008.

[12] M. G. Clarke, T. Wheatley, M. Hill, G. Werrett, and G. Sanders, "An Effective Approach to Improving Day-Case Rates following Laparoscopic Cholecystectomy," *Minimally Invasive Surgery*, vol. 2011, pp. 1–5, 2011.

[13] M. Islam, P. Deka, R. Kapur, and M. A. Ansari, "Non-bleeding spontaneous rupture of hepatocellular carcinoma," *Nigerian Journal of Surgery*, vol. 19, no. 2, pp. 82–84, 2013.

[14] N. Z. Ahmad, G. Byrnes, and S. A. Naqvi, "A meta-analysis of ambulatory versus inpatient laparoscopic cholecystectomy," *Surgical Endoscopy*, vol. 22, no. 9, pp. 1928–1934, 2008.

[15] A. Huang, C. Stinchcombe, D. Phillips, and D. L. McWhinnie, "Prospective 5-year audit for day-case laparoscopic cholecystectomy," *British Journal of Surgery*, vol. 87, no. 3, pp. 366-366, 2000.

[16] A. Kasem, A. Paix, S. Grandy-Smith, and S. El-Hasani, "Is laparoscopic cholecystectomy safe and acceptable as a day case procedure?" *Journal of Laparoendoscopic & Advanced Surgical Techniques*, vol. 16, no. 4, pp. 365–368, 2006.

[17] P. C. Leader, T. Matthews, K. Krzeminska, and T. C. B. Dehn, "Routine day-case laparoscopic cholecystectomy," *British Journal of Surgery*, vol. 91, no. 3, pp. 312–316, 2004.

[18] J. Psaila, S. Agrawal, U. Fountain et al., "Day-surgery laparoscopic cholecystectomy: Factors influencing same-day discharge," *World Journal of Surgery*, vol. 32, no. 1, pp. 76–81, 2008.

[19] J. Vaughan, K. S. Gurusamy, and B. R. Davidson, "Day-surgery versus overnight stay surgery for laparoscopic cholecystectomy.," *Cochrane Database of Systematic Reviews*, vol. 7, p. CD006798, 2013.

[20] P. K. Jain, J. D. Hayden, P. C. Sedman, C. M. S. Royston, and C. J. O'Boyle, "A prospective study of ambulatory laparoscopic cholecystectomy: Training economic, and patient benefits," *Surgical Endoscopy*, vol. 19, no. 8, pp. 1082–1085, 2005.

[21] M. S. Metcalfe, E. J. Mullin, and G. J. Maddern, "Relaxation of the criteria for day surgery laparoscopic cholecystectomy," *ANZ Journal of Surgery*, vol. 76, no. 3, pp. 142–144, 2006.

[22] J. Skattum, B. Edwin, E. Trondsen, J. Raeder, and T. Buanes, "Outpatient laparoscopic surgery: feasibility and consequences for education and health care costs," *Surgical Endoscopy*, vol. 18, no. 5, 2004.

[23] M. J. Rosen, J. A. Malm, M. Tarnoff, K. Zuccala, and J. L. Ponsky, "Cost-effectiveness of Ambulatory Laparoscopic Cholecystectomy," *Surgical Laparoscopy, Endoscopy & Percutaneous Techniques*, vol. 11, no. 3, pp. 182–184, 2001.

[24] S. M. Tenconi, L. Boni, E. M. Colombo, G. Dionigi, F. Rovera, and E. Cassinotti, "Laparoscopic cholecystectomy as day-surgery procedure: Current indications and patients' selection," *International Journal of Surgery*, vol. 6, no. 1, pp. S86–S88, 2008.

[25] J. P. Tuckey, G. N. Morris, C. J. Peden, and J. J. T. Tate, "Feasibility of day case laparoscopic cholecystectomy in unselected patients," *Anaesthesia*, vol. 51, no. 10, pp. 965–968, 1996.

[26] C. D. Briggs, G. B. Irving, C. D. Mann et al., "Introduction of a day-case laparoscopic cholecystectomy service in the UK: A critical analysis of factors influencing same-day discharge and contact with primary care providers," *Annals of the Royal College of Surgeons of England*, vol. 91, no. 7, pp. 583–590, 2009.

[27] A. Souadka, M. Naya, B. Serji et al., "Impact of seniority on operative time and short-term outcome in laparoscopic cholecystectomy: Experience of an academic Surgical Department in a developing country," *Journal of Minimal Access Surgery*, vol. 0, no. 0, p. 0, 2016.

[28] H. Lau and D. C. Brooks, "Contemporary outcomes of ambulatory laparoscopic cholecystectomy in a major teaching hospital," *World Journal of Surgery*, vol. 26, no. 9, pp. 1117–1121, 2002.

[29] W. Bugiantella, M. C. Vedovati, C. Becattini, R. C. B. Canger, N. Avenia, and F. Rondelli, "To drain or not to drain elective uncomplicated laparoscopic cholecystectomy? A systematic review and meta-analysis," *Journal of Hepato-Biliary-Pancreatic Sciences*, vol. 21, no. 11, pp. 787–794, 2014.

[30] A. M. Donatsky, F. Bjerrum, and I. Gögenur, "Surgical techniques to minimize shoulder pain after laparoscopic cholecystectomy. A systematic review," *Surgical Endoscopy*, vol. 27, no. 7, pp. 2275–2282, 2013.

[31] K. S. Gurusamy, R. Koti, and B. R. Davidson, "Routine abdominal drainage versus no abdominal drainage for uncomplicated laparoscopic cholecystectomy.," *Cochrane Database of Systematic Reviews*, vol. 9, p. CD006004, 2013.

[32] M. Picchio, P. Lucarelli, A. Di Filippo, F. De Angelis, F. Stipa, and E. Spaziani, "Meta-analysis of drainage versus no drainage after laparoscopic cholecystectomy," *JSLS : Journal of the Society of Laparoendoscopic Surgeons*, vol. 18, no. 4, 2014.

21

Effects of Fatigue Based on Electroencephalography Signal during Laparoscopic Surgical Simulation

Nyakuru Z. Ndaro and Shu-Yi Wang

Department of Biomedical Engineering, School of Medical Instrument and Food Engineering, University of Shanghai for Science and Technology, Shanghai 200093, China

Correspondence should be addressed to Nyakuru Z. Ndaro; nyakurundaro@gmail.com

Academic Editor: Isaac Kim

Background. Following recent advances in technology, there is a growing interest in studying fatigue based on electrophysiological signals as a means of monitoring brain activity. While some existing works relate fatigue to performance, others consider the two as independent entities. Therefore, we must explore this intricate issue, particularly in laparoscopic training, for the sake of patient safety. *Objective.* This paper explores and evaluates effects of fatigue on efficiency and accuracy based on laparoscopic surgical training using Electroencephalography (EEG) signal. *Materials and Methods.* 20 college students performed peg transfer task on laparoscopic simulator, with real-time recording of EEG signals for each subject. To monitor degree of fatigue, a real-time fatigue monitoring system based on fatigue analysis algorithm was designed through the use of EEG in alpha (α) and theta (θ) rhythms. We designed data acquisition and fatigue analysis modules based on MATLAB platform. BrainLink was used to record EEG signals and send them to personal computer wirelessly via Bluetooth. While artifacts from the captured EEG signals were removed using Blind Source Separation (BSS), α and θ rhythms were extracted using wavelet analysis. Fatigue was evaluated based on Regression Model and Mahalanobis Distance (D_C), and its threshold was determined from the experimental results using Receiver Operating Characteristic (ROC) curve analysis. *Results.* Completion time and number of errors behaved like a decreasing function during the first few trials while increasing afterwards with the increasing of perceived fatigue level. The results indicate that learning curve of the subjects is increasing until 13th trials when they have attained maximum learning benefits and decreases afterwards due to fatigue. *Conclusion.* Regression analysis shows that there are significant learning and fatigue effects when peg transfer task in the training is repeated in a series of trials. However, for the training to be effective and efficient, there should be monitoring during the training to observe where in the learning curve a trainee gains maximum learning benefits. Furthermore, fatigue is a significant indicator of efficiency and accuracy in terms of completion time and errors, respectively.

1. Introduction

Surgeons, particularly those in training, work for a long period of time and are often sleep deprived [1]. Such personnel may possibly experience disturbance in circadian rhythms, which may exacerbate physical or mental fatigue. Fatigue has been proved to decrease efficiency in cognitive skills [2], leading to decrease in performance as well as increasing rate of medical errors [3, 4]. However, previous studies that investigated the link between performance and fatigue are conflicting. Some studies concluded that fatigue has no impact on surgical performance [5, 6] while others link it to performance [7, 8]. Therefore, understanding the effects of fatigue, particularly in surgical training, remains an open problem.

In surgical field, virtual reality surgical simulation has been an alternative approach to examine effects of fatigue on performance [7–9] without reliance on patients for laparoscopic training. The surgical simulator is a cost-effective laparoscopic training device that uses innovative learning tools for skill acquisition and can differentiate user's level of experience. It can also evaluate surgical performance without the use of patients for skills practice [9]. A number of studies used surgical simulators to investigate effects of fatigue in laparoscopy. For example, Daruwalla et al. investigated effects of fatigue on laparoscopic skills and found that fatigue has effects on laparoscopic tasks such as peg transfer [7]. This finding was supported by Tsafrir et al. [8] who argued that efficiency and safety of residents are affected by fatigue [8]. Yet, most of the existing works are based on indirect way of measuring brain activities. These include the use of individual report scaling questionnaires [4], eye blink pattern using camera systems or Electrooculography (EOG) [10], and heart rate variability by Electrocardiography (ECG) [11]. However, an individual report questionnaire lacks sensitivity in detection of small important changes in mental fatigue. In EOG, the closure of eyelid increases with increasing fatigue while ECG holds a reflection of autonomic nerve activity. Conversely, it is very important to monitor brain activity using direct measurement technique such as Electroencephalography (EEG) [11]. This technique is regarded as a promising method for detecting mental fatigue and provides the most direct measurement of brain activity [11]. Therefore, this paper explores and evaluates effects of fatigue on efficiency and accuracy based on laparoscopic surgical simulation using Electroencephalography (EEG) as a means of monitoring brain activity. In order to study this precisely, a real-time fatigue monitoring system based on fatigue analysis algorithm was designed and 20 college students were employed to perform laparoscopic task, with real-time recording of EEG signals for each subject.

2. Materials and Methods

2.1. Subjects. 20 healthy college students in the age range of 24 to 26 with correct visual acuity of 1.0 or more were recruited from University of Shanghai for Science and Technology. A lifestyle questionnaire was administered and used as a selection criterion which required the subjects to have no medical contraindications such as history of prior brain injuries, use of prescription medication, severe concomitant disease, drug abuse, or alcoholism as well as psychological or intellectual problems, which more likely limit compliance.

All subjects filled informed agreement form and none of them had previous experience with laparoscopic simulator. Likewise, all subjects received comprehensive instructions about the task described in Section 2.3 and were given 15 minutes of hands-on introduction for orientation with the equipment until they became competent in laparoscopy simulation task. This study had the approval from the institutional ethics committee. Subjects were requested to stop cigarette smoking and consuming caffeinated drinks or any other stimulant 48 hours prior to the experiment as they may interfere with the trend of fatigue, and compliance with these instructions was reported. The experiment was performed from 13:00 to 17:00 hours in a temperature controlled room with continuous peg transfer task 20 times, in order to make the subjects into fatigue state.

2.2. Real-Time Fatigue Monitoring System. We designed a real-time monitoring system to evaluate and analyze effects of fatigue on efficiency and accuracy during laparoscopic simulation. The system consists of EEG data acquisition module, fatigue analysis module, Bluetooth communication module, and laparoscopic simulator platform. The data acquisition and fatigue analysis modules were designed based on MATLAB platform.

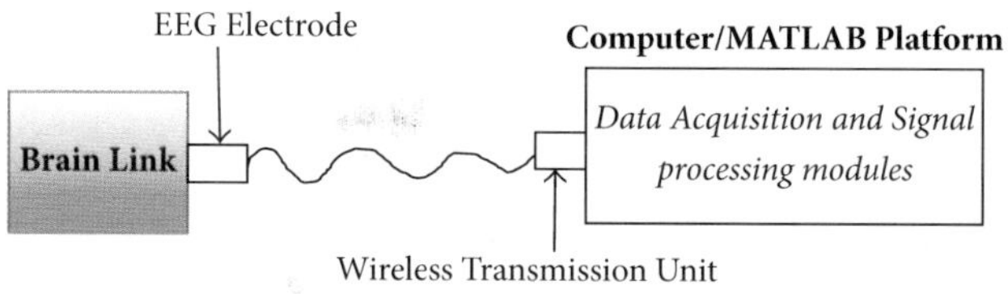

Figure 1: Schematic view of EEG fatigue monitoring system.

2.2.1. EEG Signal Recording and Acquisition Module. The experiment employed a virtual reality laparoscopic simulator (called Simbionix LAP Mentor) to perform peg transfer task. This simulator has a wide variety of modules ranging from simple to complex laparoscopic tasks such as suturing, basic operation, cholecystectomy, gastric bypass surgery, incision hernia surgery, gynecological surgery, rectal surgery, and laparoscopic assembly skills. During the experiment, BrainLink was used to record EEG signals through the use of its three forehead electrodes. The recordings of neuronal activity in the brain are identified as EEG signals [12]. Indeed, the electrodes read EEG signals from head surface and send them to personal computer wirelessly via Bluetooth module for storage and display, as demonstrated in Figure 1.

2.2.2. Signal Processing and Fatigue Analysis. Signal processing and fatigue analysis were designed to follow three steps, as demonstrated in Figure 2.

The first step is to remove artifacts from EEG signals. Although BrainLink is designed to record cerebral activity, it also records electrical activities arising from entities other than the brain. Generally, any activity that is recorded apart from cerebral origin is termed as artifact. In most cases, the artifacts can be obtained from either physiologic or extra physiologic perspectives. The former are unwanted physiological signals that arise from source other than the brain, that is, the body. For example, eye movements, heart, and muscles. The latter are technical and arise from outside the body, for example, noise in AC power line which can be reduced by decreasing electrode impedance and shorter electrode wires. In fact, any EEG signal greater than 50 μV is regarded as an artifact [13, 14]. However, many artifacts cannot be identified if their amplitude is lower than 50 μV. Therefore, a systematic approach to eliminate artifact is important to reduce chance of misinterpretation and analysis of the EEG signal. Several techniques have been proposed to remove artifacts from EEG recording. In the present study, a Blind Source Separation (BSS) method is employed to remove artifacts from EEG data. BSS is a signal processing method that includes independent component analysis. BSS technology separates interfering signal from the original. By studying distribution of the artifacts and the use of BBS technology, we obtained a pure EEG signal from the raw EEG data. The raw EEG signal obtained from the BrainLink is demonstrated in Figure 3.

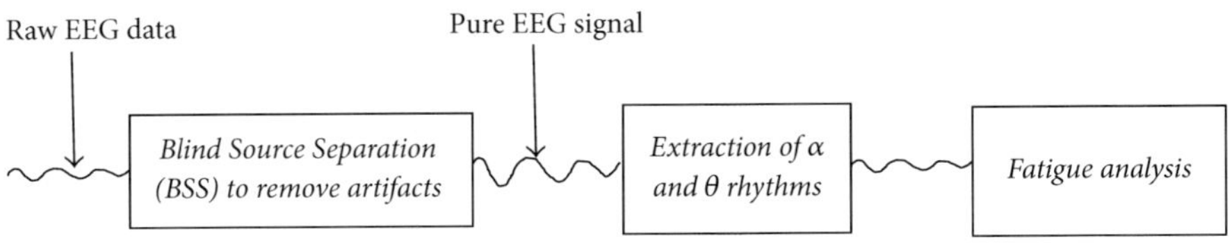

FIGURE 2: Three steps for signal processing and fatigue analysis.

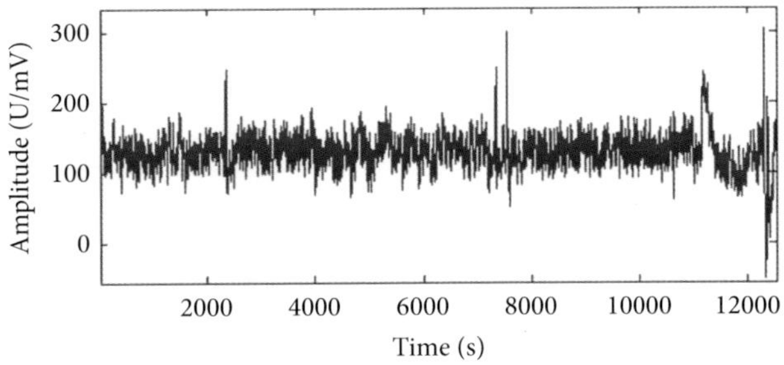

FIGURE 3: Raw EEG signal from the BrainLink.

The second step is the extraction of characteristic rhythm waves. Human brain pattern poses regular oscillations which are termed as rhythms and are differentiated on the basis of signal's frequency [15]. Rhythms of electrical activity in the brain are categorized according to frequency bands, namely, alpha (α), beta (β), theta (θ), and delta (δ) [4]. These rhythms are usually identified by frequency and amplitudes. The amplitudes recorded by scalp electrodes from the BrainLink are in the range of microvolts (μV). The present experiment employed wavelet analysis to extract two characteristic rhythms waves: alpha (α) and theta (θ), as shown in Figure 4. Since variations in the alertness state induce changes in EEG spectra, the spectra in θ rhythm (4–7 Hz) and α rhythm (8–11 Hz) will reveal changes in cognitive state and memory performance so that when mental fatigue increases, the relative power of α and θ rhythms decreases [16].

The third step is computation of deviation of EEG signals in θ and α rhythm. When fatigue occurs, both θ and α rhythms change significantly [10] and the subject's EEG spectra in them deviate from his or her alert state. Hence, his or her cognitive state and memory performance will change. This deviation was calculated using Mahalanobis Distance (D). The EEG spectra in θ and α rhythms are characterized by (μ, N), where μ is the vector of mean values and C is the covariance matrix of EEG spectra. The Mahalanobis Distance is calculated as follows:

$$D(x_\alpha) = \left[(x_\alpha - \mu)^T C^{-1} (x_\alpha - \mu)\right]^{1/2},$$
$$D(x_\theta) = \left[(x_\theta - \mu)^T N^{-1} (x_\theta - \mu)\right]^{1/2}, \tag{1}$$

where x_θ and x_α are EEG signal in θ and α rhythms, respectively. Then, the combined deviation of EEG is given by

$$D_C = \sigma * D(x_\alpha) + (1-\sigma) * D(x_\theta), \quad 0 \le \sigma \le 1. \tag{2}$$

The parameter σ is a constant. Since Mahalanobis Distance in θ and α rhythms changes with fatigue state, the weights of $D(x_\alpha)$, $D(x_\theta)$, and D_C are used as indicators of fatigue. In the present work, the threshold of fatigue was calculated from the experimental results based on Receiver Operating Characteristic (ROC) curve analysis. When the value of D_C is larger than the defined threshold, the cognitive state of the subject can be regarded as fatigue state.

2.2.3. Software Platform. The system was designed to use GUI platform which enables functions such as data processing and drawings. The system collects EEG signals and extracts characteristic rhythms wave α and θ, in order to calculate fatigue value. Since the distance between EEG and the rhythms wave increases gradually with the increase of fatigue, it is very important to determine an appropriate threshold and compare the threshold with the weighted Mahalanobis Distance of θ and α rhythm. Based on the ROC curve analysis method, the fatigue threshold was determined (6.0 μV). In the present work, when fatigue value exceeds the predefined threshold value of 6.0 μV, fatigue is detected and the system immediately rings the alarm. The system interface is shown in Figure 5.

2.3. Experimental Procedures. Peg transfer task requires pegboard (with 12 pegs) and six rubber triangles (Figure 6). Each triangle is lifted using a grasper in the subject's left hand and transferred in mid-air to a grasper in his/her right hand. Then, the triangle is placed on a peg on the opposite side of the board. After moving all the triangles on the right side, then every triangle has to be moved back to the left side of the board, using the same procedure. The number of errors is defined when a subject drops the triangle out of reach. The maximum completion time was set to 300 seconds in the simulator.

3. Results

The training was evaluated objectively by comparing efficiency (in terms of completion time), accuracy (in terms of number of errors), and fatigue level.

3.1. Objective Indicators of Effective Laparoscopic Surgical Training. In most laparoscopic surgical training, minimizing number of errors, completion time, and fatigue level is preferred in general as it would improve efficiency of the training. To get representative sample of each aforementioned quantities, we averaged the results of all subjects at each training trial. Herein, we present the results of errors made

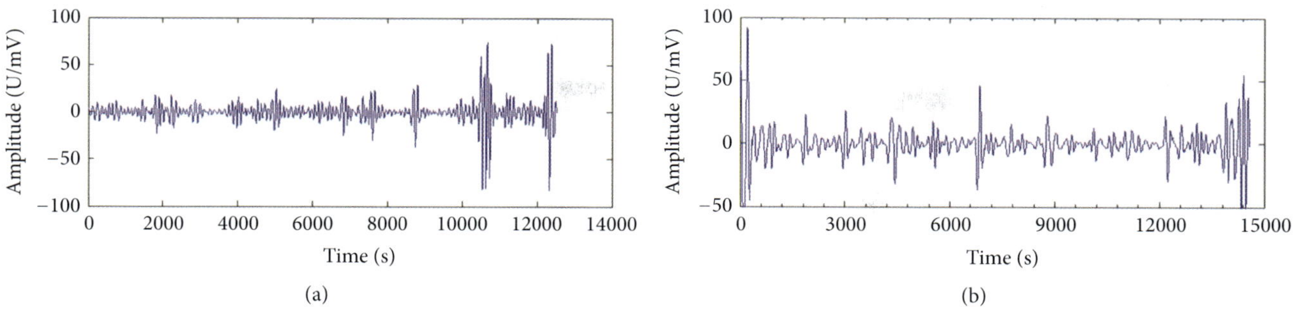

FIGURE 4: Brain waves belonging to alpha (α) and theta (θ).

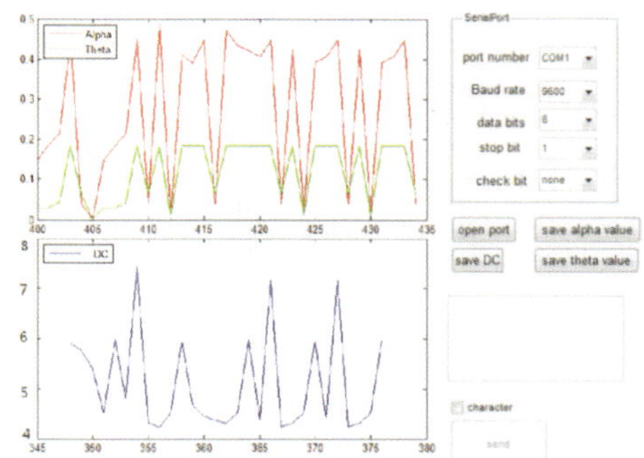

FIGURE 5: GUI platform for signal processing.

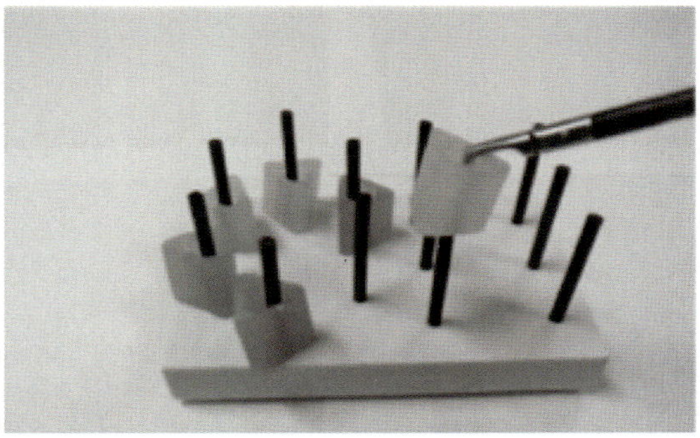

FIGURE 6: Left and right shift of six rubber triangles.

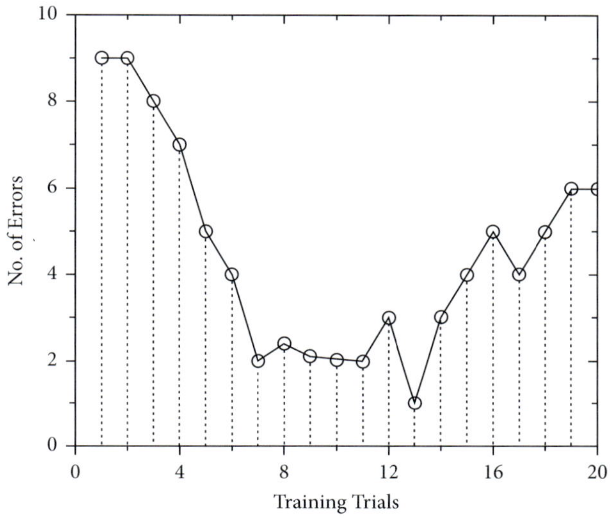

FIGURE 7: Number of errors during peg transfer task.

during peg transfer task, time to complete the task, and fatigue level.

3.1.1. Number of Errors. Regression Model predicted that the number of errors made during the first seven training trials was associated with lack of technical skills and perhaps new procedures [17], while it was associated with fatigue at the last eight trials. As predicted by the linear regression equation $y = 12.13 - 1.4 \times (R^2 = 0.98)$, the number of errors decreases until the seventh trial where it quickly attains a stable degree upon which the competency of the subject is anchored, as observed in Figure 7. This indicates that learning curve of the subjects has increased until seven trials when they have attained maximum learning benefits. During the 8th to 11th trials, the average number of errors is two, which is lower than the first seven, meaning that the subjects have acquired enough skills to cause fewer or no errors. The linear fitting equation portray $y = 3.34 - 0.13 \times (R^2 = 0.7)$, indicating a decreasing trend; however, such decrease is very scant. Between 13th and 20th trials, the number of errors is increasing and the function runs uphill, when a subject is acutely fatigued, with linear regression equation of $y = -5.96 + 0.62 \times (R^2 = 0.796)$. This means that maximum learning benefits will be gained by subjects until 13th trials and decrease afterwards due to fatigue. From the regression equation, it is shown that the slope of the regression line is 0.62 and the number of errors is expected to increase by 0.62 on average when the training proceeds to the next trial. Being fatigued significantly increases the chance of errors and decreases the learning curve. Therefore, when the same task in the training is repeated in a series of trials, there should be monitoring to observe where in the learning curve a trainee gains maximum learning benefits and then stop the training.

3.1.2. Completion Time. In terms of completion time, the laparoscopic simulator also calculated time spent for each subject to complete peg transfer task. The results show that all subjects took long time to finish the peg transfer task at the first time (around 130 seconds). However, each subsequent

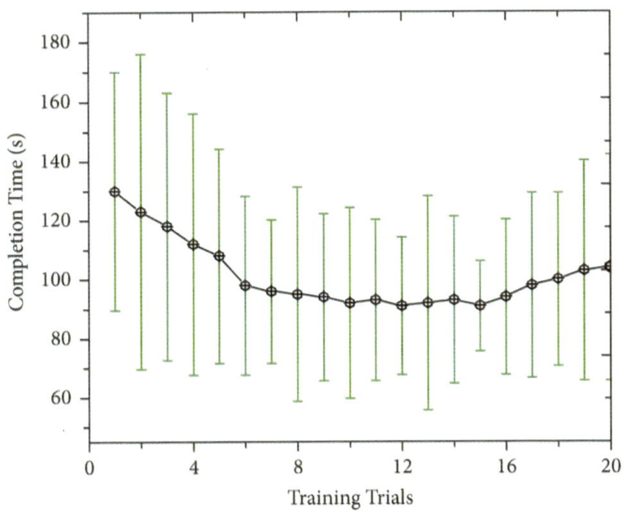

FIGURE 8: Completion time as a function of training trials.

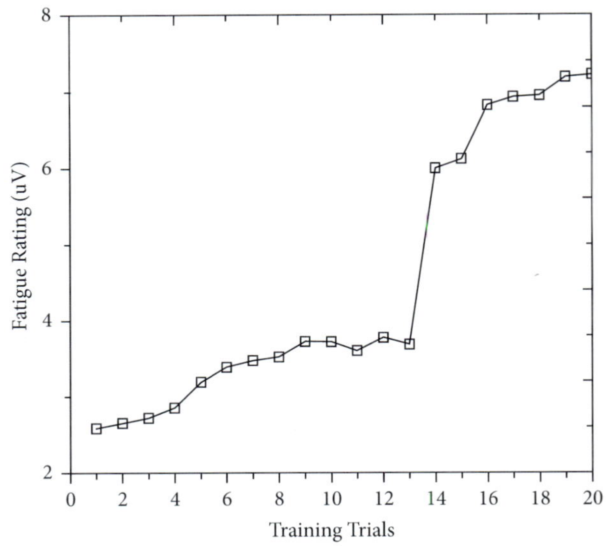

FIGURE 9: The measured rates of fatigue.

time they did the task took less time than the previous one until around 12 trials. This indicates that the subjects have learnt from doing peg transfer task and became faster each time they repeated the task. Nevertheless, the completion time started to increase at later trials due to fatigue effect. Precisely, during the first few training trials, the subjects took long time to complete the task. This is when they were acclimatized with the training. As more and more trials were conducted, significant improvement was found and the completion time decreased by 24% as predicted by the regression equation $y = 2.1 - 1.4 \times (R^2 = 0.87)$. However, the completion time remained stable at later trials until the 14th trial, which is shorter than the other trials. This is when the subjects have acquired enough skills to perform more effectively. When fatigue was drawn after 14 trials, the completion time was increased from 92 to 110 seconds, as shown in Figure 8. These results have indicated that there exists significant learning for repeated peg transfer tasks.

3.1.3. Rate of Fatigue. Fatigue exhibited different behavior, with its rate growing gradually up to around ninth training trials, as predicted by the linear regression equation $y = 2.35 + 0.15 \times (R^2 = 0.96)$, and then the trend started to fluctuate around 3.6 until 14th training where it increased sharply, as shown in Figure 9. This means that subjects are fully alerted, their self-regulatory capacities are normal, and they can concentrate on the training until 13th trials. Thereafter, the subjects undergo ego depletion and their capacities become exhausted [18]. It can be seen that the rate of fatigue was increased by 62.8% from 13th to 14th trials, which indicate that excessive number of training times reduces efficiency. During 14th to 20th trials, fatigue values behaved like an increasing function and run uphill to seven, with regression equation $y = 3.15 + 0.212 \times (R^2 = 0.84)$.

4. Discussion

Prolonged working hours and lack of sleep have been associated with loss of attention, performance decrements, and increase in errors in medical practitioners [19–21]. Following these findings, some countries had set some regulations regarding the working hours for physicians. For example, in Scandinavia the shift work is restricted to 16–24 hours and the physicians have the day off after a night shift. In United Kingdom, it is allowed to work for a maximum of 16 hours in 24 hours [22]. In United States, interns are limited to a maximum of 16 hours per shift in the 80 hours' work week [6]. The residents association in Canada (Fédération des médecins résidents du Québec) had set a limit of maximum 16 hours of consecutive working due to the fact that 24-hour continuous work endangers residents' health [23]. In the present study, regression analysis indicates that working for a long period of time induces fatigue that can increase number of errors and time to complete peg transfer task during laparoscopic simulation. These results are consistent with what was found in the previous studies [6, 9]. However, they are very different from those of Bagrodia et al. [24] and Uchal et al. [5], who detailed that fatigue and performance are covariates. Increase in errors and time to complete laparoscopic task is more likely to be caused by trainee during acclimatization; however, as more and more trials are performed, the learning curve increases, which gradually decreases errors and completion time. Yet, when fatigue is developed, the number of errors and completion time start to increase again. Nevertheless, the consequence is more severe during the acclimatization than when being fatigued after making many trials. Though, sometimes, it does not matter how long it takes the trainee to complete the task; if he/she can operate without errors, then such surgical procedure can be considered as safe. It is important to understand that subject is novice during the first few trials and learns gradually as more and more trials are performed. In fact, poor performance during the first few trials was probably a reflection of new procedures [17] and of fatigue afterwards. The results support the regulation of work hour's restrictions for surgical residents, and further they emphasize that medical educators should address these negative effects of fatigue in medical students.

5. Conclusion

This paper has explored and evaluated effects of fatigue on efficiency and accuracy during laparoscopic surgical training using direct measurement of brain activity. The findings indicate that there are significant learning and fatigue effects when peg transfer task in the training is repeated in a series of trials. However, for the training to be effective and efficient, there should be monitoring to observe where in the learning curve a trainee gains maximum learning benefits. Moreover, fatigue is a significant indicator of efficiency in terms of time to complete laparoscopic task and accuracy in terms of errors made while doing the task. Even though these results reflect laparoscopic surgical training, the principles also apply to surgeons during patient operation, which provides some useful fundamental lessons for workplace or in hospital. Future work should entail investigating effects of fatigue in surgeons during laparoscopic surgery simulation based on Electroencephalography.

References

[1] L. Lagnado, "Hospitals overwork young doctors in New York," *Wall Street Journal*, 1998.

[2] C. L. Marcus and G. M. Loughlin, "Effect of sleep deprivation on driving safety in housestaff," *Sleep*, vol. 19, no. 10, pp. 763–766, 1996.

[3] L. Kohn, J. Corrigan, and M. Donaldson, *To Err is Human: Building a Safer Health System*, National Academy Press, Washington, DC, USA, 2000.

[4] B. T. Jap, S. Lal, P. Fischer, and E. Bekiaris, "Using EEG spectral components to assess algorithms for detecting fatigue," *Expert Systems with Applications*, vol. 36, no. 2, pp. 2352–2359, 2009.

[5] M. Uchal, J. Tjugum, E. Martinsen, X. Qiu, and R. Bergamaschi, "The impact of sleep deprivation on product quality and procedure effectiveness in a laparoscopic physical simulator: A randomized controlled trial," *The American Journal of Surgery*, vol. 189, no. 6, pp. 753–757, 2005.

[6] J. Olasky, A. Chellali, G. Sankaranarayanan et al., "Effects of sleep hours and fatigue on performance in laparoscopic surgery simulators," *Surgical Endoscopy*, vol. 28, no. 9, pp. 2564–2568, 2014.

[7] J. Daruwalla, N. Marlow, J. Field et al., "Effect of fatigue on laparoscopic skills: A comparative historical cohort study," *ANZ Journal of Surgery*, vol. 84, no. 3, pp. 137–142, 2014.

[8] Z. Tsafrir, J. Korianski, B. Almog, A. Many, O. Wiesel, and I. Levin, "Effects of Fatigue on Residents' Performance in Laparoscopy," *Journal of the American College of Surgeons*, vol. 221, no. 2, pp. 564–570, 2015.

[9] S. Sikder, K. Tuwairqi, E. Al-Kahtani, W. G. Myers, and P. Banerjee, "Surgical simulators in cataract surgery training," *British Journal of Ophthalmology*, vol. 98, no. 2, pp. 154–158, 2014.

[10] B. Andreas et al., "Eye Movement Analysis for Activity Recognition Using Electrooculography," *IEEE Transactions on Pattern Analysis and Machine Intelligence*, vol. 33, no. 4, pp. 741–753.

[11] S. K. L. Lal and A. Craig, "Electroencephalography activity associated with driver fatigue: Implications for a fatigue countermeasure device," *Journal of Psychophysiology*, vol. 15, no. 3, pp. 183–189, 2001.

[12] G. V. Kondraske, "Neurophysiological measurements," in *Biomedical Engineering and Instrumentation*, J. D. Bronzino, Ed., pp. 138–179, PWS Publishing, Boston, Mass, USA, 1986.

[13] G. F. Wilson, C. R. Swain, and P. Ullsperger, "EEG power changes during a multiple level memory retention task," *International Journal of Psychophysiology*, vol. 32, no. 2, pp. 107–118, 1999.

[14] T.-P. Jung, S. Makeig, M. Stensmo, and T. J. Sejnowski, "Estimating alertness from the EEG power spectrum," *IEEE Transactions on Biomedical Engineering*, vol. 44, no. 1, pp. 60–69, 1997.

[15] S. Blanco, R. Q. Quiroga, O. A. Rosso, and S. Kochen, "Time-frequency analysis of electroencephalogram series," *Physical Review E: Statistical, Nonlinear, and Soft Matter Physics*, vol. 51, no. 3, pp. 2624–2631, 1995.

[16] G. Faramarz et al., "Detecting Driver Mental Fatigue Based on EEG Alpha Power Changes during Simulated Driving," *Iran Journal of Public Health*, vol. 44, no. 12, pp. 1693–1700, 2015.

[17] S. N. Weingart, R. M. Wilson, R. W. Gibberd, and B. Harrison, "Epidemiology of medical error," *British Medical Journal*, vol. 320, article 7237, pp. 774–777, 2000.

[18] R. F. Baumeister, "Ego Depletion and Self-Control Failure: An Energy Model of the Self's Executive Function," *Self and Identity*, vol. 1, no. 2, pp. 129–136, 2010.

[19] I. P. Olmos and M. I. Pinilla, "Night shifts, sleep deprivation, and attention performance in medical students," *International Journal of Medical Education*, vol. 5, pp. 56–62, 2014.

[20] Y. Patrick, "Effects of sleep deprivation on cognitive and physical performance in university students," *Sleep Biological Rhythms*, vol. 15, no. 3, pp. 217–225, 2017.

[21] C. Sugden, T. Athanasiou, and A. Darzi, "What are the effects of sleep deprivation and fatigue in surgical practice?" *Seminars in Thoracic and Cardiovascular Surgery*, vol. 24, no. 3, pp. 166–175, 2012.

[22] I. Amirian, "The impact of sleep deprivation on surgeons' performance during night shifts," *Danish Medical Journal*, vol. 61, no. 9, 2014.

[23] J. Temple, "Resident duty hours around the globe: Where are we now?" *BMC Medical Education*, vol. 14, no. 1, article no. S8, 2015.

[24] A. Bagrodia, V. Rachakonda, K. Delafuente et al., "Surgeon fatigue: Impact of case order on perioperative parameters and patient outcomes," *The Journal of Urology*, vol. 188, no. 4, pp. 1291–1296, 2012.

22

Fully Endoscopic Microvascular Decompression: Our Early Experience

Casey H. Halpern, Shih-Shan Lang, and John Y. K. Lee

Department of Neurosurgery, Hospital of the University of Pennsylvania, 235 South Eighth Street, Philadelphia, PA 19106, USA

Correspondence should be addressed to John Y. K. Lee; leejohn@uphs.upenn.edu

Academic Editor: Joachim Oertel

Background. Microvascular decompression (MVD) is a widely accepted treatment for neurovascular disorders associated with facial pain and spasm. The endoscope has rapidly become a standard tool in neurosurgical procedures; however, its adoption in lateral approaches to the posterior fossa has been slower. The endoscope is used primarily to assist conventional microscopic techniques. We are interested in developing fully endoscopic approaches to the cerebellopontine angle, and here, we describe our preliminary experience with this procedure for MVD. *Methods*. A retrospective review of our two-year experience from 2011 to 2012, transitioning from using conventional microscopic techniques to endoscope-assisted microsurgery to fully endoscopic MVD, is provided. We also reviewed our preliminary outcomes during this transition. *Results*. There was no difference in the surgical duration of these three procedures. In addition, the majority of procedures performed in 2012 were fully endoscopic, suggesting the ease of incorporating this solo tool into practice. Pain outcomes of fully endoscopic MVD appear to be very similar to those of both conventional and endoscope-assisted MVDs. Complications occurred in all groups at equally low rates. *Conclusion*. Fully endoscopic MVD is both safe and effective. By enhancing visualization of structures within the cerebellopontine angle, endoscopy may prove to be a valuable adjunct or alternative to conventional microscopic approaches.

1. Introduction

Microvascular decompression (MVD) is a highly effective surgical treatment of neurovascular disorders associated with facial pain and spasm (e.g., trigeminal neuralgia, hemifacial spasm) [1, 2]. However, failure to relieve symptoms associated with these conditions can occur due to poor visualization of the offending vascular contact at the root entry zone or medial vascular compression [3]. The endoscope has quickly become a standard operative tool in minimally invasive neurosurgery of the sella and ventricular system due to the panoramic views and bright illumination [4–6]. Similarly, advantages of the endoscope in visualizing structures within the cerebellopontine angle (CPA), including nerve cleavage planes and vascular anatomic features, have been noted in addition to smaller exposures and less cerebellar or brainstem retraction than conventional microscopy [7, 8]. The endoscope has been reported to be used as a standard adjunct to conventional MVD in a number of institutions, but rarely as a solo technique [9, 10]. This paper outlines our approach to fully endoscopic MVD (E-MVD) for the treatment of multiple neurovascular compression syndromes. We report our preliminary experience with this technique since incorporating the endoscope into our practice in early 2011.

2. Surgical Technique

2.1. Patient Positioning and Equipment Setup. The surgical technique has been previously described by us and others [11, 12]. Briefly, all operations are performed under general anesthesia. Prior to positioning, the patient's head is secured in a Mayfield clamp. The body is then turned in a full lateral position with an axillary role. The patient is taped down securely, and the head is flexed approximately two fingerbreadths from the sternum and rotated 70–80 degrees away from the side of the operation in order to maintain the vertex parallel to the floor. In this position, the cranial nerve 7-8 bundle is more inferior to the trigeminal nerve.

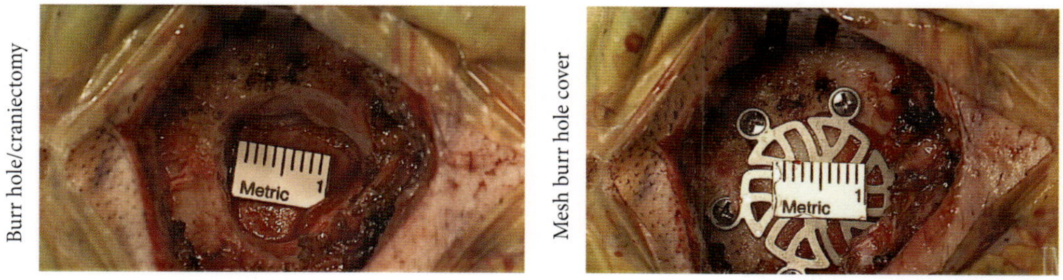

(a) (b)

FIGURE 1: Endoscopic view of burr hole/craniectomy site (a) with subsequent closure and placement of titanium mesh burr hole cover (b).

A small region of hair is shaved postauricularly, and a 4–6 cm linear incision is made just inferior to the junction of the transverse and sigmoid sinuses and approximately one centimeter behind the patient's hairline. The burr hole for the craniectomy is placed just posterior to the most superior aspect of the insertion of the digastric muscle. Once the inferior border of the transverse sinus and posterior border of the sigmoid sinus are identified following minimal craniectomy (Figures 1(a) and 1(b)), a 1 cm C-shaped dural opening is made. The dural flap is retracted anteriorly and reflected against the sinuses. None of these techniques differ from that of the conventional microscopic approach.

At this point, however, the endoscope that is attached to the Mitaka Pneumatic Arm (Mitaka Kohki Co.) is brought in. Our preference is to use the 2.7 mm zero-degree endoscope upfront (Storz; Culver City, CA, USA). This smaller diameter endoscope maximizes the amount of working space that is needed for the other instruments, thus minimizing instrument conflict and brain retraction (Figure 2). In conjunction with a high-definition camera, this system provides excellent visualization. Angled endoscopes are also utilized to facilitate identification of vascular contacts at the root entry zone and to visualize the trigeminal nerve medial to a low and prominent petrous ridge.

2.2. Endoscopic Microvascular Decompression. Next, the endoscope is inserted through the dural opening with minimal retraction on the cerebellum. The arachnoid sheath around the cranial nerve 9–11 bundle is dissected with sharp scissors, and the cerebrospinal fluid is drained, enhancing visualization of structures within the CPA. Using a combination of bipolar coagulation of minor vessels and blunt dissection, the arachnoid around the trigeminal nerve is then lysed, and the vascular anatomy is inspected. The offending vessel is then mobilized, and decompression is achieved with a Teflon pad placed between the offending vessel and trigeminal nerve. The 30-degree endoscope has been found to be the most useful in identifying occult vascular structures at the root entry zone (Figure 2), venous compression, as well as the nervus intermedius in the case of geniculate neuralgia.

3. Patient Population

From September 2010 to November 2012, 70 patients (M/F: 24/46) with the diagnosis of medically refractory trigeminal neuralgia (TGN), hemifacial spasm (HFS), glossopharyngeal neuralgia (GPN), or geniculate neuralgia (GN) were seen in the neurosurgery clinic for preoperative evaluation. Prior to this period, all patients who underwent microvascular decompression by the senior author (John Y. K. Lee) had undergone a purely microscopic surgical procedure. In the first half of this experience (9/2010 to 12/2011), 14 MVDs, 8 endoscope-assisted (EA)-MVDs, and 16 purely E-MVDs were performed. In the next half of this experience (January 2012 to November 2012,) 9 MVDs, 1 EA-MVD, and 22 purely E-MVDs were performed. Hence, the great majority of procedures performed were purely endoscopic. The decision to perform a microscopic procedure versus an endoscope-assisted procedure and purely endoscopic procedure reflected the comfort of the surgeon as well as the availability of equipment.

The great majority of procedures were performed for TGN ($n = 62$), whereas HFS ($n = 5$), geniculate neuralgia ($n = 2$), and GPN ($n = 1$) were less well represented in this cohort (see Table 1). One patient in the conventional MVD group had been treated previously with cyber knife surgery and MVD. Three patients in the EA-MVD group were previously treated with gamma knife surgery, and one surgical exploration without decompression. Three patients in the E-MVD had previous gamma knife surgery treatments, and five had prior conventional MVD.

EA-MVD procedures were performed as part of a gradual transition to a fully endoscopic procedure. Nearly 60 percent of the E-MVD, and only 1 of the 9 EA-MVD cases took place in 2012, reflecting the rapidity that this solo technique was adopted at our institution. Of interest, there was no apparent difference in surgical durations between these three treatment groups. All surgeries were performed by the senior author (John Y. K. Lee).

4. Surgical Findings

An offending vessel was identified in all cases except in one of the fully endoscopically treated patients, for which Teflon was placed between the arachnoid and nerve, and the case of geniculate neuralgia in which sectioning of the nervus intermedius was performed. Arterial compression was identified in 14 of the 23 MVD patients, 5 of the 9 EA-MVD patients, and 31 of the 38 E-MVD patients. Venous compression was identified in 12 of the MVD patients, 3 of the 9 EA-MVD

Table 1: Patient summary.

	Diagnosis (N)	Mean surgical duration (±SD)	Mean followup time	Vascular contact (N)	BNI class I to III
MVD	TGN (20) HFS (2) GPN (1),	129 ± 36	62	Artery (11) Vein (12)	19/20 (95%)
EA-MVD	TGN (7) HFS (2)	137 ± 29	77	Artery (3) Vein (6)	7/7 (100%)
E-MVD	TGN (35) HFS (1) GN (2)	130 ± 32	107	Artery (26) Vein (12)	31/35 (89%)

Microvascular decompression (MVD); endoscope-assisted microsurgery (EA-MVD); fully endoscopic microvascular decompression (E-MVD); Trigeminal neuralgia (TGN); hemifacial spasm (HFS); glossopharyngeal neuralgia (GPN); geniculate neuralgia (GN).

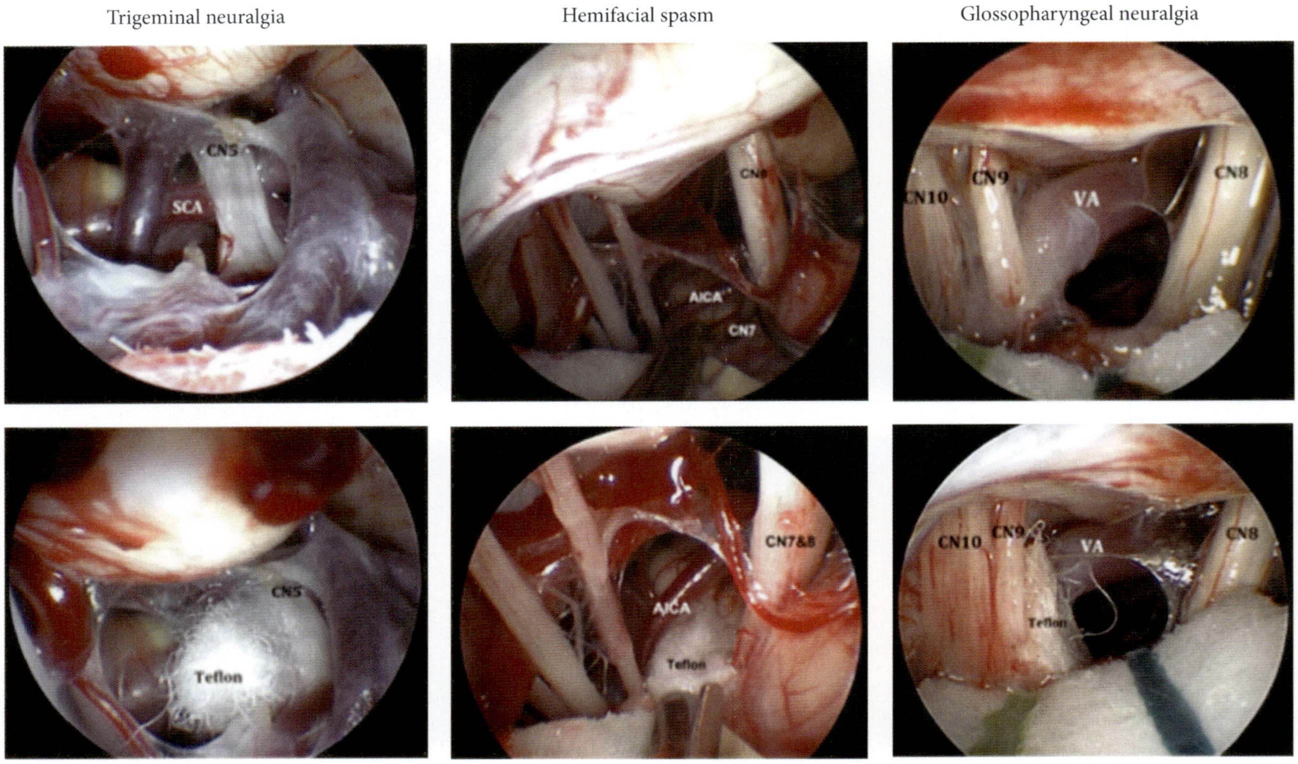

Figure 2: Endoscopic view of the vascular compression associated with cases of trigeminal neuralgia, hemifacial spasm, and glossopharyngeal neuralgia. The left panel demonstrates compression of CN 5 by the superior cerebellar artery (top) with subsequent decompression with Teflon (bottom). The middle panel illustrates compression of CN 7 by the anterior inferior cerebellar artery (top). Note that CN 7 is found on the inferior aspect of CN 8, which requires decompression deep to the CN 7-8 complex (bottom). The right panel demonstrates a case of glossopharyngeal neuralgia caused by vertebral artery contact (top) and the associated decompression (bottom). Cranial nerve (CN); superior cerebellar artery (SCA); anterior inferior cerebellar artery (AICA); vertebral artery (VA).

patients, and 12 of the E-MVD patients. Of the 62 patients with TGN, only 2 did not have any vessel identified. The rate of vascular contact was similar between the 3 groups of MVD, EA-MVD, and E-MVD. Only one patient in each group EA-MVD and E-MVD was not shown to have a vessel contact; see Figure 2.

A surgical neurolysis was performed in a minority of patients (total $n = 12$) and was undertaken either with a round knife along the fascicles of the nerve ($n = 10$) or with direct injection of 0.2 cc of glycerol ($n = 2$). This was performed at the discretion of the senior surgeon (John Y. K. Lee) based on intraoperative findings, such as insignificant vascular compression. The rate of neurolysis was 26% in the MVD group, 11% in the EA-MVD group, and 16% in the E-MVD group. Neurolysis was not performed in cases of HFS.

5. Outcomes/Followup

Patients were followed up for approximately 2–3.5 months following surgery (see Table 1). We classified pain according to the Barrow Neurological Institute scale for pain in trigeminal neuralgia, and we considered success if BNI score was between 1 (no pain, no meds), 2 (occasional pain, no meds), and 3 (some pain, adequately controlled). Using these criteria for the 62 patients with trigeminal neuralgia, we identified only 5 patients of 62 who had BNI class IV (some pain, not adequately controlled) or class V (severe pain or no relief). One of these patients was in the microscope only arm (1/20 = 5%). Four of these patients were in the endoscope only arm (4/31 = 11%), and none of the patients in the EA-MVD group were BNI class IV or V (0/7 = 0%). This was not a statistically different difference between the three groups (MVD, EA-MVD, and E-MVD), using the Kruskal Wallis test ($P = 0.5018$); see Table 1.

Of the five patients with HFS, all five had an excellent outcome with complete resolution of their hemifacial spasm. The two patients with geniculate neuralgia did not experience significant benefit and were classified as BNI class IV at last followup. The patient with glossopharyngeal neuralgia had complete relief of pain.

The conventionally treated patient who had previous cyber knife surgery did not respond to MVD. Three of the 8 E-MVD patients who had previous gamma knife surgery or MVD did report 100 percent resolution of pain. Three of the 4 EA-MVD patients who were previously treated procedurally also reported complete resolution of their symptoms.

Complications were unusual overall. In the TGN cohort, there was one wound infection (MVD), one temporary facial palsy (MVD), which required temporary gold weight but returned to normal by 9 months, and one CSF otorrhea, which required lumbar drainage for five days but sealed on its own (E-MVD). The total complication rate was 3/62 = 4.8% complication rate. None of the complications appear to have been directly related to endoscopic technique. In the hemifacial spasm cohort, there was one temporary facial palsy, which improved at six months to HB grade I (EA-MVD). This was in a patient with very severe hemifacial spasm and significant tonus, who had received prior Botox therapy. In the three patients with glossopharyngeal and geniculate neuralgia, no complications were identified.

Patients who required reoperation generally did well. The one patient in the conventional MVD group who was previously explored (no Teflon was found intraoperatively) had complete resolution of symptoms (BNI 1) following MVD. One patient in the EA-MVD who had a previous MVD without success also saw complete resolution of his symptoms. Three of the 6 patients with previous MVD who underwent E-MVD had a BNI score of 1 at followup. These data are supported by previous findings in which reoperation is both safe and frequently effective for either persistent or recurrent facial pain [3].

We performed a simple stepwise forward logistic regression analysis using the primary outcome measure of a BNI class score of three or better. We included the following variables: gender, presence of vein, artery, use of endoscope, and neurolysis. Surprisingly, the strongest predictor of success was the performance of a neurolytic procedure, although the overall P value of the model only approached statistical significance at $P = 0.0593$ (STATA 10). This finding forced us to look at the results in patients undergoing neurolysis. Although the act of neurolysis was a significant predictor in our stepwise model, it was not a predictor at face value. Two of 12 patients who underwent neurolysis had a poor outcome versus 3 of 50 patients who did not undergo a neurolysis. ($P = 0.2245$ Fisher's exact).

6. Discussion

Our preliminary experience with fully endoscopic MVD supports the safety, feasibility, and potential benefits of this approach for a wide variety of neurovascular syndromes. Although we did not demonstrate superiority of the fully endoscopic approach, we did not find any statistically significant difference when compared to the microscopic procedure. It is important to note that no difference was found despite the relatively short period of time following introduction of the endoscope into our routine practice. There was also no difference in operative time. Hence, we believe that the use of the endoscope is safe for microvascular decompression, and at least as effective as a microscopic procedure.

The use of the endoscope in the posterior fossa, however, offers additional benefits to skull base surgeons. Once the surgeon becomes accustomed to the technique of operating with the endoscope using the view from the monitor, it opens up the possibility of operating with angled scopes, which may allow safe access to structures not previously seen using the standard operative microscope. We believe that extended retrosigmoid approaches to more difficult areas of the brain will become more likely. For example, an extended retrosigmoid approach via a suprameatal approach to trigeminal schwannomas can be facilitated [13]. In addition, endoscopic supracerebellar transtentorial approaches to the medial posterior temporal lobe are a possibility [14]. This will allow the skull base surgeon improved access to regions of the brain that have traditionally required either more bone removal or intraparenchymal corridors. Facility with the simple microvascular decompression will allow the surgeon to tackle more complex pathology [15], perhaps even minimizing the morbidity associated with petroclival meningiomas in the future.

7. Conclusion

Endoscopic microvascular decompression is a safe, feasible and effective procedure for cure of TGN, hemifacial spasms and other cranial nerve disorders. Our two-year experience summarizes the transition from conventional microscopic surgery to a fully endoscopic procedure, demonstrating the ease and safety of incorporating this tool into practice as a solo instrument. Expanding this experience from neurovascular syndromes to cerebellopontine angle tumors represents the next step in the expanding era of minimally invasive endoscopic neurosurgery.

Disclosure

Casey H. Halpern and Shih-Shan Lang have nothing to disclose. John Y. K. Lee is the speaker of the bureau, Baxter.

References

[1] P. J. Jannetta, "Observations on the etiology of trigeminal neuralgia, hemifacial spasm, acoustic nerve dysfunction and glossopharyngeal neuralgia. Definitive microsurgical treatment and results in 117 patients," *Neurochirurgia*, vol. 20, no. 5, pp. 145–154, 1977.

[2] F. G. Barker II, P. J. Jannetta, D. J. Bissonette, M. V. Larkins, and H. D. Jho, "The long-term outcome of microvascular decompression for trigeminal neuralgia," *The New England Journal of Medicine*, vol. 334, no. 17, pp. 1077–1083, 1996.

[3] U. C. P. C. Ugwuanyi and N. D. Kitchen, "The operative findings in re-do microvascular decompression for recurrent trigeminal neuralgia," *British Journal of Neurosurgery*, vol. 24, no. 1, pp. 26–30, 2010.

[4] H.-D. Jho and R. L. Carrau, "Endoscopy assisted transsphenoidal surgery for pituitary adenoma," *Acta Neurochirurgica*, vol. 138, no. 12, pp. 1416–1425, 1996.

[5] F. H. Ebner, A. Koerbel, A. Kirschniak, F. Roser, J. Kaminsky, and M. Tatagiba, "Endoscope-assisted retrosigmoid intradural suprameatal approach to the middle fossa: anatomical and surgical considerations," *European Journal of Surgical Oncology*, vol. 33, no. 1, pp. 109–113, 2007.

[6] N. D. Adappa, K. O. Learned, J. N. Palmer, J. G. Newman, and J. Y. K. Lee, "Radiographic enhancement of the nasoseptal flap does not predict postoperative cerebrospinal fluid leaks in endoscopic skull base reconstruction," *The Laryngoscope*, vol. 122, no. 6, pp. 1226–1234, 2012.

[7] J. Magnan, A. Chays, F. Caces et al., "Contribution of endoscopy of the cerebellopontine angle by retrosigmoid approach. Neuroma and vasculo-nervous compression," *Annales d'Oto-Laryngologie et de Chirurgie Cervico-Faciale*, vol. 110, no. 5, pp. 259–265, 1993.

[8] W. A. King, P. A. Wackym, C. Sen, G. A. Meyer, J. Shiau, and H. Deutsch, "Adjunctive use of endoscopy during posterior fossa surgery to treat cranial neuropathies," *Neurosurgery*, vol. 49, no. 1, pp. 108–116, 2001.

[9] C. Teo, P. Nakaji, and R. J. Mobbs, "Endoscope-assisted microvascular decompression for trigeminal neuralgia: technical case report," *Neurosurgery*, vol. 59, no. 4, pp. E489–E490, 2006.

[10] J. Hae-Dong and H. J. Jho Diana, *Microvascular Decompression and the Endoscope. Trigeminal Neuralgia*, Oxford University Press, New York, NY, USA, 2010, Edit by: P. Jannetta.

[11] S. Lang, H. I. Chen, and J. Y. K. Lee, "Endoscopic microvascular decompression: a step-wise operative technique," *ORL*, vol. 74, no. 6, pp. 293–298, 2012.

[12] G. J. Artz, F. J. Hux, M. J. Larouere, D. I. Bojrab, S. Babu, and D. R. Pieper, "Endoscopic vascular decompression," *Otology & Neurotology*, vol. 29, no. 7, pp. 995–1000, 2008.

[13] A. Samii, V. Gerganov, C. Herold, A. Gharabaghi, N. Hayashi, and M. Samii, "Surgical treatment of skull base chondrosarcomas," *Neurosurgical Review*, vol. 32, no. 1, pp. 67–75, 2009.

[14] E. P. De Oliveira, ""Tangential" resection of medial temporal lobe arteriovenous malformations with the orbitozygomatic approach," *Neurosurgery*, vol. 55, no. 4, pp. 1010–1011, 2004.

[15] H. K. Shahinian, J. B. Eby, and M. Ocon, "Fully endoscopic excision of vestibular schwannomas," *Minimally Invasive Neurosurgery*, vol. 47, no. 6, pp. 329–332, 2004.

23

Robot-Assisted Myomectomy for Large Uterine Myomas: A Single Center Experience

Vinay Gunnala,[1] Robert Setton,[2] Nigel Pereira,[1] and Jian Qun Huang[3]

[1] *The Ronald O. Perelman and Claudia Cohen Center for Reproductive Medicine, Weill Cornell Medical College, New York, NY 10021, USA*
[2] *Department of Obstetrics and Gynecology, Weill Cornell Medical College, New York, NY 10021, USA*
[3] *Department of Obstetrics and Gynecology, Gynecologic Robotic Surgery, NYU Langone Medical Center, New York, NY 10016, USA*

Correspondence should be addressed to Jian Qun Huang; kathy.huang@nyumc.org

Academic Editor: Diego Cuccurullo

Objective. To determine if robot-assisted myomectomy (RAM) is feasible for women with large uterine myomas. *Methods.* Retrospective review of one gynecologic surgeon's RAM cases between May 2010 and July 2013. Large uterine myomas, defined as the largest myoma ≥9 cm by preoperative magnetic resonance imaging, was age- and time-matched to controls with the largest myoma <9 cm. Primary surgical outcomes compared were operative time and estimated blood loss (EBL). *Results.* 207 patients were included: 66 (32%) patients were in the ≥9 cm group, while 141 (68%) patients were in the <9 cm group. There was a statistically significant increase in the operative time (130 min versus 92 min) and EBL (100 mL versus 25 mL) for the ≥9 cm group compared to the <9 cm group. Ten (4.8%) patients had the largest myoma measuring ≥15 cm, and 11 (5.3%) patients had a specimen weight >900 gm, of which no major adverse outcomes were observed. All patients in the study cohort were discharged on the same day after surgery. *Conclusion.* RAM is a feasible surgical approach for patients with myomas ≥9 cm. Patients with large myomas undergoing RAM are also candidates for same-day discharge after surgery.

1. Introduction

Uterine myomas can cause menorrhagia, dysmenorrhea, pelvic pain, and infertility. Myomectomy, open or minimally invasive, is the preferred surgical modality in patients with symptomatic myomas who desire future childbearing capacity. It is well established that the laparoscopic approach is associated with shorter hospitalization, faster recovery, lesser pain, decreased blood loss, fewer surgical complications, and fewer expenses compared to the abdominal approach [1]. In recent years, as robotic technology has gained momentum in gynecology, studies have emerged indicating that surgical outcomes are similar between traditional laparoscopic and robot-assisted myomectomies [2–4]. In addition to having the same postsurgical benefits, robot-assisted myomectomy (RAM) has the advantage of three-dimensional visualization, improved dexterity, and negation of tremors, which are thought to overcome many of the surgical limitations of traditional laparoscopy. One of the lingering controversies between the two minimally invasive approaches is that, compared to conventional laparoscopy, the robotic approach has been associated with longer operative time and increased expense [2, 3].

Uterine dimensions, myoma size, and location are some of the primary factors used to determine whether an abdominal or minimally invasive surgical approach is utilized. An abdominal approach is often favored with larger, intramural, and posterior myomas, secondary to the difficulties of hemostasis, uterine closure, and tissue removal associated with minimally invasive surgery [5]. Prior studies have demonstrated that myomas measuring up to 8 cm can be safely and effectively removed using a traditional laparoscopic approach [6, 7]. While there is less data regarding RAM, there is evidence suggesting similarities to limits of myoma size compared to laparoscopic surgery [8]. As such, we selected a cutoff of 9 cm or greater to define the "large" myoma group in order to reflect a cohort of patients who may not have previously been considered appropriate candidates for minimally invasive surgery. The primary objective of the current study is to assess the surgical outcomes after RAM for uterine myomas ≥9 cm to determine if it was a feasible approach for women with large myomas. As a secondary objective, we also evaluate the feasibility of same-day discharge after RAM in the same study cohort.

2. Materials and Methods

2.1. Inclusion and Exclusion Criteria. The New York Hospital Queens institutional review board approved the study protocol. Informed consent by the patients was not required as the study was a retrospective chart review. We reviewed all RAM cases performed by one minimally invasive gynecologic surgeon (JQH) between May 5, 2010, and July 31, 2013. All patients were offered a robot-assisted approach. Other concomitant intraoperative procedures included hysteroscopy, chromotubation, ovarian cystectomy, salpingectomy, salpingo-oophorectomy, and resection of endometriosis. However, all RAM cases included in the study were performed with myomectomy as the primary indication. Patients with intraoperative findings consistent with adenomyosis rather than myomas were excluded.

2.2. Operative Technique. All procedures were performed with the patients under general endotracheal anesthesia in the dorsal lithotomy position with adjustable Allen stirrups and lower extremity compression devices for deep vein thrombosis prophylaxis. A VCare® uterine manipulator (CONMED Utica, NY, USA) was placed vaginally. A Veress needle (UNIMAX Taipei, Taiwan) was placed in the umbilicus for insufflation of the peritoneal cavity. A 5 mm bladeless ENDOPATH® XCEL® trocar (Ethicon Endo-Surgery Inc., Cincinnati, Ohio, USA) was introduced into the abdomen using a twisting motion under direct visualization with a 0° 5 mm laparoscope in the left upper quadrant. A 12 mm incision was made intra- or supraumbilically depending on the size of the uterus, through which the operative camera was placed. Three additional 8 mm incisions were made and the robotic trocars were placed under direct visualization. In general, the first 8 mm robotic trocar was placed in the patient's right lower quadrant, 2-3 cm above the anterior superior iliac spine and caudad to the camera port, along an imaginary arc centered at the pubic symphysis. The second 8 mm robotic trocar was placed similarly in the patient's left lower quadrant. The original 5 mm port in the left upper quadrant was used as the assistant port. The patient was placed in the Trendelenburg position and da Vinci robotic surgical system (Intuitive Surgical Inc., Sunnyvale, CA, USA) was side-docked, parallel to the right side of the patient regardless of number or location of myomas. Following careful intraoperative evaluation of the number, position, and size of myomas, dilute vasopressin was injected into the myoma bed for vasoconstriction, in order to minimize the blood loss during surgery. Uterine hysterotomy was made over the prominent bulge of the myoma. Myomas were enucleated intact using Plasma Kinetic (PK) dissecting forceps (Intuitive Surgical Inc., Sunnyvale, CA, USA), EndoWrist tenaculum (Intuitive Surgical Inc., Sunnyvale, CA, USA), and a monopolar cutting device. The uterine defect was repaired with 0 V-Loc suture (Covidien, Mansfield, MA, USA) in at least 2 layers. After closure of the hysterotomy, the abdomen was irrigated and suctioned and then the robot was undocked. The 12 mm incision was extended to 20 mm and the specimen was extracted with electromechanical morcellation. The 20 mm fascial incision was closed with 0 Vicryl™ suture (Ethicon Endo-Surgery Inc., Cincinnati, Ohio, USA). All skin incisions were injected with bupivacaine hydrochloride and closed with a single interrupted stitch using a 4.0 Biosyn™ Glycomer™ 631 suture (Covidien Ltd., Dublin, Ireland). All patients received intravenous ondansetron and dexamethasone for postoperative nausea and ketorolac and hydromorphone for postoperative pain. Patients were discharged home the same day after meeting immediate postoperative milestones (ambulation, pain control, and tolerating liquids orally) and a successful trial of void. Discharge medications included oral ibuprofen and combined acetaminophen/oxycodone.

2.3. Outcome Variables Assessed. Demographic characteristics including age, body mass index (kg/m^2), parity, and prior abdominopelvic surgery of patients meeting inclusion criteria were collected. Preoperative pelvic magnetic resonance imaging (MRI) was used to determine the largest myoma size. In addition, MRI was used to assess myoma characteristics including their location (submucosal, intramural, subserosal, and pedunculated) and number (> or <5 myomas). Total weight of all myomas removed was determined. Histopathologic evaluation of the excised myomas was also performed.

Patients were divided into two groups, a priori, based on the maximum dimension of the largest myoma as determined by preoperative pelvic MRI, that is, ≥9 cm versus <9 cm. The primary surgical outcomes compared between the two groups were estimated blood loss (EBL), operative time (skin-to-skin time), and duration of hospital stay (days). EBL was determined by volume in the suction canister at the end of the procedure and was concurrently agreed upon by the surgical and anesthesia teams. Major adverse outcomes assessed included injury to surrounding organs, conversion to laparotomy, requirement for transfusion of blood products, postoperative infection or abscess formation, and need for hospital readmission. All patients had a standard postoperative follow-up 2 weeks from surgery and again after 2 months.

2.4. Statistical Analysis. Data was analyzed using commercially available software (SPSS version 19.0; IBM, Armonk, NY). Student's t-test was used for comparison of means, and Mann-Whitney U test was used for nonparametric comparisons. In all cases, a P value < 0.05 was considered to be statistically significant. The normality of the data was evaluated by examining the skewness and kurtosis of scatter plots and histograms for each of the surgical outcomes.

TABLE 1: Demographic characteristics of leading myoma <9 cm versus ≥9 cm.

Parameter	Largest myoma <9 cm (n = 141)	Largest myoma ≥9 cm (n = 66)	P
Age	35.6 ± 5.8	36.9 ± 5.4	n.s.
Body mass index (kg/m^2)	26.3 ± 6.1	24.7 ± 6.0	n.s.
Parity (median)	0	0	n.s.
% with previous abdominal surgery	53.5%	25.8%	<0.001
% with >5 myomas	34.8%	26.2%	n.s.
% intramural myoma	86.5%	86.2%	n.s.
Median specimen weight (gm)	106 ± 164.5	510 ± 379.5	<0.001

n.s.: not significant.

TABLE 2: Perioperative outcomes by leading myoma <9 cm versus ≥9 cm.

Parameter	Largest myoma <9 cm (n = 141)	Largest myoma ≥9 cm (n = 66)	P
Operative time (mins) [median (IQR)]	92 (70, 141)	130 (92, 188)	<0.001
EBL (mL) [median (IQR)]	25 (15, 50)	100 (25, 200)	<0.001
Mean duration of hospital stay (days)	0	0	n.s.

n.s.: not significant.

3. Results

Two hundred and seven patients met inclusion criteria during the study period. Of those, 66 (32%) patients had the largest myoma ≥9 cm, while 141 (68%) patients had the largest myoma <9 cm. Demographic characteristics, listed in Table 1, were similar for both groups with the exception that patients in the latter group had significantly more previous abdominal surgery (53% versus 26%, $P < 0.001$). Table 1 also depicts myoma characteristics including number and location. There was no statistical difference between percentages of patients with primarily intramural fibroids and those with >5 myomas. The median specimen weight was 106 gm and 510 gm for the <9 cm and ≥9 cm group, respectively ($P < 0.001$).

Table 2 highlights the primary surgical outcomes assessed in this study. There were significant increases in operative time (130 min versus 92 min, $P < 0.001$) and EBL (100 mL versus 25 mL, $P < 0.001$) for the ≥9 cm group. However, no significant differences in the major adverse outcomes were seen between the two groups. Specifically, the mean hospital stay was zero days: that is, all patients were discharged on the same day after surgery. No RAM cases were converted to laparotomy or had intraoperative injury to surrounding organs. One patient in each group received a blood transfusion. One patient in the <9 cm group developed a postoperative pelvic abscess and was readmitted to the hospital for computed tomographic-assisted drainage and intravenous antibiotics. Of the 207 patients included in the study, 10 (4.8%) patients had the largest myoma measuring ≥15 cm by preoperative imaging, and 11 (5.3%) patients had a specimen weight >900 gm. No adverse surgical outcomes were noted in these groups either. The largest myomas excised during the study period measured 19.8 cm, for which the EBL was 100 mL and operative time was 113 min.

4. Discussion

The current study evaluates whether RAM is a feasible and safe surgical approach for large uterine myomas. Results from this study suggest that patients with larger myomas will experience an increase in EBL (100 mL versus 25 mL); however, this difference was not clinically significant, as it did not result in increased rate of blood transfusion. Patients with larger myomas also experienced a longer operative time (130 min versus 92 min). Despite these differences, we did not observe any additional adverse surgical or adverse postoperative outcomes. Furthermore, all patients in the study cohort, including those in the ≥9 cm group, were discharged on the same day of surgery after meeting immediate postoperative milestones.

Previous studies have attempted to establish criteria for candidates to determine whether laparoscopic or RAM would be an effective approach. Given that the role of RAM in gynecologic surgery is still emerging, there is limited literature on its effectiveness and safety profile; therefore, data must be extrapolated from traditional laparoscopy. Of particular concern is the rate of the conversion to laparotomy, in which fibroid size is one of the primary factors that have been shown to play a role. In one study, myomas measuring >5 cm were an independent risk factor related to the risk of conversion to laparotomy using traditional laparoscopy [9]. Conversely, another study of 51 cases with myomas measuring at least 9 cm had no conversions to laparotomy; however, one patient underwent an open hysterectomy hours after surgery due to persistent intra-abdominal hemorrhage [5]. Specific to RAM, a study analyzing 35 RAM cases had 2 cases converted to laparotomy with a conversion rate of 8.6% [10]. The mean myoma diameter was 7.9 ± 3.5 cm (95% CI 6.63–9.13) with the majority of myomas measuring greater than 5 cm [10].

Several studies, including one systematic review and meta-analysis, have also compared other surgical outcomes between abdominal, laparoscopic, and robot-assisted myomectomies [2–4, 11–14]. Studies were controlled in terms of number, diameter, and weight of myomas. Compared to abdominal myomectomy, RAM was associated with significantly lower EBL, decreased rate of blood transfusion (relative risk 0.37; 95% CI, 0.16–0.85), less postoperative fever (relative risk 0.07; 95% CI, 0.02–0.26), and decreased length of hospital stay. RAM cases were also found to have longer operating times and higher costs, but there was no difference in terms of adverse outcomes. Compared to laparoscopic myomectomy, RAM showed no differences in terms of EBL, length of hospital stay, or adverse outcomes but did show a higher cost. Notably, the conversion to laparotomy (0.4% with traditional laparoscopy and 0.5% with RAM) was similar between groups with mean myoma diameter ranging from 5 to 9 cm. All but one study included had a mean myoma diameter of 5–7 cm.

While studies investigating RAM have demonstrated efficacy with a range of myoma sizes, there has not been an evaluation of the feasibility of RAM, specifically for large myomas, to date. While previous studies have evaluated surgical outcomes based on specimen weight during histopathologic evaluation, our study, in contrast, uses preoperative imaging to define treatment groups. We speculate that this approach is more useful when counseling patients preoperatively in order to determine the best candidates for RAM. Our study also highlights that surgeries are performed by a single surgeon which limits variation in surgical technique, thereby allowing the completion of challenging surgical cases, without adversely impacting surgical outcomes. It is well established that the challenges of RAM are related to not only myoma size, but also location and number. Specifically, intramural myomas can be associated with increased EBL and often require multiple layer closure to obtain adequate hemostasis. However, given that there was no difference between percentages of patients with primarily intramural myomas or >5 myomas in either study group, we feel that our conclusions regarding myoma size are not biased by the confounding factors such as location and number.

Our study is limited by its retrospective nature and sample size. Our lack of major adverse outcomes, namely, no conversions to laparotomy, may reflect the fact that technical skill associated with RAM has improved over the past several years. Further prospective studies are needed to validate our results and help delineate recommendations for size limits of myomas amenable to robotic surgery.

In conclusion, RAM may be a feasible surgical approach for patients with myomas ≥9 cm. Although RAM is associated with greater EBL and operative time, there was no change in major adverse outcomes. Furthermore, patients with large myomas undergoing RAM can be discharged on the same day after meeting immediate postoperative milestones. Practitioners should be aware of the alternative of a minimally invasive approach, especially RAM, to avoid the known morbidities associated with the open approach. Given the improved surgical dexterity associated with robot-assisted technology over traditional laparoscopy, the robot-assisted platform may enable safe removal of large myomas that may have previously been thought to only be amenable to an abdominal approach.

References

[1] B. S. Hurst, M. L. Matthews, and P. B. Marshburn, "Laparoscopic myomectomy for symptomatic uterine myomas," *Fertility and Sterility*, vol. 83, no. 1, pp. 1–23, 2005.

[2] C. Nezhat, O. Lavie, S. Hsu, J. Watson, O. Barnett, and M. Lemyre, "Robotic-assisted laparoscopic myomectomy compared with standard laparoscopic myomectomy—a retrospective matched control study," *Fertility and Sterility*, vol. 91, no. 2, pp. 556–559, 2009.

[3] J. M. Gobern, C. J. Rosemeyer, J. F. Barter, and A. J. Steren, "Comparison of robotic, laparoscopic, and abdominal myomectomy in a community hospital," *Journal of the Society of Laparoendoscopic Surgeons*, vol. 17, no. 1, pp. 116–120, 2013.

[4] C. E. Bedient, J. F. Magrina, B. N. Noble, and R. M. Kho, "Comparison of robotic and laparoscopic myomectomy," *American Journal of Obstetrics & Gynecology*, vol. 201, no. 6, pp. 566.e1–566.e5, 2009.

[5] R. Sinha, A. Hegde, N. Warty, and N. Patil, "Laparoscopic excision of very large myomas," *The Journal of the American Association of Gynecologic Laparoscopists*, vol. 10, no. 4, pp. 461–468, 2003.

[6] J.-B. Dubuisson, C. Chapron, and L. Levy, "Difficulties and complications of laparoscopic myomectomy," *Journal of Gynecologic Surgery*, vol. 12, no. 3, pp. 159–165, 1996.

[7] P. Seinera, R. Arisio, A. Decko, C. Farina, and F. Crana, "Laparoscopic myomectomy: indications, surgical technique and complications," *Human Reproduction*, vol. 12, no. 9, pp. 1927–1930, 1997.

[8] H.-Y. Cheng, Y.-J. Chen, P.-H. Wang et al., "Robotic-assisted laparoscopic complex myomectomy: a single medical center's experience," *Taiwanese Journal of Obstetrics and Gynecology*, vol. 54, no. 1, pp. 39–42, 2015.

[9] J.-B. Dubuisson, A. Fauconnier, V. Fourchotte, K. Babaki-Fard, J. Coste, and C. Chapron, "Laparoscopic myomectomy: predicting the risk of conversion to an open procedure," *Human Reproduction*, vol. 16, no. 8, pp. 1726–1731, 2001.

[10] A. P. Advincula, A. Song, W. Burke, and R. K. Reynolds, "Preliminary experience with robot-assisted laparoscopic myomectomy," *The Journal of the American Association of Gynecologic Laparoscopists*, vol. 11, no. 4, pp. 511–518, 2004.

[11] J. Pundir, V. Pundir, R. Walavalkar, K. Omanwa, G. Lancaster, and S. Kayani, "Robotic-assisted laparoscopic vs abdominal and laparoscopic myomectomy: systematic review and meta-analysis," *Journal of Minimally Invasive Gynecology*, vol. 20, no. 3, pp. 335–345, 2013.

[12] E. E. Barakat, M. A. Bedaiwy, S. Zimberg, B. Nutter, M. Nosseir, and T. Falcone, "Robotic-assisted, laparoscopic, and abdominal myomectomy: a comparison of surgical outcomes," *Obstetrics and Gynecology*, vol. 117, no. 2, pp. 256–265, 2011.

[13] C. J. Ascher-Walsh and T. L. Capes, "Robot-assisted laparoscopic myomectomy is an improvement over laparotomy in women with a limited number of myomas," *Journal of Minimally Invasive Gynecology*, vol. 17, no. 3, pp. 306–310, 2010.

[14] N. Pluchino, P. Litta, L. Freschi et al., "Comparison of the initial surgical experience with robotic and laparoscopic myomectomy," *International Journal of Medical Robotics and Computer Assisted Surgery*, vol. 10, no. 2, pp. 208–212, 2014.

24

Analysis of a Standardized Technique for Laparoscopic Cuff Closure following 1924 Total Laparoscopic Hysterectomies

Katherine A. O'Hanlan,[1] Pamela L. Emeney,[2] Alfred Peters,[2] Margaret S. Sten,[1] Stacey P. McCutcheon,[1] Danielle M. Struck,[1] and Joseph K. Hoang[1]

[1]*Laparoscopic Institute for Gynecology and Oncology, 4370 Alpine Road, Portola Valley, CA 94028, USA*
[2]*University of California at San Francisco-Fresno, 155 North Fresno Street, Fresno, CA 93701, USA*

Correspondence should be addressed to Katherine A. O'Hanlan; kate.ohanlanmd@gmail.com

Academic Editor: Peng Hui Wang

Objective. To review the vaginal cuff complications from a large series of total laparoscopic hysterectomies in which the laparoscopic culdotomy closure was highly standardized. *Methods.* Retrospective cohort study (Canadian Task Force Classification II-3) of consecutive total and radical laparoscopic hysterectomy patients with all culdotomy closures performed laparoscopically was conducted using three guidelines: placement of all sutures 5 mm deep from the vaginal edge with a 5 mm interval, incorporation of the uterosacral ligaments with the pubocervical fascia at each angle, and, whenever possible, suturing the bladder peritoneum over the vaginal cuff edge utilizing two suture types of comparable tensile strength. Four outcomes are reviewed: dehiscence, bleeding, infection, and adhesions. *Results.* Of 1924 patients undergoing total laparoscopic hysterectomy, 44 patients (2.29%) experienced a vaginal cuff complication, with 19 (0.99%) requiring reoperation. Five patients (0.26%) had dehiscence after sexual penetration on days 30–83, with 3 requiring reoperation. Thirteen patients (0.68%) developed bleeding, with 9 (0.47%) requiring reoperation. Twenty-three (1.20%) patients developed infections, with 4 (0.21%) requiring reoperation. Three patients (0.16%) developed obstructive small bowel adhesions to the cuff requiring laparoscopic lysis. *Conclusion.* A running 5 mm deep × 5 mm apart culdotomy closure that incorporates the uterosacral ligaments with the pubocervical fascia, with reperitonealization when possible, appears to be associated with few postoperative vaginal cuff complications.

1. Introduction

Postlaparoscopic hysterectomy vaginal cuff complications, such as dehiscence, bleeding, infection, and adhesions, are infrequent but can potentially lead to more serious problems including acute anemia, evisceration, bowel injury, peritonitis, sepsis, and reoperation. A recent review of 57 cohort studies of one type of complication, cuff dehiscence, after laparoscopic hysterectomy found that transvaginal closure of the vaginal cuff was associated with the lowest dehiscence rate as compared to laparoscopic and robotic cuff closures [1]. However, variations in vaginal anatomy associated with nulliparity, obesity, and senescent vaginal constrictive changes can make transvaginal culdotomy closure difficult or impossible, underscoring the need for an effective laparoscopic approach for culdotomy closure. Additionally, other notable vaginal cuff complications, such as bleeding, infection, and postoperative adhesions, require further investigation with regard to the closure technique. Surgeon experience may also play a role and may affect the reliability of the closure.

The objective of this retrospective report and video is to review the association of the surgeon's experience and closure guidelines that include a consistent 5 mm interval with a 5mm depth from the vaginal cuff edge, incorporation of the uterosacral ligaments with the pubocervical fascia at each angle, and closure of the peritoneum over the vaginal cuff whenever possible, with the four major categories of complications: dehiscence, bleeding, infections, and adhesions.

2. Materials and Methods

With Investigational Review Board approval from Sequoia Hospital in Redwood City, CA, data for every patient undergoing total laparoscopic hysterectomy and concomitant procedures from September 1, 1996, to April 7, 2015, was abstracted from hospital and office files, anonymized, and stored on an excel spreadsheet. The patient's history and physical examination, operative report, and hospital record were reviewed to obtain age, BMI, estimated blood loss, procedure performed, and surgical duration. For this report, postoperative vaginal complications were defined as any vaginal apex or cuff-related complication, including dehiscence, bleeding, infection, or adhesions occurring up to 90 days after surgery [2]. Pelvic cellulitis was included as an infectious complication and was defined as a vague abdominal pain or the sensation of pelvic fullness, with apical vaginal induration, tenderness to palpation, and edema in the absence of abscess or peritoneal signs [3].

Surgeon experience was assessed by compiling the complications in each sequential segment of 200 cases, with 10 segments, in the series of 1924 patients.

In this practice, all patients needing hysterectomy for benign or malignant indications were scheduled for a laparoscopic approach unless they had radiologically documented metastatic disease or prior operative records documenting severe abdominal/intestinal adhesions and were excluded from this study. Every patient signed that she had read a 13-page document called "Pre-operative planning and recovery information" (available at http://www.ohanlan.com/pdf/patient_ed_planning_surgery_pdf/preoperative_instructions_and_recovery.pdf) which details the anticipated pre- and postoperative hysterectomy experience and the possible complications in this practice and provides detailed posthospital instructions. In all patients, single abdominal-vulvar-vaginal and perineal preparation with chlorhexidine was performed [4]. In each case, a simple or radical hysterectomy was performed alone or with other procedures as indicated by the patient's diagnosis, physical exam, and radiologic evaluation. The actual techniques used for the extrafascial type 7 total laparoscopic hysterectomy (TLH) [5], including the single field sterile skin preparation, and all surgical dissections are described elsewhere [4, 6]. No supracervical or vaginal hysterectomies were performed. A laparoscopic approach for closure of the vagina was performed in every case and is described in detail below, along with the supplementary video made in March 2014 (see Supplementary Material available online at http://dx.doi.org/10.1155/2016/1372685).

3. Details of Vaginal Cuff Closure Technique Incorporating Uterosacral Ligaments, Regular Placement of Sutures, and Reperitonealization

In all cases, the culdotomy was created using bipolar and monopolar electrocautery directed to a cephalad-deviated uterine manipulator cup (V-Care, ConMed, Utica, NY) to both present the cervicovaginal margin and lift that margin away from the ureters.

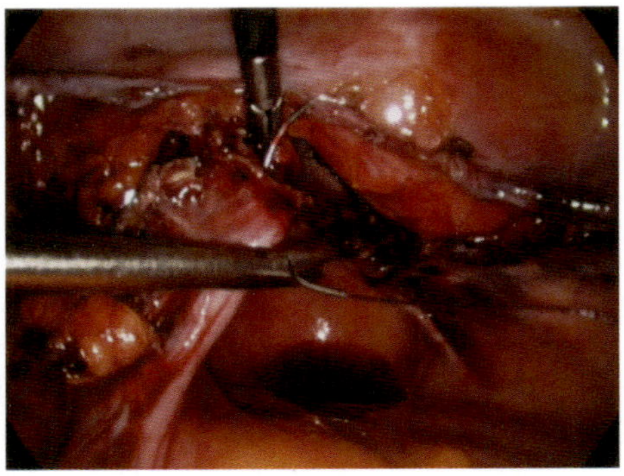

FIGURE 1: Suture is passed through the USL from about 1.5 cm posterior to the cut edge, exiting the USL fibers just proximal to the pubocervical fascia.

For culdotomy closure, two suture types were utilized. Coated braided 0-polyglactin suture on an ST-3 needle (Vicryl Endoknot, Johnson and Johnson, Cincinnati, OH, USA) was employed in the first half of the series, and monofilament 2-0 glycolide, dioxanone, and trimethylene carbonate barbed suture on a GS-22 needle (V-Loc 90, Covidien, Boulder, CO, USA) was used in the latter half. Both types of sutures have confirmed equivalent strength and absorption profiles relevant to the observation period for complications. Both sutures retain 75% of tensile strength at 14 days and are fully absorbed after a mean of 63 days (http://www.ethicon.com/healthcare-professionals/products/wound-closure/suture-assist/endoknot-suture#!description-and-specs/, http://www.covidien.com/vloc/pages.aspx?page=Materials-Guide/). The same technique for closure was used for the duration of this report and we have reviewed all cases together.

The vaginal squamous epithelial lateral-most edge (3 or 9 o'clock) is lifted anteriorly to tense and identify the uterosacral ligament (USL). The first and most lateral stitch is placed about 1.5 cm proximal to the cut edge of the USL, exiting through the posterior aspect of the transected fibers of the USL (Figure 1). Separately, it is next passed directly through the posterior vaginal cuff wall into the lumen, exiting the vaginal epithelium approximately 5 mm from the cut edge (Figure 2). The estimation of 5 mm was repeatedly based on the diameter of each of the 5 mm instruments. The suture is then passed through the lateral anterior vaginal wall, again at a depth of approximately 5 mm from the edge, exiting the tissue to be certain to include all the anterior transected fibers of the pubocervical fascia, fixing and "folding" the USL onto the posterolateral apex (Figure 3). The medial aspect of the distal uterosacral ligament is incorporated similarly into the second suture as reinforcement. Sutures are placed every 5 mm apart, at a depth of 5 mm in a noninterlocking, continuous running horizontal fashion. The contralateral USL is then incorporated in a similar fashion. The suture is run back to the contralateral side reefing through the edge of the posterior peritoneum and the anterior bladder flap

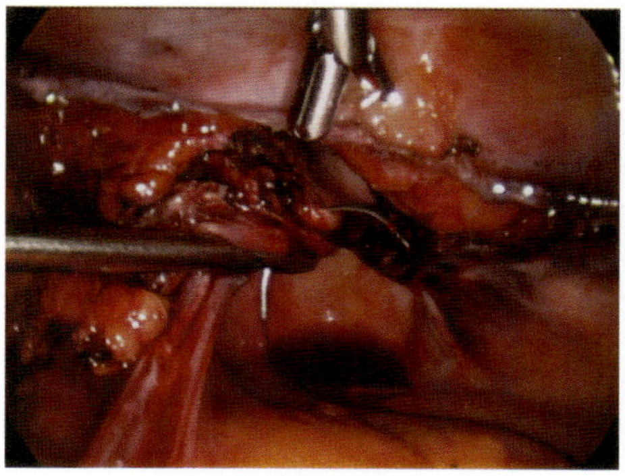

Figure 2: The suture is passed into the posterolateral vagina 5 mm deep to the cut edge.

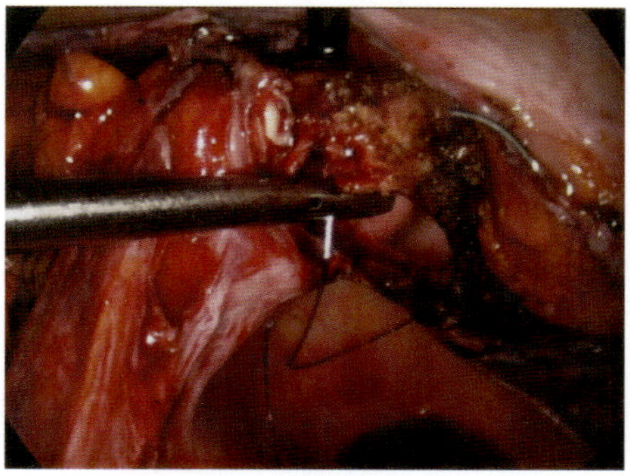

Figure 3: The anterolateral vaginal wall is pierced 5 mm deep from the cut edge and exits to include the cut fibers of the pubocervical fascia.

peritoneum to effectively cover the cut edge of the closed vagina. This reperitonealization extends from one USL to the other but leaves the sidewalls open for drainage (Figure 4). Rarely, if there is still laxity of the USL and hypermobility of the apex, a polyester suture (Ethibond Endoknot, Johnson and Johnson, Cincinnati, OH) is used to plicate the distal USLs into the posterior cervical fascia, adding further lift to the vaginal cuff [7, 8].

Following the closure, patients were normally discharged the next day, evaluated by telephone by our nurse practitioner within two days of discharge, and contacted by the surgeon within the following week to discuss pathology results. In the absence of any report of a problem with urinary, gastrointestinal, or wound healing, the patients were seen at 6 weeks for a postoperative visit and vaginal cuff exam by either the primary author or their local gynecologist. When indicated, earlier or additional postoperative visits were scheduled.

Since there was an observational study with a significant amount of skewed data, nonparametric tests were used throughout. The Kruskal-Wallis test was used to determine if a difference existed between patients with reoperative or nonreoperative complications and patients without complications against the demographic factors of age, BMI, parity, duration of surgery, days of hospitalization, and infection. The Kruskal-Wallis is a nonparametric equivalent to the ANOVA that tests equality of distributions using rank order.

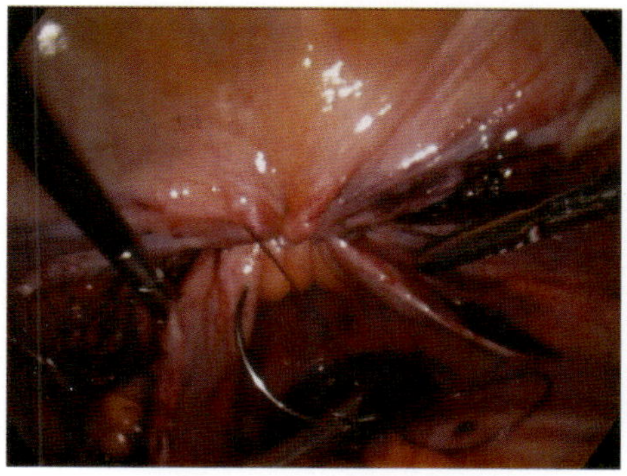

Figure 4: The bladder peritoneum has been sutured to the peritoneum of the anterior cul-de-sac so as to cover the raw cut edges of the vagina, while allowing drainage laterally. Note that the USLs are prominently providing support to the apex but not overly taught.

Spearman's rho was used to identify any linear relationships between the demographic factors and the complications of dehiscence, bleeding, and infections. Spearman's rho is a nonparametric equivalent to the Pearson Correlation.

4. Results

Over the 19-year study period, 1924 patients underwent a simple or radical laparoscopic hysterectomy. Table 1 describes the demographics of the cohort, including the preoperative diagnoses, the procedures performed, and the final pathologic diagnoses. Twenty patients had been converted to laparotomy from the planned TLH and are excluded from this analysis. Of this cohort, a total of 44 patients (2.28%) experienced a vaginal complication: 5 (.26%) had dehiscence, 13 (.68%) had bleeding, 23 (1.20%) had infection, and 3 (.16%) had adhesions (Table 2). Among the 44 patients with complications, 19 (.99%) required reoperation, while 25 (1.30%) did not require a reoperation or procedure.

There are no significant differences in demographics, operative statistics, or length of hospitalization between the patients who experienced complications and those who did not. Patients with any type of complication, reoperative or nonreoperative, were younger than those without a complication (46 versus 51 years, $p < 0.000$) and had a similar median BMI of 26.5 (range: 14.5–74.2, NS) kg/m^2 and similar median parity of 1 (range: 0–9, NS). At surgery, the median duration of surgery was 108 minutes for all patients (range: 24–556 minutes, NS); but the median estimated blood loss for patients having a reoperative complication was higher than those without any complication (100 versus 75 cc, $p = 0.049$). While the range of days of hospitalization was less in patients with any cuff complication and with both nonreoperative and reoperative complications compared to those with no complications (1–12 versus 1–13), the Kruskal-Wallis Rank Sum Test was significant for those without any complication against reoperative patients ($p < 0.000$) indicating these two sets are distinct (Table 2).

Vaginal dehiscence was observed in five patients (0.26%), all after sexual activity, on postoperative days 30, 42, 44,

Table 1: Demographics of all 1924 patients in study.

Feature	Mean	Range
Age (years)	52	(15–97)
BMI (Kg/m^2)	29	(14–74)
Parity (#)	1	(0–9)
Duration of surgery (minutes)	121	(24–556)
Uterine weight (Kg)	216	(14–3131)
Pelvic nodes (#)	23	(0–61)
Inframesenteric nodes (#)	7	(0–38)
Infrarenal nodes (#)	7	(0–37)
Transfusions (#PRBC)	0	(0–5)
Hospital stay (days)	1	(1–13)
Preoperative diagnosis	*N*	(%)
Pelvic mass	415	21.6%
Leiomyoma	400	20.8%
Endometrial carcinoma	355	18.5%
Pelvic pain	126	6.5%
BrCa+/family history	108	5.6%
Endometrial hyperplasia	100	5.2%
Transgender	94	4.9%
Adenomyosis	86	4.5%
Prolapse	68	3.5%
Cervical carcinoma	49	2.5%
Ovarian/tubal carcinoma	35	1.8%
Cervical dysplasia	31	1.6%
Menorrhagia	25	1.3%
Stress incontinence	15	0.8%
Uterine stromal/other	13	0.7%
Menstrual migraines/PCOS	3	0.2%
PID	1	0.1%
Procedure	*N*	%
TLH-BSO	1723	90%
Appendectomy	1103	57%
Any lymphadenectomy	205	11%
McCall's colposuspension	149	8%
Adhesiolysis	134	7%
Endometriosis resection	83	4%
Burch	77	4%
RLH-BSO	76	4%
TLH	68	4%
TLH-BS	48	3%
TOT	26	1%
Ureterolysis	21	1%
Herniorrhaphy	13	1%
Posterior repair	11	1%
Minilaparotomy	7	0%
Cholecystectomy	6	0%
Converted	5	0%
Tumor debulking	5	0%
RLH-BS	4	0%
Converted	3	0%
Episiotomy	2	0%
Postoperative diagnosis	*N*	%
Leiomyoma	615	32.0%
Endometrial carcinoma	368	19.1%
Benign ovarian neoplasia	363	18.9%
Adenomyosis	174	9.0%
Endometriosis	127	6.6%
Ovarian/tubal carcinoma	98	5.1%
Endometrial hyperplasia	71	3.7%
Cervical carcinoma	49	2.5%
Cervical dysplasia	26	1.4%
Adhesions	15	0.8%
Uterine stromal/other	9	0.5%
Metastatic cancer	7	0.4%
PID	2	0.1%

52, and 83. All of the vaginal dehiscence cases had benign pathology and simple hysterectomy. There were no differences in patient age, BMI, parity, blood loss, or hospital stay when compared with those not having dehiscence (Table 2). All of the vaginal dehiscence cases occurred in the first quarter of the study period and had utilized coated braided 0-polyglactin suture. Three patients (0.16%) had apical dehiscence larger than 2 cm, and the apical dehiscences were sutured closed; however, none of these patients had small bowel evisceration. Speculum examination of these three patients revealed only the fatty underside of the closed bladder peritoneum through the vaginal cuff defect.

Vaginal cuff bleeding occurred in 13 patients (0.68%), of whom 4 (0.21%) resolved spontaneously and 9 (0.47%) required suture repair. Patients with a bleeding complication were significantly younger that those without a bleeding complication (42 versus 52 years, $p = 0.001$) but had similar BMI, parity, surgical duration, blood loss, and length of hospital stay (Table 3). Five cases of cuff hemorrhage (0.26%) developed during the initial postoperative 23-hour hospitalization: 3 (0.16%) patients were taken back to the operating room from the recovery room, and 2 (0.10%) began bleeding in their hospital room the next morning. One patient had an unrecognized vaginal laceration from vaginal morcellation and the others from cuff arterioles. The other 4 (0.21%) reoperative cases all had bleeding from small cuff arterioles, which were electrocauterized or sutured vaginally in the office on postoperative days 4, 7, 7, and 18.

Infectious complications developed in 23 patients (1.2%). Pelvic cellulitis was clinically diagnosed in 18 patients during the office visit at 7–14 days postoperatively. All were treated with 5–7 days of oral antibiotics, typically doxycycline or ciprofloxacin, with resolution of pelvic induration and tenderness. Five patients had a CT-documented abscess, 4 (0.2%) of whom required drainage by computed tomography, while one resolved with antibiotics. While patients with infectious complications were younger than those without (47 versus 52 years, $p = 0.011$) and had a longer surgical duration (156 versus 120 minutes, $p = 0.013$) than those who did not, neither BMI, parity, blood loss, nor length of hospital stay was different (Table 2).

Small bowel obstruction from adhesions to the raw vaginal cuff was observed in 3 patients (0.2%), all of whom underwent laparoscopic lysis of adhesions on postoperative days 6-7 and recovered. All three had retracted or absent bladder peritoneum from anterior leiomyomas, a previous Cesarean section, or surgical treatment of endometriosis that precluded reperitonealization. A laparoscopic lysis of

TABLE 2: Comparing demographic factors of those without a cuff complication with those having any or nonreoperative or reoperative complications.

Demographics	No cuff complication $N = 1880$ (97.7)	*All* types of cuff complications $N = 44$ (2.2%)	
	Median (range)	Median (range)	p value
Age (years)	51 (15–97)	46 (25–75)	0
BMI (kg/m^2)	26.5 (14.5–74.2)	25.1 (18.2–49.1)	0.078
Parity (#)	1 (0–9)	1 (0–9)	0.94
Surgery duration (min)	108 (240–556)	121 (45–305)	0.118
Estimated blood loss (mL)	75 (24–556)	100 (5–1000)	0.06
Hospital stay (days)	1 (1–13)	1 (1–12)	0.025
Demographics	No cuff complication $N = 1880$ (97.7)	*Nonreoperative* complications $N = 25$ (1.3%)	
	Median (range)	Median (range)	p value
Age (years)	51 (15–97)	44 (27–75)	0.003
BMI (kg/m^2)	26.5 (14.5–74.2)	25.2 (19.1–49.1)	0.167
Parity (#)	1 (0–9)	1 (0–4)	0.359
Surgery duration (min)	108 (240–556)	119 (45–305)	0.446
Estimated blood loss (mL)	75 (24–556)	100 (5–400)	0.443
Hospital stay (days)	1 (1–13)	1 (1-2)	0.785
Demographics	No cuff complication $N = 1880$ (97.7)	*Reoperative* cuff complications $N = 19$ (.9%)	
	Median (range)	Median (range)	p value
Age (years)	51 (15–97)	46 (24–58)	0.007
BMI (kg/m^2)	26.5 (14.5–74.2)	24.8 (18.2–42)	0.28
Parity (#)	1 (0–9)	2 (0–9)	0.349
Surgery duration (min)	108 (240–556)	130 (50–285)	0.137
Estimated blood loss (mL)	75 (24–556)	100 (10–1000)	0.049
Hospital stay (days)	1 (1–13)	1 (1–12)	0

TABLE 3: Relationship between demographic factors and complications.

Factor	Dehiscence $N = 5$ (0.3%)		Bleeding $N = 13$ (.68%)		Infections $N = 23$ (1.2%)	
	95% CI	p value	95% CI	p value	95% CI	p value
Age (years)	40–58	0.297	33–49	0.001	43–49	0.011
BMI (kg/m^2)	15.0–27.5	0.113	12.6–30.2	0.194	23.6–28.7	0.726
Parity (#)	1, 3	0.31	50–135	0.618	0-1	0.82
Surgery duration (min)	80–180	0.732	10–200	0.175	104–195	0.013
Estimated blood loss (mL)	5–300	0.683	1, 2	0.687	100–200	0.039
Hospital stay (days)	1, 2	0.1	0-1	0.35	1, 1	0.637

the adhesion from the cuff to the small bowel was curative in all three cases.

5. Discussion

The three guidelines applied to laparoscopic vaginal closure appear to be associated with an acceptably low rate of occurrence of the four major complications. The complications and concerns are discussed separately below.

5.1. Dehiscence Complications. With regard to dehiscence, Uccella and colleagues' systematic literature review of 13,030 patients having TLH reported 91 cases of vaginal dehiscence, with 0.64% from laparoscopic culdotomy closure, 0.18% from transvaginal closure, and 1.64% from robotic closure [9]. Hur and colleagues reviewed their hospital rates of dehiscence over ten years and reported a 1.35% dehiscence rate from TLH with evidence of a learning curve, with most of the dehiscences occurring in the first two-thirds of the period of observation [10]. With all suturing performed laparoscopically, we report a dehiscence rate of 0.26%, which compares favorably with these international rates and suggests that a standard of suture placement 5 mm deep and 5 mm interval can be learned and may be safe and possibly advantageous.

This study does not support the conclusions of Uccella et al., who attributed their low dehiscence rate by the transvaginal route to more effective knots and suture type [1]. Effective knot tying and suture reliability are key features of both of the two sutures used over the duration of the study period, resulting in excellent reliability in tissue fixation for the entire period. No dehiscences occurred in the second half of the nearly one thousand patients in whom Vicryl suture with a knot pusher was used. This fact raises doubt that suture variables and knot reliability, per se, were significant [1, 11] and points more to the surgeon's suturing skill. No study has ever reported such detail as to whether the visualized sutures at the dehisced vaginal apex had broken or whether the knots had become untied, and we did not observe those features either. In the present study, all dehiscences in our series occurred exclusively early in the *first one-quarter* of the series and resolved well before any change of suture, with no dehiscence occurrence during the latter half of the use of the first type of suture. Surgeons must introspect. We believe the dehiscence complications were due to surgeon inexperience in the early part of the series and diminished only with the surgeon's growing skill, well before the change to another suture (Figure 6). The sutures were similar enough in providing reliable fixation, for example, knot pusher and barbs with an end loop that we can only conclude that suture type is not relevant to avoidance of dehiscence but reliable and consistent suture placement is extremely relevant. A randomized trial with the two sutures would confirm or negate this.

In this series, higher blood loss correlated with risk of dehiscence but no other surgical parameters. While some studies report that patients undergoing radical hysterectomy may be at higher risk of vault dehiscence because the procedure usually shortens the vagina somewhat [12], none of the patients in this study with cervical or endometrial carcinoma undergoing radical laparoscopic hysterectomy sustained a cuff complication.

Monopolar electrosurgery use for culdotomy has been implicated by some as the cause for dehiscence [13]. However, other large series have found no impact related to the method of culdotomy incision, whether by monopolar, ultrasonic shears, cold scissors, monopolar use, or its wattage [9]. Hur and colleagues endorsed use of a low-wattage, cutting monopolar current for the culdotomy to minimize charring [10]. In the current report, bipolar sealing and a proprietary monopolar blend of cut and coagulation at 40 watts were used to create all colpotomies and to achieve cuff hemostasis. This electrocautery modality was recently reviewed by Teoh and colleagues who found that the depth of thermal injury of the culdotomy using these same instruments was only 0.6–0.7 mm [14]. While avoiding excessive charring and ineffective repetitive deep electrocautery is considered standard, this report cannot implicate monopolar current or its wattage as a factor in dehiscence.

5.2. Hemorrhagic Complications. A literature search did not reveal any evidence-based standards for the depth of placement or for the interval between vaginal cuff sutures. The use of 5 mm deep and 5 mm apart suture placement in this series is originally derived from the laparoscopically magnified view of the vascularity of the cuff edge. With 5 mm interval between sutures, the vessels appeared appropriately compressed and hemostatic. With a depth of 5 mm, none of the sutures pulled through the tissue, and a consistent approximation of the edge was observed when visually inspected by speculum exam after completion. Perhaps the younger patients in this study had more bleeding complications because their vaginal skin was thicker due to higher estrogen levels, possibly making adequate suturing more difficult. It is also possible that younger women had better vascularized vaginal epithelium. Suture placement consistency during each closure was achieved by comparing the diameter of any of the 5 mm instruments to gauge suture depth and interval. In theory, the ideal closure of the culdotomy results from accurate suture placement and reliable knot tying, whether vaginally or laparoscopically. Inaccurate suture placement by any route, too shallow or too far apart, can leave gaps that do not compress the small arterioles at the cuff edge or that may pull through over time or result in postoperative bleeding or dehiscence. Sutures placed too close together can cause tissue necrosis resulting in devitalized tissue that may be more susceptible to tear or dehiscence.

Surgeons relying on suture devices to reapproximate the vaginal cuff carry risk, as these can fail or be unexpectedly unavailable. Siedhoff and colleagues reported on 387 patients, all of whom had laparoscopic culdotomy closure, and found that 4.2% of patients who underwent closure with a suture device had dehiscence, while none who were closed with a barbed suture had dehiscence [11]. We observed the same absence of dehiscence in our patients closed with the barbed suture, but, as noted previously, only a randomized trial could implicate suture type and exonerate surgeon experience. Although a transvaginal route may minimize the risk of dehiscence and bleeding by affording easier and more familiar tissue handling, with potentially more precise suture placement and more reliable knots, surgeons performing laparoscopic hysterectomy should develop the basic suturing skill to close the vaginal cuff laparoscopically because variations in patient body morphology, such as high BMI, narrow vagina, and nulliparous state, may preclude a vaginal approach to cuff closure.

5.3. Infectious Complications. Overall, infectious complications after total abdominal or vaginal hysterectomy occur in 1.6% of patients, according to a recent report from the National Surgical Quality Improvement Program [15]. Infectious complications from laparoscopic hysterectomy were very rare in the meta-analysis by Uccella and colleagues who report an occurrence rate of 0.28%. However, these were defined in their manuscript only as "vaginal infection/abscess." In the current series, 0.94% had cuff cellulitis, and 0.26% developed vaginal cuff abscesses. Among the risk factors reviewed in this study, duration of surgery correlated with risk of infectious complication, as others have historically described with total abdominal hysterectomy [16]. We confirm the findings of Lachiewicz and colleagues, who observed a correlation between increasing infection rate and increased *laparoscopic* operating time [3]. Surgical duration also relates to other complexities of the surgery beyond simply the hysterectomy. Young age was also found to be significantly associated with infectious complications, and this needs to be further studied.

5.4. Learning Curve for Culdotomy Closure Complications. Figure 6 details the occurrence of the individual categories of complications as they occurred in segments of 200 cases, demonstrating a learning curve in both the individual complication categories and in the total rate of complications. While the standards were set early in the series, it appears that surgeon experience affects the success of the applications of the guidelines. Comparing overall complications in this series with other series reveals this rate is favorable. There were no fatalities in this series as some have observed in the early years after the procedure was described [17]. However, surgeons in the 21st century now have the widely available benefit of training in advanced laparoscopic procedures in both residency and postgraduate continuing medical education courses which were not available when this series started. Learning curves now should not be as steep as they were in the 1990s [18].

5.5. Concerns about Support. It is estimated that United States women have a lifetime risk of 11% for prolapse surgery or 200,000 surgeries yearly for prolapse or incontinence [19, 20].

Surgeons have been urged to assess prolapse and continence prior to every hysterectomy and to try to prevent need for a future prolapse surgery [20]. Since 2008, it has been accepted that securing the uterosacral ligaments bilaterally to the pubocervical fascia restores and enhances level I support and decreases apical vault prolapse and may prevent subsequent prolapse surgery [21]. The baseline data from the Women's Health Initiative (WHI) of 10,727 women who had a hysterectomy by any approach, compared with 16,616 women retaining their uterus, showed very similar rates of stress incontinence (24% versus 26%), as well as cystocele (33% versus 34%) and rectocele (18% versus 19%) [22, 23]. Only parity and obesity affected prolapse in the total WHI population, not hysterectomy. While these findings offer reassurance that hysterectomy in itself does not cause prolapse or incontinence, they also suggest that we, as surgeons, are not addressing mild to moderate support issues when we perform hysterectomy for non-prolapse-related gynecologic indications [24]. Our reattachment of the uterosacral ligament replicates the first portion of the entire technique of colposuspension and at least appears to maintain and slightly enhance level 1 support. Laparoscopic approaches may provide a better opportunity for prolapse repair given that the anatomy is so well visualized. Laparoscopic uterosacral ligament suspension was shown to provide better apical support and fewer reoperations for prolapse than vaginal approach for the same procedure (Figure 5) [25, 26]. It may be that the approach from within the peritoneal cavity allows surgeons to more confidently identify the uterosacral ligament and provide better level I support [16]. Although

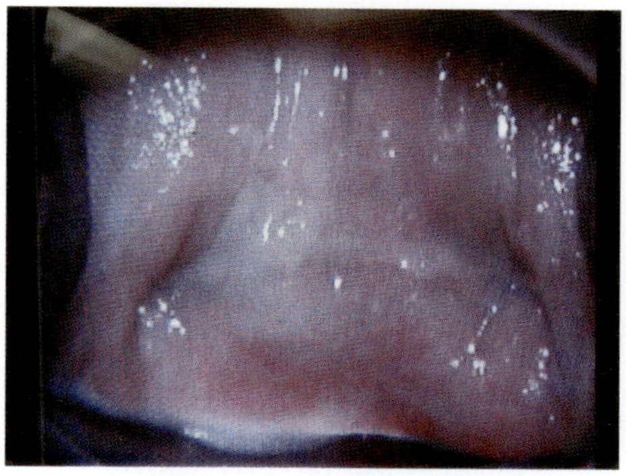

FIGURE 5: In this speculum exam photo from the six-week postoperative office check for granulation, good lateral apical support is seen bilaterally from the dimple caused by the uterosacral ligaments.

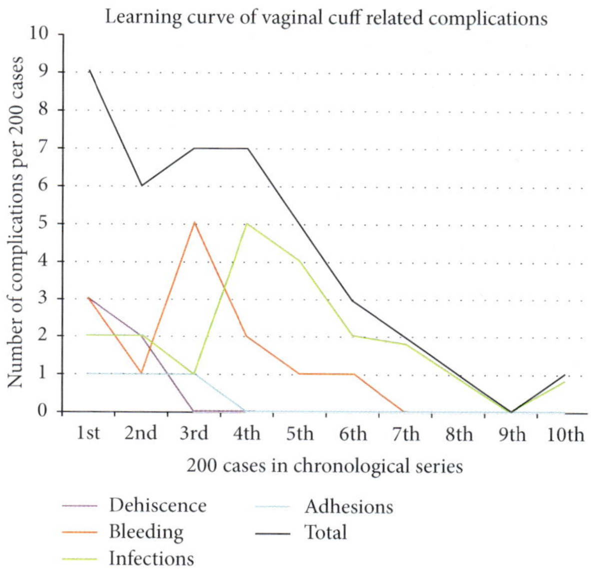

FIGURE 6: This chart reflects the complications separated in segments of 200 cases each, over the 19 years of this study. Dehiscence (purple), bleeding (red), infections (green), and adhesions (blue) show gradual decrease over time. The total decrease in complications (black) is due to a variety of factors including the surgeons' learning curve, improved surgical skills, experience, and judgment.

long-term follow-up of vaginal support issues for all patients referred from afar to this oncology-based practice is not part of this report, we can confirm that there have been six returns to our practice for prolapse issues out of 1,924. All patients were instructed to report all complications to our office for ongoing care and management, but all patients were not surveyed or brought back for exam, resulting in a possible undercount of our complications. Quality of follow-up is a major weakness of this retrospective report, and further study is needed.

5.6. Closing the Bladder Peritoneum. The technique of closing the "bladder flap," or reperitonealization of the vaginal cuff, after total abdominal hysterectomy was largely abandoned after two retrospective case cohort reports from 1983 and

1994 [27, 28]. The authors hypothesized that the peritoneum regrows quickly over the denuded pelvic tissues and that the sutures may contribute to subsequent adhesion formation. However, in a recent prospective trial of laparotomy closure in rabbits, closure of the peritoneum, regardless of suture type, reduced the amount of adhesions seen at reoperation 14 days later [29]. Parietal peritoneal closure after Cesarean section has been shown to cause fewer dense or filmy adhesions [30].

In some instances, due to anatomic limitations, the peritoneum could not be reapproximated, but the frequency of this was not recorded. This is especially true for patients with large, anterior leiomyomas, extensive endometriosis, or multiple prior Cesarean sections, which disrupt the bladder peritoneum and/or make it less pliant or adherent to the uterotomy site. The three patients in this series who developed small bowel adhesions to the raw vaginal apex all had anatomy that precluded covering the raw vaginal edges with peritoneum. While small bowel adhesions have been reported from the use of the polydioxanone barbed suture [31], in this study, none of the patients who had reperitonealization experienced a complication from adhesions.

In this series, three of the five patients with dehiscence required suture closure of the apex for a rupture larger than 2 cm, but none experienced intestinal evisceration. A literature review by Hur and colleagues in 2007 found evidence that from 30 to 95% of dehiscences were associated with evisceration [10]. While Uccella and colleagues found that peritoneal closure did not reduce dehiscence, there was no stratification of data by need for *reoperation for perforation* based on peritoneal closure over the culdotomy closure [9]. Potentially, closing the pliant bladder peritoneal layer over the raw vaginal cuff edge offers one additional layer of protection from catastrophic bowel evisceration for those few who do experience disruption of the vaginal cuff. The fact that the speculum exam in the emergency room showed the intact underside of the peritoneal layer in two of our cases of dehiscence motivates us to continue this practice until prospective studies provide more information.

There are several weaknesses in this retrospective report. First, some of the patients, living as far as nine hours away, may have experienced cuff complications and presented at another hospital for their emergency care. While all patients receive printed material describing when and how to contact the surgeon in the event of suspected complications, it is possible that they obtained local care without our knowledge, resulting in underestimation of the complication rate. The fact that one surgeon performed all the surgeries may reduce the likelihood of broader reproducibility; however, the skillset required in TLH is not beyond the certified gynecologist. Surgeon learning curve over 19 years changes in surgical practice, and specific experience with the two sutures precludes any specific conclusion about the sutures over the study period. Tissue healing is also dependent on many factors not specifically addressed herein, including comorbid medical conditions (diabetes mellitus, hypertension), steroid use, nutritional status, general health, and compliance with postoperative instructions. There was also no formal pre- or postoperative formal POP-Q assessment of level 1 support to confirm effectiveness of USL incorporation procedures.

6. Conclusions

All vaginal closures should be individualized to optimize support and avoid dehiscence, bleeding, infection, and adhesions. The low rate of the four major types of complications using these laparoscopic culdotomy closure guidelines suggests that these guidelines are safe. Our belief is that the suture material made no difference in the low rate of complications after the first-quarter of the series was completed. Rather, surgeon accuracy in suture placement with a depth of 5 mm and 5 mm interval, uterosacral ligament incorporation for apical support, and reperitonealization where possible appear most important; but a large, prospective clinical trial is needed to delineate the safest standards for laparoscopic culdotomy closure and to show which portion(s) of this technique contribute most significantly to a low rate of complications. Additionally, a large, long-term prospective analysis would be necessary to confirm any level 1 support benefit from the reattachment of the uterosacral ligament to the pubocervical fascia during the vaginal cuff closure.

Disclosure

The primary author is a gynecologic oncologist in private practice and a consultant/speaker for Applied, Baxter, and Covidien and Medical Director of the Laparoscopic Institute for Gynecology and Oncology, which produces an annual educational course on minimally invasive surgery. There is no off-label use of any medical device in this paper.

Competing Interests

The authors declare that there is no conflict of interests regarding the publication of this paper.

References

[1] S. Uccella, F. Ghezzi, A. Mariani et al., "Vaginal cuff closure after minimally invasive hysterectomy: our experience and systematic review of the literature," *American Journal of Obstetrics and Gynecology*, vol. 205, no. 2, pp. 119.e1–119.e12, 2011.

[2] C. D. Owens and K. Stoessel, "Surgical site infections: epidemiology, microbiology and prevention," *Journal of Hospital Infection*, vol. 70, supplement 2, pp. 3–10, 2008.

[3] M. P. Lachiewicz, L. J. Moulton, and O. Jaiyeoba, "Pelvic surgical site infections in gynecologic surgery," *Infectious Diseases in Obstetrics and Gynecology*, vol. 2015, Article ID 614950, 8 pages, 2015.

[4] K. A. O'Hanlan, S. P. McCutcheon, J. G. McCutcheon, and B. E. Charvonia, "Single-field sterile-scrub, preparation, and dwell for laparoscopic hysterectomy," *Journal of Minimally Invasive Gynecology*, vol. 19, no. 2, pp. 220–224, 2012.

[5] C. Nezhat, F. Nezhat, C. Nezhat, D. Admon, and A. A. Nezhat, "Proposed classification of hysterectomies involving laparoscopy," *The Journal of the American Association of Gynecologic Laparoscopists*, vol. 2, no. 4, pp. 427–429, 1995.

[6] K. A. O'Hanlan, G. S. Huang, A.-C. Garnier et al., "Total laparoscopic hysterectomy versus total abdominal hysterectomy: cohort review of patients with uterine neoplasia," *Journal*

of the Society of Laparoendoscopic Surgeons, vol. 9, no. 3, pp. 277–286, 2005.

[7] S. Uccella, F. Ghezzi, V. Bergamini et al., "Laparoscopic uterosacral ligaments plication for the treatment of uterine prolapse," *Archives of Gynecology and Obstetrics*, vol. 276, no. 3, pp. 225–229, 2007.

[8] C. P. Chung, R. Miskimins, T. J. Kuehl, P. M. Yandell, and B. L. Shull, "Permanent suture used in uterosacral ligament suspension offers better anatomical support than delayed absorbable suture," *International Urogynecology Journal and Pelvic Floor Dysfunction*, vol. 23, no. 2, pp. 223–227, 2012.

[9] S. Uccella, M. Ceccaroni, A. Cromi et al., "Vaginal cuff dehiscence in a series of 12,398 hysterectomies: effect of different types of colpotomy and vaginal closure," *Obstetrics and Gynecology*, vol. 120, no. 3, pp. 516–523, 2012.

[10] H.-C. Hur, R. S. Guido, S. M. Mansuria, M. R. Hacker, J. S. Sanfilippo, and T. T. Lee, "Incidence and patient characteristics of vaginal cuff dehiscence after different modes of hysterectomies," *Journal of Minimally Invasive Gynecology*, vol. 14, no. 3, pp. 311–317, 2007.

[11] M. T. Siedhoff, A. C. Yunker, and J. F. Steege, "Decreased incidence of vaginal cuff dehiscence after laparoscopic closure with bidirectional barbed suture," *Journal of Minimally Invasive Gynecology*, vol. 18, no. 2, pp. 218–223, 2011.

[12] A. M. Nick, J. Lange, M. Frumovitz et al., "Rate of vaginal cuff separation following laparoscopic or robotic hysterectomy," *Gynecologic Oncology*, vol. 120, no. 1, pp. 47–51, 2011.

[13] M. D. Blikkendaal, A. R. H. Twijnstra, S. C. L. Pacquee et al., "Vaginal cuff dehiscence in laparoscopic hysterectomy: influence of various suturing methods of the vaginal vault," *Gynecological Surgery*, vol. 9, no. 4, pp. 393–400, 2012.

[14] D. Teoh, W. J. Lowery, X. Jiang et al., "Vaginal cuff thermal injury by mode of colpotomy at total laparoscopic hysterectomy: a randomized clinical trial," *Journal of Minimally Invasive Gynecology*, vol. 22, no. 2, pp. 227–233, 2015.

[15] A. G. Lake, A. M. McPencow, M. A. Dick-Biascoechea, D. K. Martin, and E. A. Erekson, "Surgical site infection after hysterectomy," *American Journal of Obstetrics and Gynecology*, vol. 209, no. 5, pp. 490.e1–490.e9, 2013.

[16] M. A. Olsen, J. Higham-Kessler, D. S. Yokoe et al., "Developing a risk stratification model for surgical site infection after abdominal hysterectomy," *Infection Control and Hospital Epidemiology*, vol. 30, no. 11, pp. 1077–1083, 2009.

[17] C. Y. Liu and H. Reich, "Complications of total laparoscopic hysterectomy in 518 cases," *Gynaecological Endoscopy*, vol. 3, no. 4, pp. 203–208, 1994.

[18] C. M. Chapron, J.-B. Dubuisson, and Y. Ansquer, "Is total laparoscopic hysterectomy a safe surgical procedure?" *Human Reproduction*, vol. 11, no. 11, pp. 2422–2424, 1996.

[19] A. L. Olsen, V. J. Smith, J. O. Bergstrom, J. C. Colling, and A. L. Clark, "Epidemiology of surgically managed pelvic organ prolapse and urinary incontinence," *Obstetrics and Gynecology*, vol. 89, no. 4, pp. 501–506, 1997.

[20] J. A. Abbott, K. I. Bajzak, I. C. Green et al., "AAGL practice report: practice guidelines on the prevention of apical prolapse at the time of benign hysterectomy," *Journal of Minimally Invasive Gynecology*, vol. 21, no. 5, pp. 715–722, 2014.

[21] D. D. Rahn, R. J. Stone, A. K. Vu, A. B. White, and C. Y. Wai, "Abdominal hysterectomy with or without angle stitch: correlation with subsequent vaginal vault prolapse," *American Journal of Obstetrics & Gynecology*, vol. 199, no. 6, pp. 669e1–669.e4, 2008.

[22] S. L. Hendrix, A. Clark, I. Nygaard, A. Aragaki, V. Barnabei, and A. McTiernan, "Pelvic organ prolapse in the Women's Health Initiative: gravity and gravidity," *American Journal of Obstetrics and Gynecology*, vol. 186, no. 6, pp. 1160–1166, 2002.

[23] S. L. Hendrix, B. B. Cochrane, I. E. Nygaard et al., "Effects of estrogen with and without progestin on urinary incontinence," *Journal of the American Medical Association*, vol. 293, no. 8, pp. 935–948, 2005.

[24] K. S. Eilber, M. Alperin, A. Khan et al., "Outcomes of vaginal prolapse surgery among female medicare beneficiaries: the role of apical support," *Obstetrics and Gynecology*, vol. 122, no. 5, pp. 981–987, 2013.

[25] A. Diwan, C. R. Rardin, W. C. Strohsnitter, A. Weld, P. Rosenblatt, and N. Kohli, "Laparoscopic uterosacral ligament uterine suspension compared with vaginal hysterectomy with vaginal vault suspension for uterovaginal prolapse," *International Urogynecology Journal and Pelvic Floor Dysfunction*, vol. 17, no. 1, pp. 79–83, 2006.

[26] J. W. Barrington and G. Edwards, "Posthysterectomy vault prolapse," *International Urogynecology Journal and Pelvic Floor Dysfunction*, vol. 11, no. 4, pp. 241–245, 2000.

[27] B. Stricker, J. Blanco, and H. E. Fox, "The gynecologic contribution to intestinal obstruction in females," *Journal of the American College of Surgeons*, vol. 178, no. 6, pp. 617–620, 1994.

[28] J. B. Ratcliff, P. Kapernick, G. G. Brooks, and D. R. Dunnihoo, "Small bowel obstruction and previous gynecologic surgery," *Southern Medical Journal*, vol. 76, no. 11, pp. 1349–1360, 1983.

[29] R. R. Whitfield, H. F. Stills Jr., H. R. Huls, J. M. Crouch, and W. W. Hurd, "Effects of peritoneal closure and suture material on adhesion formation in a rabbit model," *American Journal of Obstetrics & Gynecology*, vol. 197, no. 6, pp. 644.e1–644.e5, 2007.

[30] D. J. Lyell, A. B. Caughey, E. Hu, and K. Daniels, "Peritoneal closure at primary cesarean delivery and adhesions," *Obstetrics and Gynecology*, vol. 106, no. 2, pp. 275–280, 2005.

[31] N. M. Donnellan and S. M. Mansuria, "Small bowel obstruction resulting from laparoscopic vaginal cuff closure with a barbed suture," *Journal of Minimally Invasive Gynecology*, vol. 18, no. 4, pp. 528–530, 2011.

25

Comparing Single and Dual Console Systems in the Robotic Surgical Training of Graduating OB/GYN Residents in the United States

Emad Mikhail,[1] Jason L. Salemi,[2] Stuart Hart,[1] and Anthony N. Imudia[1]

[1] *Department of Obstetrics and Gynecology, University of South Florida, Morsani College of Medicine, Tampa, FL 33606, USA*
[2] *Department of Family and Community Medicine, Baylor College of Medicine, Houston, TX 77098, USA*

Correspondence should be addressed to Emad Mikhail; emikhail@health.usf.edu

Academic Editor: Diego Cuccurullo

Objective. To assess the impact of a single versus dual console robotic system on the perceptions of program directors (PD) and residents (RES) towards robotic surgical training among graduating obstetrics and gynecology residents. *Design.* An anonymous survey was developed using *Qualtrics*, a web-based survey development and administration system, and sent to obstetrics and gynecology program directors and graduating residents. *Participants.* 39 program directors and 32 graduating residents (PGY4). *Results.* According to residents perception, dual console is utilized in about 70% of the respondents' programs. Dual console system programs were more likely to provide a robotics training certificate compared to single console programs (43.5% versus 0%, $p = 0.03$). A greater proportion of residents graduating from a dual console program perform more than 20 robotic-assisted total laparoscopic hysterectomies, 30% versus 0% ($p = 0.15$). *Conclusions.* Utilization of dual console system increased the likelihood of obtaining robotic training certification without significantly increasing the case volume of robotic-assisted total laparoscopic hysterectomy.

1. Introduction

Despite recent increases in the use of robotic surgical systems in gynecologic procedures, a trend that is expected to continue [1], incorporation of robotics into the training environment has been difficult because of the one-surgeon and one-surgery limitations of the robotic system [2]. As the transition is made into this "robotic era," in which only one surgeon at a time can perform any given operation, it is essential to provide appropriate training and ensure the competence of trainees before they literally take over the controls [3]. Some robotic surgery systems have a single surgeon console while other systems have an additional mentoring console (dual console). The dual console system has the potential to improve resident participation and training in robotic-assisted surgical cases, which is likely to translate into improved patient safety during robotic surgery [4].

Although the learning curve for robotic surgery may be less steep than for conventional laparoscopic surgery [5], the depth of residents' participation in the operating room has a strong impact on their surgical aptitude. Robotic gynecologic surgery has been associated with increased postoperative complications when compared to laparoscopic gynecologic surgery [6], which may, in part, be due to deficiencies in surgical training. In order to address the increased morbidity associated with robotic gynecologic surgeries, many residency programs across the nation have incorporated specific robotic training curriculum and some hospitals have purchased newer robotic systems with dual console. Collectively, these measures are aimed at increasing trainees' exposure and skills in robotic gynecologic surgeries. No study to date has evaluated the impact of the introduction of the dual console robotic system in residency robotic surgical training. Therefore, the objective of this study is to assess the perceptions of program directors (PD) and graduating obstetrics and gynecology residents (RES) towards robotic surgical training and to determine whether the existence of a single versus dual console robotic system as part of the residency program impacts those perceptions.

2. Materials and Methods

A survey was developed using *Qualtrics*, a web-based survey development and administration system. After obtaining exempt status from University of South Florida Institutional Review Board, the survey was pilot tested to ensure that it was easy to understand and that questions were relevant and to gauge the time required to complete the survey. The survey was sent by email to all obstetrics and gynecology residency program directors ($n = 243$). The list of emails was obtained from Association of Professors of Gynecology and Obstetrics (APGO) website. The email survey was also sent to the listserv of the obstetrics and gynecology residency program coordinators, and a request was made to forward the survey to all graduating (PGY4) obstetrics and gynecology residents in their program ($n = 1255$). After sending the initial email, two additional reminders were sent to improve the likelihood of response. The first section of the survey focused on demographics, the location and type of residency, and the number of residents in the program per year. The second section focused on aspects of individual training and surgical volume and personal perspective on robotic utilization in gynecologic surgery.

Survey responses were analyzed using SAS, version 9.4 (SAS Institute, Inc., Cary, NC). Frequencies and percentages of responses were generated overall, by type of respondent (PD, RES) and by type of robotic system (single, dual). Since the main study question sought to determine whether responses varied according to the presence of a single or dual robotic system in the program, Fisher's exact tests (characteristics with 2 groups) or Freeman-Halton tests (characteristics with >2 groups) were used to assess crude associations between each individual/program characteristic and type of robotic system. A p value of <0.05 is considered statistically significant.

3. Results

A total of 84 participants accessed the survey; 13 were missing responses for more than 50% of questions, including the type of robotic system, and were excluded from the analysis. There were 39 PD and 32 RES completed surveys. The response rates were 16% and 2.5% for the PD and RES, respectively. Nearly 94% of RES respondents were female, compared to only 66.7% of PD. The majority of RES were in a university program (71.9%) compared to 53.8% of PD. Nearly half of PD felt comfortable that residents from their program could perform robotic-assisted total laparoscopic hysterectomy (RA-TLH) upon graduation without the need for proctoring, despite their reporting that only 28.2% of their residents performed more than 20 RA-TLH before graduating. Similarly, 53.1% of RES respondents felt comfortable that residents from their program could perform RA-TLH upon graduation without proctoring even though only about 1 in 5 performed more than 20 RA-TLH before graduating. RES and PD shared the same belief that utilization of robotic surgery will increase in gynecologic oncology but probably will either decrease or stay the same in other gynecologic surgery subspecialties, Table 1.

Thirty PD (76.9%) and 23 RES (71.9%) report having a dual console in their hospital. Among PD respondents—although not statistically significant—university programs are more likely to utilize a dual console system than community or university-affiliated community programs ($p = 0.66$). Regardless of the subspecialty, programs with dual console tended to offer more subspecialty fellowships. The programs with dual console system tended to provide a robotic training certificate more frequently, 50% versus 22% ($p = 0.15$), and a bigger proportion of their graduating residents performed more than 20 RA-TLH, 33% versus 11% ($p = 0.39$). The presence of dual console did not significantly change PD perspectives on future utilization of robotics in different subspecialty of gynecologic surgery, Table 2.

According to RES responses, more university programs tend to utilize a dual console system ($p = 0.20$). The presence of dual console did not increase the proportion of the programs that offer subspecialty fellowship training. Surprisingly, 44% of single console programs offer minimally invasive gynecologic surgery fellowship compared to only 34.8 of dual console programs ($p = 0.70$). Dual console system programs were more likely to provide a robotics training certificate compared to single console programs (43.5% versus 0%, $p = 0.03$%). A greater proportion of residents graduating from a dual console program perform more than 20 RA-TLH, 30% versus 0% ($p = 0.15$). The presence of a dual console did not significantly change the RES perceptions of the future utilization of robotics in various gynecologic surgery subspecialties, Table 3.

The dual console is generally underutilized; only 30% of PD and RES report that the dual console is utilized more than 80% of the time in cases with resident involvement, while more than 50% of RES and PD report that the dual console is utilized less than 60% of the time. Moreover, only 10.7% of PD report that the residents operate through the teaching console more than 80% of the time compared to only 8.7% of RES, while about 70% of RES and PD report that the residents operate through the teaching console less than 60% of the time, Figure 1.

4. Discussion

This pilot survey study showed that robotic surgical training was comparable with and without the utilization of the dual console. As far as the graduating residents are concerned, the presence of a dual console system was influential in obtaining a postresidency training certificate. We acknowledge that our survey response rate is low regarding both PD and RES, but since this is the first study to address the perception for differences in robotic surgical training between single and dual console systems, we believe that our findings are thought provoking and stimulate the need for future studies. The da Vinci Surgical System® (Intuitive Surgical Corporations, Sunnyvale, California, USA) was first approved by the Food and Drug Administration for gynecologic surgeries in April 2005, and Intuitive Surgical introduced the da Vinci Si dual

Table 1: Characteristics of residency programs, based on perceptions of residency program directors and of graduating obstetrics and gynecology residents.

Characteristic	Survey participant: Program directors (n = 39)	Survey participant: Residents (n = 32)
Female	26 (66.7)	30 (93.8)
Age		
<35 years	0 (0.0)	31 (96.9)
35–44 years	14 (35.9)	1 (3.1)
45–54 years	15 (38.5)	0 (0.0)
55–64 years	9 (23.1)	0 (0.0)
Residency program type		
University	21 (53.8)	23 (71.9)
University-affiliated community	11 (28.2)	5 (15.6)
Community	6 (15.4)	4 (12.5)
Program has more than 5 residents per year[a]	19 (48.7)	23 (71.9)
Fellowships sponsored	20 (51.3)	22 (68.8)
Gynecologic oncology	9 (23.1)	11 (34.4)
Female pelvic medicine and reconstructive surgery	11 (28.2)	11 (34.4)
Minimally invasive gynecologic surgery	6 (15.4)	12 (37.5)
Reproductive endocrinology and infertility	10 (25.6)	10 (31.3)
Maternal fetal medicine	16 (41.0)	20 (62.5)
Robotic training certificate available	17 (43.6)	10 (31.3)
Graduating resident perform >20 RA-TLH[b]	11 (28.2)	7 (21.9)
Feeling comfortable that residents from program can perform RA-TLH upon graduation without proctoring	19 (48.7)	17 (53.1)
Future utilization of robotic surgery will increase in[c]		
Benign gynecologic surgery	12 (30.8)	9 (28.1)
Reconstructive pelvic surgery	17 (43.6)	17 (53.1)
Gynecologic oncology	26 (66.7)	27 (84.4)
Reproductive surgery	12 (30.8)	13 (40.6)

RA-TLH = robotic-assisted total laparoscopic hysterectomy.
[a]Comparison group consists of programs with 5 or fewer residents per year.
[b]Comparison group consists of programs in which residents perform 20 or fewer RA-TLH.
[c]Comparison group for each category is a response that utilization of robotic surgery will stay the same or decreases.

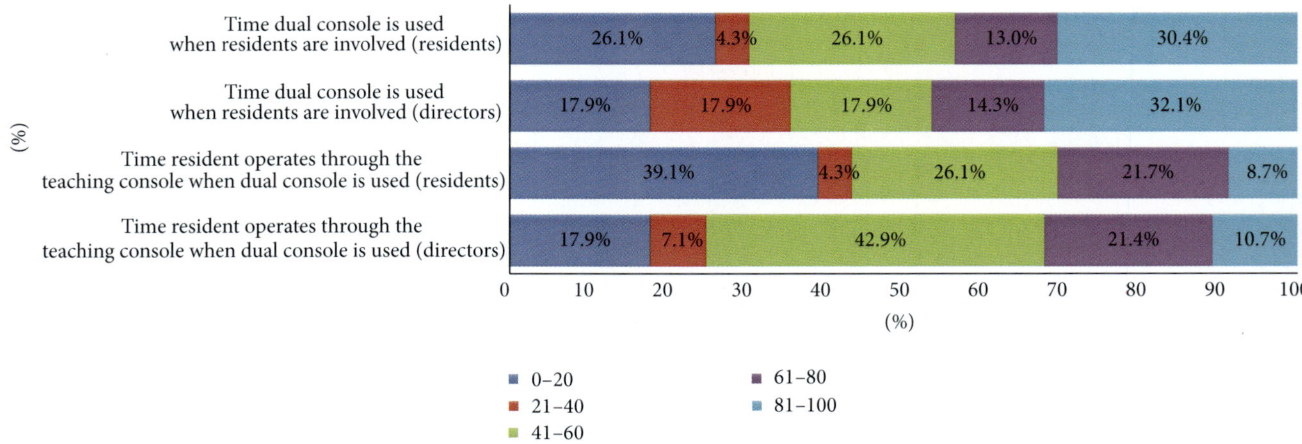

Figure 1: Involvement of residents during robotic operations using the dual console, based on perceptions of graduating obstetrics and gynecology residents and program directors.

TABLE 2: Characteristics of residency programs with single versus dual console robotic systems, based on perceptions of residency program directors.

Characteristic	Does the residency programs have a dual console robotic system?		p value[a]
	Yes ($n = 30$)	No ($n = 9$)	
Female	18 (60.0)	8 (88.9)	0.22
Age			0.26
35–44 years	11 (36.7)	3 (33.3)	
45–54 years	13 (43.3)	2 (22.2)	
55–64 years	5 (16.7)	4 (44.4)	
Residency program type			0.66
University	17 (56.7)	4 (44.4)	
University-affiliated community	8 (26.7)	3 (33.3)	
Community	4 (13.3)	2 (22.2)	
Program has more than 5 residents per year[b]	16 (53.3)	3 (33.3)	0.45
Fellowships sponsored			
Gynecologic oncology	8 (26.7)	1 (11.1)	0.65
Female pelvic medicine and reconstructive surgery	9 (30.0)	2 (22.2)	0.99
Minimally invasive gynecologic surgery	5 (16.7)	1 (11.1)	0.99
Reproductive endocrinology and infertility	9 (30.0)	1 (11.1)	0.40
Maternal fetal medicine	14 (46.7)	2 (22.2)	0.26
Robotic training certificate available	15 (50.0)	2 (22.2)	0.15
Graduating resident perform >20 RA-TLH[c]	10 (33.3)	1 (11.1)	0.39
Feeling comfortable that residents from program can perform RA-TLH upon graduation without proctoring	15 (50.0)	4 (44.4)	0.99
Future utilization of robotic surgery will increase in[d]			
Benign gynecologic surgery	10 (33.3)	2 (22.2)	0.99
Reconstructive pelvic surgery	15 (50.0)	2 (22.2)	0.42
Gynecologic oncology	21 (70.0)	5 (55.6)	0.99
Reproductive surgery	11 (36.7)	1 (11.1)	0.39

RA-TLH = robotic-assisted total laparoscopic hysterectomy.
[a] p value from Fisher's exact test (characteristics with 2 groups) or Freeman-Halton test (characteristics with >2 groups).
[b] Comparison group consists of programs with 5 or fewer residents per year.
[c] Comparison group consists of programs in which residents perform 20 or fewer RA-TLH.
[d] Comparison group for each category is a response that utilization of robotic surgery will stay the same or decreases.

console interface in April 2009, allowing 2 surgeons to sit at 2 different surgical consoles and control the same robot simultaneously [7].

This study is the first to compare residents' and program directors' perception of robotic surgical training with and without the dual console system. It is known that a major hurdle to success in robotic surgery is the associated learning curve, which applies to both the surgeon and the surgical team. Utilization of the dual console system might give a second surgeon the opportunity to gain robotic experience, which in turn may result in earlier proficiency [2]. A study by Crusco et al. concluded that there were no significant differences observed in performance time when teaching knot-tying techniques to novice medical students using the da Vinci dual console compared with the single console [7]. Although the aforementioned study focused on training medical students, its results were similar to the results of this survey. No significant difference was found regarding number of RA-TLH performed or the level of comfort performing RA-TLH without proctoring.

An advantage of dual console is that the trainee's perception of being removed from the procedure almost disappears [8]. The use of the dual console enables integrated teaching, surgical cooperation with proctoring, and supervision, without compromising operative times or patient outcomes [2]. The give or take function refers to each instrument in use, the control of which can be given singularly to the learning surgeon. The swap all function allows the master surgeon to gain full control of all the instruments at 1 time. This console also allows the learning surgeon to operate the robot in a "simplified" fashion, with 2 operating arms, while the proctor surgeon controls the third arm for retraction, exposure, or even pointing [8]. The virtual pointer is another useful tool of the dual console that facilitates surgical training. It enables the operator or proctor to point and refer to specific anatomic features on the live video image intraoperatively. Finally, there

Table 3: Characteristics of residency programs with single versus dual console robotic systems, based on perceptions of graduating obstetrics and gynecology residents.

Characteristic	Does the residency programs have a dual console robotic system? Yes ($n = 23$)	No ($n = 9$)	p value[a]
Female	21 (91.3)	9 (100)	0.99
Age < 35 years	22 (95.7)	9 (100)	0.99
Residency program type			0.20
University	18 (78.3)	5 (55.6)	
University-affiliated community	2 (8.7)	3 (33.3)	
Community	3 (13.0)	1 (11.1)	
Program has more than 5 residents per year[b]	16 (69.6)	7 (77.8)	0.99
Fellowships sponsored			
Gynecologic oncology	8 (34.8)	3 (33.3)	0.99
Female pelvic medicine and reconstructive surgery	8 (34.8)	3 (33.3)	0.99
Minimally invasive gynecologic surgery	8 (34.8)	4 (44.4)	0.70
Reproductive endocrinology and infertility	9 (39.1)	1 (11.1)	0.21
Maternal fetal medicine	15 (65.2)	5 (55.6)	0.70
Robotic training certificate available	10 (43.5)	0 (0)	**0.03**
Graduating resident perform >20 RA-TLH[c]	7 (30.4)	0 (0)	0.15
Feeling comfortable that residents from program can perform RA-TLH upon graduation without proctoring	14 (60.9)	3 (33.3)	0.41
Future utilization of robotic surgery will increase in[d]			
Benign gynecologic surgery	8 (34.8)	1 (11.1)	0.38
Reconstructive pelvic surgery	11 (47.8)	6 (66.7)	0.19
Gynecologic oncology	19 (82.6)	8 (88.9)	0.55
Reproductive surgery	9 (39.1)	4 (44.4)	0.64

RA-TLH = robotic-assisted total laparoscopic hysterectomy.
[a] p value from Fisher's exact test (characteristics with 2 groups) or Freeman-Halton test (characteristics with >2 groups).
[b] Comparison group consists of programs with 5 or fewer residents per year.
[c] Comparison group consists of programs in which residents perform 20 or fewer RA-TLH.
[d] Comparison group for each category is a response that utilization of robotic surgery will stay the same or decreases.

is also the emergency stop button, which can be pressed at any time, should the situation require a sudden cessation of activity [8]. The disadvantages of dual console include the increased cost and requirement of extra manpower, because another assistant surgeon is needed at the patient table to maneuver the instruments via the assistant ports, exchange the robotic instruments, and troubleshoot for glitches related to the robotic platform [8].

In this study, the dual console system is available in about 70% of the OBGYN residency programs that participated in the survey. A study published by Gobern et al. showed that robotic platforms were available at 82% of institutions associated with a residency program. Robotic-assisted gynecologic procedures were performed at 78% of these institutions. Resident training in robotic surgery, however, was part of the training curriculum at only 58% of those residency programs [1]. Despite that, the utilization of the dual console is variable, with 50% of our study participants reporting that the dual console is utilized less than 60% of the time.

The effect of surgical volume on perioperative outcomes and resource utilization is evident. In a study by Wallenstein et al., women treated by high-volume surgeons and at high-volume hospitals have lower morbidity; also surgical volume has a direct effect on lowering resource utilization [9]. In a study by Pitter et al., a significant improvement in operating time was noted after 20 hysterectomy and myomectomy cases were performed [10]. Despite that, defining a cutoff threshold is still difficult [11]. Surgeon volume is increasingly being used as a component in assessment of individual and hospital surgical quality [11]. Meanwhile, organizations including the American Association of Gynecologic Laparoscopists (AAGL) propose that a minimum of 20 cases per year is needed to maintain robotic privileges [12]. In this study, a greater proportion of residents graduating from a dual console program performed more than 20 RA-TLH compared to single console program, but the difference was not statistically significant [30% versus 0% ($p = 0.15$)].

It seems from this study that the availability of a dual console system does not add a significant benefit in the robotic training of the residents except that programs with a dual console tend to award more robotic training certificates to their graduating residents. However, there are some limitations such as recall, response, and research biases, which are inherent to the design of survey studies. Our response rates were 16% and 2.5% for the PD and RES, respectively, despite sending two reminder emails to encourage better response. We acknowledge that this is a major limitation of our study. Additionally, we acknowledge that this study might be underpowered to find statistically significant differences between the single and the dual console groups. Therefore, future studies with more participants and analysis of perioperative outcomes as primary endpoint between the two groups will be needed to definitely determine the utility of dual console robotic system in residency training.

Disclosure

A preliminary version of the data was presented at American Congress of Obstetrics and Gynecology-Annual Clinical Meeting, San Francisco, CA, May 2015.

References

[1] J. M. Gobern, C. M. Novak, and E. G. Lockrow, "Survey of robotic surgery training in obstetrics and gynecology residency," *Journal of Minimally Invasive Gynecology*, vol. 18, no. 6, pp. 755–760, 2011.

[2] A. L. Smith, E. M. Scott, T. C. Krivak, A. B. Olawaiye, T. Chu, and S. D. Richard, "Dual-console robotic surgery: a new teaching paradigm," *Journal of Robotic Surgery*, vol. 7, no. 2, pp. 113–118, 2013.

[3] H. S. Maniar, M. L. Council, S. M. Prasad, S. M. Prasad, C. Chu, and R. J. Damiano Jr., "Comparison of skill training with robotic systems and traditional endoscopy: implications on training and adoption," *The Journal of Surgical Research*, vol. 125, no. 1, pp. 23–29, 2005.

[4] E. J. Hanly, B. E. Miller, R. Kumar et al., "Mentoring console improves collaboration and teaching in surgical robotics," *Journal of Laparoendoscopic & Advanced Surgical Techniques Part A*, vol. 16, no. 5, pp. 445–451, 2006.

[5] P. C. Lim, E. Kang, and D. H. Park, "A comparative detail analysis of the learning curve and surgical outcome for robotic hysterectomy with lymphadenectomy versus laparoscopic hysterectomy with lymphadenectomy in treatment of endometrial cancer: a case-matched controlled study of the first one hundred twenty two patients," *Gynecologic Oncology*, vol. 120, no. 3, pp. 413–418, 2011.

[6] H. Liu, D. Lu, L. Wang, G. Shi, H. Song, and J. Clarke, "Robotic surgery for benign gynaecological disease," *Cochrane Database of Systematic Reviews*, no. 2, Article ID CD008978, 2012.

[7] S. Crusco, T. Jackson, and A. Advincula, "Comparing the da vinci si single console and dual console in teaching novice surgeons suturing techniques," *Journal of the Society of Laparoendoscopic Surgeons*, vol. 18, no. 3, 2014.

[8] E. Fernandes, E. Elli, and P. Giulianotti, "The role of the dual console in robotic surgical training," *Surgery*, vol. 155, no. 1, pp. 1–4, 2014.

[9] M. R. Wallenstein, C. V. Ananth, J. H. Kim et al., "Effect of surgical volume on outcomes for laparoscopic hysterectomy for benign indications," *Obstetrics and Gynecology*, vol. 119, no. 4, pp. 709–716, 2012.

[10] M. C. Pitter, P. Anderson, A. Blissett, and N. Pemberton, "Robotic-assisted gynaecological surgery—establishing training criteria; minimizing operative time and blood loss," *The International Journal of Medical Robotics and Computer Assisted Surgery*, vol. 4, no. 2, pp. 114–120, 2008.

[11] K. M. Doll, M. P. Milad, and D. R. Gossett, "Surgeon volume and outcomes in benign hysterectomy," *Journal of Minimally Invasive Gynecology*, vol. 20, no. 5, pp. 554–561, 2013.

[12] AAGL Advancing Minimally Invasive Gynecology Worldwide, "Guidelines for privileging for robotic-assisted gynecologic laparoscopy," *Journal of Minimally Invasive Gynecology*, vol. 21, no. 2, pp. 157–167, 2014.

26

Endovascular Recanalization for Chronic Symptomatic Intracranial Vertebral Artery Total Occlusion

Ziqi Xu,[1] Ning Ma,[1,2] Dapeng Mo,[1,2] Edward Ho chung Wong,[3] Feng Gao,[1,2] Liqun Jiao,[4] and Zhongrong Miao[1,2,4]

[1] *Department of Neurology, The First Affiliated Hospital of College of Medicine, Zhejiang University, No. 79 QingChun Road, Hangzhou, Zhejiang 310003, China*
[2] *Department of Interventional Neuroradiology, Beijing Tiantan Hospital, Capital Medical University, No. 6 Tiantan Xili, Beijing 100050, China*
[3] *Department of Medicine and Therapeutics, Chinese University of Hong Kong, Hong Kong*
[4] *Department of Neurosurgery, Xuanwu Hospital, Capital Medical University, Beijing, China*

Correspondence should be addressed to Zhongrong Miao; zhongrongm@163.com

Academic Editor: Steve Ramcharitar

Purpose. The outcome of recanalization in patients with chronic symptomatic intracranial vertebral artery (ICVA) total occlusion is poor. This paper reports the technical feasibility and long-term outcome of ICVA stenting in patients with chronic symptomatic total occlusion. *Methods.* Retrospective review of our prospectively maintained intracranial intervention database to identify patients with symptomatic total occlusion of ICVA with revascularization attempted >1 month after index ischemic event. *Results.* Eight patients (mean age 58 years) were identified. One had stroke and 7 had recurrent transient ischemic attacks. Four had bilateral ICVA total occlusion and 4 had unilateral ICVA total occlusion with severe stenosis contralaterally. Seven of 8 patients underwent endovascular recanalization, which was achieved in 6. Periprocedural complications included cerebellum hemorrhage, arterial dissection, perforation, and subacute in-stent thrombosis which occurred in 3 patients. One patient died of cerebellum hemorrhage. The other patients improved clinically after endovascular therapy. *Conclusions.* Stent-supported recanalization of ICVA total occlusion is technically feasible, and may become a viable treatment option in selected patients.

1. Introduction

Intracranial vertebral artery (ICVA) is a common site of atherosclerosis, often involved bilaterally [1, 2]. Patients with bilateral ICVA occlusion usually present with recurrent attacks of dizziness, visual disturbance, and ataxia, and some may be disabled by infarction of regions supplied by the posterior circulation [2]. While limited leptomeningeal collaterals may maintain baseline perfusion for most cases, they usually failed to provide sufficient blood flow during periods of increased oxygen demand, resulting in lifestyle-limiting symptoms. Development of endovascular intervention and improved operator experience have rendered angioplasty and stenting a potential treatment option for these patients but its safety and efficacy remains uncertain [3–5].

The incidence of the chronic ICVA occlusive disease in the Chinese patients may overweigh that of Caucasian patients [6]. To evaluate the feasibility and efficacy of the endovascular therapy for them is urgent. In this paper, we illustrated the feasibility of elective (at least 1 month after ischemic event) endovascular recanalization for symptomatic ICVA total occlusion and their long-term outcome.

2. Methods

2.1. Patient Selection and Data Collection. We retrospectively reviewed our prospectively maintained neurointerventional database from March 2007 to July 2012, to identify patients intended for ICVA recanalization. Inclusion criteria for analysis were (1) index ischemic stroke or transient ischemic attack in the posterior cerebral circulation of at least 1 month before; (2) unilateral ICVA total occlusion together with contralateral ICVA total occlusion, hypoplastic, absence, or

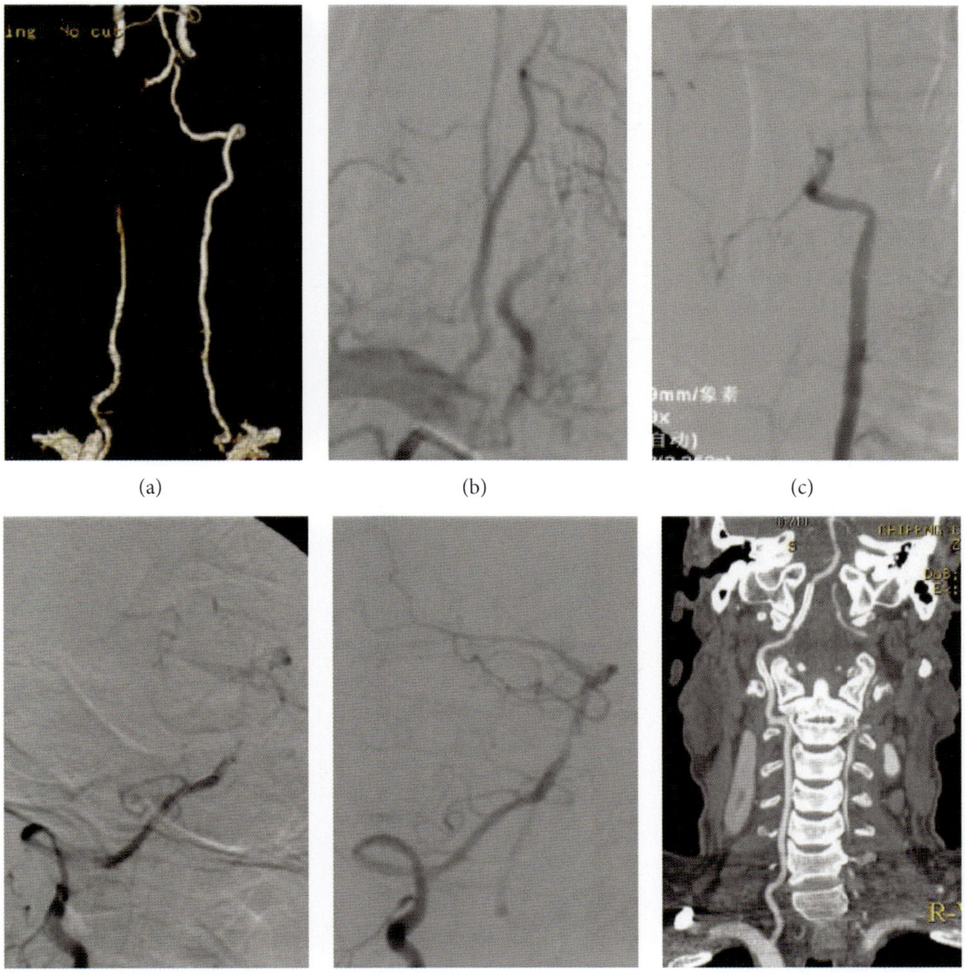

(a) (b) (c)

(d) (e) (f)

FIGURE 1: A 62-year-old man (case 3) with right intracranial vertebral artery (ICVA) total occlusion and tandem occlusion of the V3 by CTA (a) and DSA ((b), (c)). Contralateral severe stenosis of the V4 and tortuosity of the V1 were confirmed by CTA (a). The lesion was predilated with a 2 × 20 mm Invatec balloon and covered with a 3 × 18 mm Apollo stent for the V4 and a 3 × 15 mm Apollo stent for the V3 ((d), (e)). A 24-month CTA follow-up showed patency of the right V3 and V4 without in-stent stenosis (f).

severe stenosis (>70%) verified by computed tomography (CT), magnetic resonance (MR), or conventional angiography; (3) symptoms refractory to double antiplatelets (aspirin 300 mg/day and clopidogrel 75 mg/day) and strict risk factors management.

2.2. Endovascular Recanalization Protocol. Under general anesthesia, the course of the occluded ICVA was traversed and extrapolated with a coaxial assembly of Agility soft microguidewire (Cordis Corp) and Prowler 14 microcatheter (Cordis Corp). The microguidewire was withdrawn and distal patency beyond the occlusion confirmed by angiography through microcatheter. A long Transcend microguidewire (Stryker Neurovascular) was then exchanged. After withdrawing the microcatheter, the lesion was predilated with a balloon catheter and subsequently covered with a balloon-expandable stent or the Wingspan Stent System (Stryker Neurovascular) (Figures 1 and 2). The balloon and stent were sized based on measurement of the proximal ICVA as well as on the length of the occluded segment. Recanalization was defined as good antegrade perfusion of thrombolysis in cerebral ischemia (TICI) grade 3. Heparin anticoagulation therapy was maintained for the duration of the procedure. Blood pressure was tightly controlled postoperatively.

3. Results

Eight male patients (mean age, 58 years; range, 37–72 years) were analyzed in this study (Table 1). Of the 8 patients, 1 had acute stroke and 7 had recurrent transient ischemic attacks. Four had bilateral ICVA total occlusion and 4 unilateral ICVA total occlusion and contralateral severe stenosis. All patients had evidence of previous infarction in the vertebrobasilar distribution on MR imaging. Hyperlipidemia was present in all patients, 5 patients had hypertension, 4 patients had diabetes mellitus, and 5 patients had smoking history.

Seven of 8 patients underwent endovascular recanalization eventually, as procedure was abandoned in one patient

Table 1: Clinical summary of 9 patients undergoing endovascular recanalization of chronic intracranial vertebrobasilar occlusion.

No.	Age, yrs/sex	Symptoms on admission	Time between symptoms and treatment, mo	Image-documented vertebrobasilar occlusion, d	mRS score on admission	Success of recanalization	Occlusion site/balloon mm/stent mm	Periprocedural complication	Concomitant stenosis	Periprocedural complication	mRS Score at discharge	mRS score at latest follow-up	Clinical follow-up, mo	Angiography follow-up, mo	In-stent stenosis
1	52/M	Vertigo	5	8	2	Yes	LV4/ gateway 2 × 9/ Wingspan 3 × 20	None	RV4 total occlusion	None	1	0	63	60	Mild
2	59/M	Dizziness	5	14	2	Yes	LV4/ Invatec 2 × 15/ coroflex theca 3 × 13	None	RV4 total occlusion	None	1	0	47	NA	NA
3	62/M	Dizziness	6	5	1	Yes	RV4/ Invatec 2 × 20/ Apollo 3 × 18	None	RV3 total occlusion*; LV4 severe stenosis	None	0	0	44	10	None
4	61/M	Vertigo and bilateral limb weakness	4	10	2	Yes	RV4/ gateway 3 × 20/ Wingspan 4 × 20; coroflex blue, 3.5 × 13; Wingspan 4.5 × 15	Cerebellum hemorrhage	LV4 total occlusion	Cerebellum hemorrhage	6	NA	NA	NA	NA
5	52/M	Dizziness and bilateral limb weakness	6	21	2	NA	RV4/none/none	NA	LV4 total occlusion	NA	2	NA	NA	NA	NA
6	72/M	Vertigo and bilateral limb weakness	6	40	2	Yes	RV4/ Invatec 2 × 20/ Invatec 3 × 19	None	LV4 severe stenosis†	None	1	0	29	24	Mild
7	71/M	Vertigo and loss of alance	3	27	2	Partial recanalization	LV4/ gateway 2 × 15/ Wingspan 3.5 × 20, Wingspan 3.5 × 20	Dissection and perforation	LV1 moderate stenosis; RC1 moderate stenosis; RV4 severe stenosis; LC1 severe stenosis‡	Dissection; arterial perforation	1	0	1	NA	NA
8	37/M	Blurred vision and vertigo	2	31	1	Yes	LV4/ gateway 2.25 × 15/ Wingspan 3 × 20	Subacute thrombosis	RV4 severe stenosis§	Subacute thrombosis	0	0	1	NA	NA

*RV3 treated with a 3 × 15 mm Apollo stent.
†LV4 treated with a 2.5 × 10 mm Invatec balloon and placement of a 2.5 × 8 mm Apollo stent.
‡LC1 treated with a 5 × 30 mm Viatrac balloon and placement of a 9 × 30 mm precise stent.
§RV4 treated with a 2.5 × 13 mm Apollo stent.

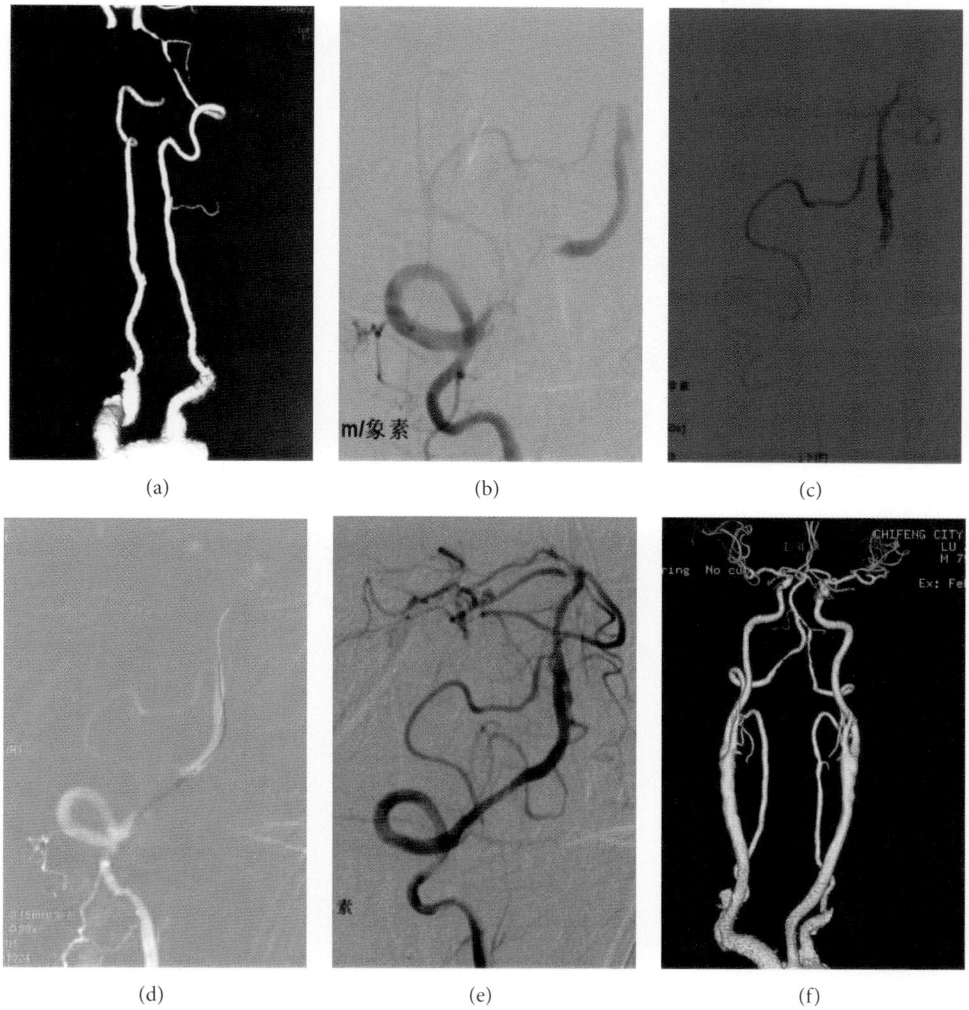

FIGURE 2: A 72-year-old man (case 6) with right intracranial vertebral artery (ICVA) total occlusion and contralateral severe stenosis confirmed by CTA (a) and DSA (b). The distal patency was confirmed by angiography through microcatheter (c). The lesion was predilated with a 2 × 20 mm Invatec balloon (d) and covered with a 3 × 19 mm Invatec balloon-expandable stent (e). A 24-month follow-up CTA showed mild in-stent stenosis (f).

(case 5) after microcatheter angiography showed complete thrombosis in the distal lumen. Recanalization was achieved in 6 of 7 patients, as 1 patient (case 7) developed dissection. Periprocedural complications included cerebellum hemorrhage due to perforation in 1 patient (case 4) (Figures 3(a)–3(c)), asymptomatic distal dissection and proximal perforation adjacent to the occlusion in 1 patient (case 7) (Figures 3(d)–3(f)), and asymptomatic subacute in-stent thrombosis one day after the procedure in another (case 8) (Figures 3(g)–3(i)). One patient (case 4) died from cerebellar hemorrhage. Other patients were stable neurologically or improved after endovascular therapy. In the 6 recanalization patients, the 3 patients with follow-up angiography (Figures 1 and 2), 2 had mild in-stent stenosis (<50%). For the 3 patients without follow-up angiography, the lumen patency was confirmed with CT angiography in 2 patients and with transcranial Doppler in 1 patient.

4. Discussion

While modern diagnostic imaging techniques demonstrate ICVA and its lesions well, treatment options of patients with ICVA disease remain limited [1]. Our series showed that direct stenting without intra-arterial thrombolysis for symptomatic chronic ICVA occlusion is technically feasible. The technical success rate of 86% (6/7) was comparable to previously reported of 89% (8/9) in subacute to chronic basilar occlusion [7]. There are several important technical issues related to this challenging procedure. Firstly, great care must be taken in advancing the microguidewire tip, with gentle rotating movement to ensure its position within the true lumen. Secondly, after traversing the microcatheter through the occlusion, segmental angiograms while withdrawing the microcatheter from the tip of basilar artery to distal end of occlusion are crucial not only to evaluate the length of lesion, but also to look for signs of distal filling defects

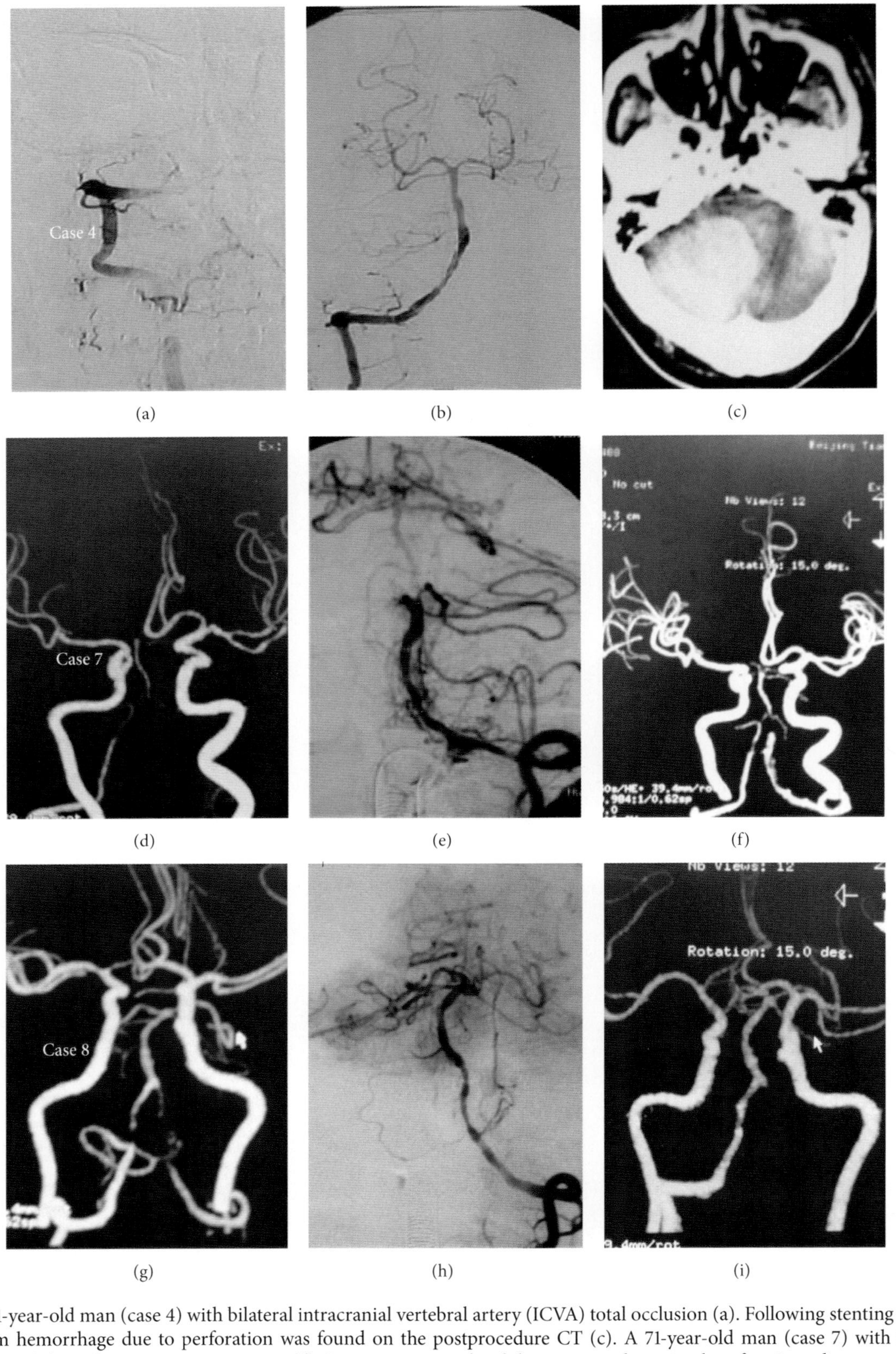

FIGURE 3: A 61-year-old man (case 4) with bilateral intracranial vertebral artery (ICVA) total occlusion (a). Following stenting of right ICVA (b), cerebellum hemorrhage due to perforation was found on the postprocedure CT (c). A 71-year-old man (case 7) with the left ICVA total occlusion and the right ICVA severe stenosis (d). D asymptomatic distal dissection and proximal perforation adjacent to the occlusion occurred during the procedure (e). The perforation resolved after balloon occlusion (f). A 37-year-old man (case 8) with the left ICVA total occlusion and the right ICVA severe stenosis (g). Both ICVA were recanalized but in-stent thrombosis occurred on the left ICVA as shown on day 1 after procedure CTA ((h), (i)).

from thrombus. Thirdly, while the balloon-expandable stent system is more rigid than Wingspan system, it is preferred for patients with suitable smooth access path as delivery of the balloon-expandable stent does not require exchanging.

Periprocedural complications of our series demonstrated the double-edge sword effect of endovascular therapy for chronic ICVA occlusion. Perforation remains a real and devastating possibility, and temporary balloon occlusion may be a solution as used in case 7. Thromboembolism and perforator stroke are other potentially serious complications which did not occur in our series. One patient succumbed from procedural-related cerebellar hemorrhage but none experienced recurrent vertebrobasilar insufficiency symptoms during follow-up, although 2 of 3 patients developed mild in-stent restenosis confirmed with follow-up angiography. For this group of patients, provided periprocedural complications can be avoided, their long-term clinical outcome appeared promising. The small sample and uncontrolled design of this study weaken its relevance so a prospective randomized trial may be warranted to evaluate the safety and efficacy of such therapy in the future.

5. Conclusions

Stent-supported recanalization of chronic total occlusion of ICVA can be a viable option with an acceptable safety profile in selected patients.

Authors' Contribution

Dr. Ziqi Xu, Ning Ma, and Dapeng Mo contributed equally to this work.

References

[1] L. R. Caplan, "The intracranial vertebral artery: a neglected species," *Cerebrovascular Diseases*, vol. 34, no. 1, pp. 20–30, 2012.

[2] H.-K. Shin, K.-M. Yoo, H. M. Chang, and L. R. Caplan, "Bilateral intracranial vertebral artery disease in the New England Medical Center Posterior Circulation Registry," *Archives of Neurology*, vol. 56, no. 11, pp. 1353–1358, 1999.

[3] A. Kansara, P. Pandey, A. Tiwari, M. Rayes, S. Narayanan, and A. R. Xavier, "Stenting of acute and subacute intracranial vertebrobasilar arterial occlusive lesions," *Journal of NeuroInterventional Surgery*, vol. 4, no. 4, pp. 274–280, 2012.

[4] R. Lin, A. Aleu, B. Jankowitz et al., "Endovascular revascularization of chronic symptomatic vertebrobasilar occlusion," *Journal of Neuroimaging*, vol. 22, no. 1, pp. 74–79, 2012.

[5] M. E. Kelly, R. D. Turner, S. I. Moskowitz et al., "Revascularization of symptomatic subacute cerebrovascular occlusions with a self-expanding intracranial stent system," *Neurosurgery*, vol. 64, no. 1, pp. 72–78, 2009.

[6] L. K. S. Wong, "Global burden of intracranial atherosclerosis," *International Journal of Stroke*, vol. 1, no. 3, pp. 158–159, 2006.

[7] S. R. Dashti, M. S. Park, M. F. Stiefel, C. G. McDougall, and F. C. Albuquerque, "Endovascular recanalization of the subacute to chronically occluded basilar artery: initial experience and technical considerations," *Neurosurgery*, vol. 66, no. 4, pp. 825–831, 2010.

27

Minimally Invasive Local Treatments for Bone and Pulmonary Metastases

Meena Bedi,[1] David M. King,[2] and Sean Tutton[3]

[1] *Department of Radiation Oncology, Medical College of Wisconsin, 8701 Watertown Plank Road, Milwaukee, WI 53045, USA*
[2] *Department of Orthopaedic Surgery, Medical College of Wisconsin, 8701 Watertown Plank Road, Milwaukee, WI 53045, USA*
[3] *Department of Interventional Radiology, Medical College of Wisconsin, 8701 Watertown Plank Road, Milwaukee, WI 53045, USA*

Correspondence should be addressed to Meena Bedi; mbedi@mcw.edu

Academic Editor: Peng Hui Wang

Surgery and chemotherapy have historically been the mainstay of treatment in patients with metastatic disease. However there are many alternative therapies available to relieve the symptoms and morbidity of metastases. In this paper, we review the role and highlight the advantages of minimally invasive techniques employed in patients with pulmonary and bone metastases.

1. Background

Multimodality therapy leads to excellent rates of local control in many malignancies. However, it is metastatic disease that usually dictates overall and disease-free survival in cancer patients. The most common sites of metastatic disease include the lung, liver, bone, and brain. Pain is the most common manifestation of osseous metastasis, whereas lung, liver, and brain metastases can lead to organ dysfunction.

Metastasis most commonly arises at the lung bases. Signs and symptoms of metastatic disease to the lung include, but are not limited to, cough, respiratory compromise, hemoptysis, dysphagia, and superior vena cava syndrome. Management is usually conducted with a palliative intent with standard treatment of chemotherapy. Although chemotherapy may lead to considerable response, side effects may be prominent and recurrence is common. Local therapy with surgery can lead to survival rates between 20 and 40% [1]. However, the number and location of metastases, as well as multiple comorbidities, make patients not always amenable to surgical resection.

Bone is the third most common site of metastasis and is a common cause of pain. Each year, it is estimated that over 100,000 patients will develop osseous metastasis, with prostate and breast cancer primaries accounting for 65–75% of these patients [2–4]. Although pain is the most common symptom of osseous metastasis, pathologic fractures secondary to cortical weakening of bone can also lead to increased morbidity with pain and dysfunction [5]. The most common location of pathologic fractures is the femur, followed by the humerus, acetabulum, tibia, and forearm [6].

Chemotherapy for painful bone metastases may be beneficial in widespread disease; however, pain response to this therapy is not well reported in the literature. Although local therapy with surgery repairs pathologic fractures and can lead to reduction of pain, improvement of function and quality of life, this management is typically not used solely for pain control.

Surgical intervention for both pulmonary and bone metastases can lead to complications such as pain, delays in wound healing, and infection. Thus, adjuvant treatment such as chemotherapy may be postponed. Minimally invasive techniques, alternatively, may be used for control of metastatic disease without the propensity for increasing complications.

The purpose of this paper is to describe the use of minimally invasive local therapies of radiation, radiopharmaceuticals, radiofrequency and cryoablation, and cementoplasty in the management of bone and pulmonary metastases.

2. Radiation Therapy

2.1. Local Field Radiation Therapy. Radiation therapy is oftentimes employed to palliate pain and other symptoms in patients with metastatic disease. Partial relief occurs in approximately 50% to 80% and complete pain relief occurs in approximately 30% to 50% of patients [7–10]. Several studies have attempted to determine the effectiveness of various dose and fractionation schemes, however, the optimal dose for pain control is not known.

RTOG 9714 was a phase III, prospective randomized control trial evaluating pain response in patients with 1 to 3 bony metastases in breast or prostate cancer [11]. Patients were randomized to a single fraction of radiation to 8 Gy versus 10 fractions of radiation to 30 Gy. Pain relief was assessed with the Brief Pain Inventory. There was no difference in the partial (50% versus 48%, resp.) and complete response (15% versus 18%, resp.). More patients required retreatment for their metastases in the single fraction arm, 18%, compared to the multi-fraction arm, 9% ($P < 0.001$). However, there was a significantly lower rate of grade-2-to-4 toxicity in the single fraction arm, 10% versus 17% ($P = 0.002$). There was no difference in late toxicities in either arm [11].

Three meta-analyses have also evaluated various fractionation schedules in patients with bony metastases [12–14]. Chow et al. reviewed 16 randomized trials, evaluating 5,000 patients, comparing radiation doses ranging from 8 Gy to 15 Gy delivered in a one fraction to 20 to 30 Gy over 3 to 10 fractions [12]. The primary outcomes examined were complete and overall response. Secondary outcomes assessed the rates of retreatment, pathological fracture, spinal cord compression, and acute toxicity [12].

Although response definitions, followup, and pain assessments varied between each study, there was no significant difference in overall response (58% versus 59%, resp.), complete response (23% versus 24%, resp.), or acute toxicity. However, there was a nonstatistically significant increase in risk of pathologic fractures and spinal cord compression in patients who underwent single fraction radiation compared to multifraction radiation. There was also an increase in the retreatment rate when radiation was delivered as a single fraction, 20%, compared to 8% when delivered over multiple fractions ($P < 0.00001$, 95% CI 1.76–3.56). The findings of comparable response rates, but higher retreatment rates, were also conferred in two other meta-analyses in patients with bony metastases [12–14].

2.2. Stereotactic Body Radiation Therapy. The development of stereotactic body radiotherapy (SBRT) originates from the use of stereotactic radiosurgery (SRS) in the treatment of CNS metastatic tumors, where a single fraction of high dose radiation using multiple beams precisely targets small intracranial tumors while minimizing radiation exposure to surrounding tissues. Due to the success in the treatment of CNS lesions, as well as the advancement in imaging, broader applications of radiosurgery have been developed to treat extracranial sites of disease.

SBRT employs conformal, high dose radiation delivery, over a limited number of fractions, for the treatment of small-to-moderate sized extracranial tumors. Advantages of SBRT include its unique radiobiological characteristics which lead to highly effective treatment of the target volume, while minimizing exposure to the surrounding tissue [15]. This is accomplished through the use of multiple beams, such that a small fraction of the total dose is administered through each beam, thereby effectively minimizing toxicity through the trajectory of the beam [15–18].

Hypofractionated SBRT is an emerging method of treatment for metastatic disease in the lungs (Figures 1(a)–1(c)). Many studies have evaluated outcomes and toxicity in patients who have undergone SBRT for pulmonary oligometastasis from various tumor primaries [15]. Lesions were usually central or peripherally located with crude local control rates between 67 and 100% and 2-year survival ranging between 32 and 87% [16, 19–23]. Toxicity is acceptable with very few developing grade 3 or 4 complications (Table 1).

Ricardi et al. evaluated 61 patients with lung metastasis treated with SBRT. Doses ranged from 26 to 45 Gy in 1 to 4 fractions. With a median followup of 20.4 months, 2-year local control, overall survival, and progression free survival were 89%, 66.5%, and 32.4%, respectively. No patient had grade 4 toxicity, and only 1 patient had grade 3 toxicity [23].

Dhakal et al. assessed 52 patients with pulmonary sarcoma metastases. Fifteen patients were treated to 74 lesions using SBRT and compared to their non-SBRT cohort. The preferred treatment regimen was delivered over 2 weeks to 50 Gy in 5 fractions using conformal arcs or multiple coplanar beams. The 3-year local control in patients managed with SBRT was 82%. The median overall survival in patients treated with SBRT was 2.1 years versus 0.6 years in those who never received SBRT [21].

2.3. Radiopharmaceuticals. Bone-seeking radiopharmaceuticals are designed to selectively deliver radiation in osteoblastic metastases in hopes of improving pain control in those with multifocal disease. The uptake of radiotracers is dependent on calcification of normal tissue and the osteoblastic activity of the tumor. The discrepancy in bone turnover between normal and metastatic sites leads to improved integration of each radionuclide into metastatic bone. Thus targeted and focal radiation therapy can be simultaneously delivered to all sites in patients with widespread metastatic disease [24–28] (Table 2). A summary of the prospective studies done on systemic radionuclides commonly used in clinical practice is located in Table 3 [29–35].

Radionuclides are typically administered in an outpatient setting through intravenous (IV) access. Authorized administers inject the radiopharmaceutical over the course of approximately 1 to 2 minutes followed by a saline flush. After the IV has been removed, patients are provided with instructions for increased fluid intake and urinary excretion. Weekly blood counts are obtained to assess any change secondary to the therapy administered.

Phosphorous-32 (^{32}P) was the first radionuclide to be consistently used in bone metastases and is available in an oral form, which allows for decreased cost and increased convenience. However, this radiotracer has fallen out of favor

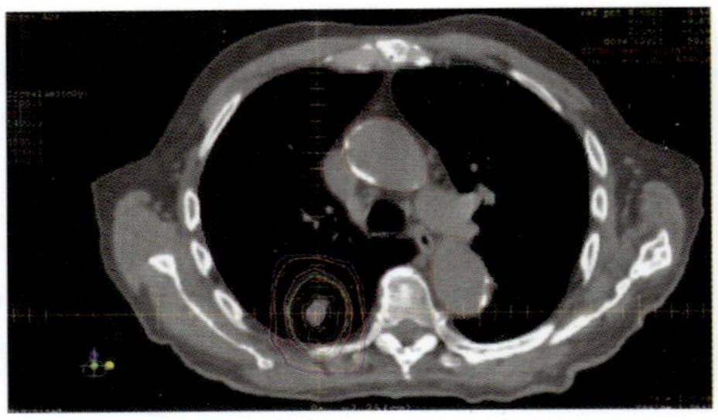

(a) Axial view of isodose distributions for SBRT of a right upper lobe metastasis

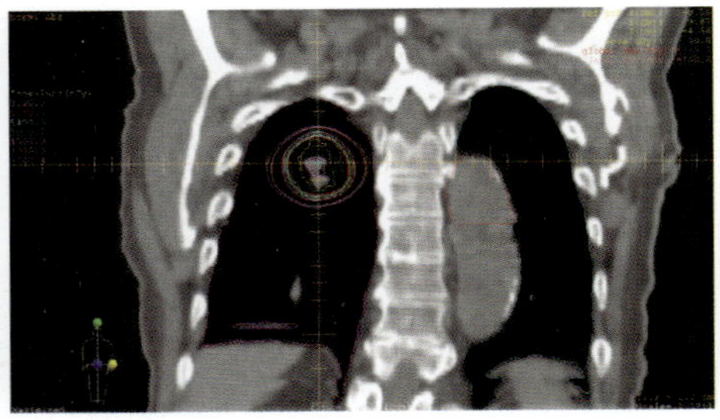

(b) Coronal view of isodose distributions for SBRT of a right upper lobe metastasis

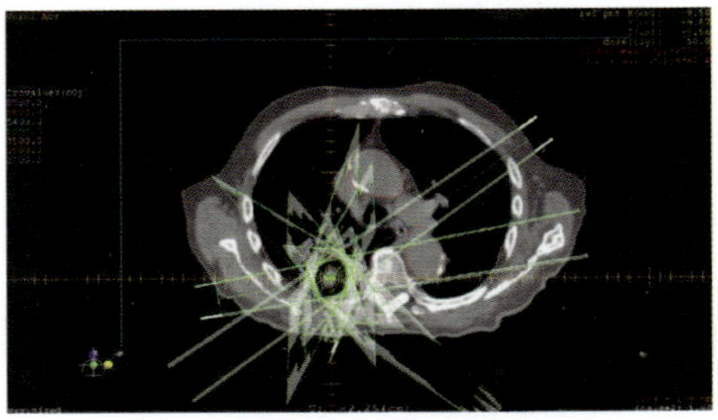

(c) Axial view of beam arrangements for SBRT of a right upper lobe metastasis

FIGURE 1: Axial view (a) and coronal view (b) of isodose distributions and beam arrangements (c) for SBRT of a right upper lobe metastasis.

TABLE 1: Summary of SBRT studies.

Author	Primary tumor	Number of patients	Median followup	Dose (median)	Outcomes	Toxicity
Le et al. [16]	Lung (91%), sarcoma (6%), and HCC (3%)	12	18 mo.	15–25 Gy in 1 fraction	LC at 15–20 Gy: 67% LC at 25 Gy: 56% 1 yr OS: 56%	19% pneumothorax (associated with fiducial placement)
Schefter et al. [19]	Colorectal (23.7%), sarcoma (18.4%), RCC (18.4%), lung (13.2%), and other (26.4%)	38	15.4 mo.	48–60 Gy in 3 fractions	1 yr LC: 100% 2 yr LC: 96% 2 yr OS: 39%	No ≥ G4 toxicity G3 toxicity: 8%
Wulf et al. [20]	Lung (45%), breast (10%), colon (8%), kidney (8%), sarcoma (8%), and other (18%)	25	14 mo.	26 Gy in 1 fraction	LC: 100% 1 yr OS: 68%	No ≥ G3 toxicity
Dhakal et al. [21]	Sarcoma (100%)	52	10.8 mo.	50 Gy in 5 fractions	2 yr LC: 88% 3 yr LC: 82% MS: 2/1 yrs	No ≥ G3 toxicity
Mehta et al. [22]	Sarcoma (100%)	16	20 mo.	54 Gy in 3-4 fractions	43 mo. LC: 94% 4 yr OS: 72%	No ≥ G2 toxicity
Ricardi et al. [23]	Lung (55.7%), colorectal (21.3%), pancreas (3.4%), HCC (3.4%), head and neck (3.4%), sarcoma (1.6%), and other (11.2%)	61	20.4 mo.	26 Gy in 1 fraction	2 yr LC: 89% 3 yr LC: 83.5% 2 yr OS: 66.5% 3 yr OS: 52.5%	G3 toxicity: 1.6%

TABLE 2: Characteristics of bone-seeking radiopharmaceuticals.

Radionuclide	Physical half-life	Energy max (MeV)	Decay	Mean range in tissue (mm)	Carrier
Phosphorous-32 (^{32}P)	14.3 days	1.71	β	7.9	Orthophosphate
Strontium-89 (^{89}P)	50.5 days	1.46	β	6.7	Chloride
Samarium-153 (^{153}Sm)	46.3 hours	0.84	β and γ	3.4	EDTMP
Radium-223 (^{223}Ra)	11.4 days	5.78	α and γ	<0.1	Chloride

TABLE 3: Summary of clinical trials evaluating radiopharmaceuticals.

Radionuclide	Cancer	Trial	Pain response	Survival
Phosphorous-32 (^{32}P)				
Nair [29]	Breast, prostate, lung, and other	^{32}P versus ^{89}Sr	>50% reduction in pain in 93.3% of pts with ^{89}Sr and 87.5% in ^{32}P	Not reported
Strontium-89 (^{89}Sr)				
Smeland et al. [30]	Prostate, breast, and other	RT + ^{89}Sr versus RT + placebo	30% versus 20% (NS)	27 weeks versus 34 weeks (P = 0.6)
Porter and McEwan [31]	Prostate	RT + ^{89}Sr versus RT + placebo	30–60% (complete response)	
Lewington et al. [32]	Prostate	^{89}Sr versus placebo	Statistically significant decrease in pain	
Samarium-153 (^{153}Sm)				
Serafini et al. [33]	Prostate, breast, lung, and other	^{153}Sm versus placebo	72%	Not reported
Collins et al. [34]	Prostate	Phase I/II for ^{153}Sm	76%	
Resche et al. [35]	Prostate, breast, lung, and other	^{153}Sm 0.5 mCi/kg versus ^{153}Sm 1.0 mCi/kg	55% versus 70% at week 4	
Radium-223 (^{223}Ra)				
Parker et al. [39]	Prostate	^{223}Ra versus placebo	Median time to first symptomatic skeletal event: 15.6 mo.	14.9 mo. versus 11.3 mo. (P < 0.001)

due to the high rates of myelotoxicity secondary to its longer range in targeted tissue and high energy decay [24–26, 28].

Strontium-89 (^{89}Sr) is administered as an IV injection and is beta emitter with a half-life of 50.5 days. Because of chemical similarities with calcium, ^{89}Sr is rapidly taken up in bony matrix, especially where active bone formation exists. ^{89}Sr was one of the first radiopharmaceuticals approved for the treatment of widespread bone metastases; thus there is abundant data reporting on outcomes and pain response to this therapy. Overall pain response to ^{89}Sr is approximately 60% to 90%, especially in patients with metastatic breast and prostate cancer [25, 36–38].

^{89}Sr use has been studied alone and in conjunction with radiation and chemotherapy. Porter and McEwan prospectively evaluated 126 patients with hormone refractory prostate cancer that were randomized to radiation therapy followed by a single injection of ^{89}Sr or radiation followed by placebo. Overall response rates were not significantly different in the two arms; however there was a decrease of the requirement for analgesics (2.4% versus 17.1%, $P < 0.05$) in favor of the combined modality group [31].

Samarium-152 ethylenediaminetetramethylenephosphonate (EDTMP) (^{153}Sm-EDTMP) is a bone-seeking radioisotope with a short half-life of 46.3 hours that is slowly administered through IV injection. ^{153}Sm is chelated to EDTMP to allow for delivery in areas of high bone turnover in patients with metastatic disease. Clinical response and experience with ^{153}Sm is somewhat limited, but published reports have indicated pain response rates of approximately 70 to 80% [25, 26, 33–35].

Collins et al. evaluated 20 patients with escalated dose regimens of 1.0, 1.5, 2.0, 2.5, and 3.0 miCi/kg ^{153}Sm EDTMP. The maximum tolerated dose was found to be 2.5 mCi/kg in this patient population. Overall pain relief occurred in 76% of patients within 1 to 2 weeks of administration [34].

Radium-223 (^{223}Ra) is a radiopharmaceutical alpha-emitter with a half-life of 11.4 days that acts as a calcium analogue. ^{223}Ra was recently approved in the use of hormone refractory metastatic prostate cancer [28]. The Alpharadin in Symptomatic Prostate Cancer Patients (ALSYMPCA) trial randomized 921 castrate resistant metastatic prostate cancer patients with 2 or more bone metastases to 6 injections of ^{223}Ra or placebo. The primary endpoint was overall survival. In the updated analysis, median survival for patients who received ^{223}Ra was 14.9 months compared to 11.3 months in the placebo group ($P < 0.001$). Time to increase in the first skeletal event ($P < 0.001$), time to increase in total alkaline phosphatase level ($P < 0.001$), and time to increase in PSA level ($P < 0.001$) were all improved with the use of ^{223}Ra. There was no significant difference in grade-3-to-4 toxicity between the ^{223}Ra and placebo groups [39].

Transient hematologic toxicity is the primary side effect of radiopharmaceuticals, especially thrombocytopenia and neutropenia. Grade-2-to-3 hematologic toxicity is not common and can occur in approximately 25% of patients. In approximately 10 to 20% of cases, a transient flare of bone pain occurs within 1 to 2 days. Less common side effects include loose stools, nausea and vomiting, hematuria, and heart palpitations [24–26].

Although conventional, stereotactic, and systemic radiation therapy may be used in the setting of metastatic disease,

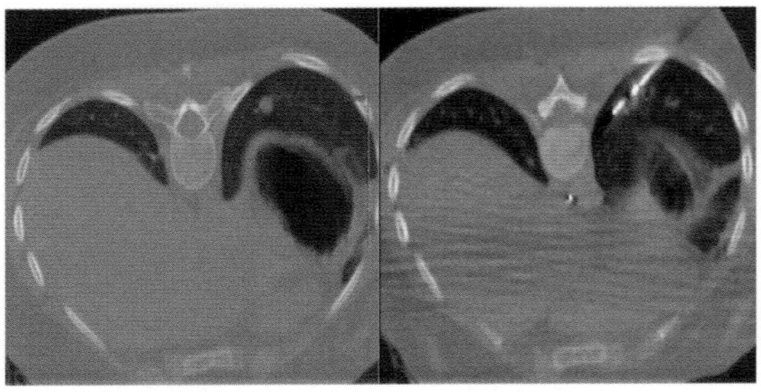

FIGURE 2: Treatment of a left lung sarcoma metastasis with radiofrequency ablation.

various histologies, such as renal cell carcinoma, are relatively radioresistant. As such, other minimally invasive methods may be used to improve local control and palliate symptoms.

3. Interventional Techniques

3.1. Radiofrequency Ablation. The susceptibility of malignant cells to extreme temperatures allows for the use of different techniques to treat metastatic disease. Radiofrequency ablation (RFA) employs temperatures as low as 41°C to cause tumor death [40, 41] and has been historically used in the treatment of unresectable tumors of the lung, liver, and kidney (Figure 2). This technique has been shown to provide excellent rates of local control and survival in patients with metastatic disease (Table 4) [42–46].

RFA is executed with the use of a percutaneously inserted electrode, typically under imaging guidance, which deposits energy in the form of an alternating electrical current to cause focal coagulation necrosis. Heat energy is distributed radially within the target tissue and a margin of normal tissue surrounding the tumor [47].

Yamakado et al. assessed 155 unresectable lung metastases from colorectal cancer in 71 patients treated with RFA. The 3-year overall survival was 46% and intrapulmonary recurrence occurred in 47% of patients in this cohort. Patients who had no extrapulmonary metastases and tumors ≤3 cm had a 3-year survival of 78%. On multivariate analysis, extrapulmonary metastasis ($P < 0.02$, CI 1.3–14.8) and tumor size >3 cm ($P < 0.001$, CI 3.4–52.6) lead to decreased survival. Pneumothorax, typically self-limited or requiring short term small bore chest tube, was the most common complication occurring in 37% of patients [42].

Nakamura et al. retrospectively reviewed 20 patients with 89 pulmonary metastases from sarcomas. The median followup was 18 months, in which the median survival was 12.9 months and the 3-year survival rate was 29%. The only prognostic indicator on univariate and multivariate analyses in this study was the ability to ablate all lung tumors. Patients with complete ablation of all tumors had a 1- and 3-year survival rate of 88.9% and 59.2%, respectively. Pneumothorax again was the most common complication, which occurred in 38% of patients. Thus, the authors concluded that RFA for pulmonary metastases was a safe and beneficial therapeutic option for appropriate candidates [43].

3.2. Cryoablation. Whereas RFA applies heat to treat the targeted tissue, cryoablation exposes tumors to freezing temperatures to treat various malignancies. Cryoablation involves the insertion of dual chamber probe(s) into the target tissue. Typically, high pressure argon gas, which is supplied by a large in-room tank, is passed through the probe. Within a few seconds, there is rapid expansion and cooling, which leads to the production of temperatures of approximately −100°C. This generates a ball of ice up to 3.5 cm in size (Figures 3(a)-3(b)). Cell death is known to occur when temperatures are below −20°C. Multiple probes can be used to allow for the creation of larger balls of ice and, thus, the treatment of larger lesions [48].

Cell death from cryoablation is due to ice formation within the cell through immediate freezing of tissue adjacent to the probe. Gradual cooling away from the probe causes osmotic variation between the cell and membrane, leading to cell dehydration and eventual death [48].

Cryoablation has been utilized in the treatment of liver metastasis, particularly from colorectal primaries. Weaver et al. reviewed 136 patients with unresectable liver metastases from colorectal primaries who underwent 158 cryoablation procedures for tumor control. The median preoperative carcinoembryonic antigen (CEA) level was 14.4 ng/dL. Median survival was 30 months. Recurrent liver disease developed in 78% of patients, with 82% of these recurrences in the liver. Complication rates were comparable to liver resection and operative mortality was 3.7%. This led the authors to conclude that hepatic cryoablation is effective and safe in treating colorectal hepatic metastases under image guidance [49].

Cryoablation has also been used to palliate primary and metastatic bone lesions. Callstrom and colleagues prospectively assessed pain outcomes in 14 patients with osseous metastases from various tumors treated with cryoablation. Posttreatment scores for pain relief, worst pain, pain interference with daily activities, and narcotic medication use decreased with the use of cryoablation [50].

Advantages of cryoablation include the large ablation zone potential using multiple probes and ease of visualizing the "iceball" with CT guidance. Tuncali et al. reported complete and partial relief of pain in 6 of 19 and 11 of 19 patients with bone and soft tissue tumors, respectively, with a mean diameter of 5.2 cm [51].

3.3. Cementoplasty. Cementoplasty refers to the percutaneous injection of polymethylmethacrylate (PMMA) to mechanically stabilize the skeletal system and provide pain relief in patients with osteolytic bony metastases. This stabilization prevents further collapse and relieves pain by mitigating stress on each vertebral body treated. Cementoplasty includes procedures such as vertebroplasty, kyphoplasty, sacroplasty, and osteoplasty, and is typically performed by trained interventional radiologists and surgeons [48].

The process of cementoplasty may be performed under general anesthesia or local anesthesia with conscious sedation

TABLE 4: Summary of RFA studies in metastatic disease.

Author	Primary tumor	Number of patients	Median followup	Outcomes	Most common toxicity
Yamakado et al. [42]	Colorectal	71	19 (mean)	3 yr OS: 46% Intrapulmonary recurrence: 47%	Pneumothorax (47%)
Nakamura et al. [43]	Sarcoma	20	18 mo.	1 yr OS: 88% 3 yr OS: 29% Incomplete ablation: 45%	Pneumothorax (65%)
Palussière et al. [44]	Sarcoma	29	50 mo.	1 yr OS: 92.2% 2 yr OS: 65.2% Incomplete ablation: 10%	Pneumothorax (67.8%)
Yan et al. [45]	Colorectal	55	24 mo.	1 yr OS: 85% 2 yr OS: 64% PFS: 15 mo.	Pneumothorax (29%)
King et al. [46]	Colorectal	19	24.3 mo.	1 yr LC: 90%	Pneumothorax (52%)

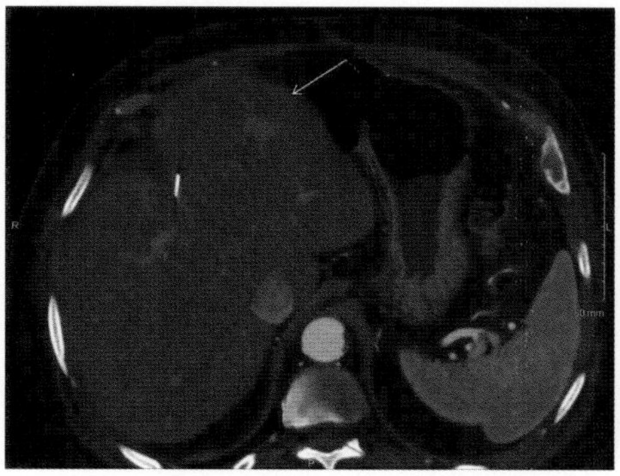

(a) Recurrent hepatocellular carcinoma after right lobe resection

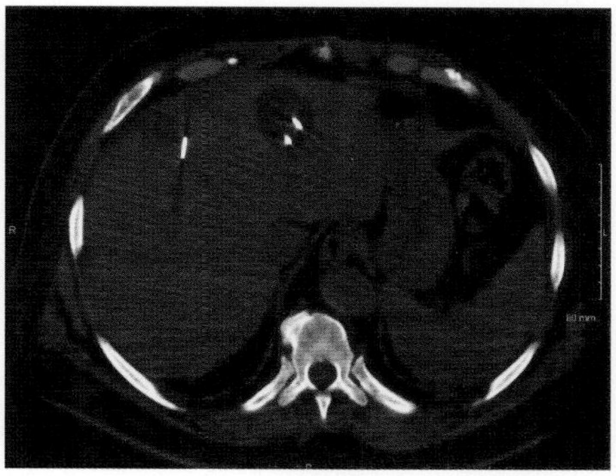

(b) CT-guided probe placement with ablation zone "iceball"

FIGURE 3: Recurrent hepatocellular carcinoma after right lobe resection (a) and ablation zone (b).

or occasionally general anesthesia. A small incision is made, and, under image guidance with fluoroscopy, CT, or less commonly MRI, a trocar or needle is passed into the affected bone. Several commercially available cement preparations of PMMA, such as barium sulfate or tantalum, are mixed with materials to enhance radio-opacity, thereby allowing for better visualization and safer delivery with fluoroscopy. Evaluation of cement filling and potential leakage is also done through real-time imaging with fluoroscopy or CT-fluoroscopy (Figures 4(a)-4(b)). Adverse effects of the procedure itself include, but are not limited to, transient radicular pain, bleeding, infection, recurrent or adjacent level fracture, and rarely symptomatic pulmonary embolus [48]. Despite these risks, clinically significant complications remain very low in the literature.

Cementoplasty has been proven to be effective in pain relief in published reports [52–54]. Kelekis and colleagues reviewed 14 inoperable patients with painful bony metastases refractory to pain medications and radiation therapy. In this study, 23 lesions were treated with percutaneous cementoplasty using PMMA cement mixed with barium powder. All 14 patients had successful stabilization with cementoplasty and symptomatic pain relief was achieved within 24 hours after procedure in 13 of the 14 patients. Moreover, mobility after procedure was improved in 13 of the 14 cases by 1 week [52]. Many other studies have evaluated the success of cementoplasty alone or in combination with other interventional procedures (Table 5).

Hoffmann et al. reviewed 22 patients with 28 metastatic lesions in the spine, pelvis, and lower extremities treated with RA followed by cementoplasty. Pain relief occurred in all patients within 24 hours and after 3 months of the performed procedure. Moreover, the amount of pain medications used was also reduced in 15 of the 22 patients. The complication rates were also low [54].

4. Conclusion

Surgery and chemotherapy have long been the mainstay of treatment in metastatic disease. However, due to medical comorbidities, intolerance of systemic drug therapy, patient preference, and progression of disease, minimally invasive methods may be utilized in these scenarios. These techniques are becoming more applicable for the treatment of patients with metastatic disease and give the option of less invasive surgical approaches for palliation and local control. With the advancement of research and technology, new and innovative

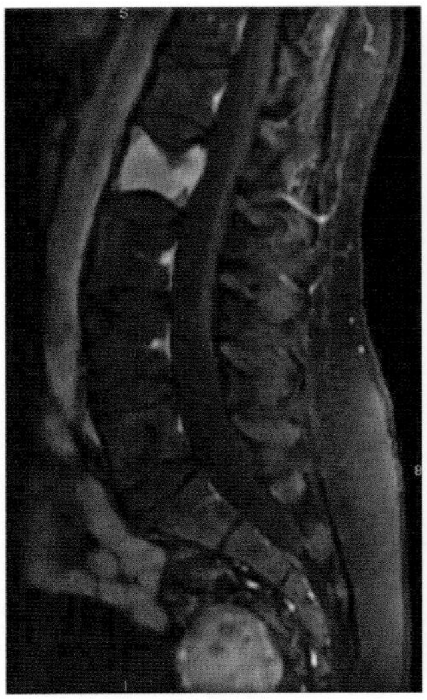

(a) Plasmacytoma of L2 on fat saturated post contrast T1 imaging

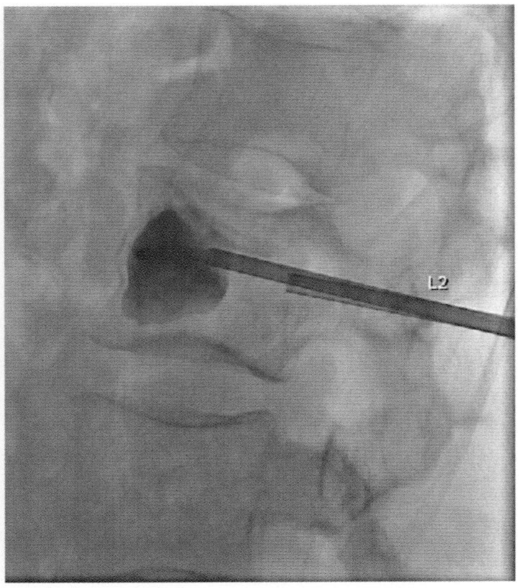

(b) Fluoroscopic guided vertebroplasty

FIGURE 4: Plasmacytoma of L2 (a) treated with vertebroplasty (b).

TABLE 5: Summary of cementoplasty studies in metastatic disease.

Author	*N*	Followup	Combination RFA	Location	Effective pain relief	Complication rate
Kelekis et al. [52]	14	9 mo. (mean)	No	Pubic rami and ischial tuberosities	92%	14.3%
Hierholzer et al. [53]	5	NR	No	Pelvis and femur	100%	0%
Hoffmann et al. [54]	25	7.7 (mean)	Yes	Spine, sacrum, acetabulum, and lower extremity	100%	0%

minimally invasive procedures are continually being developed and will benefit increasing numbers of patients with metastatic disease.

References

[1] U. Pastorino, M. Buyse, G. Friedel et al., "Long-term results of lung metastasectomy: prognostic analyses based on 5206 cases," *Journal of Thoracic and Cardiovascular Surgery*, vol. 113, no. 1, pp. 37–49, 1997.

[2] V. Ratanatharathorn, W. E. Powers, W. T. Moss, and C. A. Perez, "Bone metastasis: review and critical analysis of random allocation trials of local field treatment," *International Journal of Radiation Oncology. Biology. Physics*, vol. 44, no. 1, pp. 1–18, 1999.

[3] H. S. Smith, "Painful Osseous Metastases," *Pain Physician*, vol. 14, no. 4, pp. E373–E405, 2011.

[4] O. S. Nielsen, A. J. Munro, and I. F. Tannock, "Bone metastases: pathophysiology and management policy," *Journal of Clinical Oncology*, vol. 9, no. 3, pp. 509–524, 1991.

[5] M. Fidler, "Incidence of fracture through metastases in long bones," *Acta Orthopaedica Scandinavica*, vol. 52, no. 6, pp. 623–627, 1981.

[6] H. Mirels, "Metastatic disease in long bones: a proposed scoring system for diagnosing impending pathologic fractures," *Clinical Orthopaedics and Related Research*, vol. 249, pp. 256–264, 1989.

[7] D. Tong, L. Gillick, and F. R. Hendrickson, "The palliation of symptomatic osseous metastases. Final results of the study by the Radiation Therapy Oncology Group," *Cancer*, vol. 50, no. 5, pp. 893–899, 1982.

[8] P. Price, P. J. Hoskin, and D. Easton, "Prospective randomised trial of single and multifraction radiotherapy schedules in the treatment of painful bony metastases," *Radiotherapy and Oncology*, vol. 6, no. 4, pp. 247–255, 1986.

[9] M. Niewald, H.-J. Tkocz, U. Abel et al., "Rapid course radiation therapy vs. more standard treatment: a randomized trial for bone metastases," *International Journal of Radiation Oncology. Biology. Physics*, vol. 36, no. 5, pp. 1085–1089, 1996.

[10] D. E. Roos, S. L. Turner, P. C. O'Brien et al., "Randomized trial of 8 Gy in 1 versus 20 Gy in 5 fractions of radiotherapy for neuropathic pain due to bone metastases (Trans-Tasman Radiation Oncology Group, TROG 96.05)," *Radiotherapy and Oncology*, vol. 75, no. 1, pp. 54–63, 2005.

[11] W. F. Harstell, C. B. Scott, D. W. Bruner et al., "Randomized trial of short- versus long-course radiotherapy for palliation of painful bone metastases," *Journal of the National Cancer Institute*, vol. 97, no. 11, pp. 798–804, 2005.

[12] E. Chow, K. Harris, G. Fan, M. Tsao, and W. M. Sze, "Palliative radiotherapy trials for bone metastases: a systematic review," *Journal of Clinical Oncology*, vol. 25, no. 11, pp. 1423–1436, 2007.

[13] M. S. Wai, S. Mike, H. Ines, and M. Malcolm, "Palliation of metastatic bone pain: single fraction versus multifraction radiotherapy—a systematic review of the randomised trials," *Cochrane Database of Systematic Reviews*, no. 2, Article ID CD004721, 2004.

[14] J. S.-Y. Wu, R. Wong, M. Johnston, A. Bezjak, and T. Whelan, "Meta-analysis of dose-fractionation radiotherapy trials for the palliation of painful bone metastases," *International Journal of Radiation Oncology. Biology. Physics*, vol. 55, no. 3, pp. 594–605, 2003.

[15] S. Siva, M. MacManus, and D. Ball, "Stereotactic radiotherapy for pulmonary oligometastases: a systematic review," *Journal of Thoracic Oncology*, vol. 5, no. 7, pp. 1091–1099, 2010.

[16] Q.-T. Le, B. W. Loo, A. Ho et al., "Results of a phase I dose-escalation study using single-fraction stereotactic radiotherapy for lung tumors," *Journal of Thoracic Oncology*, vol. 1, no. 8, pp. 802–809, 2006.

[17] L. Leksell, "The stereotaxic method and radiosurgery of the brain," *Acta chirurgica Scandinavica*, vol. 102, no. 4, pp. 316–319, 1951.

[18] I. Lax, H. Blomgren, I. Naslund, and R. Svanstrom, "Stereotactic radiotherapy of malignancies in the abdomen. Methodological aspects," *Acta Oncologica*, vol. 33, no. 6, pp. 677–683, 1994.

[19] T. E. Schefter, K. E. Rusthoven, B. D. Kavanagh et al., "Multi-institutional phase I/II trial of stereotactic body radiation therapy for lung metastases," *Journal of Clinical Oncology*, vol. 27, no. 10, pp. 1579–1584, 2009.

[20] J. Wulf, K. Baier, G. Mueller, and M. P. Flentje, "Dose-response in stereotactic irradiation of lung tumors," *Radiotherapy and Oncology*, vol. 77, no. 1, pp. 83–87, 2005.

[21] S. Dhakal, K. S. Corbin, M. T. Milano et al., "Stereotactic body radiotherapy for pulmonary metastases from soft-tissue sarcomas: excellent local lesion control and improved patient survival," *International Journal of Radiation Oncology. Biology. Physics*, vol. 82, no. 2, pp. 940–945, 2012.

[22] N. Mehta, M. Selch, P. C. Wang et al., "Safety and efficacy of stereotactic body radiation therapy in the treatment of pulmonary metastases from high grade sarcoma," *Sarcoma*, vol. 2013, Article ID 360214, 6 pages, 2013.

[23] U. Ricardi, A. R. Filippi, A. Guarneri et al., "Stereotactic body radiation therapy for lung metastases," *Lung Cancer*, vol. 75, no. 1, pp. 77–81, 2012.

[24] D. J. Hillegonds, S. Franklin, D. K. Shelton, S. Vijayakumar, and V. Vijayakumar, "The management of painful bone metastases with an emphasis on radionuclide therapy," *Journal of the National Medical Association*, vol. 99, no. 7, pp. 785–794, 2007.

[25] M. Tomblyn, "The role of bone-seeking radionuclides in the palliative treatment of patients with painful osteoblastic skeletal metastases," *Cancer Control*, vol. 19, no. 2, pp. 137–144, 2012.

[26] G. Bauman, M. Charette, R. Reid, and J. Sathya, "Radiopharmaceuticals for the palliation of painful bone metastases—a systematic review," *Radiotherapy and Oncology*, vol. 75, no. 3, pp. 258.E1–258.E13, 2005.

[27] M. Fischer and W. U. Kampen, "Radionuclide therapy of bone metastases," *Breast Care*, vol. 7, no. 2, pp. 100–107, 2012.

[28] D. Brady, C. C. Parker, and J. M. O'Sullivan, "Bone-targeting radiopharmaceuticals including radium-223," *Cancer Journal*, vol. 19, no. 1, pp. 71–78, 2013.

[29] N. Nair, "Relative efficacy of 32P and 89Sr in palliation in skeletal metastases," *Journal of Nuclear Medicine*, vol. 40, no. 2, pp. 256–261, 1999.

[30] S. Smeland, B. Erikstein, M. Aas, E. Skovlund, S. L. Hess, and S. D. Fosså, "Role of strontium-89 as adjuvant to palliative external beam radiotherapy is questionable: results of a double-blind randomized study," *International Journal of Radiation Oncology. Biology. Physics*, vol. 56, no. 5, pp. 1397–1404, 2003.

[31] A. T. Porter and A. J. B. McEwan, "Strontium-89 as an adjuvant to external beam radiation improves pain relief and delays disease progression in advanced prostate cancer: results of a randomized controlled trial," *Seminars in Oncology*, vol. 20, no. 3, pp. 38–43, 1993.

[32] V. J. Lewington, A. J. McEwan, D. M. Ackery et al., "A prospective, randomised double-blind crossover study to examine the efficacy of strontium-89 in pain palliation in patients with advanced prostate cancer metastatic to bone," *European Journal of Cancer*, vol. 27, no. 8, pp. 954–958, 1991.

[33] A. N. Serafini, S. J. Houston, I. Resche et al., "Palliation of pain associated with metastatic bone cancer using samarium-153 lexidronam: a double-blind placebo-controlled clinical trial," *Journal of Clinical Oncology*, vol. 16, no. 4, pp. 1574–1581, 1998.

[34] C. Collins, J. F. Eary, G. Donaldson et al., "Samarium-153-EDTMP in bone metastases of hormone refractory prostate carcinoma: a phase I/II trial," *Journal of Nuclear Medicine*, vol. 34, no. 11, pp. 1839–1844, 1993.

[35] I. Resche, J.-F. Chatal, A. Pecking et al., "A dose-controlled study of 153Sm-ethylenediaminetetramethylenephosphonate (EDTMP) in the treatment of patients with painful bone metastases," *European Journal of Cancer*, vol. 33, no. 10, pp. 1583–1591, 1997.

[36] E. Ashayeri, A. Omogbehin, R. Sridhar, and R. A. Shankar, "Strontium 89 in the treatment of pain due to diffuse osseous metastases: a university hospital experience," *Journal of the National Medical Association*, vol. 94, no. 8, pp. 706–711, 2002.

[37] D. Fuster, R. Herranz, S. Vidal-Sicart et al., "Usefulness of strontium-89 for bone pain palliation in metastatic breast cancer patients," *Nuclear Medicine Communications*, vol. 21, no. 7, pp. 623–626, 2000.

[38] F. Kraeber-Bodere, L. Campion, C. Rousseau, S. Bourdin, J.-F. Chatal, and I. Resche, "Treatment of bone metastases of prostate cancer with strontium-89 chloride: efficacy in relation to the degree of bone involvement," *European Journal of Nuclear Medicine*, vol. 27, no. 10, pp. 1487–1493, 2000.

[39] C. Parker, S. Nilsson, D. Heinrich et al., "Alpha emitter radium-223 and survival in metastatic prostate cancer," *New England Journal of Medicine*, vol. 369, no. 3, pp. 213–223, 2013.

[40] C. J. Simon and D. E. Dupuy, "Percutaneous minimally invasive therapies in the treatment of bone tumors: thermal ablation," *Seminars in Musculoskeletal Radiology*, vol. 10, no. 2, pp. 137–144, 2006.

[41] D. E. Dupuy, W. W. Mayo-Smith, G. F. Abbott, and T. DiPetrillo, "Clinical applications of radio-frequency tumor ablation in the thorax," *Radiographics*, vol. 22, pp. s259–s269, 2002.

[42] K. Yamakado, S. Hase, T. Matsuoka et al., "Radiofrequency ablation for the treatment of unresectable lung metastases in patients with colorectal cancer: a multicenter study in Japan," *Journal of Vascular and Interventional Radiology*, vol. 18, no. 3, pp. 393–398, 2007.

[43] T. Nakamura, A. Matsumine, K. Yamakado et al., "Lung radiofrequency ablation in patients with pulmonary metastases from

musculoskeletal sarcomas," *Cancer*, vol. 115, no. 16, pp. 3774–3781, 2009.

[44] J. Palussière, A. Italiano, E. Descat et al., "Sarcoma lung metastases treated with percutaneous radiofrequency ablation: results from 29 patients," *Annals of Surgical Oncology*, vol. 18, no. 13, pp. 3771–3772, 2011.

[45] T. D. Yan, J. King, A. Sjarif, D. Glenn, K. Steinke, and D. L. Morris, "Percutaneous radiofrequency ablation of pulmonary metastases from colorectal carcinoma: prognostic determinants for survival," *Annals of Surgical Oncology*, vol. 13, no. 11, pp. 1529–1537, 2006.

[46] J. King, D. Glenn, W. Clark et al., "Percutaneous radiofrequency ablation of pulmonary metastases in patients with colorectal cancer," *British Journal of Surgery*, vol. 91, no. 2, pp. 217–223, 2004.

[47] S. C. Rose, "Radiofrequency ablation of pulmonary malignancies," *Seminars in Respiratory and Critical Care Medicine*, vol. 29, no. 4, pp. 361–383, 2008.

[48] J. S. Biermann, G. E. Holt, V. O. Lewis, H. S. Schwartz, and M. J. Yaszemski, "Metastatic bone disease: diagnosis, evaluation, and treatment," *Journal of Bone and Joint Surgery A*, vol. 91, no. 6, pp. 1518–1530, 2009.

[49] M. L. Weaver, J. G. Ashton, and R. Zemel, "Treatment of colorectal liver metastases by cryotherapy," *Seminars in Surgical Oncology*, vol. 14, no. 2, pp. 163–170, 1998.

[50] M. R. Callstrom, J. W. Charboneau, M. P. Goetz et al., "Image-guided ablation of painful metastatic bone tumors: a new and effective approach to a difficult problem," *Skeletal Radiology*, vol. 35, no. 1, pp. 1–15, 2006.

[51] K. Tuncali, P. R. Morrison, C. S. Winalski et al., "MRI-guided percutaneous cryotherapy for soft-tissue and bone metastases: initial experience," *American Journal of Roentgenology*, vol. 189, no. 1, pp. 232–239, 2007.

[52] A. Kelekis, K. O. Lovblad, A. Mehdizade et al., "Pelvic osteoplasty in osteolytic metastases: technical approach under fluoroscopic guidance and early clinical results," *Journal of Vascular and Interventional Radiology*, vol. 16, no. 1, pp. 81–88, 2005.

[53] J. Hierholzer, G. Anselmetti, H. Fuchs, C. Depriester, K. Koch, and D. Pappert, "Percutaneous osteoplasty as a treatment for painful malignant bone lesions of the pelvis and femur," *Journal of Vascular and Interventional Radiology*, vol. 14, no. 6, pp. 773–777, 2003.

[54] R. T. Hoffmann, T. F. Jakobs, C. Trumm, C. Weber, T. K. Helmberger, and M. F. Reiser, "Radiofrequency ablation in combination with osteoplasty in the treatment of painful metastatic bone disease," *Journal of Vascular and Interventional Radiology*, vol. 19, no. 3, pp. 419–425, 2008.

28

Spinal Biologics in Minimally Invasive Lumbar Surgery

Kevin Y. Chang and Wellington K. Hsu

Department of Orthopedic Surgery, Northwestern University Feinberg School of Medicine, 676 N. Saint Clair St., Suite #1350, Chicago, IL 60611, USA

Correspondence should be addressed to Wellington K. Hsu; wkhsu@yahoo.com

Academic Editor: Brian J. Dlouhy

As the use of minimally invasive spine (MIS) fusion approaches continues to grow, increased scrutiny is being placed on its outcomes and efficacies against traditional open fusion surgeries. While there are many factors that contribute to the success of achieving spinal arthrodesis, selecting the optimal fusion biologic remains a top priority. With an ever-expanding market of bone graft substitutes, it is important to evaluate each of their use as it pertains to MIS techniques. This review will summarize the important characteristics and properties of various spinal biologics used in minimally invasive lumbar surgeries and compare their fusion rates via a systematic review of published literature.

1. Introduction

Since Obenchain reported the first use of laparoscopic approach to lumbar spine discectomy in 1991, minimally invasive spine (MIS) surgery has evolved substantially over the years with the advances in robotics, imaging navigation systems, and endoscopy [1, 2]. Now more than ever, minimally invasive techniques are being applied in the treatment of a wide range of spine pathologies. With over 400,000 cases performed in the United States annually, spine fusion has become one of the most commonly performed and well-established treatment options for degenerative disorders, spine trauma, tumors, and structural deformities [3, 4].

When considering MIS fusion techniques, it is important to note that the biologic environment may differ not only from that of traditional open fusion surgeries but also among the different approaches. For example, in minimally invasive transforaminal interbody fusion (MIS-TLIF), there is limited access to the disc space for the complete removal of the disc due to surrounding neural structures [5]. On the other hand, for anterior and lateral approaches to interbody fusion such as oblique lateral interbody fusion (OLIF), extreme lateral interbody fusion (XLIF), and lateral lumbar interbody fusion (LLIF), the larger tubular access sits right on the disc space allowing for a more complete removal of the disc. This translates to an environment that is inherently more advantageous for fusion comparing to MIS-TLIF because of the greater surface area, enabling the placement of a bigger cage and more graft materials [5–9]. Nonetheless, selecting the ideal type of bone graft material for each approach is important to optimize efficacy and safety. This review will discuss and summarize the different types of fusion biologics used in minimally invasive lumbar fusions, their characteristics, properties, and efficacies.

2. Biology of Bone Regeneration, Repair, and Fusion

With a wide variety of fusion biologics available on the market, it is important to understand the basic characteristics of bone grafts in order to select the most appropriate graft material and maximize arthrodesis. The three fundamental properties of bone regeneration are osteogenesis, osteoinduction, and osteoconduction. Osteogenesis is defined as the formation of bone, and the "osteogenic" potential of a graft is its ability to provide appropriate cellular environment where the osteoprogenitor cells could survive transplantation and proliferate and differentiate into osteoblasts and osteocytes [10]. Osteoinductive properties of a graft refer to its ability to recruit immature cells and induce their proliferation and differentiation into bone-forming cells [11]. Lastly, osteoconduction describes the physical property of a graft material that allows bone cells such as osteoblasts and osteoclasts to attach, migrate, and grow in order to form viable bone [11, 12]. It is the interplay between all three of these properties of orthobiologics that leads to bone formation and regeneration.

Similarly, incorporation of bone grafts in spine fusion is highly dependent on these same principles. This process relies on many factors both systemically and locally between the graft and the host bed. Based on our current understanding, this process occurs in three distinct stages: (1) the inflammatory stage, (2) the repair stage, and (3) the late remodeling stage [12]. During the inflammatory stage (initial hours to days), osteoinduction drives chemotaxis and differentiation of host osteoprogenitor cells [78]. Inflammatory cells and fibroblasts are recruited through prostaglandin mediation into the graft where granulation and vascular tissues are formed. Osteoblasts also begin to form. The repair stage (weeks to months) is dominated by fibroblasts leading to the formation of a stroma supporting vascular ingrowth, as well as the deposition of a collagen matrix where osteoids are secreted and mineralization occurs [12]. This vascular growth also provides osteoclasts that could resorb the surfaces of the graft. Finally, the remodeling stage (months to years) is characterized by the restoration of the bone to its original structure and strength through mechanical stress placed on the bone over time [12]. During this time, the osteoconductive properties of the bone graft leads to the resorption and replacement of the graft tissue with new bone in a process called "creeping substitution" [78].

3. Method for Review of the Literature

MEDLINE was used to search for publications in English from 2005 through November 2017 with the keyword "minimally invasive" and combinations of the following: "posterior lumbar interbody fusion," "transforaminal lumbar interbody fusion," "anterior lumbar interbody fusion," "extreme lateral interbody fusion," "oblique lateral interbody fusion," "direct lateral lumbar interobdy fusion," and "lateral lumbar interbody fusion" (Figure 1). While this search yielded a total of 710 papers, additional articles were hand-retrieved from respective bibliographies. Inclusion criteria used were as follows: (1) clinical studies and case series with a minimum of 10 patients (2) adult patients with a minimum age of 18 years old, (3) studies explicitly stating the type of graft material used for fusion, and (4) studies reporting fusion rates by computed tomography (CT) or plain radiograph evaluation. For studies utilizing more than one type of bone graft, patients may be categorized into more than one group. A total of 66 studies met the inclusion criteria, and patients from each study were grouped based on the bone graft used (Table 3).

4. Bone Graft Materials

4.1. Autologous Graft: Iliac Crest Bone Graft and Local Bone Graft. An autologous bone graft is defined as bone harvested from one part of the body and transplanted to a different site in the same individual. Two of the most common sites where autologous bone grafts are derived from are the iliac crest or local spinous processes, lamina or facets. Iliac crest bone graft (ICBG) has historically been considered as the gold standard for spinal fusion due to its osteogenic, osteoinductive, and osteoconductive properties as well as its biocompatibility and mechanically stability [79, 80]. Furthermore, it also possesses minimal antigenic factors and no risk of disease transmission, eliminating risk of rejection [12]. However, this procedure has become less popular among spine surgeons in recent years due to the need for an additional surgical site, increased surgical time and blood loss, limited quantity, postoperative pain, and donor site complications [12, 79, 81]. These rates have been reported between 9 and 49% in the literature and ranged from minor superficial infections and seromas to major neurovascular injuries, deep infections, or herniation of abdominal contents through the harvest site [81, 82]. Of the six studies that met our inclusion criteria and utilized ICBG in MIS fusion procedures, two of them reported donor site complications. Ohtori et al. reported donor site pain at the location of the iliac crest in eight out of twelve patients [41]. In the prospective study by Peng et al., there were two cases (out of 29) of ICBG site infections that required wound debridement and antibiotic treatment postoperatively. Due to these drawbacks of ICBG, local bone harvest has become a more popular and viable option and, when available, is a common bone graft of choice in minimally invasive spine fusion procedures.

Regardless of where the autologous bone is harvested from, it is important to understand that the biomechanical properties of autografts vary between different types of autograft: cancellous versus cortical grafts [78, 80]. Cancellous bone grafts exhibit a much higher porosity than cortical grafts, which translates to significantly lower initial mechanical strength [78]. However, a higher porosity allows for easy revascularization and greater cellular diversity and biological activity allowing osteoblasts to form new bone. As remodeling occurs and the new graft is successfully incorporated, the mechanical strength of cancellous bone gradually increases [78, 80]. On the other hand, cortical bone is extremely dense and has a limited biologic profile. Even though it provides good initial strength and mechanical stability, vascular ingrowth is challenging. Therefore, osteoclasts must initiate the process of resorption first, leading to a transient decrease in mechanical strength, before revascularization could occur and new bone could be formed [80].

The efficacies of autografts have been widely reported in the literature. Based on our review, a total of 23 studies involving 1209 patients met our inclusion criteria and utilized autologous local bone without additional extenders and achieved a fusion rate of 91% (68–100%). Similarly, when ICBG was used alone, a fusion rate of 96% (90–100%) was calculated across 3 studies and 101 patients. Not surprisingly secondary to availability, no studies were found using only local autografts or combination of local and ICBG in lateral approaches. Ohtori et al. was the only study that utilized ICBG alone in OLIF with 12 patients, reporting a fusion rate of 90% [41].

4.2. Autologous: Bone Marrow Aspirate. Bone Marrow Aspirate (BMA) is a cell-based bone graft that can be harvested from either the iliac crest or the pedicle and utilized as an alternative to ICBG [83]. It provides an autogenic source of

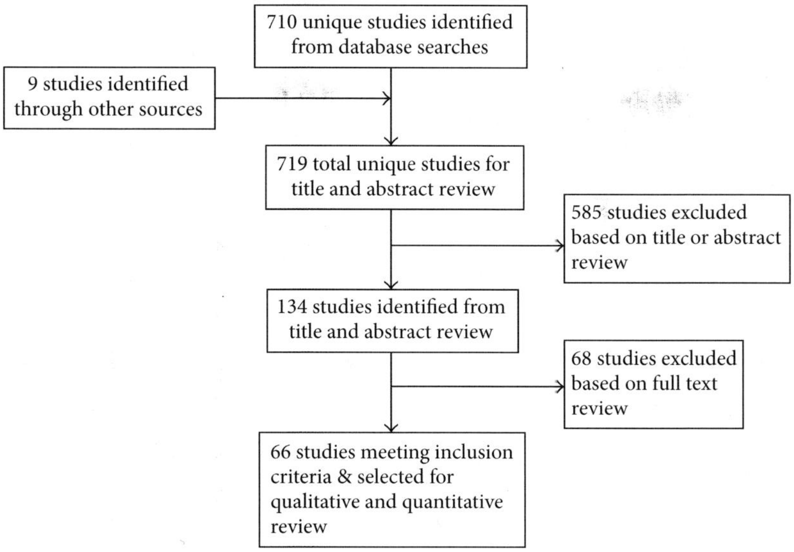

FIGURE 1: Systematic literature review and selection flowchart used to assess efficacies of various bone grafts.

osteogenic precursor cells that have the potential to differentiate into osteoblasts to synthesize new bone tissues [79, 84]. While BMA also possesses other pluripotent mesenchymal stem cells and less donor site morbidity than ICBG, disadvantages include variability in processing, difficulty obtaining enough bone marrow with sufficient progenitors cells, and age-related decline in osteoprogenitor cells [79, 84–86].

Due to the lack of structural support and osteoconductive properties, BMAs are often combined with scaffolds including autografts, allografts, ceramics, and implants to achieve spinal fusion. BMAs can be harvested from the iliac crest or the vertebral body pedicles using needle suction prior to mixing with other bone graft materials [49–51, 53, 87]. For example, Nandyala et al. described filling an interbody cage with 5 mL of BMA from cannulated pedicles, local bone autograft, and rhBMP-2 in an MIS-TLIF [49]. In another application, Abbasi et al. combined tricalcium phosphate soaked in autologous BMAs aspirated from the pedicles using a Jamshidi needle before packing into the disc space in treatment of scoliosis with oblique lateral lumbar interbody fusion (OLLIF) [51]. Additionally, other studies have reported mixing BMAs harvested from the iliac crest with (1) β-tricalcium phosphate and hydroxyapatite (HA) in an extreme lateral interbody fusion (XLIF), (2) demineralized bone matrix (DBM) and rhBMP-2 packed in a polyether ether ketone (PEEK) cage in an oblique lateral interbody fusion (OLIF), and (3) local autograft, DBM, and cancellous allograft in XLIF procedure (Table 3) [50, 53, 87].

A total of 109 patients from 2 studies utilized BMAs as bone graft extenders (Table 1) in MIS-TLIF and achieved a fusion rate of 93% (93-94%) [49]. Furthermore, 271 patients were enrolled across 4 studies in retroperitoneal approaches to interbody fusions such as OLIF, XLIF, or OLLIF and achieved a fusion rate of 97% (93–100%) (Table 2).

4.3. Allograft. Human allograft is a type of bone graft that is transferred from an individual to another and may be obtained from either a cadaverous tissue or a donor patient following an operation such as the femoral head after a hip-replacement surgery. The mechanism of action of allografts is thought to be due to its osteoconductive properties as it provides a scaffold for bone formation and weakly osteoinductive depending on the preservation of growth factors after its processing [88]. It is important to note that these grafts do not possess any osteogenic potential because they do not contain any viable cells [89]. Compared to autologous bone graft, allografts are readily available at low costs and avoid additional donor site morbidity and mortality, making them a popular alternative [79]. Complications related to allograft use have been reported in the literature primarily concerning the potential risk of viral infection and disease transmission. Even though such transmission is extremely rare, there have been reported cases of human immunodeficiency virus (HIV), hepatitis B virus (HBV), hepatitis C virus (HCV), and certain bacterial infections [88, 89]. After proper screening and processing of the blood products, the reported risk of transmission is 1 in 63,000 for HBV, 1 in 100,000 for HCB, and less than 1 in 1,000,000 [90]. Not surprisingly, of all the studies included in this review that utilized allografts, there were no reports of allograft-related complications.

Allografts have rarely been used alone and almost always in combination with autografts, BMAs, DBMs, or rhBMP-2 for minimally invasive procedures (Table 3). From the 5 studies that used allograft as an extender to autografts in MIS-TLIF, a fusion rate of 96% was calculated (Table 1). Ahmadian et al. was the only study that used allograft alone in a lateral interbody fusion reporting a fusion rate of 90% (Table 2) [47].

4.4. Demineralized Bone Matrix. Demineralized Bone Matrix (DBM) is a human allograft-derived bone graft first introduced in 1991 as a substitute or additive to autologous bone grafts [91]. After its procurement from human cadaveric bone, it is treated with acid that removes the mineralized portion while maintaining the collagens (mostly type I with

TABLE 1: Fusion rates for various bone grafts in posterior approaches to minimally invasive interbody fusions.

Bone grafts material	Posterior approaches to MIS interbody fusion			
	Number of studies	Number of patients	Fusion rate (%)	Range (%)
Autograft (local and iliac crest)	2	29	86	83–91
Autograft (local) alone	23	1209	91	68–100
Autograft (iliac crest) alone	3	101	96[a]	90–100
Autograft + allograft	5	178	96[a]	92–100
BMA (as extender)	2	109	93[a]	93-94
DBM (as extender)	5	264	85	77–97
Ceramics (as extender)	3	217	86	83–88
Ceramics alone	1	57	76	76
rhBMP-2 (with another bone graft)	7	486	95[a]	65–100
rhBMP-2 alone	1	36	94[a]	94

[a]There are no significant differences in fusion rates among these groups; however, they do demonstrate significantly higher fusion rates when compared to the rest ($P < 0.05$).

TABLE 2: Fusion rates for various bone grafts in anterior/lateral approaches to minimally invasive interbody fusions.

Bone graft materials	Anterior/lateral approaches to mis interbody fusion			
	Number of studies	Number of patients	Fusion rate (%)	Range (%)
Autograft (iliac crest) alone	1	12	90	90
Allograft alone	1	40	90	90
BMA (as extender)	4	271	97[b]	93–100
DBM (as extender)	2	203	98[a]	97-98
Ceramics (as extender)	5	149	95	80–100
Ceramics alone	5	206	88	80–100
rhBMP-2 (with another bone graft)	7	308	96[b]	80–100
rhBMP-2 alone	2	122	97[b]	96–100

[a]DBM (as extender) demonstrates significantly higher fusion rates than all bone grafts ($P < 0.05$), except for BMA (as extender) and rhBMP-2 alone. [b]These three types of bone grafts (BMA as extender, rhBMP-2 with another bone graft, and rhBMP-2 alone) are no different from each other and DBM in terms of fusion rate but significantly better than the rest ($P < 0.05$).

some types IV and X), the noncollagenous proteins, and certain growth factors (GF) [92]. The organic matrix (collagens and noncollagenous proteins) provides osteoconductive properties while the growth factors, which consist of bone morphogenetic proteins (BMP), transforming growth factor-β, and fibroblast growth factors among other GFs, contribute to its osteoinductive potential [93]. While the advantages of DBM include its unlimited availability and avoidance of an additional donor site comparing to autografts, its disadvantages have been well documented in the literature, most important of which are the significant variability in composition and efficacy not only between different products from different manufacturers but also within the same product from the same manufacturer [79, 94].

With over 35 commercially available products, DBM comes in a variety of different forms, such as dry powder, granules, injectable gels, putties, pastes, strips, flexible sheets, or blocks [92, 95]. Because DBM becomes particulate powder or fibers after initial processing that is difficult to manage clinically for surgeons, DBM is often combined with various biocompatible carriers such as sodium hyaluronate, carboxymethylcellulose, or glycerol into the form of moldable putty, thereby improving its handling properties [92].

Due to the lack of mechanical strength and ability to hold its structure intact, DBM is rarely used alone. The outcome of DBM use as an extender in lumbar fusion is widely reported in the literature. Kang et al. compared the efficacies of commercial DBM graft (Grafton™) with local autograft versus ICBG in patients who received a single-level posterior lumbar fusion and found that the fusion rates were comparable between the two groups (86% versus 92%) [96]. They also reported that the DBM group had a better clinical outcome with significantly less mean intraoperative blood loss and a higher physical function scores (though not statistically significant) at 24 months postoperatively [96]. In another study by Cammisa et al., 120 patients received ICBG implant on one side of the spine and DBM (Grafton)/autograft composite on the other side of the same patient. At 24-month follow-up, radiographic evidence showed similar fusion rates (ICBG, 54%; DBM, 52%), which suggests the efficacy of DBM as a bone graft extender is equally successful as autologous. Similar to the fusion rates reported by Kang et al., a fusion rate of 85% (77–97%) was calculated out of 264 patients (Table 1) in the 5 studies that we identified using DBM as an graft extender in MIS posterior interbody fusion procedures. In minimally invasive anterior and lateral interbody fusions,

TABLE 3: Published peer-reviewed studies utilizing various bone grafts in MIS interbody fusion procedures identified through our literature search.

Bone graft material	Author and year	Type of procedure	Type of material used in disc space	Type of material used in the cage	Method of fusion evaluation	Number of patients	Fusion rate (%)
Autograft (local and ICBG)	Yoo et al. 2015 [13]	MIS-TLIF	NA	Autograft (local + ICBG)	X-ray + CT	11	90.9
	Schizas et al. 2009 [14]	MIS-TLIF	Autograft (local + ICBG)	Autograft (local + ICBG)	X-ray	18	83.3
Autograft (local) alone	Zhang et al. 2017 [15]	MIS-TLIF	NA	Autograft (local)	X-ray + CT	26	100
	Rajakumar et al. 2017 [16]	MIS-TLIF	NA	Autograft (local)	X-ray	36	97.2
	Yang et al. 2017 [17]	MIS-TLIF	Autograft (local)	Autograft (local)	NA	21	85.7
	Huang et al. 2017 [18]	MIS-TLIF	Autograft (local)	Autograft (local)	X-ray	58	87.9
	Choi et al. 2017 [19]	MIS-TLIF	Autograft (local)	Autograft (local)	CT	44	95.2
	Choi et al. 201 7[19]	MIS-TLIF	Autograft (local)	Autograft (local)	CT	40	96.6
	Lv et al. 2017 [20]	MIS-TLIF	NA	Autograft (local)	CT	50	96.0
	Fan et al. 2016 [21]	MIS-TLIF	NA	Autograft (local)	X-ray	41	92.7
	Fan et al. 2016 [21]	MIS-TLIF	NA	Autograft (local)	X-ray	37	81.1
	Tian and Liu 2016 [22]	MIS-TLIF	Autograft (local)	NA	CT	47	90.0
	Tian and Liu 2016 [22]	W-TLIF	Autograft (local)	NA	CT	50	88.9
	Fan et al. 2016 [23]	MIS-TLIF	Autograft (local)	Autograft (local)	X-ray	24	91.7
	Fan et al. 2016 [23]	MIS-TLIF	Autograft (local)	Autograft (local)	X-ray	21	85.7
	Yang et al. 2015 [24]	MIS-TLIF	Autograft (local)	Autograft (local)	X-ray	50	88.0
	Liu et al. 2015 [25]	MIS-TLIF	Autograft (local)	NA	X-ray	42	81.0
	Liu et al. 2015 [25]	MIS-TLIF	Autograft (local)	NA	X-ray	42	95.2
	Lee et al. 2016 [26]	MIS-TLIF	NA	Autograft (local)	X-ray + CT	27	81.5
	Chen et al. 2015 [27]	MIS-TLIF	Autograft (local)	NA	CT	42	100
	Chen et al. 2015 [27]	MIS-TLIF	Autograft (local)	NA	CT	36	100
	Kim et al. 2015 [28]	MIS-TLIF	NA	Autograft (local)	CT	18	88.9
	Kim et al. 2015[28]	MIS-TLIF	NA	Autograft (local)	CT	23	87.0
	Zhang et al. 2015 [29]	MMI-TLIF	Autograft (local)	NA	NA	49	81.7
	Gu et al. 2015 [30]	MIS-TLIF	Autograft (local)	Autograft (local)	X-ray	35	94.3
	Gu et al. 2015 [30]	MIS-TLIF	Autograft (local)	Autograft (local)	X-ray	39	94.9
	Shen et al. 2014 [31]	MIS-TLIF	Autograft (local)	NA	CT	31	96.8
	Shen et al. 2014 [31]	MIS-TLIF	Autograft (local)	NA	CT	34	100.0
	Gu et al. 2014 [32]	MIS-TLIF	Autograft (local)	Autograft (local)	X-ray	44	93.2
	Choi et al. 2013 [33]	MIS-TLIF	NA	Autograft (local)	X-ray + CT	26	84.6
	Choi et al. 2013 [33]	MIS-TLIF	NA	Autograft (local)	X-ray + CT	27	96.3
	Sonmez et al. 2013 [34]	MIS-TLIF	Autograft (local)	Autograft (local)	X-ray	10	80.0
	Sonmez et al. 2013 [34]	MIS-TLIF	Autograft (local)	Autograft (local)	X-ray	10	90.0

Table 3: Continued.

Bone graft material	Author and year	Type of procedure	Type of material used in disc space	Type of material used in the cage	Method of fusion evaluation	Number of patients	Fusion rate (%)
	Wang et al. 2014 [35]	MIS-TLIF	Autograft (local)	NA	X-ray + CT	43	97.7
	Kasliwal and Deutsch 2012 [36]	MIS-TLIF	Autograft (local)	Autograft (local)	CT	40	67.5
	Scheufler et al. 2007 [37]	MIS-TLIF	Autograft (local)	Autograft (local)	CT	46	93.5
Autograft (ICBG) alone	Serban et al. 2017 [38]	MIS-TLIF	Autograft (ICBG)	NA	CT	40	90
	Fan et al. 2010 [39]	MIS-TLIF	Autograft (ICBG)	Autograft (ICBG)	X-ray	32	100
	Peng et al. 2009 [40]	MIS-TLIF	Autograft (ICBG)	NA	X-ray	29	100
	Ohtori et al. 2015 [41]	OLIF	NA	Autograft (ICBG)	CT	12	90
Autograft + allograft	He et al. 2017 [42]	MIS-TLIF	Autograft (local) + Allograft	Autograft (local) + Allograft	CT	42	92.9
	Lee et al. 2016 [43]	MIS-TLIF	NA	Autograft (local) + Allograft	X-ray	38	100
	Lim and Kim 2013 [44]	MIS-TLIF	Autograft (local) + Allograft	NA	X-ray + CT	19	100
	Kim et al. 2011 [45]	MIS-TLIF	Autograft (local) + Allograft	Autograft (local) + Allograft	X-ray	56	96.4
	Jang and Lee 2005 [46]	MIS-TLIF	NA	Autograft (local +/− ICBG) + Allograft	X-ray	23	91.7
Allograft alone	Ahmadian et al. 2015 [47]	MIS-LIF	Allograft (unclear interbody or in cage)		X-rays +/− CT	40	89.7
BMA (as extender)	Hawasli et al. 2017 [48]	MIS-TLIF	Allograft + bma	Autograft (local) + BMA	X-ray +/− CT	44	93.2
	Nandyala et al. 2014 [49]	MIS-TLIF	Autograft (local) + rhBMP-2 + BMA	Autograft (local)	CT	65	93.8
	Woods et al. 2017 [50]	OLIF	DBM + BMA + rhBMP-2	DBM + BMA + rhBMP-2	CT	137	97.9
	Abbasi et al. 2017 [51]	OLLIF	β-TCP + BMA	NA	NA	24	100
	Rodgers et al. 2012 [52]	XLIF	Formagraft (β-TCP + HA) + BMA (unclear interbody or in cage)		X-ray + CT	44	93.2
	Rodgers et al. 2010 [53]	Mini-ALIF XLIF	Autograft (local) + Allograft + DBM + BMA		CT	66	97.0

Table 3: Continued.

Bone graft material	Author and year	Type of procedure	Type of material used in disc space	Type of material used in the cage	Method of fusion evaluation	Number of patients	Fusion rate (%)
DBM (as extender)	Choi et al. 2016 [54]	MIS-TLIF	Autograft (local) + DBM	Autograft (local) + DBM	CT	21	95.2
	Kuo et al. 2016 [55]	MIS-TLIF	NA	Autograft (local) + DBM	X-ray + CT	22	77.3
	Park et al. 2014 [56]	MIS-TLIF	Autograft (local) + DBM	NA		83	80.7
	Lee et al. 2012 [57]	MIS-TLIF	Autograft (local) + DBM	NA	X-ray	72	97.0
	Park et al. 2011 [58]	MIS-TLIF	Autograft (local) + DBM	NA	CT	66	77.3
	Woods et al. 2017 [50]	OLIF	DBM + BMA + rhBMP-2	DBM + BMA + rhBMP-2	CT	137	97.9
	Rodgers et al. 2010 [53]	Mini-ALIF/XLIF	Autograft (local) + Allograft + DBM + BMA		CT	66	97.0
Ceramic (as extender)	Yoo et al. 2014 [59]	MIS-TLIF	NA	Autograft (local) + HA	X-ray + CT	92	87.0
	Yoo et al. 2015 [13]	MIS-TLIF	Autograft (local) + HA	Autograft (local)	X-ray + CT	49	87.8
	Yoo et al. 2015 [13]	MIS-TLIF	Autograft (local) + HA	Autograft (local)	X-ray + CT	28	85.7
	Lin and Chiang 2014 [60]	MIS-TLIF	Autograft (local) + SinboneHT (60% HA, 40% TCP)	NA	X-ray	48	83.3
	Malham et al. 2017 [61]	XLIF	NA	Mastergraft (β-TCP + HA) + rhBMP-2	CT	21	95.2
	Malham et al. 2017 [61]	XLIF	NA	Mastergraft (β-TCP + HA) + rhBMP-2	CT	19	80.0
	Abbasi et al. 2017 [51]	OLLIF	β-TCP + BMA	NA	NA	24	100
	Waddell et al. 2014 [62]	LLIF	NA	Mastergraft (β-TCP + HA) + rhBMP-2	CT	21	98.0
	Rodgers et al. 2012 [52]	XLIF	Formagraft (β-TCP + HA) + BMA (unclear interbody or in cage)		X-ray + CT	44	93.2
	Dakwar et al. 2010 [63]	XLIF	NA	TCP + HA + rhBMP-2	X-ray +/− CT	20	100.0

TABLE 3: Continued.

Bone graft material	Author and year	Type of procedure	Type of material used in disc space	Type of material used in the cage	Method of fusion evaluation	Number of patients	Fusion rate (%)
Ceramics alone	Alimi et al. 2017 [64]	MIS-TLIF	NA	Si-CaP	CT	57	76.3
	Parker and Malham 2017 [65]	XLIF	NA	AttraX (β-TCP + HA)	CT	25	80.0
	Alimi et al. 2017 [64]	XLIF	NA	Si-CaP	CT	44	82.1
	Berjano et al. 2015 [66]	XLIF	NA	AttraX (β-TCP + HA)	X-ray + CT	13	83.0
	Berjano et al. 2015 [66]	XLIF	NA	Calcium Triphosphate	X-ray + CT	35	89.0
	Marchi et al. 2013 [67]	XLIF	Calcium Phosphate (unclear interbody or in cage)		CT	74	91.0
	Pimenta et al. 2013 [68]	XLIF	Si-CaP (unclear interbody or in cage)		X-ray + CT	15	100.0
rhBMP-2 (with another graft)	Wang and Grossman 2016 [69]	MIS-TLIF	rhBMP-2	Allograft	X-ray	10	87.5
	Siddiqui et al. 2016 [70]	MIS-TLIF	Autograft (local) + rhBMP-2	Autograft (local)	X-ray	148	98.5
	Nandyala et al. 2013 [49]	MIS-TLIF	Autograft (local) + rhBMP-2 + BMA	Autograft (local)	CT	65	93.8
	Tsahtsarlis and Wood 2012 [71]	MIS-TLIF	NA	Autograft (local) + rhBMP-2	CT	34	97.1
	Rouben et al. 2011 [72]	MIS-TLIF	NA	Autograft (local) + rhBMP-2	X-ray + CT	169	96.0
	Park and Foley 2008 [73]	MIS-TLIF	Autograft (local) + rhBMP-2	Autograft (local) + rhBMP-2	CT	40	100
	Deutsch and Musacchio Jr. 2006 [74]	MIS-TLIF	Autograft (local) + rhBMP-2	Autograft (local) + rhBMP-2	CT	20	65.0
	Malham et al. 2017 [61]	XLIF	NA	Mastergraft (β-TCP + HA) + rhBMP-2	CT	21	95.2
	Malham et al. 2017 [61]	XLIF	NA	Mastergraft (β-TCP + HA) + rhBMP-2	CT	19	80.0
	Woods et al. 2017 [50]	OLIF	DBM + BMA + rhBMP-2	DBM + BMA + rhBMP-2	CT	137	97.9
	Ahmadian et al. 2015 [47]	MIS-LIF	Allograft + rhBMP-2 (unclear interbody or in cage)		X-rays +/− CT	19	100.0
	Waddell et al. 2014 [62]	LLIF	NA	Mastergraft (β-TCP + HA) + rhBMP-2	CT	21	98.0
	Castellvi et al. 2014 [75]	LLIF	NA	Allograft + rhBMP-2	CT	36	100.0
	Dakwar et al. 2010 [63]	XLIF	NA	TCP + HA + rhBMP-2	X-ray +/− CT	20	100.0
	Aryan et al. 2008 [76]	AxiaLIF	Autograft (local) + rhBMP-2		X-ray +/− CT	35	91.4

Table 3: Continued.

Bone graft material	Author and year	Type of procedure	Type of material used in disc space	Type of material used in the cage	Method of fusion evaluation	Number of patients	Fusion rate (%)
rhBMP-2 alone	Dahdaleh et al. 2013 [77]	MIS-TLIF	NA	rhBMP-2	X-ray	20	95.0
	Dahdaleh et al. 2013 [77]	MIS-TLIF	NA	rhBMP-2	X-ray	16	93.8
	Parker and Malham 2017 [65]	XLIF	NA	rhBMP-2	CT	107	96.3
	Pimenta et al. 2013 [68]	XLIF	rhBMP-2 (unclear interbody or in cage)		X-ray + CT	15	100.0

MIS, minimally invasive spine; TLIF, transforaminal lumbar interbody fusion; ALIF, anterior lumbar interbody fusion; XLIF, extreme lateral interbody fusion; OLIF, oblique lumbar interbody fusion; OLLIF, oblique lateral lumbar interbody fusion; ICBG, iliac crest bone graft; BMA, bone marrow aspirate; DBM, demineralized bone graft; rhBMP-2, recombinant morphogenetic protein 2; HA, hydroxyapatite; TCP, tricalcium phosphate; Si-CaP, silicated calcium phosphate; CT, computed tomography; NA, not available.

a total of 203 patients received DBM in addition to other biologics and achieved a fusion rate of 98% (97-98%), which is significantly higher than any bone graft material ($P < 0.05$) except for BMA as extender and rhBMP-2 alone for anterior/lateral approach to interbody fusion (Table 2).

4.5. Ceramics. Ceramics are calcium-based synthetic bone grafts that are used primarily as bone graft extenders because they possess only osteoconductive properties without any osteogenic or osteoinductive properties [89]. They are made from a process called "sintering," which essentially uses high temperatures to force various chemical compounds to bond together [97]. Because they are manufactured through a controlled chemical process, their forms, compositions, porosities, biodegradability, and other characteristics can be modified. Some advantages of ceramics include immediate strength, no risk of disease transmission, unlimited supply, long-shelf life, and availability in many different forms and compositions, while its disadvantages include its brittleness and lack of cortical stability [79, 89].

Materials that are commonly found in ceramics include hydroxyapatite (HA), tricalcium phosphate (TCP), calcium phosphate, and calcium sulfate. Commercially, they come in various preparations and are either found alone or in compositions with one another to provide different properties of biodegradability, porosity, and utility [98]. One of the most important properties to understand when using ceramics in orthopedic procedures is the porosity of different types of ceramics and how it contributes to the biomechanical strength of the graft. β-TCP has a higher porosity and pore size than HA, leading to a larger surface area and lower compressive strength. However, this allows for a higher biologic response, faster osteoclastic resorption, and the subsequent osteoblastic bone formation. HA, on the other hand, is more dense and undergoes a slow resorption but provides a much stronger biomechanical stability [10]. Considering these factors, HA and β-TCP are often modified and combined with each other to enhance the functionality and take advantage of strengths of each material [10, 99]. Multiple studies have also reported using HA, β-TCP, or calcium phosphate alone as a supplement to an osteoinductive source in anterior/lateral or posterior approach to MIS fusion [13, 51, 59].

A total of 4 studies that met our inclusion criteria used ceramics either alone or as bone graft extenders. In the 3 studies that used ceramics as extenders to osteoinductive local autograft, a fusion rate of 86% (83–88%) was observed (Table 1), which is consistent with the literature for open spine procedures [98]. In the only study that reported using ceramics alone, Alimi et al. reported a fusion rate of 76.3% in MIS-TLIF when silicate substituted calcium phosphate (Si-CaP) was used [64]. Despite the lower fusion rate in MIS-TLIF, the authors concluded that Si-CaP alone is still a viable option as a bone graft substitute because the overall fusion rate was 82.9% when all fusion procedures in the study were considered [64]. In retroperitoneal approaches, the collective fusion rates are 95% (80–100%) and 88% (80–100%) corresponding to ceramics used as an extender and alone, respectively (Table 2). The lower fusion rate seen with ceramics alone may be due to the lack of osteoinductive agents.

4.6. Bone Morphogenetic Protein 2. Bone morphogenetic proteins (BMPs) are endogenous, soluble proteins that are members of the transforming growth factor-β (TFG-β) family found in the human body [79]. They are growth factors that are involved in a myriad of cellular responses including the differentiation, maturation, and proliferation of mesenchymal stem cells (MSCs) into mature cartilage- and bone-forming cells [79, 100]. BMPs are thought to possess osteoinductive properties by binding serine-threonine kinase receptors on cell surfaces and activating Smad (Smad1/5) complex proteins, leading to their translocation into the nucleus and inducing expression of genes related to osteoblast phenotypes [101]. After its discovery by Marshall Urist through partially purified extract of DBM in 1965, over 20 BMPs have since been identified to play an active role in fracture healing and formation of new bone [102, 103]. With the advent of genomic technology, they have become commercially available in the form of recombinant proteins and have become one of the most popular bone graft substitutes in MIS fusion procedures [103].

However, its limitations include a potential side effect profile of seroma/hematoma formation, prevertebral swelling, radiculitis, retrograde ejaculation, osteolysis, and heterotopic ossification [79, 100, 104]. In a retrospective review of 610 patients who has underwent MIS-TLIF, Singh et al. have shown that heterotopic ossification and osteolysis are both complications associated with rhBMP-2 use [104]. Heterotopic ossification is characterized by bone formation at an abnormal anatomical site, usually the soft tissue, where bone normally does not exist. Osteolysis, on the other hand, describes the opposite process where there is a pathological destruction of bone tissue. In addition, rhBMP-2 use in the cervical spine has been linked to life-threatening complications such as airway edema and dysphagia, leading to the FDA issuing a warning its use in cervical spine procedures in 2008 [105–107]. Furthermore, there have been multiple studies, most notably the study published from the Yale University Open Data Access (YODA) collaboration with Medtronic, linking the use of rhBMP-2 to an increase in incidence of cancer [108, 109]. However, two large-scale retrospective studies with a combined cohort of over 600,000 patients concluded that there is no evidence of increased malignancy with the use of rhBMP-2 [110, 111]. From the 8 studies that met our inclusion criteria utilizing rhBMP-2 in MIS-TLIF, Nandyala et al. documented a case of rhBMP-2 related neuroforaminal bone growth and cage migration/osteolysis and Siddiqui et al. reported two cases of bone overgrowth with radiculopathy, a case of osteolysis, and two cases of radiculitis [49, 70].

Surgical technique involving rhBMP-2 (INFUSE) in MIS procedures have been described within the implant, disc space, or both. For example, Tsahtsarlis and Wood and Rouben et al. both described inserting a cage filled with local autograft and rhBMP-2 after end-plate preparation, whereas Wang and Grossman and Siddiqui et al. packed rhBMP-2 into the anterior disc space [69–72]. Two other MIS-TLIF studies inserted local autograft and rhBMP-2 soaked collagen sponge anteriorly within the disc space as well as inside the interbody implant (Table 3) [73, 74]. While the site of rhBMP-2 insertion can vary based on surgeon preference and the pathologies, the relative dose of rhBMP-2 also differed. Of all the MIS-TLIF studies we included, Tsahtsarlis and Wood, Siddiqui et al., and Nandyala et al. reported using 1.4 mg, 4.2 mg, and either 4.2 mg or 12 mg, respectively [49, 70, 71]. Notably, the majority of these studies used CT scans as the method of evaluation for fusion during their postoperative follow-ups (Table 3).

In patients utilizing rhBMP-2 as a bone graft substitute in addition to autografts or allografts in minimally invasive posterior interbody fusion approaches, a collective fusion rate of 95% (65–100%) was reported (Table 1). This rate is consistent with those reported by the meta-analysis performed by Parajón in MIS-TLIF [112]. In the only study that used rhBMP-2 alone, Dahdaleh et al. concluded that there was no significant difference in unilateral and bilateral instrumentation in patients undergoing MIS-TLIF with fusion rates of 93.8% and 95%, respectively [77]. The combined fusion rate for those two groups is 94.4% (Table 1). While these fusion rates are robust, it is not statistically significant compared to ICBG alone, autograft plus allograft, and BMA in posterior approaches. When rhBMP-2 is used in anterior/lateral interbody fusion techniques alone and with other fusion biologics, fusion rates of 97% (96–100%) and 97% (80–100%) were calculated, respectively (Table 2).

5. Conclusion

With an ever-expanding arena of fusion biologics and bone graft materials, it is important to understand each of their properties, advantages, and disadvantages, as well as their applications. While ICBG remains the gold standard for spine fusion surgeries, local autologous bone graft is by far the predominant bone graft material utilized in minimally invasive posterior approach to interbody fusion. In anterior/lateral techniques, ceramics and rhBMP-2 are the most common, likely due to the need for the mechanical properties of ceramics as well as rhBMP-2s strong osteoinductivity in treating more severe structural deformities. Overall, fusion rates were high with over 90% and 95% calculated for MIS posterior and MIS anterior/lateral approaches to interbody fusion, respectively, regardless of bone grafts used.

References

[1] S. Jaikumar, D. H. Kim, and A. C. Kam, "History of minimally invasive spine surgery," *Neurosurgery*, vol. 51, no. 5, pp. 1–14, 2002.

[2] T. G. Obenchain, "Laparoscopic Lumbar Discectomy: Case Report," *World Journal of Laparoscopic Surgery*, vol. 1, no. 3, pp. 145–149, 1991.

[3] S. S. Rajaee, H. W. Bae, L. E. A. Kanim, and R. B. Delamarter, "Spinal fusion in the United States: analysis of trends from 1998 to 2008," *The Spine Journal*, vol. 37, no. 1, pp. 67–76, 2012.

[4] F. M. Phillips, I. Cheng, Y. R. Rampersaud et al., "Breaking through the 'glass ceiling' of minimally invasive spine surgery," *The Spine Journal*, vol. 41, S8, pp. S39–S43, 2016.

[5] A. F. Cannestra, M. D. Peterson, S. R. Parker, T. F. Roush, J. V. Bundy, and A. W. Turner, "MIS Expandable Interbody Spacers," *The Spine Journal*, p. 1, 2016.

[6] R. J. Mobbs et al., "Lumbar interbody fusion: techniques, indications and comparison of interbody fusion options including PLIF, TLIF, MI-TLIF, OLIF/ATP, LLIF and ALIF," *Journal of Spine Surgery*, vol. 1, no. 1, p. 18, 2015.

[7] M. Mica, L. Voronov, G. Carandang, R. Havey, B. Wojewnik, and A. Patwardhan, "Biomechanics of an Expandable Lumbar Interbody Fusion Cage Deployed Through Transforaminal Approach," *International Journal of Spine Surgery*, vol. 11, no. 4, pp. 193–200, 2017.

[8] R. J. Mobbs, A. Loganathan, V. Yeung, and P. J. Rao, "Indications for Anterior Lumbar Interbody Fusion," *Orthopaedic Surgery*, vol. 5, no. 3, pp. 153–163, 2013.

[9] L. Pimenta, A. W. L. Turner, Z. A. Dooley, R. D. Parikh, and M. D. Peterson, "Biomechanics of lateral interbody spacers: Going wider for going stiffer," *The Scientific World Journal*, vol. 2012, Article ID 381814, 2012.

[10] P. V. Giannoudis, H. Dinopoulos, and E. Tsiridis, "Bone substitutes: an update," *Injury*, vol. 36, supplement 3, pp. S20–S27, 2005.

[11] T. Albrektsson and C. Johansson, "Osteoinduction, osteoconduction and osseointegration," *European Spine Journal*, vol. 10, no. 2, pp. S96–S101, 2001.

[12] I. H. Kalfas, "Principles of bone healing," *Neurosurgical Focus*, vol. 10, no. 4, p. E1, 2001.

[13] J.-S. Yoo, S.-H. Min, and S.-H. Yoon, "Fusion rate according to mixture ratio and volumes of bone graft in minimally invasive transforaminal lumbar interbody fusion: minimum 2-year follow-up," *European Journal of Orthopaedic Surgery and Traumatology*, vol. 25, pp. 183–189, 2015.

[14] C. Schizas, N. Tzinieris, E. Tsiridis, and V. Kosmopoulos, "Minimally invasive versus open transforaminal lumbar interbody fusion: Evaluating initial experience," *International Orthopaedics*, vol. 33, no. 6, pp. 1683–1688, 2009.

[15] D. Zhang, K. Mao, and X. Qiang, "Comparing minimally invasive transforaminal lumbar interbody fusion and posterior lumbar interbody fusion for spondylolisthesis," *Medicine (United States)*, vol. 96, no. 37, Article ID e8011, 2017.

[16] D. V. Rajakumar, A. Hari, M. Krishna, A. Sharma, and M. Reddy, "Complete anatomic reduction and monosegmental fusion for lumbar spondylolisthesis of Grade II and higher: Use of the minimally invasive "rocking" technique," *Neurosurgical Focus*, vol. 43, no. 2, article no. E12, 2017.

[17] Y. Yang, L. Zhang, B. Liu et al., "Hidden and overall haemorrhage following minimally invasive and open transforaminal lumbar interbody fusion," *Journal of Orthopaedics and Traumatology*, pp. 1–6, 2017.

[18] P. Huang, Y. Wang, J. Xu et al., "Minimally invasive unilateral pedicle screws and a translaminar facet screw fixation and interbody fusion for treatment of single-segment lower lumbar vertebral disease: Surgical technique and preliminary clinical results," *Journal of Orthopaedic Surgery and Research*, vol. 12, no. 1, article no. 117, 2017.

[19] W. Choi, J. Kim, J. Hur, and J. Seong, "Minimally invasive transforaminal lumbar interbody fusion using banana-shaped and straight cages: radiological and clinical results from a

prospective randomized clinical trial," *Neurosurgery*, vol. 82, no. 3, pp. 289–298, 2018.

[20] Y. Lv, J. Chen, J. Chen et al., "Three-year postoperative outcomes between MIS and conventional TLIF in1-segment lumbar disc herniation," *Minimally Invasive Therapy & Allied Technologies*, vol. 26, no. 3, pp. 168–176, 2017.

[21] G. Fan, H. Zhang, X. Guan et al., "Patient-reported and radiographic outcomes of minimally invasive transforaminal lumbar interbody fusion for degenerative spondylolisthesis with or without reduction: A comparative study," *Journal of Clinical Neuroscience*, vol. 33, pp. 111–118, 2016.

[22] Y. Tian and X. Liu, "Clinical outcomes of two minimally invasive transforaminal lumbar interbody fusion (TLIF) for lumbar degenerative diseases," *European Journal of Orthopaedic Surgery and Traumatology*, vol. 26, no. 7, pp. 745–751, 2016.

[23] G. Fan, G. Gu, Y. Zhu et al., "Minimally invasive transforaminal lumbar interbody fusion for isthmic spondylolisthesis: in situ versus reduction," *World Neurosurgery*, vol. 90, pp. 580–587.E1, 2016.

[24] Y. Yang et al., "Microendoscopy-assisted minimally invasive transforaminal lumbar interbody fusion for lumbar degenerative disease: short-term and medium-term outcomes," *International Journal of Clinical and Experimental Medicine*, vol. 8, no. 11, pp. 21319-26, 2015.

[25] X. Liu, G. Li, J. Wang, and H. Zhang, "Minimally invasive unilateral vs. bilateral pedicle screw fixation and lumbar interbody fusion in treatment of multi-segment lumbar degenerative disorders," *Medical Science Monitor*, vol. 21, article no. A494, pp. 3652–3657, 2015.

[26] W.-C. Lee, J.-Y. Park, K. H. Kim et al., "Minimally Invasive Transforaminal Lumbar Interbody Fusion in Multilevel: Comparison with Conventional Transforaminal Interbody Fusion," *World Neurosurgery*, vol. 85, pp. 236–243, 2016.

[27] C. Chen, X. Cao, L. Zou, G. Hao, Z. Zhou, and G. Zhang, "Minimally invasive unilateral versus bilateral technique in performing single-segment pedicle screw fixation and lumbar interbody fusion," *Journal of Orthopaedic Surgery and Research*, vol. 10, no. 1, article no. 112, 2015.

[28] J. Y. Kim, J. Y. Park, K. H. Kim et al., "Minimally invasive transforaminal lumbar interbody fusion for spondylolisthesis: comparison between isthmic and degenerative spondylolisthesis," *World Neurosurgery*, vol. 84, no. 5, pp. 1284–1293, 2015.

[29] W. Zhang, X. Li, X. Shang et al., "Modified minimally invasive transforaminal lumbar interbody fusion using a transmultifidus approach: A safe and effective alternative to open-TLIF," *Journal of Orthopaedic Surgery and Research*, vol. 10, no. 1, article no. 93, 2015.

[30] G. Gu, H. Zhang, G. Fan et al., "Clinical and radiological outcomes of unilateral versus bilateral instrumentation in two-level degenerative lumbar diseases," *European Spine Journal*, vol. 24, no. 8, pp. 1640–1648, 2015.

[31] X. Shen, H. Zhang, X. Gu, G. Gu, X. Zhou, and S. He, "Unilateral versus bilateral pedicle screw instrumentation for single-level minimally invasive transforaminal lumbar interbody fusion," *Journal of Clinical Neuroscience*, vol. 21, no. 9, pp. 1612–1616, 2014.

[32] G. Gu, H. Zhang, G. Fan et al., "Comparison of minimally invasive versus open transforaminal lumbar interbody fusion in two-level degenerative lumbar disease," *International Orthopaedics*, vol. 38, no. 4, pp. 817–824, 2014.

[33] U. Y. Choi, J. Y. Park, K. H. Kim et al., "Unilateral versus bilateral percutaneous pedicle screw fixation in minimally invasive transforaminal lumbar interbody fusion," *Neurosurgical Focus*, vol. 35, no. 2, article no. E11, 2013.

[34] E. Sonmez, I. Coven, F. Sahinturk, C. Yilmaz, and H. Caner, "Unilateral percutaneous pedicle screw instrumentation with minimally invasive tlif for the treatment of recurrent lumbar disk disease: 2 years follow-up," *Turkish Neurosurgery*, vol. 23, no. 3, pp. 372–378, 2013.

[35] J. Wang, Y. Zhou, Z. Feng Zhang, C. Qing Li, W. Jie Zheng, and J. Liu, "Comparison of the clinical outcome in overweight or obese patients after minimally invasive versus open transforaminal lumbar interbody fusion," *Journal of Spinal Disorders & Techniques*, vol. 27, no. 4, pp. 202–206, 2014.

[36] M. K. Kasliwal and H. Deutsch, "Clinical and radiographic outcomes using local bone shavings as autograft in minimally invasive transforaminal lumbar interbody fusion," *World Neurosurgery*, vol. 78, no. 1-2, pp. 185–190, 2012.

[37] K.-M. Scheufler, H. Dohmen, and V. I. Vougioukas, "Percutaneous transforaminal lumbar interbody fusion for the treatment of degenerative lumbar instability," *Neurosurgery*, vol. 60, 2, no. 4, pp. 203–212, 2007.

[38] D. Serban, N. Calina, and G. Tender, "Standard versus Minimally Invasive Transforaminal Lumbar Interbody Fusion: A Prospective Randomized Study," *BioMed Research International*, vol. 2017, Article ID 7236970, 2017.

[39] S. Fan, X. Zhao, F. Zhao, and X. Fang, "Minimally invasive transforaminal lumbar interbody fusion for the treatment of degenerative lumbar diseases," *The Spine Journal*, vol. 35, no. 17, pp. 1615–1620, 2010.

[40] C. W. B. Peng, W. M. Yue, S. Y. Poh, W. Yeo, and S. B. Tan, "Clinical and radiological outcomes of minimally invasive versus open transforaminal lumbar interbody fusion," *The Spine Journal*, vol. 34, no. 13, pp. 1385–1389, 2009.

[41] S. Ohtori, C. Mannoji, S. Orita et al., "Mini-open anterior retroperitoneal lumbar interbody fusion: Oblique lateral interbody fusion for degenerated lumbar spinal kyphoscoliosis," *Asian Spine Journal*, vol. 9, no. 4, pp. 565–572, 2015.

[42] E.-X. He, J. Guo, Q.-J. Ling, Z.-X. Yin, Y. Wang, and M. Li, "Application of a narrow-surface cage in full endoscopic minimally invasive transforaminal lumbar interbody fusion," *International Journal of Surgery*, vol. 42, pp. 83–89, 2017.

[43] H.-J. Lee, J.-S. Kim, and K.-S. Ryu, "Minimally Invasive TLIF Using Unilateral Approach and Single Cage at Single Level in Patients over 65," *BioMed Research International*, vol. 2016, Article ID 4679865, 2016.

[44] J. K. Lim and S. M. Kim, "Radiographic Results of Minimally Invasive (MIS) Lumbar Interbody Fusion (LIF) Compared with Conventional Lumbar Interbody Fusion," *Korean Journal of Spine*, vol. 10, no. 2, p. 65, 2013.

[45] M.-C. Kim, H.-T. Chung, D.-J. Kim, S.-H. Kim, and S.-H. Jeon, "The clinical and radiological outcomes of minimally invasive transforaminal lumbar interbody single level fusion," *Asian Spine Journal*, vol. 5, no. 2, pp. 111–116, 2011.

[46] J.-S. Jang and S.-H. Lee, "Minimally invasive transforaminal lumbar interbody fusion with ipsilateral pedicle screw and contralateral facet screw fixation.," *Journal of Neurosurgery: Spine*, vol. 3, no. 3, pp. 218–223, 2005.

[47] A. Ahmadian, K. Bach, B. Bolinger et al., "Stand-alone minimally invasive lateral lumbar interbody fusion: Multicenter clinical outcomes," *Journal of Clinical Neuroscience*, vol. 22, no. 4, pp. 740–746, 2015.

[48] A. H. Hawasli, J. M. Khalifeh, A. Chatrath, C. K. Yarbrough, and W. Z. Ray, "Minimally invasive transforaminal lumbar

interbody fusion with expandable versus static interbody devices: Radiographic assessment of sagittal segmental and pelvic parameters," *Neurosurgical Focus*, vol. 43, no. 2, article no. E10, 2017.

[49] S. V. Nandyala, S. J. Fineberg, M. Pelton, and K. Singh, "Minimally invasive transforaminal lumbar interbody fusion: one surgeon's learning curve," *The Spine Journal*, vol. 14, no. 8, pp. 1460–1465, 2014.

[50] K. R. M. Woods, J. B. Billys, and R. A. Hynes, "Technical description of oblique lateral interbody fusion at L1–L5 (OLIF25) and at L5–S1 (OLIF51) and evaluation of complication and fusion rates," *The Spine Journal*, vol. 17, no. 4, pp. 545–553, 2017.

[51] H. Abbasi, L. Miller, A. Abbasi, V. Orandi, and K. Khaghany, "Minimally Invasive Scoliosis Surgery with Oblique Lateral Lumbar Interbody Fusion: Single Surgeon Feasibility Study," *Cureus*, vol. 9, no. 6, article e1389, 2017.

[52] W. B. Rodgers, E. J. Gerber, and J. A. Rodgers, "Clinical and radiographic outcomes of extreme lateral approach to interbody fusion with β-tricalcium phosphate and hydroxyapatite composite for lumbar degenerative conditions," *International Journal of Spine Surgery*, vol. 6, no. 1, pp. 24–28, 2012.

[53] W. B. Rodgers, E. J. Gerber, and J. R. Patterson, "Fusion after minimally disruptive anterior lumbar interbody fusion: Analysis of extreme lateral interbody fusion by computed tomography," *SAS Journal*, vol. 4, no. 2, pp. 63–66, 2010.

[54] W.-S. Choi, J.-S. Kim, K.-S. Ryu, J.-W. Hur, and J.-H. Seong, "Minimally invasive transforaminal lumbar interbody fusion at L5-S1 through a unilateral approach: technical feasibility and outcomes," *BioMed Research International*, vol. 2016, Article ID 2518394, 8 pages, 2016.

[55] C.-H. Kuo, P.-Y. Chang, J.-C. Wu et al., "Dynamic stabilization for L4-5 spondylolisthesis: Comparison with minimally invasive transforaminal lumbar interbody fusion with more than 2 years of follow-up," *Neurosurgical Focus*, vol. 40, no. 1, article no. E3, 2016.

[56] Y. Park, J. W. Ha, Y. T. Lee, and N. Y. Sung, "Minimally invasive transforaminal lumbar interbody fusion for spondylolisthesis and degenerative spondylosis: 5-year results," *Clinical Orthopaedics and Related Research*, vol. 472, no. 6, pp. 1813–1823, 2014.

[57] K. H. Lee, W. M. Yue, W. Yeo, H. Soeharno, and S. B. Tan, "Clinical and radiological outcomes of open versus minimally invasive transforaminal lumbar interbody fusion," *European Spine Journal*, vol. 21, no. 11, pp. 2265–2270, 2012.

[58] Y. Park, J. W. Ha, Y. T. Lee, H. C. Oh, J. H. Yoo, and H. B. Kim, "Surgical outcomes of minimally invasive transforaminal lumbar interbody fusion for the treatment of spondylolisthesis and degenerative segmental instability," *Asian Spine Journal*, vol. 5, no. 4, pp. 228–236, 2011.

[59] J.-S. Yoo, S.-H. Min, S.-H. Yoon, and C.-H. Hwang, "Paraspinal muscle changes of unilateral multilevel minimally invasive transforaminal interbody fusion," *Journal of Orthopaedic Surgery and Research*, vol. 9, p. 130, 2014.

[60] J.-H. Lin and Y.-H. Chiang, "Unilateral approach for bilateral foramen decompression in minimally invasive transforaminal interbody fusion," *World Neurosurgery*, vol. 82, no. 5, pp. 891–896, 2014.

[61] G. M. Malham, N. J. Ellis, R. M. Parker et al., "Maintenance of segmental lordosis and disk height in stand-alone and instrumented extreme lateral interbody fusion (XLIF)," *Clinical Spine Surgery*, vol. 30, no. 2, pp. E90–E98, 2017.

[62] B. Waddell, D. Briski, R. Qadir et al., "Lateral lumbar interbody fusion for the correction of spondylolisthesis and adult degenerative scoliosis in high-risk patients: early radiographic results and complications," *The Ochsner Journal*, vol. 14, no. 1, pp. 23–31, 2014.

[63] E. Dakwar, R. F. Cardona, D. A. Smith, and J. S. Uribe, "Early outcomes and safety of the minimally invasive, lateral retroperitoneal transpsoas approach for adult degenerative scoliosis.," *Neurosurgical Focus*, vol. 28, no. 3, p. E8, 2010.

[64] M. Alimi et al., "Radiographic and clinical outcome of silicate-substituted calcium phosphate (si-cap) ceramic bone graft in spinal fusion procedures," *Clinical Spine Surgery*, vol. 30, no. 6, pp. E845–e852, 2017.

[65] R. M. Parker and G. M. Malham, "Comparison of a calcium phosphate bone substitute with recombinant human bone morphogenetic protein-2: a prospective study of fusion rates, clinical outcomes and complications with 24-month follow-up," *European Spine Journal*, vol. 26, no. 3, pp. 754–763, 2017.

[66] P. Berjano, F. Langella, M. Damilano et al., "Fusion rate following extreme lateral lumbar interbody fusion," *European Spine Journal*, vol. 24, supplement 3, pp. 369–371, 2015.

[67] L. Marchi, N. Abdala, L. Oliveira, R. Amaral, E. Coutinho, and L. Pimenta, "Radiographic and clinical evaluation of cage subsidence after stand-alone lateral interbody fusion," *Journal of Neurosurgery: Spine*, vol. 19, no. 1, pp. 110–118, 2013.

[68] L. Pimenta, L. Marchi, L. Oliveira, E. Coutinho, and R. Amaral, "A prospective, randomized, controlled trial comparing radiographic and clinical outcomes between stand-alone lateral interbody lumbar fusion with either silicate calcium phosphate or rh-BMP2," *Journal of Neurological Surgery Part A: Central European Neurosurgery*, vol. 74, no. 6, pp. 343–350, 2013.

[69] M. Y. Wang and J. Grossman, "Endoscopic minimally invasive transforaminal interbody fusion without general anesthesia: initial clinical experience with 1-year follow-up," *Neurosurgical Focus*, vol. 40, no. 2, p. E13, 2016.

[70] M. M. A. Siddiqui, A. R. P. Sta Ana, W. Yeo, and W.-M. Yue, "Bone morphogenic protein is a viable adjunct for fusion in minimally invasive transforaminal lumbar interbody fusion," *Asian Spine Journal*, vol. 10, no. 6, pp. 1091–1099, 2016.

[71] A. Tsahtsarlis and M. Wood, "Minimally invasive transforaminal lumber interbody fusion and degenerative lumbar spine disease," *European Spine Journal*, vol. 21, no. 11, pp. 2300–2305, 2012.

[72] D. Rouben, M. Casnellie, and M. Ferguson, "Long-term durability of minimal invasive posterior transforaminal lumbar interbody fusion: A clinical and radiographic follow-up," *Journal of Spinal Disorders & Techniques*, vol. 24, no. 5, pp. 288–296, 2011.

[73] P. Park and K. T. Foley, "Minimally invasive transforaminal lumbar interbody fusion with reduction of spondylolisthesis: technique and outcomes after a minimum of 2 years' follow-up," *Neurosurgical Focus*, vol. 25, no. 2, article no. E16, 2008.

[74] H. Deutsch and M. J. Musacchio Jr., "Minimally invasive transforaminal lumbar interbody fusion with unilateral pedicle screw fixation.," *Neurosurgical Focus*, vol. 20, no. 3, p. E10, 2006.

[75] A. E. Castellvi, T. W. Nienke, G. A. Marulanda, R. D. Murtagh, and B. G. Santoni, "Indirect decompression of lumbar stenosis with transpsoas interbody cages and percutaneous posterior instrumentation," *Clinical Orthopaedics and Related Research*, vol. 472 no. 6, pp. 1784–1791, 2014.

[76] H. E. Aryan, C. B. Newman, J. J. Gold, F. L. Acosta Jr., C. Coover, and C. P. Ames, "Percutaneous axial lumbar interbody fusion

(AxiaLIF) of the L5-S1 segment: Initial clinical and radiographic experience," *Minimally Invasive Neurosurgery*, vol. 51, no. 4, pp. 225–230, 2008.

[77] N. S. Dahdaleh, A. T. Nixon, C. D. Lawton, A. P. Wong, Z. A. Smith, and R. G. Fessler, "Outcome following unilateral versus bilateral instrumentation in patients undergoing minimally invasive transforaminal lumbar interbody fusion: A single-center randomized prospective study," *Neurosurgical Focus*, vol. 35, no. 2, article no. E13, 2013.

[78] V. M. Goldberg and S. Akhavan, "Biology of Bone Grafts," in *in Bone Regeneration and Repair: Biology and Clinical Applications*, J. R. Lieberman and and G. E. Friedlaender, Eds., pp. 57–65, Humana Press, 2005.

[79] A. Kannan, S.-N. M. Dodwad, and W. K. Hsu, "Biologics in spine arthrodesis," *Journal of Spinal Disorders & Techniques*, vol. 28, no. 5, pp. 163–170, 2015.

[80] H. C. Pape, A. Evans, and P. Kobbe, "Autologous bone graft: properties and techniques," *Journal of Orthopaedic Trauma*, vol. 24, supplement 1, pp. S36–S40, 2010.

[81] E. D. Arrington, W. J. Smith, H. G. Chambers, A. L. Bucknell, and N. A. Davino, "Complications of Iliac Crest Bone Graft Harvesting," *Clinical Orthopaedics & Related Research*, vol. 329, pp. 300–309, 1996.

[82] C. E. Schwartz, J. F. Martha, P. Kowalski et al., "Prospective evaluation of chronic pain associated with posterior autologous iliac crest bone graft harvest and its effect on postoperative outcome," *Health and Quality of Life Outcomes*, vol. 7, article 49, 2009.

[83] M. Khashan, S. Inoue, and S. H. Berven, "Cell based therapies as compared to autologous bone grafts for spinal arthrodesis," *The Spine Journal*, vol. 38, no. 21, pp. 1885–1891, 2013.

[84] R. M. Ajiboye, J. T. Hamamoto, M. A. Eckardt, and J. C. Wang, "Clinical and radiographic outcomes of concentrated bone marrow aspirate with allograft and demineralized bone matrix for posterolateral and interbody lumbar fusion in elderly patients," *European Spine Journal*, vol. 24, no. 11, pp. 2567–2572, 2015.

[85] G. F. Muschler, H. Nitto, C. A. Boehm, and K. A. Easley, "Age- and gender-related changes in the cellularity of human bone marrow and the prevalence of osteoblastic progenitors," *Journal of Orthopaedic Research*, vol. 19, no. 1, pp. 117–125, 2001.

[86] S. M. Mueller and J. Glowacki, "Age-related decline in the osteogenic potential of human bone marrow cells cultured in three-dimensional collagen sponges," *Journal of Cellular Biochemistry*, vol. 82, no. 4, pp. 583–590, 2001.

[87] W. B. Rodgers, J. A. Lehmen, E. J. Gerber, and J. A. Rodgers, "Grade 2 spondylolisthesis at L4-5 treated by XLIF: Safety and midterm results in the worst case scenario," *The Scientific World Journal*, vol. 2012, Article ID 356712, 2012.

[88] V. Campana, G. Milano, E. Pagano et al., "Bone substitutes in orthopaedic surgery: from basic science to clinical practice," *Journal of Materials Science: Materials in Medicine*, vol. 25, no. 10, pp. 2445–2461, 2014.

[89] G. Zimmermann and A. Moghaddam, "Allograft bone matrix versus synthetic bone graft substitutes," *Injury*, vol. 42, no. 2, pp. S16–S21, 2011.

[90] T. T. Roberts and A. J. Rosenbaum, "Bone grafts, bone substitutes and orthobiologics the bridge between basic science and clinical advancements in fracture healing," *Organogenesis*, vol. 8, no. 4, pp. 114–124, 2012.

[91] R. M. Duarte, P. Varanda, R. L. Reis, A. R. Duarte, and J. Correia-Pinto, "Biomaterials and Bioactive Agents in Spinal Fusion," *Tissue Engineering Part B: Reviews*, vol. 23, no. 6, pp. 540–551, 2017.

[92] E. Gruskin, B. A. Doll, F. W. Futrell, J. P. Schmitz, and J. O. Hollinger, "Demineralized bone matrix in bone repair: history and use," *Advanced Drug Delivery Reviews*, vol. 64, no. 12, pp. 1063–1077, 2012.

[93] K. Tilkeridis, P. Touzopoulos, A. Ververidis, S. Christodoulou, K. Kazakos, and G. I. Drosos, "Use of demineralized bone matrix in spinal fusion," *World Journal of Orthopedics*, vol. 5, no. 1, pp. 30–37, 2014.

[94] H. W. Bae, L. Zhao, L. E. A. Kanim, P. Wong, R. B. Delamarter, and E. G. Dawson, "Intervariability and intravariability of bone morphogenetic proteins in commercially available demineralized bone matrix products," *The Spine Journal*, vol. 31, no. 12, pp. 1299–1306, 2006.

[95] A. Kadam, P. W. Millhouse, C. K. Kepler et al., "Bone substitutes and expanders in spine surgery: A review of their fusion efficacies," *International Journal of Spine Surgery*, vol. 10, no. 2016, article no. 3033, 2016.

[96] J. Kang, H. An, A. Hilibrand, S. T. Yoon, E. Kavanagh, and S. Boden, "Grafton and local bone have comparable outcomes to iliac crest bone in instrumented single-level lumbar fusions," *The Spine Journal*, vol. 37, no. 12, pp. 1083–1091, 2012.

[97] W. K. Hsu, M. S. Nickoli, J. C. Wang et al., "Improving the Clinical Evidence of Bone Graft Substitute Technology in Lumbar Spine Surgery," *Global Spine Journal*, vol. 2, no. 4, pp. 239–248, 2012.

[98] M. S. Nickoli and W. K. Hsu, "Ceramic-Based Bone Grafts as a Bone Grafts Extender for Lumbar Spine Arthrodesis: A Systematic Review," *Global Spine Journal*, vol. 4, no. 3, pp. 211–216, 2014.

[99] G. Grabowski and C. A. Cornett, "Bone graft and bone graft substitutes in spine surgery: Current concepts and controversies," *Journal of the American Academy of OrthopaedicSurgeons*, vol. 21, no. 1, pp. 51–60, 2013.

[100] W. K. Hsu, C. L. Goldstein, M. F. Shamji et al., "Novel Osteobiologics and Biomaterials in the Treatment of Spinal Disorders," *Neurosurgery*, vol. 80, no. 3, pp. S100–S107, 2017.

[101] S. Ebara and K. Nakayama, "Mechanism for the action of bone morphogenetic proteins and regulation of their activity," *The Spine Journal*, vol. 27, no. 16, supplement 1, pp. S10–S15, 2002.

[102] K. L. Ong, M. L. Villarraga, E. Lau, L. Y. Carreon, S. M. Kurtz, and S. D. Glassman, "Off-label use of bone morphogenetic proteins in the United States using administrative data," *The Spine Journal*, vol. 35, no. 19, pp. 1794–1800, 2010.

[103] A. Faundez, C. Tournier, M. Garcia, S. Aunoble, and J.-C. Le Huec, "Bone morphogenetic protein use in spine surgery—complications and outcomes: a systematic review," *International Orthopaedics*, vol. 40, no. 6, pp. 1309–1319, 2016.

[104] K. Singh, S. V. Nandyala, A. Marquez-Lara et al., "Clinical sequelae after rhBMP-2 use in a minimally invasive transforaminal lumbar interbody fusion," *The Spine Journal*, vol. 13, no. 9, pp. 1118–1125, 2013.

[105] E. J. Carragee, E. L. Hurwitz, and B. K. Weiner, "A critical review of recombinant human bone morphogenetic protein-2 trials in spinal surgery: emerging safety concerns and lessons learned," *The Spine Journal*, vol. 11, pp. 471–491, 2011.

[106] O. R. Oliveira, S. P. Martins, W. G. Lima, and M. M. Gomes, "The use of bone morphogenetic proteins (BMP) and pseudarthrosis, a literature review," *Revista Brasileira de Ortopedia (English Edition)*, vol. 52, no. 2, pp. 124–140, 2017.

[107] C. P. Hofstetter, A. S. Hofer, and A. D. Levi, "Exploratory meta-analysis on dose-related efficacy and morbidity of bone morphogenetic protein in spinal arthrodesis surgery," *Journal of Neurosurgery: Spine*, vol. 24, no. 3, pp. 457–475, 2016.

[108] M. C. Simmonds, J. V. E. Brown, M. K. Heirs et al., "Safety and effectiveness of recombinant human bone morphogenetic protein-2 for spinal fusion: a meta-analysis of individual-participant data," *Annals of Internal Medicine*, vol. 158, no. 12, pp. 877–889, 2013.

[109] R. Fu et al., "Effectiveness and harms of recombinant human bone morphogenetic protein-2 in spine fusion: a systematic review and meta-analysis," *Annals of Internal Medicine*, vol. 158, no. 12, pp. 890–902, 2013.

[110] G. S. Cooper and T. D. Kou, "Risk of cancer after lumbar fusion surgery with recombinant human bone morphogenic protein-2 (rh-BMP-2)," *The Spine Journal*, vol. 38, no. 21, pp. 1862–1868, 2013.

[111] M. P. Kelly, J. W. Savage, S. M. Bentzen, W. K. Hsu, S. A. Ellison, and P. A. Anderson, "Cancer risk from bone morphogenetic protein exposure in spinal arthrodesis," *Journal of Bone and Joint Surgery - American Volume*, vol. 96, no. 17, pp. 1417–1422, 2014.

[112] A. Parajón, M. Alimi, R. Navarro-Ramirez et al., "Minimally invasive transforaminal lumbar interbody fusion: meta-analysis of the fusion rates. what is the optimal graft material?" *Neurosurgery*, vol. 81, no. 6, pp. 958–971, 2017.

Interspinous Process Decompression Improves Quality of Life in Patients with Lumbar Spinal Stenosis

Pierce D. Nunley,[1] Vikas V. Patel,[2] Douglas G. Orndorff,[3] William F. Lavelle,[4] Jon E. Block,[5] and Fred H. Geisler[6]

[1]*Spine Institute of Louisiana, Shreveport, LA, USA*
[2]*The Spine Center, University of Colorado Hospital, Denver, CO, USA*
[3]*Spine Colorado, Mercy Regional Hospital, Durango, CO, USA*
[4]*Upstate Bone and Joint Center, East Syracuse, NY, USA*
[5]*San Francisco, CA, USA*
[6]*Chicago, IL, USA*

Correspondence should be addressed to Jon E. Block; jb@drjonblock.com

Academic Editor: Nader S. Dahdaleh

Lumbar spinal stenosis has been shown to negatively impact health-related quality of life. Interspinous process decompression (IPD) is a minimally invasive procedure that utilizes a stand-alone spacer to serve as a joint extension blocker to relieve neural compression in patients with spinal stenosis. Using the 5-year results from an FDA randomized controlled trial of IPD, the quality of life in 189 patients treated with the Superion® spacer was evaluated with the SF-12. Physical and mental component summary (PCS, MCS) scores were computed preoperatively and at annual intervals. For the PCS, mean scores improved from 29.4 ± 8.1 preoperatively to 41.2 ± 12.4 at 2 years (40%) and to 43.8 ± 11.6 at 5 years (49%) ($p<0.001$ for both comparisons). At 2 years, 81% (103 of 128) of subjects demonstrated maintenance or improvement in PCS scores. The mean MCS score improved from 50.0 ± 12.7 preoperatively to 54.4 ± 10.6 and 54.7 ± 8.6 at 2 and 5 years, respectively ($p>0.10$ for both comparisons). These results demonstrate that the significant impairment in physical well-being found in patients with lumbar spinal stenosis can be ameliorated, in large part, by IPD treatment.

1. Introduction

The classic clinical feature of lumbar spinal stenosis is neurogenic claudication which causes intermittent lower extremity pain and diminished functional abilities [1]. As symptoms progressively grow more chronic and refractory to conservative measures, spinal stenosis inevitably leads to systemic impairment of overall well-being and quality of life [2].

Interspinous process decompression (IPD) devices (aka "spacers") were developed to address a distinct therapeutic gap in the continuum of care of lumbar spinal stenosis treatment [3]. Interspinous spacers effectively bridge the often lengthy interval between failed conservative care and the point where surgical decompression becomes necessary to manage intractable symptoms. These devices are inserted posteriorly via a minimally invasive procedure without disruption of osseous or ligamentous tissues. Spacers provide immediate symptom amelioration by serving as a spinal extension blocker to prevent the repetitive compression of neural elements during back extension that is the primary source of claudicant symptoms.

The Superion spacer is the only stand-alone IPD device available on the US market. There is an extensive body of published research supporting the safety and effectiveness of this device for treatment of moderate lumbar spinal stenosis [4–9]. Importantly, IPD has also been shown to offer similar symptom relief as operative decompressive laminectomy [10, 11]. Herein, we described the results of long-term IPD treatment on generic health-related quality of life.

2. Materials and Methods

Health-related quality of life outcomes through 5 years of postoperative follow-up were obtained from the Superion (Vertiflex, Carlsbad, CA USA) treatment arm of a randomized controlled FDA noninferiority trial comparing two interspinous spacers. This multicenter trial evaluated the use of stand-alone IPD in the treatment of subjects aged 45 or older with moderate symptoms of intermittent neurogenic claudication, secondary to a diagnosis of moderate degenerative lumbar spinal stenosis at one or two contiguous levels from L1 to L5. Three hundred ninety-one subjects met the trial eligibility criteria and were randomized to treatment. The Superion was approved by the FDA in 2015 for commercial distribution based on the 2-year primary endpoint analysis [8]. Additionally, the condition-specific clinical outcomes have been reported through 5 years of follow-up [5–7]. The current quality of life analysis was restricted exclusively to the Superion arm of the trial.

This investigational device exemption (IDE) trial complied with all US regulatory requirements and was approved by the Institutional Review Board at each participating site, and patients provided written informed consent before any study-related procedures were performed. The trial was prospectively registered at ClinicalTrials.gov (NCT00692276).

As assessment of health-related quality of life was included as an ancillary clinical measurement in this trial. It was not included as component of the primary study composite endpoint or as a secondary condition-specific outcome such as the Zurich Claudication Questionnaire (ZCQ), leg and back pain severity by visual analog scale, or the Oswestry Disability Index (ODI). Prior to surgery as well as at annual intervals, quality of life was evaluated in study subjects using the SF-12® Health Survey, version 2 (SF-12) [12]. The SF-12 is a 12-item questionnaire used to assess patient-reported generic health outcomes, such as general health and well-being, including the impact of any and all illnesses on a broad range of functional domains. The SF-12 consists of a subset of 12 items from the SF-36® Health Survey (SF-36) covering the same eight domains of health outcomes, including physical functioning, role-physical, bodily pain, general health, vitality, social functioning, role emotional, and mental health [13]. The SF-12 provides two composite scores: the physical component summary (PCS) and the mental component summary (MCS). These summary scores are computed using the scores of the twelve questions and range from 0 to 100, where zero indicates the lowest level of health and 100 indicates the highest level of health. Based on a general US population sample, both the PCS and MCS scores are linearly transformed to adjust scores to a mean of 50 and standard deviation of 10 [14].

The percentage improvement in PCS and MCS at the 2-year primary trial endpoint and the 5-year follow-up interval compared to preoperative values was computed and the results were displayed graphically. The degree of improvement was analyzed using the paired t-test, 2-tailed. We also computed the percentage of subjects that maintained or improved in PCS and MCS score over baseline at the same follow-up intervals.

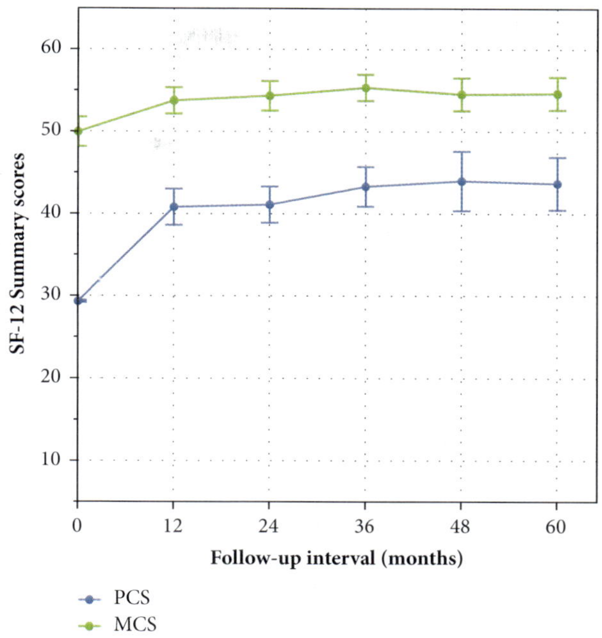

FIGURE 1: Time course of results for the physical component summary (PCS) and mental component summary (MCS) scores through 5 years of follow-up. Results presented as mean (95% CIs).

Of 189 patients initially randomized to Superion treatment, SF-12 questionnaire responses were captured in 144, 128, 96, 55, and 68 study subjects at 1, 2, 3, 4, and 5 years, respectively.

3. Results

Longitudinal changes in PCS and MCS scores through 5 years of follow-up are illustrated in Figure 1. The mean PCS score improved from 29.4 ± 8.1 preoperatively to 41.2 ± 12.4 at the 2-year primary trial endpoint and to 43.8 ± 11.6 at 5 years, representing average percentage improvements of 40% and 49%, respectively ($p<0.001$ for both comparisons). At 2 years, 81% (103 of 128) of subjects demonstrated maintenance or improvement in PCS scores. Similarly, 87% (59 of 68) of subjects who provided 5-year SF-12 responses continued to maintain or improve their PCS score.

The mean MCS score improved from 50.0 ± 12.7 preoperatively to 54.4 ± 10.6 and 54.7 ± 8.6 at 2 and 5 years, respectively, representing a 9% improvement at both follow-up intervals ($p>0.10$ for both comparisons). At 2 and 5 years, 60% (77 of 128) and 57% (39 of 68) of subjects showed maintenance or improvement in PCS scores.

4. Discussion

IPD treatment has been shown to provide durable condition-specific symptom amelioration through 5 years of follow-up [6]. The current findings extend these previous results and demonstrate significant improvement in overall well-being following IPD, particularly in the physical function domains of quality of life.

There has been a limited number of previous reports of the association between IPD and quality of life outcomes. Using a first-generation IPD spacer compared with conservative care in a randomized trial, Hsu et al. [15] evaluated quality of life using the SF-36 questionnaire instrument in patients with moderate lumbar spinal stenosis. At all posttreatment time points, mean SF-36 domain scores in IPD-treated patients were significantly greater than those in patients treated conservatively, with the exception of the mean general health (GH), role emotional, and MCS scores at 2 years. Additionally, mean posttreatment domain scores in IPD-treated patients were significantly greater than mean pretreatment scores, with the exception of mean GH scores. The results of this study demonstrated that IPD was significantly more effective than conservative care in improving the quality of life in patients with lumbar spinal stenosis.

Previously reported feasibility studies with the Superion spacer reported strikingly similar results to the current study in terms of improvements realized in physical functioning. In a pre-IDE study, Bini et al. [16] reported on a total of 121 patients with moderate lumbar spinal stenosis treated with IPD and followed for 12 months. Using the SF-36 questionnaire instrument, these authors reported a percentage improvement of 41% over preoperative scores for the PCS. Also employing the SF-36, Shabat et al. [17] found a PCS improvement of 40% in 53 IPD-treated patients with intermittent neurogenic claudication followed for 2 years.

Preoperatively, we noted significant impairment in the PCS scores of patients enrolled in this FDA-IDE trial, with an average value (29.4) that was more than 2 standard deviations below normal. Conversely, the mean preoperative MCS score (50.0) was identical to the US norm-based average, showing no impairment. These findings corroborate results reported from a large community-based sample of patients with lumbar spinal stenosis evaluated with the SF-36 [2]. In this observational study of 1,862 individuals, the presence of symptomatic lumbar spinal stenosis had a strong negative impact on the PCS, but not the MCS.

In a randomized trial comparing laminectomy with laminectomy plus fusion, Ghogawala et al. [18] also noted depressed preoperative PCS scores in patients with lumbar spinal stenosis (e.g., 34.7, laminectomy; 31.5, laminectomy/fusion). At 2 years postoperatively, percentage improvements in PCS were 27% and 48% for laminectomy and laminectomy plus fusion, respectively.

We demonstrated that IPD treatment improves PCS scores by > 40% through 5 years of postoperative follow-up. Importantly, mean posttreatment PCS scores increased to and remained consistently in the low-normal range, within one standard deviation of the US norm.

Because the IPD implantation procedure is performed in a minimally invasive fashion and causes only minor anatomical disruption, the full range of surgical options remains available if a revision becomes necessary to manage reemergence of symptoms. Thus, with simplicity of the operative procedure, rapid patient recovery, low surgical risk of complications, and long-term clinical durability, IPD remains a viable treatment option for stenosis patients.

5. Conclusions

In addition to its documented benefits on condition-specific efficacy outcomes, interspinous process decompression with a stand-alone spacer also offers significant improvement in overall health-related quality of life, particularly in areas of physical functioning.

Acknowledgments

The authors thank Terry Meredith for graphical assistance.

References

[1] S. Genevay and S. J. Atlas, "Lumbar spinal stenosis," *Best Practice & Research Clinical Rheumatology*, vol. 24, no. 2, pp. 253–265, 2010.

[2] K. Otani, S. Kikuchi, S. Yabuki et al., "Lumbar spinal stenosis has a negative impact on quality of life compared with other comorbidities: An epidemiological cross-sectional study of 1862 community-dwelling individuals," *The Scientific World Journal*, vol. 2013, Article ID 590652, 9 pages, 2013.

[3] V. Loguidice, W. Bini, S. Shabat, L. E. Miller, and J. E. Block, "Rationale, design and clinical performance of the Superion® Interspinous Spacer: a minimally invasive implant for treatment of lumbar spinal stenosis," *Expert Review of Medical Devices*, vol. 8, no. 4, pp. 419–426, 2011.

[4] L. E. Miller and J. E. Block, "Interspinous spacer implant in patients with lumbar spinal stenosis: preliminary results of a multicenter, randomized, controlled trial," *Pain Research & Management*, vol. 2012, Article ID 823509, 10 pages, 2012.

[5] P. D. Nunley, V. V. Patel, D. G. Orndorff, W. F. Lavelle, J. E. Block, and F. H. Geisler, "Superion Interspinous Spacer Treatment of Moderate Spinal Stenosis: 4-Year Results," *World Neurosurgery*, vol. 104, pp. 279–283, 2017.

[6] P. D. Nunley, V. V. Patel, D. Gorndorff, W. F. Lavelle, J. E. Block, and F. H. Geisler, "Five-year durability of stand-alone interspinous process decompression for lumbar spinal stenosis," *Clinical Interventions in Aging*, vol. 12, pp. 1409–1417, 2017.

[7] V. V. Patel, P. D. Nunley, P. G. Whang et al., "Superion® Interspinous spacer for treatment of moderate degenerative lumbar spinal stenosis: durable three-year results of a randomized controlled trial," *Journal of Pain Research*, vol. 8, pp. 657–662, 2015.

[8] V. V. Patel, P. G. Whang, T. R. Haley et al., "Superion interspinous process spacer for intermittent neurogenic claudication secondary to moderate lumbar spinal stenosis: two-year results from a randomized controlled FDA-IDE pivotal trial," *The Spine Journal*, vol. 40, no. 5, pp. 275–282, 2015.

[9] V. V. Patel, P. G. Whang, T. R. Haley et al., "Two-year clinical outcomes of a multicenter randomized controlled trial comparing two interspinous spacers for treatment of moderate lumbar spinal stenosis," *BMC Musculoskeletal Disorders*, vol. 15, no. 1, article 221, 2014.

[10] C. Lauryssen, R. J. Jackson, J. M. Baron et al., "Stand-alone interspinous spacer versus decompressive laminectomy for treatment of lumbar spinal stenosis," *Expert Review of Medical Devices*, vol. 12, no. 6, pp. 763–769, 2015.

[11] P. D. Nunley, A. N. Shamie, S. L. Blumenthal, D. Orndorff, J. E. Block, and F. H. Geisler, "Interspinous Process Decompression: Expanding Treatment Options for Lumbar Spinal Stenosis," *BioMed Research International*, vol. 2016, Article ID 3267307, 5 pages, 2016.

[12] J. E. Ware Jr., M. Kosinski, and S. D. Keller, "A 12-Item short-form health survey: construction of scales and preliminary tests of reliability and validity," *Medical Care*, vol. 34, no. 3, pp. 220–233, 1996.

[13] J. E. Ware, "SF-36 health survey update," *The Spine Journal*, vol. 25, no. 24, pp. 3130–3139, 2000.

[14] L. Busija, E. Pausenberger, T. P. Haines, S. Haymes, R. Buchbinder, and R. H. Osborne, "Adult measures of general health and health-related quality of life: Medical Outcomes Study Short Form 36-Item (SF-36) and Short Form 12-Item (SF-12) Health Surveys, Nottingham Health Profile (NHP), Sickness Impact Profile (SIP), Medical Outcomes Study Short Form 6D (SF-6D), Health Utilities Index Mark 3 (HUI3), Quality of Well-Being Scale (QWB), and Assessment of Quality of Life (AQ O L)," *Arthritis Care & Research*, vol. 63, no. 11, pp. S383–S412, 2011.

[15] K. Y. Hsu, J. F. Zucherman, C. A. Hartjen et al., "Quality of life of lumbar stenosis-treated patients in whom the X STOP interspinous device was implanted," *Journal of Neurosurgery: Spine*, vol. 5, no. 6, pp. 500–507, 2006.

[16] J. E. Block, "Minimally Invasive Treatment of Moderate Lumbar Spinal Stenosis with the Superion® Interspinous Spacer," *The Open Orthopaedics Journal* , vol. 5, no. 1, pp. 361–367, 2011.

[17] S. Shabat, L. E. Miller, J. E. Block, and R. Gepstein, "Minimally invasive treatment of lumbar spinal stenosis with a novel interspinous spacer," *Clinical Interventions in Aging*, vol. 6, no. 1, pp. 227–233, 2011.

[18] Z. Ghogawala, J. Dziura, W. E. Butler et al., "Laminectomy plus fusion versus laminectomy alone for lumbar spondylolisthesis," *The New England Journal of Medicine*, vol. 374, no. 15, pp. 1424–1434, 2016.

Differences in Epidural and Analgesic Use in Patients with Apparent Stage I Endometrial Cancer Treated by Open versus Laparoscopic Surgery: Results from the Randomised LACE Trial

Jannah Baker,[1] Monika Janda,[1] David Belavy,[2] and Andreas Obermair[3]

[1] *Queensland University of Technology, School of Public Health, Institute of Health and Biomedical Innovation, Brisbane, QLD 4059, Australia*
[2] *University of Queensland, School of Medicine, Brisbane, QLD 4072, Australia*
[3] *Queensland Centre for Gynaecological Cancer, Ned Hanlon Building, Butterfield St. Herston, Brisbane, QLD 4029, Australia*

Correspondence should be addressed to Andreas Obermair; andreas_obermair@health.qld.gov.au

Academic Editor: Diego Cuccurullo

Objectives. We compared postoperative analgesic requirements between women with early stage endometrial cancer treated by total abdominal hysterectomy (TAH) or total laparoscopic hysterectomy (TLH). *Methods.* 760 patients with apparent stage I endometrial cancer were treated in the international, multicentre, prospective randomised trial (LACE) by TAH ($n = 353$) or TLH ($n = 407$) (2005–2010). Epidural, opioid, and nonopioid analgesic requirements were collected until ten months after surgery. *Results.* Baseline demographics and analgesic use were comparable between treatment arms. TAH patients were more likely to receive epidural analgesia than TLH patients (33% versus 0.5%, $P < 0.001$) during the early postoperative phase. Although opioid use was comparable in the TAH versus TLH groups during postoperative 0–2 days (99.7% versus 98.5%, $P = 0.09$), a significantly higher proportion of TAH patients required opioids 3–5 days (70% versus 22%, $P < 0.0001$), 6–14 days (35% versus 15%, $P < 0.0001$), and 15–60 days (15% versus 9%, $P = 0.02$) after surgery. Mean pain scores were significantly higher in the TAH versus TLH group one (2.48 versus 1.62, $P < 0.0001$) and four weeks (0.89 versus 0.63, $P = 0.01$) following surgery. *Conclusion.* Treatment of early stage endometrial cancer with TLH is associated with less frequent use of epidural, lower post-operative opioid requirements, and better pain scores than TAH.

1. Introduction

Endometrial cancer is the most common gynaecological cancer in developed countries and the current standard of treatment is hysterectomy and bilateral salpingectomy using an open abdominal surgical approach [1]. Three recent clinical trials have shown that a laparoscopic approach to surgery results in shorter hospital stay and fewer adverse events compared with open surgery [2–5] and two of these trials found better quality of life outcomes [3, 5]. Epidural and nonepidural opioid analgesia may be used for pain management following both, open or laparoscopic surgery, and guidelines are available for anaesthetic prescription and monitoring [6]. Although epidural analgesia may decrease the risk of cardiovascular and pulmonary complications in high-risk patients undergoing major surgery, it is invasive, costly, time consuming, and labour intensive [7]. There is developing evidence that other forms of regional analgesia may be more cost effective without sacrificing efficacy [7, 8].

Minimally invasive procedures have been found to be associated with smaller postoperative analgesia requirements compared with open surgery in patients treated for gynaecological cancers [9–12] and in ovarian metastasectomy from gastric cancer [13]. There is also evidence that total laparoscopic hysterectomy (TLH) offers benefits over vaginal hysterectomy in terms of reduced opioid and NSAID analgesic requirements following surgery [14].

Minimally invasive procedures for endometrial cancer, including total laparoscopic, laparoscopic-assisted vaginal, or robotic-assisted laparoscopic hysterectomy, are associated with significantly reduced postoperative analgesic use compared with open abdominal laparotomic hysterectomy [5, 15–18]; however, these studies only followed patients' perioperative analgesic requirements and there is a lack of randomised clinical trials comparing postoperative analgesic use between open and minimally invasive treatment arms during a more extended period of time after surgery and a lack of data from the Australian context.

This report examines differences in postoperative opioid and analgesic prescription between patients with apparent stage I endometrial cancer undergoing TLH or total abdominal hysterectomy (TAH) and outcomes of these patients up to ten months after surgery.

2. Methods

The LACE trial (laparoscopic approach to cancer of the endometrium) commenced recruitment in October 2005, and a total of 760 women with apparent stage I endometrial cancer were enrolled by June 2010 through one of 20 participating tertiary gynaecological oncology centres in Australia, New Zealand, Switzerland, and Hong Kong. The trial design and methodology, as well as QOL and AE outcomes, have been previously described [3, 4]. Women were eligible if they were 18 years or older and had a histologically confirmed endometrioid adenocarcinoma of the endometrium of any grade, an Eastern Cooperative Oncology Group (ECOG) score of less than two, and imaging studies (computed tomography (CT) of the abdomen and pelvis and chest radiograph or chest CT) suggesting the absence of extrauterine disease. Patients were excluded if they had histological cell type other than endometrioid on curettage, clinically advanced disease (stage II–IV) or bulky lymph nodes on imaging, uterine size greater than 10 weeks of gestation, estimated life expectancy of less than 6 months, medically unfit for surgery, or patient compliance or geographic proximity preventing adequate followup or if they are unfit to complete quality of life questionnaires. FIGO 2009 staging criteria were used.

Overall, 407 patients were randomised to TLH and 353 to TAH using block randomisation stratified by centre and grade of differentiation. Surgeons involved in the trial were all accredited gynaecological oncologists who had completed at least 20 TLHs, submitted video footage of a TLH, and performed a TLH live in the presence of a senior accredited surgeon. Seven patients withdrew before completing six weeks followup and were included in baseline and perioperative analyses but excluded from long-term comparison of analgesic use.

Details of medication use including medication name, dose, frequency, unit, route of administration, start date, and end date of prescription were recorded for each patient by the trial nurses at each hospital. Information was collected in detail during the perioperative period and then during the patients' postoperative one-week, four-weeks, three-month and six-month data clinical followup. Recorded start dates and end dates of analgesic prescription were used to categorise analgesic use into more distinct periods of time, up to a maximum record of 310 days (ten months) postoperatively.

Free-text entries of all medication names were scanned and classified into drug classes by one medical professional. All drugs classified as analgesics were further categorised by one of the authors (J. Baker) in consultation with anaesthetists, into opioid and nonopioid analgesia, and opioid analgesics further classified by route of administration (epidural, parenteral, or oral).

2.1. Statistical Analysis. Intention-to-treat analysis was used. Baseline demographic and clinical characteristics were compared between treatment arms using descriptive statistics. Descriptive statistics and chi-squared tests of heterogeneity were used to compare epidural, parenteral, or oral opioid requirements within two days of surgery and postoperative opioid and nonopioid analgesic requirements up to 10 months following surgery between treatment arms, based on comparisons of prescription start and end dates to date of surgery. Perioperative opioid use within two days of surgery was categorized by the most invasive route of administration for each patient. Long-term use of analgesics was explored by counting each patient in more than one analgesic category if they were prescribed more than one type of analgesic class. t-tests were used to compare postoperative pain scores between treatment arms.

3. Results

Within the TAH group ($N = 353$), 247 patients underwent a vertical midline incision, and 99 had a low abdominal transverse incisions. Among the TLH group, 24 patients needed to be converted and 11 of these underwent a vertical midline incision. Five patients randomised to TAH requested and received a TLH procedure (overall conversion rate 3.8%). Baseline characteristics and analgesic use were comparable between treatment arms, with 67% of patients overall not taking any analgesia, 29% taking nonopioid, and 3% taking opioid analgesia (Table 1).

Overall, 121/353 (34%) TAH and 2/407 (0.5%) TLH patients received pain relief through an epidural during the study period ($P < 0.0001$). At data collection two days after surgery, significantly more patients with TAH (116/353; 33%) had received an epidural compared with 2/407 (0.5%) of TLH patients ($P < 0.0001$, Table 2). Mean pain scores were significantly higher in the TAH versus TLH group at one week (2.48 versus 1.62, $P < 0.0001$), four weeks (0.89 versus 0.63, $P = 0.01$), and six months (0.45 versus 0.27, $P = 0.04$), but not at three months following surgery (Table 2).

During the first two postoperative days, although a similar proportion of patients in the TAH or TLH groups were prescribed opioid analgesia (99.7% versus 98.5%, $P = 0.09$) and NSAIDS (61% versus 60%, $P = 0.7$), a significantly higher proportion of TAH patients required Paracetamol (98% versus 95%, $P = 0.03$). At 3–5 days after surgery, significantly higher proportions of patients allocated to TAH required opioid analgesia (70% versus 22%, $P < 0.0001$),

TABLE 1

	TLH (N = 407)	TAH (N = 353)
Age in years, mean (SD)	63 (10)	63 (11)
BMI category†	n (%)	n (%)
Normal (18.50–24.99)	47 (12)	46 (14)
Overweight (25.00–29.99)	98 (25)	72 (21)
Obesity class I (30.00–34.99)	77 (20)	87 (26)
Obesity class II (35.00–39.99)	81 (21)	61 (18)
Obesity class III (≥40)	86 (22)	74 (22)
Education		
Completed ≤12 years of school	270 (70)	232 (70)
Completed >12 years of school	118 (30)	99 (30)
Employment		
Retired	170 (44)	134 (40)
Employed full time	55 (14)	42 (13)
Employed part time or casual	44 (11)	54 (16)
Other	119 (31)	101 (31)
Marital status		
Married or living together	243 (63)	212 (64)
Other	145 (37)	119 (36)
Private health insurance		
Yes	101 (26)	90 (27)
No	287 (74)	241 (73)
Income		
Less than AUS$40,000	261 (67)	207 (62)
AUS$40,000+	83 (21)	82 (25)
Not answered	44 (11)	42 (13)
Birth country		
Australia	249 (64)	219 (66)
Other	139 (36)	112 (34)
ECOG performance status		
0	352 (86)	303 (86)
1	55 (14)	50 (14)
Baseline analgesic use (pts categorised by strongest class taken)		
No analgesia	273 (67)	239 (68)
Nonopioid analgesia	120 (29)	103 (29)
Opioid analgesia	14 (3)	11 (3)

Data are number of patients (%). TLH: total laparoscopic hysterectomy. TAH: total abdominal hysterectomy. BMI: body mass index. ECOG: Eastern Cooperative Oncology Group. Numbers do not always add up to 760 because of missing demographic data. †Based on WHO categories.

NSAIDs (38% versus 21%, $P < 0.0001$), and Paracetamol (91% versus 62%, $P < 0.0001$). This effect persisted at 6–14 days after surgery, with significantly higher proportions of patients allocated to TAH still requiring opioid analgesia (35% versus 15%, $P < 0.0001$), NSAIDs (24% versus 15%, $P = 0.003$), and Paracetamol (65% versus 46%, $P < 0.0001$). At 15–60 days after surgery, a significantly higher proportion in the TAH group still required opioid analgesia (15% versus 9%, $P = 0.02$) and Paracetamol (40% versus 28%, $P = 0.0004$), but a similar proportion in both treatment arms required NSAIDs (13% versus 9%, $P = 0.2$). Analgesic use was comparable between groups after 60 days after surgery (Table 3).

TABLE 2: Opioid use ≤2 days after surgery.

	TLH (N = 407) n (%)	TAH (N = 353) n (%)	P value
Route of postoperative opioid use*			
Epidural	2 (0.5)	116 (33)	
Parenteral	392 (96)	230 (65)	
Oral	5 (1)	2 (0.6)	
Nil	8 (2)	5 (1)	
	Mean (SD)	Mean (SD)	
Painscore			
Week 1	1.62 (2.01)	2.48 (2.13)	<0.0001
Week 4	0.63 (1.34)	0.89 (1.5)	0.01
Month 3	0.48 (1.39)	0.54 (1.26)	0.59
Month 6	0.27 (0.98)	0.45 (1.27)	0.04

*Patients categorised by the most invasive route of administration.

4. Discussion

Although patients undergoing TAH or TLH required narcotic analgesia for the first two days after surgery, those undergoing TLH recovered faster and fewer required analgesia by day three after surgery. This difference in analgesic requirements between the treatment groups persisted until after two months following surgery. Both the surgical approach and the epidural procedure could have contributed to these findings, as well as the greater prevalence of adverse surgical events observed among the TAH group [4]. Despite advances in the aftercare for patients with TAH, such as through fast-track surgical care [19], a significantly greater number of women require epidural analgesia for open abdominal compared to laparoscopic surgery for stage I endometrial cancer. As the LACE trial was unblinded, the anaesthetic prescription choices of the anaesthetists can be influenced by the planned procedure. As TAH patients require hospital care for a significantly longer time than TLH patients [4, 5, 20] providing an epidural conforms with recommendations to lessen the risk of prolonged immobilisation and the subsequent risk of thromboembolism in oncology patients [6, 21]. On the other hand, there is little evidence of decreased perioperative morbidity or mortality with epidural analgesia, particularly in the low to medium risk surgical population [7].

Our study is in agreement with a smaller Phase III trial conducted in the Netherlands which compared clinical and postoperative outcomes in 283 patients treated within 21 hospitals who were assigned to either laparoscopic or the standard procedure of open surgery for early stage endometrial cancer. Similar to the present study, this trial found the duration of pain after surgery to be significantly

TABLE 3: Postoperative analgesic use, excluding 7 pts without 6-week followup*.

	TLH (N = 404) n (%)	TAH (N = 349) n (%)	P value
Analgesic classes 0–2 days after surgery			
Opioid	398 (98.5)	348 (99.7)	0.09
NSAID	242 (60)	214 (61)	0.69
Paracetamol	384 (95)	342 (98)	0.03
No analgesia	—	—	
Analgesic classes 3–5 days after surgery			
Opioid	87 (22)	246 (70)	<0.0001
NSAID	86 (21)	132 (38)	<0.0001
Paracetamol	252 (62)	317 (91)	<0.0001
No analgesia	125 (31)	14 (4)	
Analgesic classes 6–14 days after surgery			
Opioid	60 (15)	121 (35)	<0.0001
NSAID	61 (15)	82 (24)	0.0034
Paracetamol	187 (46)	227 (65)	<0.0001
No analgesia	190 (47)	86 (25)	
Analgesic classes 15–60 days after surgery			
Opioid	37 (9)	52 (15)	0.015
NSAID	37 (9)	44 (13)	0.24
Paracetamol	112 (28)	139 (40)	0.0004
No analgesia	271 (67)	180 (52)	
Analgesic classes 61–150 days after surgery			
Opioid	23 (6)	20 (6)	0.98
NSAID	20 (5)	20 (6)	0.63
Paracetamol	42 (10)	48 (14)	0.16
No analgesia	342 (85)	282 (81)	
Analgesic classes 151–310 days after surgery			
Opioid	13 (3)	10 (3)	0.78
NSAID	12 (3)	11 (3)	0.89
Paracetamol	19 (5)	16 (5)	0.94
No analgesia	369 (91)	319 (91)	

NSAID: nonsteroidal anti-inflammatory drugs.
*Patients counted more than once if taking more than one analgesic class.

shorter for TLH versus TAH patients (median 3 (0–7) versus 5 days (0–7), $P < 0.0001$) [22]. However, this smaller trial followed analgesic outcomes perioperatively only, did not compare epidural use between treatment arms, did not distinguish between different classes of analgesia, and did not use or report pain score outcomes.

Our study findings are also similar to those of a prospective cohort study which found that women undergoing either laparoscopic or robotic surgery for endometrial cancer reported little need for opioid analgesia (45% did not require any analgesia, 34% required nonopioid analgesia, and only 21% required opioid analgesia) at 3-4 weeks after surgery [23]. In our study, during the comparable time period of 15–60 days after surgery, few patients undergoing TLH surgery had requirement for opioids (67% did not require analgesia, 28% required Paracetamol, 9% required NSAIDs, and 9% required opioid analgesia). Our study also supports findings from a prospective cohort study comparing minimally invasive surgery to open surgery [15]. This study involved 182 consecutive patients undergoing surgery for early endometrial cancer or endometrial hyperplasia with atypia and found that the patients receiving laparoscopically assisted vaginal hysterectomy (LAVH) (N = 74) had less need for analgesia than those receiving TAH (N = 108). Postoperatively, the laparotomy surgery group also had more frequent prolonged use of epidural analgesia than the LAVH group (72% versus 49%, $P < 0.01$).

A retrospective analysis compared 181 consecutive patients with endometrial cancer undergoing open (N = 97) or minimally invasive staging hysterectomy (N = 84) including LAVH, TLH, or robotic-assisted laparoscopic hysterectomy using the da Vinci Surgical System, with or without lymphadenectomy [16]. This study found that in the open group, median surgery time was shorter (197 versus 288 minutes, $P < 0.0001$). Median narcotic (13 versus 43 mg morphine equivalents; $P < 0.0001$) and antiemetic (43% versus 25%; $P = 0.01$) needs, however, were lower for minimally invasive surgery already in the first 24 hours postoperatively.

A systematic review summarised the safety and efficacy of TLH versus open surgery in women with endometrial cancer and included 4 randomised clinical trials. This review specifically highlighted the reduced need for analgesia among women as one of the benefits of laparoscopic surgery [14, 17].

Besides the specific evidence related to endometrial cancer surgery to which the present study adds, there is also evidence that analgesic requirements and pain are reduced when minimally invasive surgery is applied to other gynaecological malignant conditions [11, 12] and are also less for women undergoing laparoscopic surgery for benign gynaecological conditions compared with an open surgical approach [10, 20]. For example, a review article examining surgical treatment for obese women with endometrial, cervical, and ovarian cancer found evidence that laparoscopic surgery was associated with less postoperative pain compared with open surgery [9].

Strengths of the present study include the fact that analgesic prescription can be compared between treatment arms within the context of a randomised clinical trial, a long follow-up period, distinction between different analgesic classes, inclusion of pain score comparisons, and the fact that a lower conversion rate than previous trials allows clearer inferences to be made regarding treatment arms. Limitations include the fact that the trial was unblinded, biasing decision-making for epidural and analgesic prescription.

In summary, the results of this study show that laparoscopic surgery for endometrial cancer is associated with less need for epidural and postoperative analgesic prescription compared with open surgery, saving on costs of analgesia and highlighting a further significant benefit to patients and the healthcare system of laparoscopic treatment over traditional open abdominal surgery.

Acknowledgments

The authors thankfully acknowledge Drs. Sue Lawrence and Hau Tan for their assistance with analgesic classification and comments on previous versions of this paper.

References

[1] W. T. Creasman, C. P. Morrow, B. N. Bundy, H. D. Homesley, J. E. Graham, and P. B. Heller, "Surgical pathologic spread patterns of endometrial cancer. A gynecologic oncology group study," *Cancer*, vol. 60, no. 8, supplement, pp. 2035–2041, 1987.

[2] J. L. Walker, M. R. Piedmonte, N. M. Spirtos et al., "Laparoscopy compared with laparotomy for comprehensive surgical staging of uterine cancer: Gynecologic Oncology Group Study LAP2," *Journal of Clinical Oncology*, vol. 27, no. 32, pp. 5331–5336, 2009.

[3] M. Janda, V. Gebski, A. Brand et al., "Quality of life after total laparoscopic hysterectomy versus total abdominal hysterectomy for stage I endometrial cancer (LACE): a randomised trial," *The Lancet Oncology*, vol. 11, no. 8, pp. 772–780, 2010.

[4] A. Obermair, M. Janda, J. Baker et al., "Improved surgical safety after laparoscopic compared to open surgery for apparent early stage endometrial cancer: results from a randomised controlled trial," *European Journal of Cancer*, vol. 48, no. 8, pp. 1147–1153, 2012.

[5] M. J. E. Mourits, C. B. Bijen, H. J. Arts et al., "Safety of laparoscopy versus laparotomy in early-stage endometrial cancer: a randomised trial," *The Lancet Oncology*, vol. 11, no. 8, pp. 763–771, 2010.

[6] L. Powell and J. M. Garfield, "Anesthetic considerations for gynecologic cancer surgery," *Seminars in Surgical Oncology*, vol. 6, no. 3, pp. 194–198, 1990.

[7] N. Rawal, "Epidural technique for postoperative pain: gold standard no more?" *Regional Anesthesia and Pain Medicine*, vol. 37, no. 3, pp. 310–317, 2012.

[8] P. Tilleul, M. Aissou, F. Bocquet, N. Thiriat, O. le Grelle, M. Burke et al., "Cost-effectiveness analysis comparing epidural, patient-controlled intravenous morphine, and continuous wound infiltration for postoperative pain management after open abdominal surgery," *British Journal of Anaesthesia*, vol. 108, no. 6, pp. 998–1005, 2012.

[9] I. E. Martinek, K. Haldar, and R. Tozzi, "Laparoscopic surgery for gynaecological cancers in obese women," *Maturitas*, vol. 65, no. 4, pp. 320–324, 2010.

[10] L. R. Medeiros, A. T. Stein, J. Fachel, R. Garry, and S. Furness, "Laparoscopy versus laparotomy for benign ovarian tumor: a systematic review and meta-analysis," *International Journal of Gynecological Cancer*, vol. 18, no. 3, pp. 387–399, 2008.

[11] R. Naik, K. S. Jackson, A. Lopes, P. Cross, and J. A. Henry, "Laparoscopic assisted radical vaginal hysterectomy versus radical abdominal hysterectomy—a randomised phase II trial: perioperative outcomes and surgicopathological measurements," *British Journal of Obstetrics and Gynaecology*, vol. 117, no. 6, pp. 746–751, 2010.

[12] M. Lee, W. S. Kim, J. Paek et al., "Comparisons of surgical outcomes, complications, and costs between laparotomy and laparoscopy in early-stage ovarian cancer," *International Journal of Gynecological Cancer*, vol. 21, no. 2, pp. 251–256, 2011.

[13] M. Lee, J. Paek, S. H. Lee et al., "Feasibility and surgical outcomes of laparoscopic metastasectomy in the treatment of ovarian metastases from gastric cancer," *International Journal of Gynecological Cancer*, vol. 21, no. 7, pp. 1306–1311, 2011.

[14] M. C. Nascimento, A. Kelley, C. Martitsch, I. Weidner, and A. Obermair, "Postoperative analgesic requirements—total laparoscopic hysterectomy versus vaginal hysterectomy," *Australian and New Zealand Journal of Obstetrics and Gynaecology*, vol. 45, no. 2, pp. 140–143, 2005.

[15] O. Devaja, I. Samara, and A. J. Papadopoulos, "Laparoscopically assisted vaginal hysterectomy (LAVH) versus total abdominal hysterectomy (TAH) in endometrial carcinoma: prospective cohort study," *International Journal of Gynecological Cancer*, vol. 20, no. 4, pp. 570–575, 2010.

[16] N. D. Fleming, L. J. Havrilesky, F. A. Valea et al., "Analgesic and antiemetic needs following minimally invasive vs open staging for endometrial cancer," *American Journal of Obstetrics and Gynecology*, vol. 204, no. 1, pp. 65.el–65.e6, 2011.

[17] S. G. de la Orden, M. M. Reza, J. A. Blasco, E. Andradas, D. Callejo, and T. Pérez, "Laparoscopic hysterectomy in the treatment of endometrial cancer: a systematic review," *Journal of Minimally Invasive Gynecology*, vol. 15, no. 4, pp. 395–401, 2008.

[18] M. A. Martino, J. Shubella, M. B. Thomas et al., "A cost analysis of postoperative management in endometrial cancer patients treated by robotics versus laparoscopic approach," *Gynecologic Oncology*, vol. 123, no. 3, pp. 528–531, 2011.

[19] J. Carter and R. Szabo, "Fast track surgery: a clinical audit," *Australian and New Zealand Journal of Obstetrics and Gynaecology*, vol. 50, no. 2, pp. 159–163, 2010.

[20] T. E. Nieboer, N. Johnson, A. Lethaby et al., "Surgical approach to hysterectomy for benign gynaecological disease," *Cochrane Database of Systematic Reviews*, no. 3, Article ID CD003677, 2009.

[21] C. B. M. Bijen, J. M. Briët, G. H. de Bock, H. J. G. Arts, J. A. Bergsma-Kadijk, and M. J. E. Mourits, "Total laparoscopic hysterectomy versus abdominal hysterectomy in the treatment of patients with early stage endometrial cancer: a randomized multi center study," *BMC Cancer*, vol. 9, article 23, 2009.

[22] M. J. E. Mourits, C. B. Bijen, H. J. Arts et al., "Safety of laparoscopy versus laparotomy in early-stage endometrial cancer: a randomised trial," *The Lancet Oncology*, vol. 11, no. 8, pp. 763–771, 2010.

[23] S. Lau, K. Buzaglo, Z. Vaknin et al., "Relationship between body mass index and robotic surgery outcomes of women diagnosed with endometrial cancer," *International Journal of Gynecological Cancer*, vol. 21, no. 4, pp. 722–729, 2011.

31

Challenges and Results of Laparoscopic Splenectomy for Hematological Diseases in a Developing Country

Vikal Chandra Shakya,[1] Bikram Byanjankar,[1] Rabin Pandit,[1] Anang Pangeni,[1] Anir Ram Moh Shrestha,[1] and Bishesh Poudyal[2]

[1] *Department of Surgery, Civil Service Hospital of Nepal, Kathmandu, Nepal*
[2] *Clinical Hematology and Bone Marrow Transplant Unit, Department of Medicine, Civil Service Hospital of Nepal, Kathmandu, Nepal*

Correspondence should be addressed to Vikal Chandra Shakya; vikalcsh@yahoo.com

Academic Editor: Diego Cuccurullo

Introduction. Though, in developed countries, laparoscopy is now a gold standard for splenectomy, we are lacking in this aspect in the eastern world. Splenectomy has mostly been performed by open surgery in our region. This is our effort to introduce laparoscopic splenectomy in our country. *Methods.* This is a retrospective cohort study done in patients presenting to hematology and surgery department of our hospital who underwent laparoscopic splenectomy for hematological diseases from January 2013 to December 2016. *Results.* There were 50 patients (38 females, 12 males). The diagnoses were idiopathic thrombocytopenic purpura in 31, (steroid/azathioprine-resistant, steroid dependent), hereditary spherocytosis in 9, alpha-thalassemia in 3, beta-thalassemia in 2, autoimmune hemolytic anemia in 4, and isolated splenic tuberculosis in 1. Average platelet counts preoperatively were 62000 ± 11000/mm3 (range 52000-325000/mm3). The mean operative time was 130 ± 49 minutes (range 108-224 min). The mean postoperative stay was 4 ± 2.11 days (range 3-9 days). Laparoscopic splenectomy could be completed in 45 (90%) patients. *Conclusion.* Laparoscopic splenectomy could be successfully contemplated in patients with hematological diseases, especially if spleen is normal or only mildly enlarged, and is an advantageous alternative to open splenectomy. Absence of ideal resources has not limited our progress in minimal access approach.

1. Introduction

After the first report of laparoscopic splenectomy in 1991, this technique has been rapidly established to be a safe and effective treatment for a range of benign and malignant hematological conditions [1, 2]. It is associated with low morbidity rates of 18–26% [2–4] and zero mortality in some series [5–7], with others recently reporting mortality of up to 4% [2, 4, 8–12]. The hospital stay is also shorter [7, 13], and the conversion rate to open operation is reported at 0–15% in recent series [14–19]. Though laparoscopic splenectomy has been well accepted in the developed countries, advanced laparoscopic surgeries have been largely eluded in a country like ours. However, we have ventured to perform laparoscopic splenectomy in our country. The aim of this study was to evaluate the results of a single-center single-surgeon experience of laparoscopic splenectomy in patients with hematological diseases.

2. Methods

This is a retrospective cohort study done of prospective maintained data of all patients undergoing laparoscopic splenectomy for hematological diseases between January 2013 and December 2016 at Civil Service Hospital of Nepal, a government hospital at our capital Kathmandu, by a single surgeon. The methodology has been adapted from personal series by Paddenden et al. [20]. The data included patient age, hematological diagnosis, duration of operation, operative blood loss, size of spleen, conversion to open, postoperative complications, length of hospital stay, mortality, and the duration of follow-up.

Table 1: Operative characteristics.

	Mean	Median	Standard deviation	Range
Operating time (in min)	130	130	49	108-224
Blood loss (in ml)	456	253	120	Negligible to 1600
Time of orally allowing (in hrs)	8	8	3.2	6-24
Total postoperative stay (in days)	4	4	2.1	3-9
Total hospital stay (in days)	6	7	2.52	4-12

Exclusion criteria were as follows:

(1) Traumatic splenic injury

(2) Splenectomy when combined with other operations as distal pancreatectomy, gastrectomy, and cholecystectomy

(3) Massive splenomegaly: a spleen palpable inferior and to the right of the umbilicus

(4) Preoperative low platelet counts <50000/ml.

The patients were also evaluated with radiological investigations to determine the size of the spleen, usually by ultrasonography, and computed tomography in case of large spleens and doubtful diagnosis. Vaccinations and antibiotic prophylaxis were given in accordance with the guidelines of the British Committee for Standards in Hematology; all patients were immunized against pneumococcus, hemophilus, and meningococcus at least 2 weeks preoperatively and influenza vaccine annually [21]. Antithrombotic prophylaxis was not given to patients with ITP which is an inherent bleeding disorder; in all other patients with normal platelet counts like in thalassemia, antithrombotic prophylaxis was given.

Patients were subjected to general anesthesia, paralyzed, and ventilated. Prophylactic antibiotic Ceftriaxone 1gm stat was given during induction of the anesthesia. They were positioned in a right, lateral, semisupine (60°) position [3]. A 10-mm umbilical port was inserted with an open technique using a blunt Hassan trocar at the midclavicular line. The remaining ports were inserted under direct vision. These consisted of three further ports, two in the left flank (10 mm and 5 mm ports), and one 5-mm port in the epigastrium, just inferior to the xiphoid process. A 30° scope was used in all cases. The spleens were mobilized with a combination of monopolar, bipolar cautery (Valleylab cautery machine), and ultrasonic energy source (Ethicon Harmonic, USA) when available. After opening the gastrocolic ligament by dividing the short gastric vessels, the hilar vessels and short gastric vessels were individually identified and divided between Hem-o-lok clips (Weg, UK). Staplers or mass ligation has not been used. The lienorenal ligament and lienophrenic ligament are divided with a combination of monopolar diathermy hook and scissors. The spleens were placed in endogenous bags made of urobags (Romo-10, India) with mouth sutured with retractable silk suture and morcellated intracorporeally with help of sponge-holding forceps, and Yankauer suction tip through the 10 mm port; and the spleen was retracted piecemeal through the midclavicular port with the urobag intact protecting the wound as well. Depending upon subjective assessment of the hemostasis, occasionally, 14-Fr suction drains (Romovac-Romson, India) were placed in the splenic beds. For large spleen, when the spleen was not possible to be kept in a bag and in which splenectomy was performed for diagnostic purposes, the spleen was delivered through transverse left lumbar or Pfannenstiel incision. The patients were transferred to a surgical postoperative ward for 4-hourly observations of pulse, blood pressure, and temperature. The following morning, the hemoglobin and platelet count were checked. The drains, if present, were removed provided the drainage was less than 50 ml over 24 hours. They were monitored for consequent hemoglobin and platelet increases daily and chest x-rays and ultrasound of the abdomen if any problems. Patients were discharged with oral analgesia once they were sufficiently comfortable, antibiotics for 7 days postoperatively, and their observations were satisfactory. The patients were seen once in general surgical outpatients to ensure good healing of wounds. The hematological follow-up depended upon the underlying diagnosis.

3. Results

During the study period, there were 50 consecutive laparoscopic splenectomies performed. There were 50 patients (38 females, 12 males). The mean age of presentation was 28 ± 10 years (range 14-56). The mean duration of symptoms was 4.65 ± 2.78 years (range 1.3-12.23 years). The average splenic size determined preoperatively was 13.45 ± 6.26 cm (range 10-23.5 cm). The diagnosis was Idiopathic Thrombocytopenic Purpura in 31 (steroid/azathioprine-resistant, steroid dependent), hereditary spherocytosis in 9, alpha-thalassemia in 3, beta-thalassemia in 2, autoimmune hemolytic anemia in 4, and isolated splenic TB in 1. Average platelet counts preoperatively was 62000 ± 11000/mm3 (range 52000-325000/mm3). The mean operative time was 130 ± 49 minutes (range 108-224 min) (Table 1). Average blood loss was 456 ml (from negligible to 1600 ml). Laparoscopic splenectomy could be completed in 45 (90%) patients. The remaining 5 (10%) needed conversion to open (causes being excessive bleeding from the splenic vein, splenic capsular tear and excessively low platelet counts with gross oozing) (Table 2). Five patients needed an additional Pfannenstiel or lumbar incision to retrieve the spleen after completion of procedure laparoscopically. Splenunculi (accessory spleens) were noted and excised from 3 patients in this series (6%). Postoperative morbidities were seen in 8 patients (16%). Postoperatively, one patient developed splenic and partial portal vein thrombosis and started on heparin and later warfarin; he was monitored with repeat Doppler ultrasonography of the abdomen; his

TABLE 2: Postoperative complications.

	Complications	n	%
1	Mortality	0	0
2	Pneumonia	2	4
3	Splenic and portal vein thrombosis	1	4
4	Subcutaneous hematoma	1	2
5.	Intraoperative hemorrhage	5	10

vessels recanalized at 1.5 years of follow-up without any symptoms, and he is presently off warfarin. Packed cell transfusion was needed in 7 (18.52%) patients. Postoperative pneumonia occurred in 2 of the converted ones, none in the laparoscopic group (4%). The mean postoperative stay was 4 ± 2.11 days (range 3-9 days). One patient developed small hematoma at one 10 mm port site, which required opening of the skin sutures. No patients developed a pancreatic fistula. Rise of platelet counts could be seen up to 12 lakhs/mm3. Steroids and/or azathioprine could be stopped in all patients except one; he still needed low-dose steroids to keep platelet count around 50,000/mm3 at 2.47 years of follow-up. Rise of hemoglobin was seen up to 16gm/dl. The 30-day mortality rate was zero. No other long-term complications were noted.

4. Discussion

Advanced laparoscopic surgery has largely been eluded in Nepal due to lack of resources and poverty. Earlier reports have mostly been of laparoscopic cholecystectomy and appendectomy and one of laparoscopic hernia [22–25]. Although laparoscopic splenectomy had been introduced in 2010 in Nepal with a laparoscopic-assisted splenectomy [22], this is the first attempt of contribution to advanced laparoscopic surgery such as splenectomy in largest volume from any center in Nepal. This series of 50 laparoscopic splenectomies by a single surgeon is a step to introduction and establishment of advanced laparoscopic surgery in the region.

Regarding the epidemiology of the diseases for which splenectomy was done, beta-thalassemia trait is the most common hemoglobinopathy in Nepal, hemoglobinopathy being found in 6.66% of the normal population in a screening study in Nepal [26]. Though, in our series, hereditary spherocytosis is the most common cause of anemia for which splenectomy was done. Other than hemoglobinopathies, ITP is also a common blood disorder in Nepalese population and is frequently seen in young women [27]. Poudyal et al. have studied azathioprine as second-line modality for ITP patients; we have studied in those patients who were both azathioprine and steroid refractory/dependent [27]. Shrestha et al. have established open splenectomy to have significant response for these patients before; we have ventured via minimally invasive approach [28]. Most patients due to their inability to afford other expensive options as IVIG and Rituximab accept splenectomy relatively readily.

Splenectomy is not without morbidity and mortalities, and laparoscopic splenectomy is one of the advanced laparoscopic surgeries. We always had an inhibition as whether we would be successful in stepping up from basic laparoscopic surgery. However, we dared to progress, with acquirement of some expensive resources like ultrasonic energy. And here we are, with acceptable morbidity rates of 16% and zero mortality, which is comparable to other studies in the literature [2, 5, 7–10]. However, these resources are still far from ideal as in developed countries, like the endocatch bag, morcellators, and endostaplers which add to the cost of the surgeries, though their use has been reported to decrease the operative time. Ultrasonic energy could be used when the hand shears were available; in about half of all cases, they were not available and dissection was done with the help of monopolar and bipolar diathermy. In addition, the mean operating time of 130 min compares favorably and the mean hospital stay of 7 days is comparable to the majority of other series [11–15]. The conversion rate to open splenectomy was 10% for this series, again comparing favorably to results in the literature [2–6, 9, 10, 14, 15, 18, 19].

There are two approaches to laparoscopic splenectomy: anterior and lateral [3]. We learnt the lateral approach; we still have not attempted laparoscopy in very large spleens (which reach below the umbilicus), in which the anterior approach is more appropriate. In lateral approach the large spleen hanging would obliterate the operative space. Laparoscopic splenectomy for such massive splenomegaly still remains controversial and has traditionally been contraindicated [7]. Data in the literature have demonstrated an increased risk of hemorrhage, morbidity, and conversion to open procedure [29–31]. However, it is well proven from literature that laparoscopic splenectomy is now universally accepted due to low postsurgical pain, hospital stay, low incidence of postoperative pulmonary complications, and wound related complications. Like other solid organs laparoscopy procedures, it possesses specific technical challenges like lack of tactile feedback, difficult assessment of accessory spleens, need of advanced energy sources like harmonic scalpel and endostapler because of inherent possibility of bleeding especially in low platelet counts, and finally the technically demanding manipulation for removal of spleen without breaking the capsule of the spleen [32–34]. All these reasons make this a technically difficult procedure with steep learning curve. However, these can be overcome with continuing experience of the surgeon and persistent perseverance towards continuation of the procedure.

5. Conclusion

This case series is one of a series of totally laparoscopic splenectomy in a developing country, which could be successfully contemplated in patients with hematological diseases, especially if the spleen is normal or mildly enlarged. Absence of ideal resources has not limited our progress in minimal access approach. This initial report highlights the safety of laparoscopic splenectomy and expands the horizons of laparoscopic splenectomy and advanced laparoscopic surgery in a developing country like ours.

Abbreviations

mm: Millimeter
Fr: French
ml: Milliliter
ITP: Idiopathic thrombocytopenic purpura.

Consent

All participants provided written informed consent to participate in this study.

Authors' Contributions

Anang Pangeni, Vikal Chandra Shakya, and Bishesh Poudyal made substantial contributions to concept and design of the article and acquisition of materials. Bikram Byanjankar, Anir Ram Moh Shrestha, and Rabin Pandit contributed significantly to critical revision and drafting the manuscript. All authors read and approved the final version of the manuscript

References

[1] B. Delaitre and B. Maignien, "Splenectomy by the laparoscopic approach. Report of a case," *La Presse Médicale*, vol. 20, no. 44, article 2263, 1991.

[2] M. Casaccia, P. Torelli, S. Squarcia et al., "Laparoscopic splenectomy for hematologic diseases: a preliminary analysis performed on the Italian Registry of Laparoscopic Surgery of the Spleen (IRLSS)," *Surgical Endoscopy*, vol. 20, no. 8, pp. 1214–1220, 2006.

[3] C. Palanivelu, K. Jani, V. Malladi, R. Shetty, R. Senthilkumar, and G. Maheshkumar, "Early ligation of the splenic artery in the leaning spleen approach to laparoscopic splenectomy," *Journal of Laparoendoscopic & Advanced Surgical Techniques*, vol. 16, no. 4, pp. 339–344, 2006.

[4] G. Silecchia, C. E. Boru, A. Fantini et al., "Laparoscopic splenectomy in the management of benign and malignant hematologic diseases.," *JSLS : Journal of the Society of Laparoendoscopic Surgeons / Society of Laparoendoscopic Surgeons*, vol. 10, no. 2, pp. 199–205, 2006.

[5] T. Sammour, G. Poole, A. Bartlett, and H. Blacklock, "Laparoscopic splenectomy at Middlemore Hospital, New Zealand: A safe procedure with heterogeneous indications," *The New Zealand Medical Journal*, vol. 119, no. 1230, 2006.

[6] F. G. Qureshi, O. Ergun, V. C. Sandulache, E. P. Nadler, H. R. Ford, and D. J. Hackam, "Laparoscopic splenectomy in children," *Journal of the Society of Laparoendoscopic Surgeons*, vol. 9, pp. 389–392, 2005.

[7] A. Owera, A. M. Hamade, O. I. Bani Hani, and B. J. Ammori, "Laparoscopic versus open splenectomy for massive splenomegaly: A comparative study," *Journal of Laparoendoscopic & Advanced Surgical Techniques*, vol. 16, no. 3, pp. 241–246, 2006.

[8] J.-M. Wu, I.-R. Lai, R.-H. Yuan, and S.-C. Yu, "Laparoscopic splenectomy for idiopathic thrombocytopenic purpura," *The American Journal of Surgery*, vol. 187, no. 6, pp. 720–723, 2004.

[9] R. Pugliese, F. Sansonna, I. Scandroglio et al., "Laparoscopic splenectomy: A retrospective review of 75 cases," *International Surgery*, vol. 91, no. 2, pp. 82–86, 2006.

[10] A. E. Canda, Y. Ozsoy, and S. Yuksel, "Laparoscopic Splenectomy Using LigaSure in Benign Hematologic Diseases," *Surgical Laparoscopy, Endoscopy & Percutaneous Techniques*, vol. 19, no. 1, pp. 69–71, 2009.

[11] V. Mahatharadol and S. Meesiri, "Results of laparoscopic splenectomy for immune thrombocytopenic purpura," *Journal of the Medical Association of Thailand*, vol. 89, no. 6, pp. 821–825, 2006.

[12] A. Pomp, M. Gagner, B. Salky et al., "Laparoscopic Splenectomy: A Selected Retrospective Review," *Surgical Laparoscopy, Endoscopy & Percutaneous Techniques*, vol. 15, no. 3, pp. 139–143, 2005.

[13] S. W. Grahn, J. Alvarez III, and K. Kirkwood, "Trends in laparoscopic splenectomy for massive splenomegaly," *JAMA Surgery*, vol. 141, no. 8, pp. 755–761, 2006.

[14] A. Bedirli, E. M. Sozuer, A. Saglam et al., "Grasper-Assisted versus Traditional Laparoscopic Splenectomy in the Management of Hematologic Disorders," *Journal of Laparoendoscopic & Advanced Surgical Techniques A*, vol. 13, no. 6, pp. 359–363, 2003.

[15] R. M. Walsh, F. Brody, and N. Brown, "Laparoscopic splenectomy for lymphoproliferative disease," *Surgical Endoscopy*, vol. 18, no. 2, pp. 272–275, 2004.

[16] B. Edwin, X. Skattum, J. Ræder, E. Trondsen, and T. Buanes, "Outpatient laparoscopic splenectomy: Patient safety and satisfaction," *Surgical Endoscopy*, vol. 18, no. 9, pp. 1331–1334, 2004.

[17] S. Sampath, A. T. Meneghetti, J. K. MacFarlane, N. H. Nguyen, W. B. Benny, and O. N. M. Panton, "An 18-year review of open and laparoscopic splenectomy for idiopathic thrombocytopenic purpura," *The American Journal of Surgery*, vol. 193, no. 5, pp. 580–584, 2007.

[18] R. L. Bell, K. E. Reinhardt, E. Cho, and J. L. Flowers, "A ten-year, single institution experience with laparoscopic splenectomy," *Journal of the Society of Laparoendoscopic Surgeons*, vol. 9, pp. 163–168, 2005.

[19] P. K. Chowbey, A. Goel, R. Panse et al., "Laparoscopic splenectomy for hematologic disorders: Experience with the first fifty patients," *Journal of Laparoendoscopic & Advanced Surgical Techniques A*, vol. 15, no. 1, pp. 28–32, 2005.

[20] C. J. Pattenden, C. D. Mann, M. S. Metcalfe, M. Dyer, and D. M. Lloyd, "Laparoscopic splenectomy: A personal series of 140 consecutive cases," *Annals of the Royal College of Surgeons of England*, vol. 92, no. 5, pp. 398–402, 2010.

[21] J. Davies, R. Barnes, and D. Milligan, "Update of guidelines for the prevention and treatment of infection in patients with an absent or dysfunctional spleen," *Clinical Medicine*, vol. 2, no. 5, pp. 440–443, 2002.

[22] P. B. Thapa, "Initiating advanced laparoscopic surgery in a medical college hospital with basic laparoscopic set up: Is it feasible and safe?" *Kathmandu University Medical Journal*, vol. 8, no. 30, pp. 261–264, 2010.

[23] V. C. Shakya, S. Sood, B. K. Bhattarai, C. S. Agrawal, and S. Adhikary, "Laparoscopic inguinal hernia repair: a prospective evaluation at Eastern Nepal," *The Pan African Medical Journal*, vol. 17, p. 241, 2014.

[24] R. Koirala, V. C. Shakya, S. Khania, S. Adhikary, and C. S. Agrawal, "Rise in liver enzymes after laproscopic cholecystectomy: a transient phenomenon.," *Nepal Medical College journal : NMCJ*, vol. 14, no. 3, pp. 223–226, 2012.

[25] S. K. Shrestha, U. M. Singh Dongol, P. B. Thapa, and S. K. Sharma, "A 5 year clinical experience of laparoscopic appendicectomy," *Journal of Nepal Health Research Council*, vol. 8, pp. 91–94, 2010.

[26] R. Jha, "Distribution of hemoglobinopathies in patients presenting for electrophoresis and comparison of result with High performance liquid chromatography," *Journal of Pathology of Nepal*, vol. 5, no. 10, p. 850, 2015.

[27] B. S. Poudyal, B. Sapkota, G. S. Shrestha, S. Thapalia, B. Gyawali, and S. Tuladhar, "Safety and efficacy of azathioprine as a second line therapy for primary immune thrombocytopenic purpura," *Journal of Nepal Medical Association*, vol. 55, no. 203, pp. 16–21, 2016.

[28] S. Shrestha, G. B. Pradhan, R. Shrestha, and R. Singh, "Study on responses after splenectomy for idiopathic thrombocytopenic purpura patients, Kathmandu, Nepal.," *Nepal Medical College journal : NMCJ*, vol. 14, no. 4, pp. 328–330, 2012.

[29] A. P. Boddy, D. Mahon, and M. Rhodes, "Does open surgery continue to have a role in elective splenectomy?" *Surgical Endoscopy*, vol. 20, no. 7, pp. 1094–1098, 2006.

[30] D. Mahon and M. Rhodes, "Laparoscopic splenectomy: Size matters," *Annals of the Royal College of Surgeons of England*, vol. 85, no. 4, pp. 248–251, 2003.

[31] A. G. Patel, J. E. Parker, B. Wallwork et al., "Massive Splenomegaly Is Associated with Significant Morbidity after Laparoscopic Splenectomy," *Annals of Surgery*, vol. 238, no. 2, pp. 235–240, 2003.

[32] B. Delaitre and B. Maignien, "Laparoscopic splenectomy - technical aspects," *Surgical Endoscopy*, vol. 6, no. 6, pp. 305–308, 1992.

[33] J. L. Flowers, A. T. Lefor, J. Steers, M. Heyman, S. M. Graham, and A. L. Imbembo, "Laparoscopic splenectomy in patients with hematologic diseases," *Annals of Surgery*, vol. 224, no. 1, pp. 19–28, 1996.

[34] J. Gigot, F. Jamar, A. Ferrant et al., "Inadequate detection of accessory spleens and splenosis with laparoscopic splenectomy A shortcoming of the laparoscopic approach in hematologic diseases," *Surgical Endoscopy*, vol. 12, no. 2, pp. 101–106, 1998.

32

Ureteral Stenting after Uncomplicated Ureteroscopy for Distal Ureteral Stones

Y. El Harrech, N. Abakka, J. El Anzaoui, O. Ghoundale, and D. Touiti

Department of Urology, Hospital Avicenne, Marrakech 40000, Morocco

Correspondence should be addressed to Y. El Harrech; youness.elharrech@gmail.com

Academic Editor: Peng Hui Wang

Objectives. We compared outcome and complications after uncomplicated ureteroscopic treatment of distal ureteral calculi with or without the use of ureteral stents. *Materials and Methods.* 117 patients, prospectively divided into three groups to receive a double j stent (group 1, 42 patients), ureteral stent (group 2, 37 patients), or no stent (group 3, 38 patients), underwent ureteroscopic treatment of distal ureteral calculi. Stone characteristics, operative time, postoperative pain, lower urinary tract symptoms (LUTS), analgesia need, rehospitalization, stone-free rate, and late postoperative complications were all studied. *Results.* There were no significant differences in preoperative data. There was no significant difference between the three groups regarding hematuria, fever, flank pain, urinary tract infection, and rehospitalisation. At 48 hours and 1 week, frequency/urgency and dysuria were significantly less in the nonstented group. When comparing group 1 and group 3, patients with double j stents had statistically significantly more bladder pain ($P = 0.003$), frequency/urgency ($P = 0.002$), dysuria ($P = 0.001$), and need of analgesics ($P = 0.001$). All patients who underwent imaging postoperatively were without evidence of obstruction or ureteral stricture. *Conclusions.* Uncomplicated ureteroscopy for distal ureteral calculi without intraoperative ureteral dilation can safely be performed without placement of a ureteral stent.

1. Introduction

Nowadays ureteroscopy has become the treatment of choice for managing ureteral stones, specially mid and distal ones [1].

There is no consensus on placing a ureteral catheter after uncomplicated ureteroscopy and it is still controversial. It is a routine justified by the belief that this practice decreases ureteral stricture formation, protects the kidney, and minimizes postoperative pain [2]. However the use of stents is accompanied by significant morbidity, including pain, infection, and irritative voiding symptoms [3, 4].

The aim of our study was to assess the need for routine ureteral stenting after uncomplicated ureteroscopic stone removal, evaluating the patient characteristics, stone features, complications, and treatment outcome among stented and unstented patients.

2. Materials and Methods

From January 2009 to January 2011, a total of 117 patients treated with successful ureteroscopy for distal ureteral stones were prospectively randomized to 3 groups. Group 1 included 42 patients in whom a double j stent was inserted, group 2 comprised 37 in whom a ureteral stent was inserted, and group 3 included 38 patients in whom no stent was inserted after stone removal.

Informed consent was obtained from all patients. Patients were excluded from the study when stone size was greater than 2 cm.

The mean age was, respectively, 44.1, 39.6, and 43.2 for group 1, group 2, and group 3.

Preoperative imaging consisted of KUB and renal ultrasonography with NCCT or IVP.

TABLE 1: Patient's characteristics and results.

	Double j stent (group 1, 42 patients)	Ureteral stent (group 2, 37 patients)	No stent (group 3, 38 patients) stent	P
Mean patient age (y, range)	44.1 (22–72)	39.6 (27–72)	43.2 (20–76)	0.24
Side of stone: R/L	16/26	17/20	20/18	0.12
Mean stone size (mm)	8.6 ± 3.4	10.1 ± 2.7	9.6 ± 3.6	0.18
Mean operative time (min)	36 ± 4	34 ± 5	31 ± 9	0.17
Success rate (%)	100	100	100	0.69

All procedures were performed under epidural anesthesia after discussion with patients.

Ureteroscopy was done with a 7.5 Fr semirigid ureteroscope. One 0.038-inch guide wire was inserted via cystoscopy under fluoroscopic guidance. The cystoscope was removed and a semirigid ureteroscope was passed into the ureter over the working guide wire with nonprior ureteral dilation. The pneumatic lithoclast (Swiss LithoClast) was used to fragment the offending calculus into pieces in all cases requiring lithotripsy.

The stents used in the study were 7 Fr in diameter.

In the patients of group 2, the ureteral stent was left for 24 hours. All patients in group 1 were rehospitalized after 3 weeks for double j stent removal.

All patients were closely followed up.

Procedures were considered a success if either a solitary calculus was removed in its entirety or all fragments were absent on radiographic followup. Radiographic followup typically consisted of a plain radiograph and renal ultrasound 1 month after the procedure.

Age, gender, stone characteristics, total operating time, the mean operative time, and mean hospital stay were all recorded.

For postoperative symptoms and the complications, a special questionnaire and a precise clinical exam were used, looking for flank pain, hematuria, dysuria, urgency, fever, and urinary tract infection. Postoperative pain and dysuria were measured using a 10 cm visual analog scale.

We also studied, the need of analgesics in postoperative time, the rate of rehospitalisation, and the appearence of an ureteral stricture.

Patients were followed up postoperatively with a minimum of 3 months (the mean follow-up was 12 months).

Differences in percentages (qualitative variables) were analyzed by the χ^2 test. Kruskal-Wallis and Mann-Whitney U test were used for comparison of treatment groups. Statistical analyses were performed using the SPSS 15.0. The P value < 0.05 was considered statistically significant.

3. Results

The 3 study groups were comparable regarding patients and stone characteristics (Table 1). Overall mean stone size in the study was 8.7 ± 3.1 mm. Moreover, the ureteroscopy technique, type of intracorporeal lithotripsy, and method of stone retrieval were not significantly different between the treatment groups.

Ureteroscopy was successfully achieved in the three groups and the stone-free rate at 4 weeks was 100% in each group.

Mean operative time plus or minus standard deviation in group 1 was 36 ± 4 minutes, 34 ± 5 in group 2, and 31 ± 9 in group 3. Thus, operative time was not significantly longer when a ureteral stent or double j stent was placed.

Table 2 shows the mean visual analog pain scores at 48 hours and 1 week after ureteroscopy and other postoperative symptoms and complications in the three groups.

At 48 hours and 1 week, symptoms like frequency/urgency, dysuria were significantly less in the non stented group comparing to other groups.

When comparing group 1 and group 3, patients with double j stents had statistically significantly more bladder pain ($P = 0.003$), frequency/urgency ($P = 0.002$), dysuria ($P = 0.001$), and need of analgesics ($P = 0.001$) compared to those without stents.

There was no significant difference between the three groups regarding hematuria, fever, flank pain, urinary tract infection, and rehospitalisation.

When taking into consideration all LUTS and the need of analgesics, they were significantly more important in the first group using a double pigtail stent (group 1 versus group 2: $P = 0.002$; group 1 versus group 3: $P = 0.001$).

Readmission to the hospital for unremitting pain was necessary in 1 of 117 patients. No patients in the stented group required postoperative readmission to the hospital.

All complications were easily and successfully managed by conservative measures.

All patients (75%) who underwent imaging postoperatively were without evidence of obstruction or ureteral stricture on followup imaging.

4. Discussion

Ureteral stents are commonly placed after ureteroscopic stone extraction. The rationale for the routine use of ureteral stents after ureteroscopy originates from supposition, rather than from evidence-based medicine. However, the placement of a ureteral stent may be associated with significant morbidity.

Joshi et al. identified patient morbidity associated with ureteral stents as a significant health problem and investigated it in detail [5]. They found that ureteral stents are associated with significant symptoms, such as pain affecting daily activities (80%), urinary symptoms (73%), and reduced work capacity (58%), which reduce quality of life. During

TABLE 2: Postoperative symptoms and complications.

	Double j stent (group 1; 42 patients)	Ureteral stent (group 2; 37 patients)	No stent (group 3; 38 patients) stent	P
Mean flank pain score at 48 hours (0–10) ± S.D.	4.3 ± 2.1	4.3 ± 2.3	4.7 ± 1.9	0.14
Mean flank pain score on day 7 (0–10) ± S.D.	2.6 ± 1.4	2.1 ± 1.2	2.1 ± 1.4	0.09
Mean bladder pain score at 48 hours (0–10) ± S.D.	5.3 ± 2.6	4.9 ± 1.9	2.2 ± 1.4	0.004
Mean bladder pain score on day 7 (0–10) ± S.D.	4.8 ± 2.5	2.5 ± 1.7	1.9 ± 1.1	0.003
Dysuria number (%)	11 (26.1)	8 (21.6)	5 (13.1)	0.002
Hematuria number (%)	3 (7.1)	3 (8.1)	2 (5.2)	0.67
Frequency/urgency number (%)	17 (40.4)	10 (27.0)	7 (18.4)	<0.001
Need of analgesics in follow-up	11 (26.1)	4 (10.8)	3 (7.8)	<0.001
Fever number (%)	3 (7.1)	2 (5.4)	3 (7.8)	0.50
Urinary tract infection number (%)	3 (7.1)	2 (5.4)	3 (7.8)	0.39
Rehospitalization number (%)	0	0	1	0.34
Ureteral stricture number (%)	0	0	0	0.70
Mean hospital stay (hours)	26	26	25	0.48

the research, it became clear that stents profoundly affect physical and psychosocial health and have a negative impact on functional capacity and work performance [3, 5].

In our present study involving 117 patients, we did not find significant difference between the three groups concerning flank pain, hematuria, fever, and urinary tract infection.

Several trials have demonstrated similar postoperative complication rates among stented and unstented patient populations. These trials have several similarities with our study including a preponderance of patients with distal ureteral calculi, uncomplicated procedure, and absence of ureteral dilation.

In the study of Ibrahim et al. [6], early postoperative complications, including low grade fever, hematuria, and urinary tract infection, were observed in 22 patients (20%) in nonstented patients and 19 (19%) in stented ones, a difference of no significant value. Mean initial hospitalization and time to return to normal physical activity were not different between the 2 groups. At 48 hours and 1 week there was no significant difference in flank pain between the 2 groups.

Borboroglu et al. [7] in a multi-institutional prospective randomized controlled study were surprised to find a statistically significant lower incidence in flank pain in their patients without stents and explained it by the fact that perhaps the patients with stents had so much overall pain that they reflected this in response to the flank pain question.

The main significant difference that was found in our study concerned dysuria, bladder pain, frequency, and the need of analgesics after the ureteroscopy.

Nabi et al. [8] reported the results of a meta-analysis of 9 randomized, controlled trials of stenting following uncomplicated ureteroscopy. The incidence of lower urinary tract symptoms was significantly higher in participants who had a stent inserted after ureteroscopy.

The same results were confirmed by Ibrahim et al. [6] and Borboroglu et al. [7] who found that patients without stents had significantly less bladder pain, urinary symptoms, and narcotic use postoperatively.

In a recent meta-analysis [9] studying the effect of ureteral stent placement on postureteroscopy complications, the authors concluded that the published evidence supports the practice of omitting a ureteral stent after an uncomplicated ureteroscopic procedure. This meta-analysis attests that there is a slightly lower absolute risk of complication associated with the placement of a ureteral stent after ureteroscopy but does not detect a significant difference in outcome between patients who undergo ureteral stent placement after ureteroscopy and those who do not.

In the stented group, a cystoscopy is needed to remove the double pig tail stent. Richter et al. [10] claimed that placement of a ureteral stent is "a friendly procedure with unfriendly high morbidity." The additional cystoscopy for stent removal is a cause of discomfort and overall cost.

Netto Jr. et al. [11] assessed the cost-effectiveness of routine ureteral stenting after ureteroscopic stone removal. The cost per patient in patients with a stent was $9,900.95 versus $3,661.78 for patients without, about 30% the cost of using a stent. They concluded that routine catheter placement after ureteroscopic stone removal increased operative time and the cost of procedure and did not seem to improve patient outcome.

Some authors [12] sought to identify significant clinical characteristics affecting postoperative morbidity in unstented patients. They found that patients undergoing bilateral stentless ureteroscopy, those with recent or recurrent urinary tract infections, and those with a history of urolithiasis are at greater risk for a postoperative complication. Other factors such as operative time and renal stone location may have a role as well. This will help to select patients suitable for stentless procedure.

An advantage of the current series is the prospective and randomized comparison of three arms. To our knowledge, there have been no published studies of outcomes and results among three different groups including patients with double j stent, ureteral stent, and no stent.

The current study has some limitations, including the absence of a validated symptom score for proper assessment of pain and lower urinary tract symptoms. Another limitation is the absence of a precise assessment of the amount of analgesia used and the absence of assessment of cost.

5. Conclusion

The ureteral stent has become an integral part of the urological armamentarium. However, stent related morbidity is a reality in the majority of patients.

Uncomplicated ureteroscopy for distal ureteral calculi without intraoperative ureteral dilation can safely be performed without placement of a ureteral stent.

Patients without stents had significantly less pain, fewer urinary symptoms, and decreased analgesic use postoperatively and are not at risk of increased late complications.

The other potential benefits to leaving patients without stents after ureteroscopy are cost savings and the avoidance of followup cystoscopy for stent removal.

References

[1] G. M. Preminger, H. G. Tiselius, D. G. Assimos et al., "2007 guideline for the management of ureteral calculi," *European Urology*, vol. 52, no. 6, pp. 1610–1631, 2007.

[2] D. H. Hosking, S. E. McColm, and W. E. Smith, "Is stenting following ureteroscopy for removal of distal ureteral calculi necessary?" *Journal of Urology*, vol. 161, no. 1, pp. 48–50, 1999.

[3] H. B. Joshi, N. Newns, A. Stainthorpe, R. P. MacDonagh, F. X. Keeley Jr., and A. G. Timoney, "Ureteral stent symptom questionnaire: development and validation of a multidimensional quality of life measure," *Journal of Urology*, vol. 169, no. 3, pp. 1060–1064, 2003.

[4] M. Duvdevani, B. H. Chew, and J. D. Denstedt, "Minimizing symptoms in patients with ureteric stents," *Current Opinion in Urology*, vol. 16, no. 2, pp. 77–82, 2006.

[5] H. B. Joshi, A. Stainthorpe, R. P. MacDonagh, F. X. Keeley Jr., and A. G. Timoney, "Indwelling ureteral stents: evaluation of symptoms, quality of life and utility," *Journal of Urology*, vol. 169, no. 3, pp. 1065–1069, 2003.

[6] H. M. Ibrahim, A. M. Al-Kandari, H. S. Shaaban, Y. H. Elshebini, and A. A. Shokeir, "Role of ureteral stenting after uncomplicated ureteroscopy for distal ureteral stones: a randomized, controlled trial," *Journal of Urology*, vol. 180, no. 3, pp. 961–965, 2008.

[7] P. G. Borboroglu, C. L. Amling, N. S. Schenkman et al., "Ureteral stenting after ureteroscopy for distal ureteral calculi : a multi-institutional prospective randomized controlled study assessing pain, outcomes and complications," *Journal of Urology*, vol. 166, no. 5, pp. 1651–1657, 2001.

[8] G. Nabi, J. Cook, J. N'Dow, and S. McClinton, "Outcomes of stenting after uncomplicated ureteroscopy: systematic review and meta-analysis," *British Medical Journal*, vol. 334, no. 7593, pp. 572–575, 2007.

[9] D. V. Makarov, B. J. Trock, M. E. Allaf, and B. R. Matlaga, "The effect of ureteral stent placement on post-ureteroscopy complications: a meta-analysis," *Urology*, vol. 71, no. 5, pp. 796–800, 2008.

[10] S. Richter, A. Ringel, M. Shalev, and I. Nissenkorn, "The indwelling ureteric stent: a "friendly" procedure with unfriendly high morbidity," *BJU International*, vol. 85, no. 4, pp. 408–411, 2000.

[11] N. R. Netto Jr., J. Ikonomidis, and C. Zillo, "Routine ureteral stenting after ureteroscopy for ureteral lithiasis: is it really necessary?" *Journal of Urology*, vol. 166, no. 4, pp. 1252–1254, 2001.

[12] B. K. Hollenbeck, T. G. Schuster, B. D. Seifman, G. J. Faerber, and J. S. Wolf Jr., "Identifying patients who are suitable for stentless ureteroscopy following treatment of urolithiasis," *The Journal of Urology*, vol. 170, no. 1, pp. 103–106, 2003.

Association between Fellowship Training, SurgicalVolume, and Laparoscopic Sutur ing Techniques among Members of the American Association of Gynecologic Laparoscopists

Emad Mikhail,[1] Lauren Scott,[1] Branko Miladinovic,[2] Anthony N. Imudia,[1] and Stuart Hart[1]

[1]*Department of Obstetrics and Gynecology, University of South Florida, Morsani College of Medicine, Tampa, FL 33606, USA*
[2]*Center for Comparative Effectiveness Research and Evidence-Based Medicine, University of South Florida, Morsani College of Medicine, Tampa, FL 33612, USA*

Correspondence should be addressed to Emad Mikhail; emikhail@health.usf.edu

Academic Editor: Peng Hui Wang

Study Objective. To compare surgical volume and techniques including laparoscopic suturing among members of the American Association of Gynecologic Laparoscopists (AAGL) according to fellowship training status. *Design.* A web-based survey was designed using Qualtrics and sent to AAGL members. *Results.* Minimally invasive gynecologic surgery (FMIGS) trained surgeons were more likely to perform more than 8 major conventional laparoscopic cases per month (63% versus 38%, $P < 0.001$, OR [95% CI] = 2.78 [1.54–5.06]) and were more likely to perform laparoscopic suturing during these cases (32% versus 16%, $P < 0.004$, OR [95% CI] = 2.44 [1.25–4.71]). The non-fellowship trained (NFT) surgeons in private practice were less likely to perform over 8 conventional laparoscopic cases (34% versus 51%, $P = 0.03$, OR [95% CI] = 0.50 [0.25–0.99]) and laparoscopic suturing during these cases (13% versus 27%, $P = 0.01$, OR [95% CI] = 0.39 [0.17–0.92]) compared to NFT surgeons in academic practice. *Conclusion.* The surgical volume and utilization of laparoscopic suturing of FMIGS trained surgeons are significantly increased compared to NFT surgeons. Academic practice setting had a positive impact on surgical volume of NFT surgeons but not on FMIGS trained surgeons.

1. Introduction

The depth and complexity of gynecologic surgery are continually increasing due to surgical innovation and a trend towards minimally invasive surgical approaches. Due to this increasing intricacy of laparoscopic and hysteroscopic procedures and conflicting obligations during residency training, gynecology residents are frequently uncomfortable performing a variety of advanced endoscopic procedures at the completion of their training [1, 2]. In 2001, the American Association of Gynecologic Laparoscopists (AAGL) and the Society of Reproductive Surgeons (SRS) collaborated to establish the first fellowship in minimally invasive gynecologic surgery (FMIGS), which standardized a MIGS curriculum and a research requirement [3]. The goal of the fellowship is to provide a standardized training program for gynecologists who have completed their residency so that they may acquire additional skills in minimally invasive gynecologic surgery and serve as a scholarly and surgical resource for the community in which they practice [4].

It has been shown that operative outcomes are directly related to surgical volumes, yet there has been a continual decline over the last several decades in the annual number of procedures performed by gynecologists [5, 6]. From 1979 to 2006, there was an 81% decline in the number of gynecologic surgeries performed by ACOG fellows, from 132 to 25 gynecologic cases per year [5]. This trend has also impacted the rate of hysterectomies performed, the most common major gynecologic procedure performed on women in the United States. The number of hysterectomies performed annually by practicing gynecologists has decreased from 28 in 1980 to 8.5 in 2010. This decrease has occurred despite the increased number of methods available to perform a hysterectomy, which now includes a robotic and laparoscopic approach [4].

There have not been any previous studies comparing surgical volumes for FMIGS graduates to other gynecologic surgeons. Given this void in knowledge on the impact of a formal fellowship training program on surgical volume and laparoscopic surgical techniques, we sought to compare fellowship training status, surgical volume, and the surgical techniques of laparoscopic suturing among members of the American Association of Gynecologic Laparoscopists (AAGL).

2. Material and Methods

The AAGL is the leading association promoting minimally invasive gynecologic surgery among physicians worldwide. Its membership extends to over 110 countries, with over 7000 members [4]. Given the mission of AAGL, their members were thought to be the most appropriate sample for this study.

A survey was developed using Qualtrics (Qualtrics, Provo, UT) [7] web-based survey platform. After obtaining exempt status from University of South Florida Institutional Review Board, the survey was sent to the AAGL scientific review committee for approval. The survey was pilot tested to ensure that it was easy to understand and the questions were relevant and to gauge the time needed to complete the survey. Upon approval, the survey was sent to all AAGL members through the AAGL Digital Member Bulletin. Following the initial email, two additional reminders were sent to all members to enhance the response rate. The survey was divided into different sections. The first section focused on demographics, the location and type of residency, and the number of residents per year. The second section focused on individual training and surgical volume while the last section focused on individual preferences and technique of laparoscopic suturing. Performance of a total laparoscopic hysterectomy (TLH) was used as a minimum reference point to allow study participants to proceed into the survey. As TLH is a commonly performed minimally invasive gynecologic procedure that requires advanced laparoscopic and suturing skills, it was considered a good reference surgery for this study. Only study participants who perform TLH were included in this study. We focused on conventional laparoscopic cases and conventional laparoscopic suturing in this survey.

A total of 521 respondents accessed the survey, and 163 respondents were excluded from the final analysis because they do not perform conventional total laparoscopic hysterectomy procedures ($n = 100$), are currently in training ($n = 35$, 5 residents and 30 fellows), listed multiple responses ($n = 28$), or had missing information in their responses ($n = 28$). The remaining 330 respondents were categorized into one of the following groups: (1) non-fellowship trained (NFT) ($n = 219$), (2) minimally invasive gynecologic surgery (FMIGS) trained ($n = 74$), and (3) other training (OT) ($n = 37$). The respondents from other training group were Gynecologic Oncology ($n = 13$), Female Pelvic Medicine and Reconstructive Surgery ($n = 10$), and Reproductive Endocrinology and Infertility ($n = 14$). Given that the emphasis of the study was on non-fellowship trained and FMIGS surgeons, these two groups were the basis of our comparison for this study. Regarding questions comparing laparoscopic suturing zones, any combination of vertical alignment of the needle driver and the assistant instrument was considered as suturing in the vertical zone, and any combination of horizontal alignment of the needle driver and the assistant instrument was considered as suturing in the horizontal zone, and any combination that uses the suprapubic port site was considered utilization of the suprapubic site for suturing.

All data was analyzed using Stata 13.1 (StataCorp LP, College Station, TX) SVY survey data analysis module. SVY module incorporates survey design features such as probability weights, stratification, and clustering. Results were expressed as mean ± SD or median (range) for continuous variables and as frequencies and percentages for categorical variables. For comparisons between groups, mean difference for continuous data or odds ratios for categorical data were used. A P value of < 0.05 is considered statistically significant.

3. Results

A total of 330 respondents were included in the final analysis, over 66% ($n = 219$) of these were NFT, and 22% ($n = 74$) were FMIGS trained while the remaining 18% ($n = 37$) were trained in other types of fellowships (Gynecologic Oncology, Reproductive Endocrinology and Infertility and Female Pelvic Medicine and Reconstructive Surgery) (Table 1).

The vast majority of NFT and FMIGS trained surgeons were male (78% versus 55%, resp.), and over 50% of the respondents (NFT and FMIGS) were between the ages of 35 and 55 years. About 68% of NFT and 52% of FMIGS surgeons practice in the US and predominately in private practice (75% versus 55%, resp.). A greater proportion of FMIGS surgeons work in academic practice (37.9%) versus private practice (19.9%), $P < 0.001$, Table 1.

Most of the NFT and FMIGS respondents were trained at a university residency program (54% versus 72%, $P = 0.011$) with 1–5 residents per year (61% versus 45%, $P = 0.07$) and over three-quarters of the respondents attended a laparoscopic suturing course (78% versus 87%, $P = 0.13$), Table 2.

Minimally invasive gynecologic surgery fellowship trained physicians were more likely to perform more than 8 major conventional laparoscopic cases a month (63% versus 38%, $P < 0.001$, OR [95% CI] = 2.78 [1.54–5.06]) and they were more likely to perform laparoscopic suturing during these cases (32% versus 16%, $P < 0.004$, OR [95% CI] = 2.44 [1.25–4.71]), Table 3.

The NFT surgeons in private practice were less likely to perform over 8 conventional laparoscopic cases (34% versus 51%, $P = 0.03$, OR [95% CI] = 0.50 [0.25–0.99]) and laparoscopic suturing in these cases (13% versus 27%, $P = 0.01$, OR [95% CI] = 0.39 [0.17–0.92]) compared with NFT surgeons in academic practice. The surgical volume and proportion of conventional laparoscopic cases in which suturing is performed among FMIGS surgeons in academic and private practices were not significantly different (Table 4).

Table 1: Demographics of study participants.

	Non-fellowship trained $n = 219$	FMIGS $n = 74$	Gynecologic Oncology $n = 13$	FMPRS $n = 10$	REI $n = 14$	P value
Male	171 (78%)	41 (55%)	10 (77%)	5 (56%)	14 (100%)	<0.001
Female	48 (22%)	33 (45%)	3 (23%)	4 (44%)	0 (0%)	
Age						
25–34	9 (4%)	11 (15%)	0 (0%)	0 (0%)	0 (0%)	<0.001
35–44	49 (22%)	37 (50%)	3 (13%)	4 (40%)	3 (21%)	
45–55	65 (30%)	19 (26%)	6 (46%)	3 (30%)	2 (14%)	
>55	96 (44%)	7 (10%)	4 (31%)	3 (30%)	9 (65%)	
Geographical location						
US	146 (68%)	38 (52%)	6 (50%)	6 (60%)	7 (54%)	0.10
International	69 (32%)	35 (48%)	6 (50%)	4 (40%)	6 (46%)	
Practice type						
Academic practice	54 (25%)	33 (45%)	9 (69%)	5 (50%)	5 (36%)	<0.001
Private practice	165 (75%)	41 (55%)	4 (31%)	5 (50%)	9 (64%)	

Table 2: Training background for study participants.

	Non-fellowship trained (219)	FMIGS trained (74)	P value
Residency training			
University	117 (54%)	53 (72%)	0.011
Community-university affiliated	58 (27%)	16 (22%)	
Community	41 (19%)	5 (6%)	
Residency program size			
1–5	130 (61%)	33 (45%)	0.07
6–10	59 (27%)	28 (38%)	
>10	25 (12%)	12 (7%)	
Attended laparoscopic suturing training courses			
Yes	169 (78%)	64 (87%)	0.13
No	49 (22%)	10 (13%)	

Specific analysis of surgical techniques for TLH between NFT and FMIGS surgeons revealed overall similarities in the two groups except in the use of a curved laparoscopic needle driver, which was more common in FMIGS trained surgeons (66% versus 52%, $P = 0.03$) compared to NFT surgeons. Additionally, NFT surgeons were more likely to utilize self-righting needle driver (22% versus 7%, $P = 0.003$) and less likely to perform continuous vaginal cuff closure during TLH (52 versus 66%, $P = 0.03$).

Comparison of the different laparoscopic suturing zones between NFT and FMIGS surgeons showed no statistically significant difference. However, the most commonly utilized one was the transverse zone suturing used by 71 (45%) of NFT and 25 (45%) of FMIGS surgeons, followed by vertical zone suturing and then suprapubic port utilization.

4. Discussion

The findings from this survey amongst AGGL members reveal that surgical volume and utilization of laparoscopic suturing in FMIGS trained gynecologists are significantly higher than those of NFT gynecologists. Interestingly, regardless of training though, the TLH surgical technique between the two groups (FMIGS and NFT) of gynecologic surgeons was generally similar.

Several studies have found that surgical residents perceive a need for additional training in advanced laparoscopic procedures after residency [8–10]. This is also true in obstetrics and gynecology residency training programs. In a study by Burkett et al., it was found that only 28.6% of US obstetrics and gynecology residency program directors, and 22.2% of graduating residents from these programs, reported graduating residents as "completely prepared" to perform a laparoscopic hysterectomy procedure [2]. A study by Kolkman et al. found that 73% of recent graduates from a residency training program in obstetrics and gynecology felt they were adequately trained in basic laparoscopic skills, but 82% felt they were not adequately trained to perform more advanced laparoscopic procedures. A lack of an adequate case load was listed as a significant reason for these findings [11].

Obtaining adequate surgical training has now become even more challenging with residency training work week restrictions, combined with the declining rate of gynecologic surgical volume including hysterectomy procedures, which may result in gynecologists in practice altering their practice patterns and even referring relatively uncomplicated procedures to gynecologists with higher volumes [12]. This may cause the practicing gynecologist to be at a serious competitive disadvantage if they are not proficient in the growing repertoire of endoscopic surgeries [13]. As many OB/GYNs have busy schedules, moving between the office and taking care of obstetric patients, the ability to learn and integrate advanced laparoscopic procedures successfully into daily practice is a major hurdle in the implementation of laparoscopy not learned during residency training [11].

Table 3: Case volume of study participants.

	Non-fellowship trained	FMIGS trained	P value	OR (95% CI)
Major gynecologic conventional laparoscopic surgical cases/month				
>8	81 (38%)	45 (63%)	<0.001	2.78 (1.54–5.06)
Monthly cases with conventional laparoscopic suturing				
>8	34 (16%)	23 (32%)	0.004	2.44 (1.25–4.71)

Table 4: Case volume of non-fellowship trained participants according to practice setting.

	Non-fellowship trained		P value	OR (95% CI)
	Academic practice	Private practice		
Major gynecologic conventional laparoscopic surgical cases/month				
>8	26 (51%)	55 (34%)	0.03	0.50 (0.25, 0.99)
Monthly cases with conventional laparoscopic suturing				
>8	14 (27%)	20 (13%)	0.01	0.39 (0.17, 0.92)
	FMIGS trained		P value	OR (95% CI)
	Academic practice	Private practice		
Major gynecologic conventional laparoscopic surgical cases/month				
>8	23 (72%)	22 (56%)	0.18	0.51 (0.16, 1.52)
Monthly cases with conventional laparoscopic suturing				
>8	8 (24%)	15 (38%)	0.2	1.95 (0.63, 6.31)

In 2012, according to the American Council for Graduate Medical Education, the average graduating resident in obstetrics and gynecology performed 38 laparoscopic hysterectomies. Considering that the learning curve for a laparoscopic hysterectomy is between 30 and 80 procedures and a US gynecologist only performs an average of 8.5 hysterectomies per year in practice, it could take several years after residency training before proficiency is fully achieved [5, 14–16]. Additionally, two decades ago the graduating resident in obstetrics and gynecology was only required to learn two routes for hysterectomy, open and vaginal, but today the graduating resident and the practicing gynecologic surgeon are required to master multiple approaches to the same procedure: abdominal, vaginal, laparoscopic, and robotic hysterectomy [17]. The above-mentioned numbers also do not take into account the volume of surgery needed to maintain proficiency since performance can deteriorate over time, including laparoscopic suturing skills if not practiced regularly to maintain those skills. Therefore maintenance training has been proposed to ensure better skill retention [18].

In this study, FMIGS trained surgeons in both an academic and private practice perform more complex cases with higher utilization of laparoscopic suturing. This presents a significant challenge for the low volume gynecologic surgeons as surgical volume is increasingly being used as a component in assessment of individual and hospital surgical quality [19]. Recently, surgeon volume requirements have been incorporated into maintenance of certification for cardiothoracic surgery [20]. It is evident from this study that the surgical volume of FMIGS trained surgeons is significantly more than that of NFT surgeons. The effect of surgical volume on perioperative outcomes and resource utilization has also been demonstrated in the literature. In a study by Wallenstein et al., it was found that women operated on by high volume surgeons (>14.10 operations per year) were 25% less likely to experience a complication, while women undergoing a surgical procedure at a high volume center (>105 laparoscopic hysterectomies per year) were 18% less likely to experience a complication. Procedure costs were also lower for high volume surgeons ($867 lower costs) and when the procedure was performed at a high volume center ($966 lower costs) [6]. There appears to be a dose-response relationship between surgical volume and outcomes more than a strict cutoff level [6, 19, 21].

This study showed that not only does additional postresidency laparoscopic training enhance a gynecologist's surgical volume, but also the type of practice setting plays an important role. We found that NFT gynecologists practicing in an academic setting had an increase in their surgical volume compared to their peers in private practice, a finding that was not found in the FMIGS group since they had a higher surgical volume regardless of their practice. The hybrid obstetrician-gynecologist career can be uniquely vulnerable to available surgical volume, which could ultimately limit major operative cases to select surgeons [19]. On the other hand, gynecologic surgeons who have a high surgical volume are more likely to feel comfortable offering a minimally invasive hysterectomy to their patients [22]. Laparoscopic suturing and knot tying require development of a significant skillset requiring patience and a long learning curve, which can be difficult to achieve despite many advances made in the field [23]. This study shows that postresidency FMIGS training enhances the surgical volume of practicing gynecologist, including those cases requiring laparoscopic suturing. While this study emphasizes the importance of MIGS fellowship training in our specialty, survey studies such as this have some inherent limitations such as recall, response, and researcher biases.

Certain limitations were obvious in this study, including low sample size due to low response rate (10%), despite sending 2 reminder emails to encourage members to respond.

5. Conclusion

In summary, this study analyzed surgical volume between FMIGS and NFT surgeons and showed that surgeon volume among FMIGS trained gynecologists is higher and they are more likely to perform advanced laparoscopic cases involving laparoscopic suturing. Further prospective studies evaluating the benefits of postresidency advanced laparoscopic training on enhancement of perioperative outcomes are needed.

Disclosure

A preliminary version of the analyses used in this paper was presented at 43th AAGL Annual Global Congress on Minimally Invasive Gynecology, Vancouver, British Columbia, November 2014.

References

[1] J. I. Einarsson, A. Young, L. Tsien, and H. Sangi-Haghpeykar, "Perceived proficiency in endoscopic techniques among senior obstetrics and gynecology residents," *The Journal of the American Association of Gynecologic Laparoscopists*, vol. 9, no. 2, pp. 158–164, 2002.

[2] D. Burkett, J. Horwitz, V. Kennedy, D. Murphy, S. Graziano, and K. Kenton, "Assessing current trends in resident hysterectomy training," *Female Pelvic Medicine & Reconstructive Surgery*, vol. 17, no. 5, pp. 210–214, 2011.

[3] M. W. Dassel, M. A. Daw, M. R. Adelman, T. R. Bardsley, J. Kim, and R. K. Zurawin, "Compensation among graduated fellowship in minimally invasive gynecologic surgery fellows," *Journal of Minimally Invasive Gynecology*, vol. 22, no. 3, pp. 469–474, 2015.

[4] AAGL, "AAGL; Advancing Minimally Invasive Gynecology Worldwide," 2014, http://www.aagl.com/.

[5] J. F. Magrina, "Isn't it time to separate the O from the G?" *Journal of Minimally Invasive Gynecology*, vol. 21, no. 4, pp. 501–503, 2014.

[6] M. R. Wallenstein, C. V. Ananth, J. H. Kim et al., "Effect of surgical volume on outcomes for laparoscopic hysterectomy for benign indications," *Obstetrics and Gynecology*, vol. 119, no. 4, pp. 709–716, 2012.

[7] Qualtrics, 2005, http://www.qualtrics.com/.

[8] Society of American Gastrointestinal Endoscopic Surgeons (SAGES), "Integrating advanced laparoscopy into surgical residency training," *Surgical Endoscopy*, vol. 12, no. 4, pp. 374–376, 1998.

[9] D. W. Rattner, K. N. Apelgren, and W. S. Eubanks, "The need for training opportunities in advanced laparoscopic surgery," *Surgical Endoscopy*, vol. 15, no. 10, pp. 1066–1070, 2001.

[10] P. M. Chiasson, D. E. Pace, C. M. Schlachta, J. Mamazza, and E. C. Poulin, "Minimally invasive surgery training in Canada: a survey of general surgery," *Surgical Endoscopy and Other Interventional Techniques*, vol. 17, no. 3, pp. 371–377, 2003.

[11] W. Kolkman, R. Wolterbeek, and F. W. Jansen, "Implementation of advanced laparoscopy into daily gynecologic practice: difficulties and solutions," *Journal of Minimally Invasive Gynecology*, vol. 13, no. 1, pp. 4–9, 2006.

[12] J. D. Wright, T. J. Herzog, J. Tsui et al., "Nationwide trends in the performance of inpatient hysterectomy in the United States," *Obstetrics and Gynecology*, vol. 122, no. 2, part 1, pp. 233–241, 2013.

[13] D. L. Olive, W. W. Hurd, G. M. Janik, A. A. Luciano, and J. S. Sanfillippo, "Legitimizing the stepchild: organizing and expanding fellowship opportunities in endoscopic surgery," *The Journal of the American Association of Gynecologic Laparoscopists*, vol. 7, no. 3, pp. 299–300, 2000.

[14] Education ACfGM, *Data Resource Book*, American Council for Graduate Medical Education, 2012-2013.

[15] R. M. Kho, "Comparison of robotic-assisted laparoscopy versus conventional laparoscopy on skill acquisition and performance," *Clinical Obstetrics and Gynecology*, vol. 54, no. 3, pp. 376–381, 2011.

[16] A. Perino, G. Cucinella, R. Venezia, A. Castelli, and E. Cittadini, "Total laparoscopic hysterectomy versus total abdominal hysterectomy: an assessment of the learning curve in a prospective randomized study," *Human Reproduction*, vol. 14, no. 12, pp. 2996–2999, 1999.

[17] M. Moen, A. Walter, O. Harmanli et al., "Considerations to improve the evidence-based use of vaginal hysterectomy in benign gynecology," *Obstetrics & Gynecology*, vol. 124, no. 3, pp. 585–588, 2014.

[18] S. Van Bruwaene, M. P. Schijven, and M. Miserez, "Maintenance training for laparoscopic suturing: the quest for the perfect timing and training model: a randomized trial," *Surgical Endoscopy and Other Interventional Techniques*, vol. 27, no. 10, pp. 3823–3829, 2013.

[19] K. M. Doll, M. P. Milad, and D. R. Gossett, "Surgeon volume and outcomes in benign hysterectomy," *Journal of Minimally Invasive Gynecology*, vol. 20, no. 5, pp. 554–561, 2013.

[20] Surgery ABoT, "Certification: operative requirements," 2012, https://www.abts.org/root/home/certification/operative-requirements.aspx.

[21] L. J. Rogo-Gupta, S. N. Lewin, J. H. Kim et al., "The effect of surgeon volume on outcomes and resource use for vaginal hysterectomy," *Obstetrics and Gynecology*, vol. 116, no. 6, pp. 1341–1347, 2010.

[22] J. I. Einarsson, K. A. Matteson, J. Schulkin, N. R. Chavan, and H. Sangi-Haghpeykar, "Minimally invasive hysterectomies-a survey on attitudes and barriers among practicing gynecologists," *Journal of Minimally Invasive Gynecology*, vol. 17, no. 2, pp. 167–175, 2010.

[23] R. B. Jagad, "A new technique for intracorporeal knot tying in laparoscopic surgery," *Journal of Laparoendoscopic & Advanced Surgical Techniques, Part A*, vol. 18, no. 4, pp. 626–628, 2008.

34

Trends in Route of Hysterectomy after the Implementation of a Comprehensive Robotic Training Program

Eleni Papalekas and Jay Fisher

Department of Obstetrics and Gynecology, Beaumont Hospital, Royal Oak, MI, USA

Correspondence should be addressed to Eleni Papalekas; eleni.papalekas@beaumont.edu

Academic Editor: Peng Hui Wang

Objective. To evaluate trends in surgical approach for hysterectomy following the introduction and implementation of a comprehensive robotic surgery program. *Methods*. A retrospective review of all hysterectomies done at two institutions, a community hospital and a suburban, tertiary-care teaching hospital, in the same health system over a five-year period, January 2010 through December 2014. A robotic surgery training program was implemented during the first year of the study and trends in route of hysterectomy were evaluated in the subsequent years. *Results*. A total of 5175 patients undergoing hysterectomy, for both benign and malignant indications, were included in the study. There was a significant decrease in the percent of cases performed through an abdominal approach at both the community and teaching hospitals (19.3% decline at each institution). There was an inversely related significant increase in the percent of robotic procedures at both the community and teaching hospitals (44.5% and 17%, respectively). A decrease in number of cases performed vaginally over this period was only noted in the community hospital site (25.2% decrease), and there was a slightly higher rate of vaginal hysterectomies at the teaching hospital over this study period (21.9% in 2010, 24.1% in 2014). *Conclusion*. The decrease in number of abdominal and laparoscopic hysterectomies and increase in number of robotic hysterectomies that was seen are consistent with national trends. The initiation of a robotic training program did not prevent the proliferation of use of the robot but did aim to ensure proficiency on the robot prior to gaining privileges for patient use. This type of comprehensive training and monitoring program could be applied to future technologic advances to ensure a standard level of surgical proficiency. Trends in route of hysterectomy are clearly multifactorial and involve patient, provider, and location-specific factors that are likely to continue to change.

1. Introduction

Hysterectomies are the most common gynecologic surgical procedures in the United States with an estimated number of 600,000 cases performed annually [1, 2]. While the procedure has traditionally been performed either by laparotomy or straight-stick (also known as "traditional") laparoscopy or vaginally, the introduction of the robotic-assisted hysterectomy offers patients another minimally invasive option. With the US Food and Drug Administration approval of a robotic mode of hysterectomy in 2005, the da Vinci surgical platform was introduced [3], offering women smaller incisions, shorter hospital stays, and the potential for fewer complications when compared to abdominal hysterectomy. However, the translation of this technology into practice leaves providers responsible for determining the optimal patients for each surgical approach. According to ACOG, a vaginal hysterectomy should be performed "whenever feasible" [1, 4]. When it is not feasible, surgeons are left to choose a different surgical approach.

Prior to the introduction of the robotic mode of hysterectomy, if the vaginal approach was not possible, a traditional laparoscopic approach was often considered. However, traditional laparoscopy requires the development of very specific surgical skills associated with a steep learning curve. The main complaints about traditional laparoscopy include counter-intuitive hand movements, 2D visualization, and limited degrees of instrument motion within the body [5].

Robotic gynecologic surgery has generated a great deal of excitement: offering more "wrist-like" motions and 3D visualization and enabling the surgeon to be seated at a console remote from the patient. However, existing data on outcomes of robotic-assisted hysterectomies is limited. A

2014 Cochrane review of robotic surgery for gynecologic disease found six RCTs with 371 women undergoing hysterectomy via either robotic-assisted or conventional laparoscopic techniques. According to this study, there were no measurable differences in either of the primary outcomes, which included intraoperative complications and postoperative complications [4, 6, 7]. Based on these systematic reviews and other available data, there is not enough evidence to make definitive conclusions regarding robotic-assisted compared to conventional laparoscopic hysterectomy [3–5, 8, 9]. Nonetheless, gynecologists have incorporated this technology into their armamentarium at a much greater rate than traditional laparoscopic procedures which were adopted, and they are left to choose the route of hysterectomy using current research, personal surgical expertise, and individual patient characteristics to guide their decision.

2. Materials and Methods

This was a retrospective repeated cross-sectional study. In this multisite study, information was collected from two separate hospitals within the Beaumont Health System. The first site is Beaumont Royal Oak, a 1,070-bed tertiary-care center that performs approximately 48,000 surgeries per year. It is considered a teaching hospital with 24 Ob/Gyn residents and full subspecialty services. The second site is Beaumont Troy, a 458-bed private community hospital without residents and with limited subspecialty consulting services. The two hospitals are very similar in terms of demographic and socioeconomic patient populations. Subjects undergoing hysterectomy between January 1, 2010, and December 31, 2014, were included in the study. 2010 was chosen as the first year of the study because this was when the robotic surgery training program and eligibility guidelines were initially implemented. A study period of five years was then chosen to adequately track the effects of these changes, represented by the rates in route of hysterectomy, comparing the first year, prior to full implementation, to the subsequent years.

Subjects to be included in the study were identified by Current Procedural Terminology (CPT) codes. All codes containing the word "hysterectomy" were used to generate the list of patients. Patients who underwent hysterectomy for any indication were included.

Hysterectomy is defined as the surgical removal of the uterus. In this study the types of hysterectomy were categorized as follows:

(i) Abdominal hysterectomy (AH) is accomplished by creating an incision in the abdomen through which the entire surgery is carried out and uterus removed.

(ii) Vaginal hysterectomy denotes a procedure mainly performed transvaginally, including the removal of the uterus. The two subtypes are as follows:

   (a) Vaginal hysterectomy (VH), where the entire procedure is performed transvaginally without the assistance of any abdominal incisions.

   (b) Laparoscopic-assisted vaginal hysterectomy (LAVH), where the division of the uterine vessels is performed transvaginally but laparoscopy assists in the procedure to some extent. In the vast majority of cases, laparoscopy was utilized to perform unilateral or bilateral salpingooophorectomy. Thus the surgical skills needed to perform a vaginal hysterectomy were still employed, making it most appropriate to categorize them amongst the other vaginal hysterectomies.

(iii) Laparoscopic hysterectomy refers to a procedure that is largely carried out via conventional (straight-stick) laparoscopy. The subtypes are as follows:

   (a) Laparoscopic supracervical hysterectomy in which the uterine vessels are ligated laparoscopically and the cervix is amputated at the level of the uterine vessels.

   (b) Total laparoscopic hysterectomy (TLH) where the entire procedure, including the suturing of the vaginal cuff, is carried out with conventional laparoscopy.

(iv) Robotic-assisted hysterectomy, both subtypes below are utilizing the da Vinci surgical platform as the mode of laparoscopy. Subtypes include the following:

   (a) Robotic-assisted total laparoscopic hysterectomy (RATLH), which consists of removal of cervix, uterus, and bilateral adnexal structures using the robot.

   (b) Robotic-assisted supracervical hysterectomy (RASCH), which consists of removal of uterus and adnexal structures above the level of the cervix

A comprehensive robotic surgery training and monitoring program was initiated during the first year of the study. Because full implementation did not occur until the end of the first year, 2010 served as an index year to compare to subsequent years during which the training program was fully functional. The program entailed robotic simulation, mentoring, proctoring, and maintenance of skills (Box 1). More specifically, surgeons with a projected volume of > 15 robotic or advanced laparoscopic (which could include hysterectomy, myomectomy, sacrocolpopexy, and extensive excision of endometriosis) cases per year were eligible for the program. The first step in training was to complete online learning modules. These modules are found on the da Vinci website and are designed to teach about the robot and its components, setting up the equipment and using/understanding basic principles of electrosurgery. Once completed, trainees had to complete simulation modules on the da Vinci or Mimic consoles. Each module had to be completed with a passing rate of 70% or higher. Next, trainees had to observe at least two robotic-assisted hysterectomies. The proctor and training physician then performed three to five cases jointly with shared time on the robotic console. The last step in the training program was three or more monitored

Criteria for Obtaining Robotic Surgery Privileges include completing the following steps:

- (i) Completing the da Vinci® didactic and on-line training
  - (a) Complete online e-learning module www.selectroboticsurgery.com
  - (b) Complete da Vinci® online module www.davincisurgerycommunity.com
- (ii) Problem Based Learning/Improvement
  - (a) Simulation/Skills and drills on simulator (20 hrs)
    - (1) It is expected that all required simulation modules will have a passing score of 70% or better before moving on to bedside assisting.
- (iii) Case observations (2)
- (iv) Training cases (3-5) - co-managed by proctor and training physician
  - (a) Expectation of shared time on console
  - (b) Emphasis on teaching
- (v) Monitored cases (≥3)
  - (a) Expectation that physician requesting credentialing will perform case in its entirety within a reasonable amount of time and with efficiency
  - (b) Meet or exceed objective skill set necessary for full privileging

It is expected that the surgeon in training will complete the above requirements within 6 months from the time the initial Intuitive da Vinci® training takes place.

Box 1: Robotics curriculum.

Table 1: Percent of hysterectomies by route-by hospital.

	Hospital Type	2010 (n)	2011 (n)	2012 (n)	2013 (n)	2014 (n)	% Change 2010- 2014
Abdominal	Community	37.1 (147)	21.9 (102)	13.5 (58)	17.3 (69)	17.9 (84)	-19.3 (*)
	Teaching	50.2 (321)	37.1 (225)	34 (212)	28.6 (172)	30.9 (169)	-19.3 (*)
Vaginal[a]	Community	41.2 (163)	26.6 (124)	23.9 (99)	22.9 (91)	16.0 (75)	-25.2 (*)
	Teaching	21.9 (140)	21.8 (132)	20.1 (125)	24.8 (149)	24.1 (132)	+2.3
Laparoscopic[b]	Community	16.7 (66)	11.2 (52)	5.8 (25)	5.3 (21)	1.5 (7)	-15.2 (*)
	Teaching	12.5 (80)	10.4 (63)	9 (56)	9.2 (55)	7.3 (40)	-5.2 (*)
Robotic	Community	5.1 (20)	40.3 (188)	57.5 (249)	54.5 (217)	64.7 (304)	+59.6 (*)
	Teaching	15.5 (99)	30.7 (186)	36.9 (230)	37.4 (225)	37.7 (206)	+22.2 (*)
All Minimally Invasive[c]	Community	21.7 (86)	51.5 (240)	63.6 (274)	59.8 (238)	66.2 (311)	+44.5 (*)
	Teaching	28.0 (179)	41.4 (249)	45.9 (286)	46.6 (280)	45.0 (246)	+17.0 (*)

Percentages are rounded up to the nearest tenth place; a includes laparoscopic-assisted vaginal hysterectomy; b includes total laparoscopic hysterectomy and laparoscopic supracervical hysterectomy both via traditional laparoscopy; c combined robotic and laparoscopic cases; *statistical significance, $p < 0.05$.

cases. Training physicians were expected to complete all steps of training within a six-month time period. After successful completion, surgeons were granted probationary privileges for one year. After the first year, a QA committee reviewed the surgeon's case volume and patient outcomes and subsequently granted or denied continued privileges.

3. Results

Patients who had a hysterectomy for any indication were identified and included in the study. Combining data from both hospitals, there were 5175 cases total: 1036 cases in 2010, 1072 cases in 2011, 1054 cases in 2012, 999 cases in 2013, and 1014 cases in 2014. These patients were stratified into a category based on type of hysterectomy performed and percentages were calculated and trended for further analysis.

Over the five-year study period there was a significant decrease in the percent of cases performed via an abdominal approach. In the community hospital the percent of abdominal hysterectomies went from 37.1% in 2010 to 17.9% in 2014 (Table 1, Figure 1(a)). In the teaching hospital the rate of abdominal hysterectomies went from 50.2% in 2010 to 30.9% in 2014 (Table 1, Figure 1(b)). Looking at the hospitals together, there was 20.2% overall decline in the rate of abdominal hysterectomies over the study period (Table 2, Figure 1(c)).

The rate of nonrobotic laparoscopic cases also decreased. In the community and academic hospitals only 16.7% and 12.5% (respectively) of hysterectomies were done via this method at the beginning of the study period. Despite already being the least commonly used method of hysterectomy, rates of "straight-stick" laparoscopy were seen to further decline. In the community hospital, the rate fell by 15.2%, with this route making up less than 2% of hysterectomies in 2014 (Table 1, Figure 1(a)). In the academic hospital the rate of this approach decreased by 5.2% (Table 1, Figure 1(b)). In both hospitals together, there was a 9.4% decline (Table 2, Figure 1(c)).

There was a concurrent, inversely related, significant increase in the rate of robotic cases. This was seen in both the community hospital, where robotic cases rose by 59.6%

TABLE 2: Percent of hysterectomies by route-both hospitals.

Type of Hysterectomy	2010 (n)	2011 (n)	2012 (n)	2013 (n)	2014 (n)	% Change 2010-2014
Abdominal	45.2 (468)	30.5 (327)	25.6 (270)	24.1 (241)	25.0 (253)	-20.2 (∗)
Vaginal[a]	29.3 (303)	23.9 (256)	21.3 (224)	24.0 (240)	20.4 (207)	-8.8 (∗)
Laparoscopic[b]	14.1 (146)	12 (115)	7.7 (81)	7.6 (76)	4.7 (47)	-9.4 (∗)
Robotic	11.5 (119)	34.9 (374)	45.5 (479)	44.2 (442)	49.9 (506)	+38.4 (∗)
All Minimally Invasive[c]	25.6 (265)	46.9 (489)	53.1 (560)	51.9 (518)	54.6 (554)	+29.1 (∗)

Percentages are rounded up to the nearest tenth place; a includes laparoscopic-assisted vaginal hysterectomy; b includes total laparoscopic hysterectomy and laparoscopic supracervical hysterectomy both via traditional laparoscopy; c combined robotic and laparoscopic cases; ∗statistical significance, $p < 0.05$.

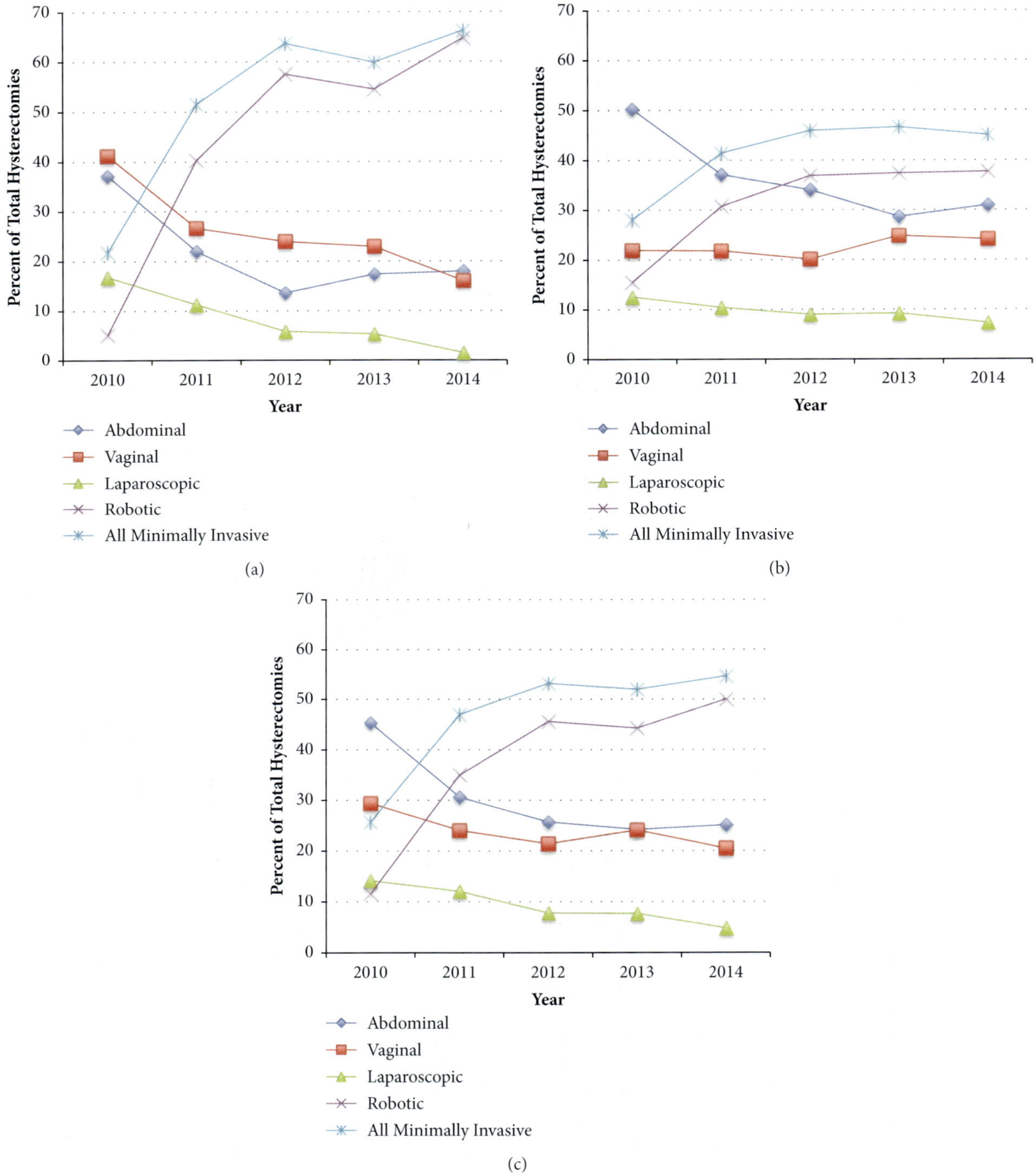

FIGURE 1: (a) Percent of hysterectomies by route-community hospital. (b) Percent of hysterectomies by route-teaching hospital. (c) Percent of hysterectomies by route-both hospitals.

(Table 1, Figure 1(a)), and the teaching hospital, where robotic cases rose by 22.2% (Table 1, Figure 1(b)). Combining the data from both hospitals, the rate of robotic cases rose by 38.4% (Table 2, Figure 1(c)).

A decrease in the number of cases done vaginally was noted at the community hospital only, where there was a 25.2% decline during the study period (Table 1, Figure 1(a)). In the teaching hospital, the percent of cases performed vaginally was 21.9% in 2010 and increased (although not achieving statistical significance) to 24.1% of cases in 2014 (Table 1, Figure 1(b)).

4. Discussion

The introduction of robotic surgery has had a significant impact on trends in route of hysterectomy. In this hospital system, the implementation of a comprehensive robotic training and monitoring program aimed to ensure proficiency prior to its use. There was a significant decline in percent of abdominal hysterectomies performed, with an inversely related increase in laparoscopic hysterectomies, specifically robotic-assisted, over the same time period. These results are consistent with a study published in JAMA in 2013 that gathered data from 441 hospitals across the US (N = 264,758) [3]. This study had a four-year study period, from 2007-2010, and found that there was a substantial increase in both laparoscopic and robotic-assisted hysterectomies, and a decrease in both vaginal and abdominal hysterectomies. While the results of our study are similar to previously published data, it also gives us insight as to how different hospital settings may impact these trends [3, 10–13]. One unique strength of our study is the inclusion of data from a large teaching hospital in addition to a smaller community hospital. As a result, our data can be extrapolated to larger patient populations. This also helps to ensure that observed trends are not unique to an academic center that may reflect a different rate of adoption than that of community hospitals. In addition, this study also provides a relatively long study period of five years over which to monitor these trends.

The ability to analyze data from the two hospitals separately has its own advantages. In the community hospital the rates of vaginal hysterectomy decreased over the study period, whereas in the academic hospital the rates increased. One plausible explanation is that practice is more influenced by consumer demand in the private hospital setting. Advertisements and publicity permeate the minds of the general public, seemingly insinuating that robotic surgery is the current standard of practice. Vaginal hysterectomies are simultaneously viewed as less desirable and outdated. On the contrary, an academic center has a strong emphasis on education and evidence-based practice standards. In this setting, surgical technique is taught and generally performed in accordance with current practice guidelines. The rate of vaginal hysterectomies remained unchanged over the study period in keeping with ACOG recommendations to do so whenever feasible. In addition, full subspecialty services at the academic center, including urogynecology, are available to assist and proctor surgeons performing vaginal cases. All of these factors help explain the disparity in rates of vaginal hysterectomies in the different hospital settings.

A weakness of the study is that the design type is observational in nature and does not provide causality for the observed trends. Deciding upon a route of hysterectomy involves both surgeon and patient-specific factors. The main surgeon-specific factor addressed in this study is the surgeon's skill set and comfort level with traditional laparoscopic and/or robotic surgery, compared to conventional vaginal approach. The robotic training and certification program in this study allowed surgeons to learn and subsequently elect to perform robotic hysterectomy if they were interested in doing so. Conversely, practitioners who do not routinely perform vaginal hysterectomies may not be comfortable employing this approach even when surgically indicated. Other surgeon-specific factors, such as access to laparoscopic equipment and compensation for different routes of hysterectomy, add an additional layer of complexity in surgical planning. Patient-specific factors include pathology and patient-specific characteristics (i.e., obesity) and how they have changed over time. Finally, cost is a driving force in all aspects of healthcare and greatly impact trends in surgical methods. Some insurance companies require preauthorization for any nonvaginal hysterectomy [14]. While this study investigated overall trends in route of hysterectomy, the next step may be to further analyze causation and stratify the impact of these recognized factors.

An interesting implication of the changing rates in route of hysterectomy is how this will affect future Ob/Gyn resident training. From 2003 to 2011, the American Council of Graduate Medical Education (ACGME) reported a decline in the mean number of abdominal and vaginal hysterectomies per resident, by 27.4% and 43%, respectively [15, 16]. This trend is consistent with the data from the community hospital, where a decline in both vaginal and abdominal hysterectomies was observed. This translates into fewer open abdominal and vaginal hysterectomies, which subsequently threatens the development of broad-based surgical skills in training gynecologists. However, we found no change in the rate of vaginal hysterectomies performed at the academic center during the study period. Despite the national trend, it is clearly possible to maintain numbers of vaginal cases alongside the increasing popularity of the robot. It is the responsibility of practicing gynecologists to acknowledge vaginal hysterectomy as the ACOG-endorsed standard of care so it does not get underutilized or forgotten. While not feasible in every patient, this route should be discussed and offered when possible. If current trends continue undeterred, development of vaginal and abdominal surgical skills in training gynecologists will be significantly affected.

5. Conclusion

Whether viewed from a patient, resident, or attending perspective, the introduction of the robotic-assisted hysterectomy has significantly impacted the field of gynecology. How this skill set will ultimately fit into the toolbox of the practicing gynecologist is yet to be determined. The robotic training and monitoring program detailed in this study offers an effective way to ensure surgical proficiency of providers offering robotic services. Perhaps more significantly, in a teaching hospital setting, it is more feasible to address the appropriate application of new technologies while offering support for less experienced surgeons. This would include subspecialty support, such as urogynecology, for potential vaginal hysterectomy candidates. Trends in route of hysterectomy are clearly multifactorial and involve patient, provider, and location-specific factors that are likely to continue to change.

Disclosure

Some of the data in this paper was presented in a poster at the 2015 AAGL Global Congress.

Acknowledgments

The authors would like to acknowledge Dr. John Leahy for his help in presenting the information in this study as a poster presentation at the 2015 AAGL Global Conference. Additionally, they would like to thank Dr. Katherine Betcher for her help in presenting it in the form of an abstract at the 2016 ACOG Annual Clinical and Scientific Meeting.

References

[1] The American College of Obstetricians and Gynecologists, "ACOG Committee Opinion no. 444: choosing the route of hysterectomy for benign disease," *Obstetrics & Gynecology*, vol. 114, no. 5, pp. 1156–1158, 2009.

[2] "AAGL Position Statement: Robotic-Assisted Laparoscopic Surgery in Benign Gynecology," *Journal of Minimally Invasive Gynecology*, vol. 20, no. 1, pp. 2–9, 2013.

[3] J. D. Wright, C. V. Ananth, S. N. Lewin et al., "Robotically assisted vs laparoscopic hysterectomy among women with benign gynecologic disease," *Journal of the American Medical Association*, vol. 309, no. 7, pp. 689–698, 2013.

[4] J. W. M. Aarts, T. E. Nieboer, N. Johnson et al., "Surgical approach to hysterectomy for benign gynaecological disease," *Cochrane Database of Systematic Reviews*, vol. 8, Article ID CD003677, 2015.

[5] A. P. Advincula and A. Song, "The role of robotic surgery in gynecology," *Current Opinion in Obstetrics and Gynecology*, vol. 19, no. 4, pp. 331–336, 2007.

[6] H. Liu, D. Lu, L. Wang, G. Shi, H. Song, and J. Clarke, "Robotic surgery for benign gynaecological disease," *Cochrane Database of Systematic Reviews*, no. 2, Article ID CD008978, 2012.

[7] J. A. N. Dorresteijn, D. M. W. Kriegsman, W. J. J. Assendelft, and G. D. Valk, "Patient education for preventing diabetic foot ulceration," *Cochrane Database of Systematic Reviews*, vol. 12, Article ID CD001488, 2014.

[8] T. N. Payne and F. R. Dauterive, "A Comparison of Total Laparoscopic Hysterectomy to Robotically Assisted Hysterectomy: Surgical Outcomes in a Community Practice," *Journal of Minimally Invasive Gynecology*, vol. 15, no. 3, pp. 286–291, 2008.

[9] C. C. G. Chen and T. Falcone, "Robotic gynecologic surgery: Past, present, and future," *Clinical Obstetrics and Gynecology*, vol. 52, no. 3, pp. 335–343, 2009.

[10] C. A. Walsh, S. R. Walsh, T. Y. Tang, and M. Slack, "Total abdominal hysterectomy versus total laparoscopic hysterectomy for benign disease: A meta-analysis," *European Journal of Obstetrics & Gynecology and Reproductive Biology*, vol. 144, no. 1, pp. 3–7, 2009.

[11] M. Loring, S. N. Morris, and K. B. Isaacson, "Minimally invasive specialists and rates of laparoscopic hysterectomy," *Journal of the Society of Laparoendoscopic Surgeons*, vol. 19, no. 1, Article ID e2014.00221, pp. 1–6, 2015.

[12] E. B. Rosero, K. A. Kho, G. P. Joshi, M. Giesecke, and J. I. Schaffer, "Comparison of robotic and laparoscopic hysterectomy for benign gynecologic disease," *Obstetrics & Gynecology*, vol. 122, no. 4, pp. 778–786, 2013.

[13] L. C. Turner, J. P. Shepherd, L. Wang, C. H. Bunker, and J. L. Lowder, "Hysterectomy surgery trends: a more accurate depiction of the last decade?" *American Journal of Obstetrics & Gynecology*, vol. 277, no. 2, pp. e1–e7, 2013.

[14] T. L. Beck, C. B. Morse, H. J. Gray, B. A. Goff, R. R. Urban, and J. B. Liao, "Route of hysterectomy and surgical outcomes from a statewide gynecologic oncology population: Is there a role for vaginal hysterectomy?" *American Journal of Obstetrics & Gynecology*, vol. 214, no. 3, pp. 348–348.e9, 2016.

[15] D. Moola, L. B. Westermann, R. Pauls, M. Eschenbacher, and C. Crisp, "The impact of robotic-assisted surgery on training gynecology residents," *Female Pelvic Medicine & Reconstructive Surgery*, vol. 22, no. 1, pp. 11–15, 2016.

[16] E. E. Washburn, S. L. Cohen, E. Manoucheri, R. K. Zurawin, and J. I. Einarsson, "Trends in reported resident surgical experience in hysterectomy," *Journal of Minimally Invasive Gynecology*, vol. 21, no. 6, pp. 1067–1070, 2014.

35

Microvascular Anastomosis Training in Neurosurgery

Vadim A. Byvaltsev,[1,2,3,4] Serik K. Akshulakov,[5] Roman A. Polkin,[1] Sergey V. Ochkal,[1] Ivan A. Stepanov,[1] Yerbol T. Makhambetov,[5] Talgat T. Kerimbayev,[5] Michael Staren,[6] Evgenii Belykh,[1,6] and Mark C. Preul[6]

[1] *Irkutsk State Medical University, Krasnogo Vosstaniya St. 1, Irkutsk, Russia*
[2] *Irkutsk Scientific Center of Surgery and Traumatology, Bortsov Revolutsii St. 1, Irkutsk, Russia*
[3] *Railway Clinical Hospital, Irkutsk-Passazhirskiy of Russian Railways Ltd., Botkina St. 10, Irkutsk, Russia*
[4] *Irkutsk State Medical Academy of Postgraduate Education, Jubileiniyi 100, Irkutsk, Russia*
[5] *National Center of Neurosurgery, 34/1 Turan Av., Astana, Kazakhstan*
[6] *Department of Neurosurgery Research, Barrow Neurological Institute, St. Joseph's Hospital and Medical Center, 350 West Thomas Road, Phoenix, AZ 85013, USA*

Correspondence should be addressed to Vadim A. Byvaltsev; byval75vadim@yandex.ru

Academic Editor: Peng Hui Wang

Cerebrovascular diseases are among the most widespread diseases in the world, which largely determine the structure of morbidity and mortality rates. Microvascular anastomosis techniques are important for revascularization surgeries on brachiocephalic and carotid arteries and complex cerebral aneurysms and even during resection of brain tumors that obstruct major cerebral arteries. Training in microvascular surgery became even more difficult with less case exposure and growth of the use of endovascular techniques. In this text we will briefly discuss the history of microvascular surgery, review current literature on simulation models with the emphasis on their merits and shortcomings, and describe the views and opinions on the future of the microvascular training in neurosurgery. In "dry" microsurgical training, various models created from artificial materials that simulate biological tissues are used. The next stage in training more experienced surgeons is to work with nonliving tissue models. Microvascular training using live models is considered to be the most relevant due to presence of the blood flow. Training on laboratory animals has high indicators of face and constructive validity. One of the future directions in the development of microsurgical techniques is the use of robotic systems. Robotic systems may play a role in teaching future generations of microsurgeons. Modern technologies allow access to highly accurate learning environments that are extremely similar to real environment. Additionally, assessment of microsurgical skills should become a fundamental part of the current evaluation of competence within a microneurosurgical training program. Such an assessment tool could be utilized to ensure a constant level of surgical competence within the recertification process. It is important that this evaluation be based on validated models.

1. Introduction

Cerebrovascular diseases are among the most widespread diseases in the world, which largely determine the structure of morbidity and mortality rates. Cerebral vascular pathology comprises the major part of neurology and neurosurgery. Today, significant progress has been made in the field of preventative revascularization of strokes due to the introduction of new technologies of microneurosurgery into clinical practice, contributing to the improvement of safety of treatment. It was shown that cerebral revascularization using extracranial to intracranial bypass may result in neurological symptoms improvement and an objective increase in regional cerebral blood flow in a selective cohort of patients with symptomatic chronic cerebrovascular ischemia [1]. But at the same time, several randomized controlled trials have shown no benefit of surgical revascularization compared to the best medical treatments to prevent stroke [2]. Bypass techniques are still valuable for the surgical treatment of complex cerebral aneurysms by reducing the risk of temporary and constant brain ischemia due to the alteration in blood flow.

Microvascular anastomosis techniques are important for revascularization surgeries on brachiocephalic and carotid arteries, complex cerebral aneurysms, and even during resection of brain tumors that obstruct major cerebral arteries. Successful performance of such complex procedures necessitates advanced requirements for neurosurgical training programs. Such training should include anastomosis practice in the depth of operative wound in conditions of limited vascular mobility and limited time periods.

Because of its complexity, the microanastomosis technique cannot be acquired by observing more experienced surgeons. Training in microsurgery requires considerable time and training resources. Surgeons develop microsurgical skills during training courses or in local hospital laboratories by practicing on various simulation models, using both synthetic and biological materials [3]. Analysis of the training of neurosurgery residents revealed a growing dissatisfaction with the quality of training as forty percent of young surgeons rated their microsurgical training as inadequate [4]. In this regard, neurosurgical training programs may benefit from an increased focus on hands-on microsurgical training.

In this text we will briefly discuss the history of microvascular surgery, review current literature on the simulation models with the emphasis on their merits and shortcomings, and describe the views and opinions on the future of the microvascular training in neurosurgery.

2. History of Microanastomosis Techniques Development

Modern surgery cannot be imagined without the vascular suture. The history of surgical interventions on the vessels goes back to at least ancient Hindu civilization, Greece, and Rome [24]. Instructions and experience to perform ligature procedures to locally arrest hemorrhage can be traced from Celsus through Galen, Oribasius, Rhases, Avicenna, Averroes, Guy of Cauliac, Lanfrancus, and Ambrose Pare. Ancient and medieval skilled surgeons or trained medical personnel traveling with the army frequently placed ligatures around bleeding vessels. They knew how to use tourniquets, arterial clamps, and ligatures to stem blood flow. It was common knowledge among ancient surgeons that veins and arteries carried blood; it was obvious to those dealing with horrendous injuries of weapons such as swords, knives, and spears which caused catastrophic peripheral injuries to soldiers and gladiators. The Roman surgeon was highly motivated to keep as many soldiers as functional as possible and had many delicate instruments for dealing with bleeding vessels. Hooks, probes, and other long thin metal instruments allowed efficient and effective maneuvering of small pieces of tissue. Such instruments were primarily used for dissection and for identifying and isolating blood vessels.

The first documented case of vessel recovery was an operation conducted by Hallowell in 1759, in which the patient was sutured with a lateral lesion of the wall of the brachial artery [25]. In 1877 Russian surgeon Eck first performed the anastomosis "side-by-side" between two vessels: the portal and the inferior vena cava [26]. In 1889 Jassinowski used thin nodular sutures when sewing a damaged vessel in a person, suggesting that vascular sutures should not penetrate through the intima of the vessel [27]. However, the most significant technical breakthrough occurred in 1902, when Carrel reported [28] the triangulation technique of anastomosing the vessel for which in part he was awarded the Nobel Prize in 1912. It is this technique of anastomosis developed by Alexis Carrel that is still used today. The following year, Hopfner reported a successful limb replantation in a dog [29]. The work of these pioneers laid the foundation for the subsequent development of microvascular surgery.

Introduction to clinical practice of anticoagulants was one of the key events in vascular surgery. Heparin was discovered by McLean in 1916 and the first successful clinical trials were published in the 1930s [30, 31]. The ability to control clotting was an important step in the development of microvascular surgery.

The final innovation that prompted the beginning of microvascular surgery was the introduction of an operating microscope into clinical practice. In 1954, in Sweden, Nylean experimented on a rabbit fenestration of the ear labyrinth fistula under a microscope with an increase of 10–15 magnification [32]. In 1922, his supervisor Holmgren invented the world's first binocular microscope and introduced its use in otology [33].

In 1963, American neurosurgeon Kurze introduced a microscope into neurosurgical practice to remove the neuroma of the seventh nerve [33, 34]. Then, in 1960 Jacobson and Suarez first described the technique of performing vascular microanastomoses using an operating microscope, which marked the beginning of microvascular surgery [35].

In 1962 Jacobson together with Donaghy reported the first endarterectomy from the middle cerebral artery, using microsurgical reconstruction [36]. In 1965 Potts performed an anastomosis between the superficial temporal artery and the anterior cerebral artery, using a synthetic prosthesis as a shunt [37]. The era of widespread development of revascularization surgery began on October 30, 1967. After a year of training at the Donaghy Microsurgical Laboratory, Yasargil first performed the superposition of an extra-intracranial (EC-IC) microanastomosis between the superficial temporal artery and the cortical branch of middle cerebral artery in a patient with occlusion of the internal carotid artery [38].

Since the 1970s, reconstructive vascular surgeries have begun in the vertebrobasilar basin. Sundt performed EC-IC bypass between occipital artery and posterior cerebral artery in patients with cerebral circulation disorder [39]. Further development of vascular microneurosurgery led to the development of intra-intracranial (IC-IC) microanastomosis techniques. In 1979 Miller et al. conducted a microanastomosis between the middle meningeal artery and the cortical branch of the middle cerebral artery in a 61-year-old patient with parasagittal meningioma [40]. This technique has been intensively developed since the early 1990s and has found its application in reconstructive interventions in the treatment of complex cerebral aneurysms.

TABLE 1: Validated models for microvascular anastomosis practice.

Type	Author	Model	Approximate cost, availability, logistics	Validity
Non-animal	Meier et al., 2004 [5]	Silicone and polymer microtubes	$10–100 cost, no need for coordination with the ethics committee, simple technical equipment	High constructive validity, low face validity
	Guler and Rao, 1990 [6]	Surgical glove	No cost, no need for coordination with the ethics committee, simple technical equipment	High constructive validity, low face validity
Animal	Bates et al., 2013 [7]	Poultry blood vessels	Little to moderate cost, no need for coordination with the ethics committee, simple technical equipment	High constructive validity, low face validity
	Shurey et al., 2014 [8]	Live laboratory animals (rat)	Average cost $120, requires protocol approval by the Institutional Animal Care and Use Committee, requires vivarium and animal care staff, requires pharmaceuticals and training for administration of anesthesia	High face and constructive validity
	Belykh et al., 2016 [9]	Bovine placental arteries	No to little cost, anatomical relevance, requires coordination with local dairy. Does not require approval from ethics committee	High construct, content, and constructive validity
Human	Aboud et al., 2002 [10]	Perfused cadavers	High cost of cadaveric material, requires special laboratory space to work with cadaver material, normal vessel structure and feel usually disrupted by preservation techniques	No formal validation performed
	Tellioglu et al., 2009 [11]	Human cadaveric vessels	High cost of cadaveric material, preservation techniques, time or temperature changes may damage vessel structure and feel, requires special laboratory space to work with cadaver material	No formal validation performed
	Belykh et al., 2016 [9]	Human placental arteries	No cost, anatomical relevance, requires coordination with obstetrics department, requires protocol approval from the ethics committee	High construct, content, and constructive validity
Technical	Alrasheed et al., 2014 [12]	Robotic systems	High cost of equipment and services	No formal validity of microscope or robot

3. Overview of Definitions

The term validity is borrowed from literature on the problems of knowledge assessment and attestation. Its use in the context of simulation differs from the traditional one. In the context of knowledge assessment, in the simplest form, validity reflects the adequacy of the methodology in measuring outcomes. With respect to simulation, validity is the ability to teach higher cognitive, emotional, and psychomotor skills as much as is expected by the degree of realism achieved.

To assess the simulation models, several types of validity are distinguished [3]. "Face validity" is used to determine the realism of the situation and shows how well the experimental model reflects the actual operation; "content validity" is an assessment of the adequacy of the simulation, to what extent the model estimates a specific skill, and not other aspects, for example, anatomical knowledge; "construct validity" determines whether the successful passage of the model correlates with real operational skills, thus differentiating beginners and experts; "predictive validity" determines that the skills acquired in the simulator training process reflect the skill level in the real operating theater and are translated into clinical practice [41].

4. Simulation Models of Microanastomosis for a "Dry" Training

Among the various models used for the training of the microanastomosis skills (Table 1), dry models are the simplest ones.

In "dry" microsurgical training, simulation models simulating biological tissues created from various materials are used. Such models are useful for beginning surgeons, since they are economically viable and do not require sophisticated technical equipment or coordination with an ethical committee. Disadvantages include low face and content validity. Thus, such models are only suitable for practicing basic skills of microscopy, training beginning surgeons with the subsequent transition to living models, and maintaining the skill of more experienced surgeons [42].

At the initial stage of the microvascular training, silicone tubes are used, which allow for the explanation of the basic principles of superposition of different types of anastomoses [43]. They are available in the form of cards with a set of tubes of different diameters: 2.0 mm, 1.0 mm, and 0.7 mm. In addition to silicone, the tubes can also be made of polyurethane [5], a thin latex [44], or hydrogel based on polyvinyl alcohol [45]. A simple model of microanastomosis can also be made from a conventional surgical glove [6]. This model is created by two longitudinal incisions of the glove strip, in which the glove site is then sewn by nodal seams. The obtained tube of glove rubber is suitable for testing anastomosing technique.

Such models can have potentially high construct validity. However, they have low face validity in view of the lack of similarity with living tissues since the elastic properties of the tubes do not correspond to the properties of living vessels. Thus, they cannot fully replace the "wet" training. With silicone tubes, it is best to train counter-pressure technique, suturing, and knotting in different directions.

To develop skills of anastomosing in a deep field, advanced synthetic models with an artificial skull and brain can be used, allowing for the use of brain retractors [46]. Modeling of the topographic location of arteries and cranial structures is carried out with computed tomography data and may be produced for a specific patient. Such models are excellent for sharpening the skills of working with microinstruments in the deep surgical field, handholding techniques with the hand rest against the cranial structures, and exercising suturing on vessels located with variable depths [47].

5. Tissue Simulation Models for a "Wet" Training

The next stage in training more experienced surgeons is to work with nonliving biological tissue models. Similarly to artificial models, nonliving biological models do not require complex technical equipment, coordination with the ethics committee (except for human tissues), and the availability of laboratories and have a relatively low cost. They have a potentially high face and construct validities, as they provide experience of handling of biological tissue. The main drawback of such models is the absence of living tissues and functioning blood flow.

The simplest tissue model is the use of chicken blood vessels taken from the wing [48]. Some authors reported that the use of chicken wing arteries reduced the use of live models by 80–100% [49]. The average size of the cortical branch of the middle cerebral artery is 1 mm (range 0.6–1.4 mm), which corresponds to the size of the radial arteries of the chicken wings [50]. A more efficient alternative to a chicken vessels can be the use of turkey wings [7]. Comparative studies show the superiority of turkey vessels due to the larger size of the vessels and decreased variability [51]. Other vessels exist such as in the thigh, but these require dissection, and such sections of the chicken or turkey are more expensive as they are more preferred food grade product. Chicken and turkey wings are seldom preferred for consumption and thus are much less cost to obtain. The vessels at the top of the wing are easily identified and dissected, and many wings can be stored in the freezer and then thawed and used by the student when convenient for practice.

The technique of microvascular anastomosis can also be reproduced using human or bovine placentas [9]. Human placenta anastomosis model includes cleaning of the fetal surface of the placenta, isolation of a second, or third-order arterial branch of 2-3 mm in diameter and more than 30 mm in length. This branch is then dissected free, cut distally, and moved towards the adjacent 1-2 mm arterial branch to perform an end-to-side anastomosis. Human placental arteries and bovine placental veins are convenient, are anatomically relevant material, and are a useful model for microneurosurgical training. Bovine placental vessels have some structural differences compared to human placentas, but they can be easily and continuously obtained from local dairies. Both human and bovine placentas are expansive, allowing several students to work at once on various sizes of vessels. They can be stored unperfused in normal saline in the refrigerator for up to at least a week. These models have a high face, content, and constructive validity. Models of cadaveric vessels have also been described [11]. The advantage of human cadaveric models is the possibility to practice the relevant human vessels of various sizes and diameters. However, this advantage comes with a risk of infections and need for appropriate infrastructure for acquisition and work with cadaveric material.

All of the above-mentioned models can be augmented by creating artificial perfusion using a closed system that mimics the circulation, using silicone tubes for intravenous infusion [52]. Standard infusion pumps can be connected to the system to simulate arterial pressure and pulsation may be simulated with these pumps. The system is filled with normal saline and can be tinted to achieve a resemblance to blood. A disadvantage of dyes is their frequent staining of the walls of the vessels. Blood perfusion most accurately simulates a living model due to the correspondence of viscosity and fluidity in living models, but may be impractical [53].

Perfused cadaver brain is a laborious model to set-up but is most similar to the real operative environment [54]. The opening of the arachnoid cisterns, vascular dissection, and microanastomosis can be performed very realistically in such a model although the actual "feel" of the vessel is usually altered (i.e., stiffened) as it is affected by the perfusate.

6. "Wet" Training Using Live Models

Microvascular training using live models could be considered as one of the best substrates for training of microvascular anastomoses due to the presence of natural blood flow. Despite the huge variety of models designed to replace training using animals, live models remain to be an indispensable part of microsurgical courses around the world.

Training conducted on laboratory animals has high indicators of face and constructive validity [8]. Working with animal vessels allows feasible rehearsal of the main stage of reconstructive vascular brain surgeries, the direct microanastomosis [55]. The presence of natural blood flow,

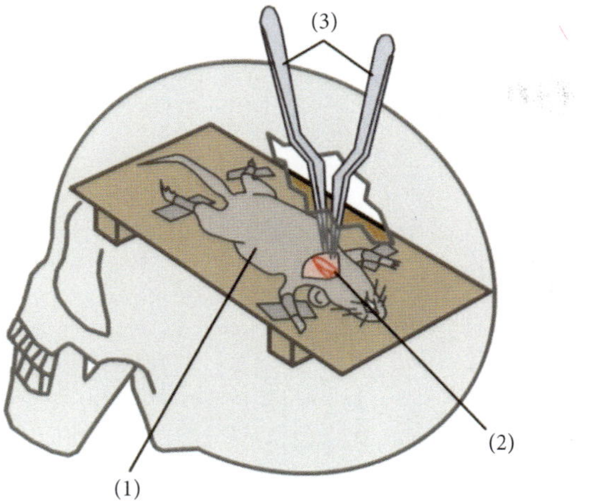

Figure 1: Microsurgical training on rat carotid arteries using an artificial skull with craniotomy as a simulation of surgical approach: (1) rat, (2) rat carotid arteries, and (3) microsurgical instruments.

the potential for thrombosis, and relative similarity of live animal tissues to human allow trainees to practice technique with great viability and realism.

A Wistar rat is the most commonly used laboratory animal in microvascular laboratories (Figure 1).

Microvascular suturing can be practiced on multiple large animal vessels including femoral, iliac, and carotid arteries and veins, aorta, and vena cava. Multiple types of anastomoses can be performed on the rat vessels including end-to-end, end-to-side, and side-to-side anastomoses and various arterial loops [8]. Venous [56], arterial, and synthetic vascular grafts [57] can also be used for practice on live animals.

Performance of anastomosis in the deep confined surgical field can be simulated with a plastic hand-rest that is placed above the operated area of the rat. This gives an open field about 3 cm wide and 3 cm deep. An anastomosis of the arteries and veins is then carried out through this opening [8].

Vessels of the rat are also suitable for submillimeter microanastomoses, like on the distal femoral neurovascular bundle with vessel diameter of 0.5 to 0.8 mm [58]. Vessels of such small diameter may be used for the treatment of moyamoya disease in children. However, otherwise, submillimeter vessels are rarely anastomosed in neurosurgery.

Working with living tissues provides great opportunities for training and assessing the skills of the surgeon. One of the most serious complications of the EC-IC bypass operations is cerebral ischemia associated with vascular thrombosis. The frequency of thrombosis has been reported to be as low as 1.7% in specialized centers [59]. The presence of thrombosis cannot be estimated on a nonliving model; therefore laboratory animal models give the opportunity to identify and analyze the causes of errors and develop methods to prevent their further occurrence.

Another advantage of working with animals is the ability to fully assess the damage to surrounding tissues during the operation. During training with nonliving models, the smallest damage that the surgeon does to surrounding tissues is not always noticeable. Live models can reveal such imperfections and provide valuable feedback to the operator. Also, the limitation of time is an important condition when working on anesthetized laboratory animal.

However, when working with laboratory animals, there are additional requirements for equipping the laboratory, coordinating logistics and training with procurement and handling of animals, acquiring ethical committee approval, ensuring adequate pharmaceutical control, and caring for animals during the surgery. The purchase and maintenance of laboratory animals impose serious material costs for the organization of a microvascular training laboratory. In order to minimize economic losses, various methods are being used: reducing work with animals on the initial stages and replacing them with synthetic or using tissue models from cryopreserved animal vessels left after training by more experienced trainees [60]. Trainees working with live animals should be required to practice on as many appropriate vessels as possible, not only on carotid arteries, but also on various accessible arteries and veins in the body as mentioned, even to include the vas deferens.

Despite the economic difficulties in their organization, microsurgery courses using live models have many advantages. They provide an excellent substrate to improve surgical skills and provide high accuracy of simulating clinical operations. The use of live models at advanced courses within the training program for microsurgeons is an excellent simulation model for complex procedures for microsurgical reconstruction. The live rat is one of the most universal models of microsurgery courses around the world, and 50 years after microsurgery was first developed, the laboratory rat model is still valid for developing microsurgery skills.

7. New Horizons in the Evolution of Microanastomosis Simulation Models

Training in microsurgery has always been conducted in the modeled environment, and the use of laboratory rat as a teaching model became standard, despite being without objective evidence of advantage over other models. The ex vivo simulation environment is becoming increasingly appealing on the basis of research that indicates reduced economic costs and limiting the use of animals. The experimental ex vivo training offers an economically efficient means to master microsurgical skills and it is in this environment that learning curves for specific exercises can be established [61]. Modern microsurgical training is often based on theories of acquiring and developing skills. As a result, validation and modeling have become increasingly important components of the microsurgical simulation.

As we proceed towards standardization of the microsurgical simulation models, there is a need to choose reliable assessment tools that adequately assess microsurgical competence (Table 2).

Requirements for objective methods for evaluating microsurgical techniques led to the development of several global rating scales. These scales split the process of microsurgery into the relevant components, which are found to

TABLE 2: Tools for microvascular anastomosis performance assessment.

Author	Assessment Tool	Comments
Martin et al., 1997 [13]	Objective structured assessment of technical skills	Established validity for general surgery and microsurgery, this is one of the first and most reliable assessment tools
Grober et al., 2003 [14]	Imperial College surgical assessment device	Motion tracking device attached to the surgeon's hands for objective assessment of the motions during surgical training
Moulton et al., 2006 [15]	Modified objective structured assessment of technical skills	A video based modified version of the objective structured assessment of technical skills
Chan et al., 2010 [16]	Structured assessment of microsurgery skills	Validated tool for microanastomosis assessment validated in clinical setting
Temple and Ross, 2011 [17]	University of Western Ontario microsurgical skills acquisition/assessment instrument	Validated tool for microvascular performance assessment
Ghanem et al., 2013 [18]	Anastomotic patency assessment tool	This tool uses qualitative photogrammetry for the assessment of anastomosis quality with a special attention to the intimal surface
Alrasheed et al., 2014 [12]	Structured assessment of robotic microsurgical skills	Tool was developed to assess microsurgical skills using the Da-Vinci surgical robot while performing a 3-mm vessel diameter microanastomosis
Satterwhite et al., 2014 [19]	The Stanford microsurgery and resident training scale	This tool was validated on latex and chicken vessels
Aoun et al., 2015 [20]	Northwestern objective microanastomosis assessment tool	Face and construct validity has been established for this tool
Harada et al., 2015 [21]	Instrument motion tracking	Infrared motion tracking camera has been use for objective measurement of the instrument movements in experienced and novice surgeons during microanastomosis training
Ghanem et al., 2016 [22]	Anastomosis lapse index	A list of possible errors could be used for quantitative assessment
Belykh et al., 2017 [23]	Objective structured assessment of aneurysm clipping skills	Tool was validated on the human placenta aneurysm models

contribute to the overall effectiveness of the task accomplishment [62]. Video recording allows one to assess skills in a controlled environment [63], and, as technology developed, various methods for assessing competence became available, such as hand motion analysis. For example, the Imperial College of Surgeons capture device uses motion sensors attached to hands to assess hand movements and the length of time to complete a task [64]. It was shown that this device has applications for the evaluation of trainees microsurgeons [65].

One of the future directions in the development of microsurgical techniques is the use of robotic systems. Performing operations using these devices has several advantages. For example, the presence of hand tremor during surgical procedures is completely eliminated with robots, which is important when working under high magnification [66]. Furthermore, the precision of manipulation can be increased to the level that surpass free-hand human abilities [67]. These advantages provide great promise for using robotics in microsurgical manipulations. However, the main current limitation of robotic systems is an increase in the time spent for manipulations compared to standard techniques by 24–60% [67, 68]. Robotic systems attached to the arm or hand may limit the normal movement of the hand, thus significantly slowing the procedure. When using the Zeus® robotic surgery system, the increase in the time to complete anastomosis is also associated with the large size of the needle holder installed on this device [68].

The use of robotic systems to teach microsurgical skills may play a role in the education of the future generations of microsurgeons. The advantage includes familiarization with the methods of remote robotic manipulation of the instruments at the early stage of training. With the use of a robotic system, the goal is to bridge the gap in the quality and speed of anastomoses between the experienced surgeon and a specialist who does not possess special skills in microsurgery [67]. However, the fact that anastomosis completion time is still shorter with conventional method when compared to a robotic one [68] indicates the need of substantial improvements in robotic microsurgery before its use in surgical practice or training could be approved. Incorporation of various microvascular anastomotic devices such as Precise (3M, St. Paul, MN) for end-to-end anastomosis and Elana (Elana bv, Utrecht, Netherlands) for end-to-side anastomosis would result in decrease of the anastomosis time and could advance the field.

During microsurgical procedures, the operator is visually immersed in the operative environment with a microscope thorough the eyepieces; therefore this type of surgery is well suited for developing virtual reality simulation technologies [69]. Stanford University has developed a system that consists of a graphical workstation connected to a stereoscopic display. Real microsurgical instruments, to which motion sensors are connected, are used as input devices. Traceable tools allow the user to perform microanastomoses, and the system evaluates the effectiveness of the surgeon based on a set of objective variables [70]. Further research is necessary in this area to assess the role of virtual reality in surgical education, especially for the manual skill development. However, with the rapid advances in the three-dimensional visualization and tactile feedback sensors, there is a high likelihood that such simulators would play an increasing role in surgical learning of microanastomosis techniques.

8. Conclusions

In this article, we reviewed several models for the study and training of vascular microsurgery. Although very few of these models have been validated, such become an increasingly important component of surgical education. Additionally, evaluation of microsurgical skills is becoming an important part of the current evaluation of the trainee's competence in a training program. At more advanced levels, simulation models can be utilized to assess the level of competence of surgeons within the recertification process. It is important that such evaluation be based on validated models.

Modern technologies provide highly accurate and extremely realistic learning environments. Microsurgery, over the past decades, has made significant progress in the field of materials, technologies, and the scope of reconstructive methods. However, efforts are yet to be made to establish appropriate tools and models for training and assessment of competence. Evidence of reliability and validity must be obtained before models can be included in training and accreditation programs. The ideal model should be one that can combine being highly relevant and meaningful, having high constructive and predictive validity, and being economically efficient. Implementation of validated realistic training models and modern objective assessment tools will further advance the microsurgical training.

References

[1] P. Jabbour and N. Chalouhi, "Simulation-based neurosurgical training for the presigmoid approach with a physical model," *Neurosurgery*, vol. 73, no. 4, pp. S81–S84, 2013.

[2] R. L. Grubb, W. J. Powers, W. R. Clarke, T. O. Videen, H. P. Adams, and C. P. Derdeyn, "Surgical results of the Carotid Occlusion Surgery Study," *Journal of Neurosurgery*, vol. 118, no. 1, pp. 25–33, 2013.

[3] W.-Y. Chan, P. Matteucci, and S. J. Southern, "Validation of microsurgical models in microsurgery training and competence: A review," *Microsurgery*, vol. 27, no. 5, pp. 494–499, 2007.

[4] J. Regelsberger, O. Heese, P. Horn et al., "Training Microneurosurgery – Four Years Experiences with an in vivo Model," *Central European Neurosurgery*, vol. 72, no. 04, pp. 192–195, 2011.

[5] S. A. Meier, A. Lang, and G. M. Beer, "Training von Mikrogefässanastomosen an Polyurethangefässen zur Reduktion von Tierversuchen," in *ALTEX 21.3/04*, vol. 135, 2004.

[6] M. M. Guler and G. S. Rao, "Canniesburn 'ever-ready' model to practise microsurgery," *British Journal of Plastic Surgery*, vol. 43, no. 3, pp. 381-382, 1990.

[7] B. J. Bates, S. M. Wimalawansa, B. Monson, M. C. Rymer, R. Shapiro, and R. M. Johnson, "A simple cost-effective method of microsurgical simulation training: The turkey wing model," *Journal of Reconstructive Microsurgery*, vol. 29, no. 9, pp. 615–618, 2013.

[8] S. Shurey, Y. Akelina, J. Legagneux, G. Malzone, L. Jiga, and A. M. Ghanem, "The rat model in microsurgery education: Classical exercises and new horizons," *Archives of Plastic Surgery*, vol. 41, no. 3, pp. 201–208, 2014.

[9] E. Belykh, T. Lei, S. Safavi-Abbasi et al., "Low-flow and high-flow neurosurgical bypass and anastomosis training models using human and bovine placental vessels: A histological analysis and validation study," *Journal of Neurosurgery*, vol. 125, no. 4, pp. 915–928, 2016.

[10] E. Aboud, O. Al-Mefty, and M. G. Yaşargil, "New laboratory model for neurosurgical training that simulates live surgery," *Journal of Neurosurgery*, vol. 97, no. 6, pp. 1367–1372, 2002.

[11] A. T. Tellioglu, E. Eker, K. Cimen, A. Comert, G. Karaeminogullari, and I. Tekdemir, "Training Model for Microvascular Anastomosis," *The Journal of Craniofacial Surgery*, vol. 20, no. 1, pp. 238-239, 2009.

[12] T. Alrasheed, J. Liu, M. M. Hanasono, C. E. Butler, and J. C. Selber, "Robotic microsurgery: Validating an assessment tool and plotting the learning curve," *Plastic and Reconstructive Surgery*, vol. 134, no. 4, pp. 794–803, 2014.

[13] J. A. Martin, G. Regehr, R. Reznick et al., "Objective structured assessment of technical skill (OSATS) for surgical residents," *British Journal of Surgery*, vol. 84, no. 2, pp. 273–278, 1997.

[14] E. D. Grober, S. J. Hamstra, R. K. Reznick, E. D. Matsumoto, R. S. Sidhu, and K. A. Jarvi, "Validation of novel and objective measures of microsurgical skill: Hand-motion analysis and stereoscopic visual acuity," *Microsurgery*, vol. 23, no. 4, pp. 317–322, 2003.

[15] C.-A. E. Moulton, A. Dubrowski, H. MacRae, B. Graham, E. Grober, and R. Reznick, "Teaching surgical skills: What kind of practice makes perfect? A randomized, controlled trial," *Annals of Surgery*, vol. 244, no. 3, pp. 400–407, 2006.

[16] W. Y. Chan, N. Niranjan, and V. Ramakrishnan, "Structured assessment of microsurgery skills in the clinical setting," *Journal of Plastic, Reconstructive & Aesthetic Surgery*, vol. 63, no. 8, pp. 1329–1334, 2010.

[17] C. L. F. Temple and D. C. Ross, "A new, validated instrument to evaluate competency in microsurgery: The University of Western Ontario microsurgical skills acquisition/assessment instrument" *Plastic and Reconstructive Surgery*, vol. 127, no. 1, pp. 215–222, 2011.

[18] A. Ghanem, A. E. Kim, M. Singh, and S. Myers, "Trauma'12 Winning Abstract - End Product Assessment in Microsurgery Simulation Training - A New Insider View," *Annals of Medicine and Surgery*, vol. 2, no. 1, p. 36, 2013.

[19] T. Satterwhite, J. Son, J. Carey et al., "The stanford microsurgery and resident training (SMaRT) scale: Validation of an on-line global rating scale for technical assessment," *Annals of Plastic Surgery*, vol. 72, no. 1, pp. S84–S88, 2014.

[20] S. G. Aoun, T. Y. El Ahmadieh, N. E. El Tecle et al., "A pilot study to assess the construct and face validity of the Northwestern Objective Microanastomosis Assessment Tool," *Journal of Neurosurgery*, vol. 123, no. 1, pp. 103–109, 2015.

[21] K. Harada, A. Morita, Y. Minakawa et al., "Assessing Microneurosurgical Skill with Medico-Engineering Technology," *World Neurosurgery*, vol. 84, no. 4, pp. 964–971, 2015.

[22] A. M. Ghanem, Y. Al Omran, B. Shatta, E. Kim, and S. Myers, "Anastomosis Lapse Index (ALI): A Validated End Product Assessment Tool for Simulation Microsurgery Training," *Journal of Reconstructive Microsurgery*, vol. 32, no. 3, pp. 233–241, 2016.

[23] E. Belykh, E. J. Miller, T. Lei et al., "Face, Content, and Construct Validity of an Aneurysm Clipping Model Using Human Placenta," *World Neurosurgery*, vol. 105, pp. 952–960, 2017.

[24] "The Battle of Ligatures," in *The Lancet*, vol. 15, p. 889, London, UK, 1877.

[25] Shumacker Jr. and B. Harris, "Authority, research and publication. Reflections based upon some historical aspects of vascular surgery," *Annals of Surgery*, vol. 168, no. 2, pp. 169–182, 1968.

[26] N. V. Eck, "On the question of ligature of the portal vein," *Voenno Med J*, vol. 130, pp. 1-2, 1877.

[27] A. Jassinowski, "Die Arteriennhat: Eine experimentelle Studie," *Inaug Diss Dorpat*, 1889.

[28] A. Carrel, "La technique operatoire des anastomoses vasculaires et la transplantation des visceres," *Lyon méd*, vol. 98, no. 859, 1902.

[29] E. Hopfner, "Uber Gefassnhaht, Gefasstransplantationen und Replantation von amputierten Extremitaten," *Arch Klin Chir*, vol. 70, pp. 417–471, 1903.

[30] A. F. Charles and D. A. Scott, "Studies on heparin I. The preparation of heparin," *Journal of Biological Chemistry*, vol. 102, no. 2, pp. 425–429, 1933.

[31] J. McLean, "The discovery of heparin," *Circulation*, vol. 19, no. 1, pp. 75–78, 1959.

[32] C. O. Nylean, "The microscope in aural surgery, its first use and later development," *Acta Oto-Laryngologica*, vol. 43, no. 116, pp. 226–240, 1954.

[33] V. A. Byvaltsev, "Operating microscope for vertebrologic and cranial operations: from monocular to 3-D imaging," *Sib. med. Zhurn*, vol. 8, 2015.

[34] T. Kurze, "Microtechniques in Neurological Surgery," *Clinical neurosurgery*, vol. 11, pp. 128–137, 1963.

[35] J. H. Jacobson and E. L. Suarez, "Microsurgery in anastomosis of small vessels," *Surgical forum*, vol. 11, 1960.

[36] J. H. Jacobson, L. J. Wallman, G. A. Schumacher, M. Flanagan, E. L. Suarez, and R. M. Peardon Donaghy, "Microsurgery as an Aid to Middle Cerebral Artery Endarterectomy," *Journal of Neurosurgery*, vol. 19, no. 2, pp. 108–115, 1962.

[37] D. G. Potts, "Aneurysms and arteriovenous anomalies of the brain: diagnosis and treatment," *Hoeber Medical Division: Harper & Row*, 1965.

[38] R. M. Donaghy, "The history of microsurgery in neurosurgery," *Clinical Neurosurgery*, vol. 26, pp. 619–625, 1979.

[39] T. M. Sundt Jr., J. P. Whisnant, D. G. Piepgras, J. K. Campbell, and C. B. Holman, "Intracranial bypass grafts for vertebral-basilar ischemia," *Mayo Clinic Proceedings*, vol. 53, no. 1, pp. 12–18, 1978.

[40] C. F. Miller, R. F. Spetzler, and D. J. Kopaniky, "Middle meningeal to middle cerebral arterial bypass for cerebral revascularization. Case report," *Journal of Neurosurgery*, vol. 50, no. 6, pp. 802–804, 1979.

[41] R. K. Reznick, "Teaching and testing technical skills," *The American Journal of Surgery*, vol. 165, no. 3, pp. 358–361, 1993.

[42] N. Matsumura, N. Hayashi, H. Kamiyama et al., "Microvascular anastomosis at 30-50 magnifications (super-microvascular anastomosis) in neurosurgery," *Surgical Neurology International*, vol. 2, no. 1, article no. 6, 2011.

[43] B. J. Kim, S. Kim, Y. Jeong, W. Lee, K. Lee, and S. Paeng, "An Efficient Microvascular Anastomosis Training Model Based on Chicken Wings and Simple Instruments," *Journal of Cerebrovascular and Endovascular Neurosurgery*, vol. 15, no. 1, pp. 20–25, 2013.

[44] H. Tehrani, J. McPhail, and K. Graham, "A simple training model for microvascular repair," *Journal of Plastic, Reconstructive & Aesthetic Surgery*, vol. 63, no. 6, article 1063, 2010.

[45] T. Mutoh, T. Ishikawa, H. Ono, and N. Yasui, "A new polyvinyl alcohol hydrogel vascular model (KEZLEX) for microvascular anastomosis training," *Surgical Neurology International*, vol. 1, no. 74, 2010.

[46] T. Ishikawa, N. Yasui, and H. Ono, "Novel brain model for training of deep microvascular anastomosis," *Neurologia medico-chirurgica*, vol. 50, no. 8, pp. 627–629, 2010.

[47] M. Takeuchi, N. Hayashi, H. Hamada, N. Matsumura, H. Nishijo, and S. Endo, "A new training method to improve deep microsurgical skills using a mannequin head," *Microsurgery*, vol. 28, no. 3, pp. 168–170, 2008.

[48] J. K. Byeong et al., "An efficient microvascular anastomosis training model based on chicken wings and simple instruments," *Journal of cerebrovascular and endovascular neurosurgery*, vol. 15, no. 1, pp. 20–25, 2013.

[49] H. Schoffl et al., "Strategies for the reduction of live animal use in microsurgical training and education," *ATLA-Alternatives to Laboratory Animals*, vol. 36, no. 2, article 153, 2008.

[50] P. A. S. Kadri, A. F. Krisht, and G. K. Gandhi, "An anatomic mathematical measurement to find an adequate recipient M4 branch for superficial temporal artery to middle cerebral artery bypass surgery," *Operative Neurosurgery*, vol. 61, no. 3, pp. S-74–S-78, 2007.

[51] A. A. Abla, T. Uschold, M. C. Preul, and J. M. Zabramski, "Comparative use of turkey and chicken wing brachial artery models for microvascular anastomosis training: Laboratory investigation," *Journal of Neurosurgery*, vol. 115, no. 6, pp. 1231–1235, 2011.

[52] M. E. Colpan, K. V. Slavin, S. Amin-Hanjani, M. Calderon-Arnuphi, and F. T. Charbel, "Microvascular anastomosis training model based on a turkey neck with perfused arteries," *Operative Neurosurgery*, vol. 62, 5, pp. ONS407–ONS411, 2008.

[53] K. G. Krishnan, P. Dramm, and G. Schackert, "Simple and viable in vitro perfusion model for training microvascular anastomoses," *Microsurgery*, vol. 24, no. 4, pp. 335–338, 2004.

[54] J. Olabe, J. Olabe, and V. Sancho, "Human cadaver brain infusion model for neurosurgical training," *World Neurosurgery*, vol. 72, no. 6, pp. 700–702, 2009.

[55] B. Mathon, "Apprentissage des techniques microchirurgicales vasculaires sur un modèle animal," *Neurochirurgie*, vol. 60, no. 5, pp. 227–233, 2014.

[56] R. Sooppan, S. J. Paulsen, J. Han et al., "In vivo anastomosis and perfusion of a threedimensionally-printed construct containing microchannel networks," *Tissue Engineering Part C: Methods*, vol. 22, no. 1, pp. 1–7, 2015.

[57] N. Lee, R. A. Daley, and B. C. Cooley, "Rat posterior facial vein interpositional graft: A more relevant training model," *Microsurgery*, vol. 34, no. 8, pp. 653–656, 2014.

[58] H. L. Liu, "Microvascular Anastomosis of Submillimeter Vessels—A Training Model in Rats," *Journal of Hand and Microsurgery*, vol. 05, no. 1, pp. 14–17, 2013.

[59] V. A. Byvaltsev, E. G. Belykh, and I. A. Stepanov, "The choice of the treatment method for cerebral aneurysms of different locations in the era of advanced endovascular technologies: A meta-analysis," *Vestnik Rossiĭskoĭ akademii meditsinskikh nauk*, vol. 71, no. 1, pp. 31–40, 2016.

[60] N. R. Lausada, E. Escudero, R. Lamonega, E. Dreizzen, and J. C. Raimondi, "Use of cryopreserved rat arteries for microsurgical training," *Microsurgery*, vol. 25, no. 6, pp. 500-501, 2005.

[61] J. C. Selber, E. I. Chang, J. Liu et al., "Tracking the Learning Curve in Microsurgical Skill Acquisition," *Plastic and Reconstructive Surgery*, vol. 130, no. 4, pp. 550e–557e, 2012.

[62] A. Mehta and P. S. Li, "Male infertility microsurgical training," *Asian Journal of Andrology*, vol. 15, no. 1, pp. 61–66, 2013.

[63] N. Jabbour and J. Sidman, "Assessing instrument handling and operative consequences simultaneously: A simple method for creating synced multicamera videos for endosurgical or microsurgical skills assessments," *Simulation in Healthcare*, vol. 6, no. 5, pp. 299–303, 2011.

[64] V. Datta, S. Mackay, M. Mandalia, and A. Darzi, "The use of electromagnetic motion tracking analysis to objectively measure open surgical skill in the laboratory-based model," *Journal of the American College of Surgeons*, vol. 193, no. 5, pp. 479–485, 2001.

[65] I. Balasundaram, R. Aggarwal, and L. A. Darzi, "Development of a training curriculum for microsurgery," *British Journal of Oral and Maxillofacial Surgery*, vol. 48, no. 8, pp. 598–606, 2010.

[66] C. G. Knight et al., "Computer-assisted, robot-enhanced open microsurgery in an animal model," *Journal of Laparoendoscopic & Advanced Surgical Techniques*, vol. 15, no. 2, pp. 182–185, 2005.

[67] J. Lee, T. Mattar, T. Parisi, B. Carlsen, A. Bishop, and A. Shin, "Learning Curve of Robotic-Assisted Microvascular Anastomosis in the Rat," *Journal of Reconstructive Microsurgery*, vol. 28, no. 07, pp. 451–456, 2012.

[68] R. A. Li, J. Jensen, and J. C. Bowersox, "Microvascular anastomoses performed in rats using a microsurgical telemanipulator," *Computer Aided Surgery*, vol. 5, no. 5, pp. 326–332, 2000.

[69] R. S. Haluck and T. M. Krummel, "Computers and virtual reality for surgical education in the 21st century," *JAMA Surgery*, vol. 135, no. 7, pp. 786–792, 2000.

[70] K. Montgomery et al., "Virtual reality in microsurgery training," *Medicine meets virtual reality*, vol. 41, 1999.

TULAA: A Minimally Invasive Appendicectomy Technique for the Paediatric Patient

Giordano Perin and Maria Grazia Scarpa

Paediatric Surgery and Urology, Institute of Maternal and Child Health, IRCCS Burlo Garofolo, Trieste, Italy

Correspondence should be addressed to Giordano Perin; giordanoperin87@gmail.com

Academic Editor: Stephen Kavic

TULAA or Transumbilical Laparoscopic Assisted Appendicectomy is a minimally invasive technique described by Pelosi in 1992 for the removal of the inflamed appendix. Its main advantage is the possibility of exploring the peritoneal cavity and performing a simple and safe extracorporeal appendicectomy. Since its first description, different authors reported their experience with such technique. The aim of this review is to summarise the surgical outcomes currently reported in the literature for this minimally invasive surgical approach and compare it with standard open and laparoscopic appendicectomy.

1. Introduction

The first literature report of a technique for the removal of the inflamed appendix dates back to Amyand in 1735 [1]: the surgeon removed the inflamed appendix of a young child that swallowed a pin. The appendix was found in an inguinal hernia sac and was perforated by the swallowed pin. In 1889, once made professor of Surgery [2], Charles McBurney highlighted the importance of early diagnosis and early surgical treatment of such a condition. Since then, many different techniques have been described. The first description of a laparoscopic appendicectomy in an adult population dates back to Semm in 1983 [3]. Such a technique became widely popular in the following years and is now considered a standard treatment for acute appendicitis. In 1992, Pelosi described an innovative surgical approach [4]: a Transumbilical Laparoscopic Assisted Appendicectomy (TULAA). This technique requires the use of an initial laparoscopic approach with pneumoperitoneum via a single umbilical port, the externalisation of the inflamed appendix via that port, and the removal of the appendix itself via a standard extracorporeal appendicectomy. Since then, this technique became quite popular especially in some European countries and has been shown to be particularly effective in the paediatric population. The main advantage of this approach is combining the possibility of exploring the peritoneal cavity and performing a simple and safe extracorporeal appendicectomy with a single small umbilical incision. The aim of this review is to summarise the results reported in the literature especially concerning the surgical outcomes (surgical time, hospital stay, and complications) and compare such results with what is reported for open and laparoscopic appendicectomy.

2. Materials and Methods

We searched PubMed and Google Scholar using the keywords "Transumbilical Laparoscopic assisted Appendicectomy", "Transumbilical Laparoscopic assisted Appendectomy", "Single Port Appendicectomy", and "Single Port Appendectomy". After analysing the available abstracts, we selected only the papers reporting results related to a laparoscopic assisted extracorporeal appendicectomy technique with umbilical access (initial laparoscopic approach via a single umbilical port and pneumoperitoneum, minimal dissection of the identified appendix with or without the insertion of a second port, externalisation of the inflamed appendix via the umbilical port and deflation of the pneumoperitoneum, and removal of the appendix itself via a standard extracorporeal technique and closure). A total of 24 papers, published between 1998 and 2015, were finally selected and reviewed. All the papers analysed were in English language. Seven were available in the form of abstracts; the remaining 17 were available in full text. Only 2 papers comparing Transumbilical Laparoscopic Assisted Appendicectomy with a standard open appendicectomy were found. Only 3 papers comparing Transumbilical Laparoscopic Assisted Appendicectomy with a standard laparoscopic appendicectomy were retrieved. Only 2 papers comparing outcomes between Transumbilical Laparoscopic Assisted Extracorporeal Appendicectomy, open appendicectomy, and laparoscopic appendicectomy were found.

3. Results

24 studies were found and analysed. Four involved a mixed population of adults and children; 20 described only paediatric cases. Inclusion and exclusion criteria were extremely variable and not always available (see Table 1). The specific technique in terms of equipment used (laparoscope, type of port, and number of ports used) is variable across the analysed studies; a detailed report can be found in Table 1. The number of patients enrolled ranged from 11 to 500. Only retrospective analyses were available; no prospective cohort studies were found.

The overall operating time reported in the literature ranges from 10 to 196 minutes. The use of descriptive statistic methods varies across the analysed literature; some authors prefer to report their outcome as mean operating time, and some authors prefer to use a median value. Overall, the mean/median operating time reported ranges from 15 to 58.6 minutes (see Table 2 for details). The overall hospital stay reported ranges from 1 to 89 days. Again, the use of descriptive statistic methods varies across the analysed papers; the mean/median hospital stay reported ranges from 2 to 7.9 days.

The need to use one or more additional ports to complete the appendicectomy ranges from 0 to 26.9%. The rate of conversion to open appendicectomy ranges from 0 to 15%.

The surgical wound infection rate ranges from 0 to 13.7% and the rate of intra-abdominal abscess ranges from 0 to 3.8%.

A full summary of the analysed literature is available in Table 1 (selection criteria, technique, and laparoscope used) and Table 2 (surgical time, hospital stay, and complication rate).

Only two studies comparing Transumbilical Laparoscopic Assisted Appendicectomy with a standard open technique were identified. Pappalepore and colleagues in 2002 [8] retrospectively analysed the records of 65 children undergoing a standard extracorporeal appendectomy and 58 patients undergoing a two-port Transumbilical Laparoscopic Assisted Extracorporeal Appendicectomy: 1 surgical wound infection was recorded in the first group, and no complications were recorded in the second group. Koizumi and colleagues in 2015 [22] retrospectively compared 64 patients undergoing open appendicectomy with 62 patients undergoing a single port Transumbilical Laparoscopic Assisted Extracorporeal Appendicectomy. 8/64 patients developed a complication in the first group (5 surgical wound infections, 1 intra-abdominal abscess, and 2 cases of ileus); 12/62 patients developed a complication in the second group (9 surgical wound infections, 1 abscess, and 2 cases of ileus).

Only three studies comparing Transumbilical Laparoscopic Assisted Appendicectomy with a standard laparoscopic approach were found. Visnjic [13] compared their outcomes with three different appendicectomy techniques: laparoscopic appendicectomy with staplers (34), laparoscopic appendicectomy with loops (9), and Transumbilical Laparoscopic Assisted Appendicectomy (29). 43 patients underwent one of the two laparoscopic technique appendicectomies and 3 developed a complication (2 wound infections and 1 intra-abdominal abscess). 29 patients underwent a Transumbilical Laparoscopic Assisted Appendicectomy and 4 developed a wound infection. Ostlie [19] in 2011 compared two groups of 180 patients undergoing a standard laparoscopic appendicectomy and Transumbilical Laparoscopic Assisted Extracorporeal Appendicectomy. 1.7% of the patients in the first group and 3.3% of the patients in the second group developed a wound infection. Finally, Kulaylat and colleagues [26] compared 132 patients that underwent Transumbilical Laparoscopic Assisted Appendicectomy with 240 patients treated with a standard laparoscopic multiport appendicectomy. Median operating time was shorter for Transumbilical Laparoscopic Assisted Appendicectomy (1 h versus 0.6 h, $p < 0.0001$). Hospital stay was comparable in the two groups. Fourteen out of 240 (5.8%) patients in the laparoscopic appendicectomy group and 9/132 (6.8%) patients in the Transumbilical Laparoscopic Assisted Appendicectomy group required a readmission. In each group, one case of surgical wound infection was recorded (resp., 0.42% in the laparoscopic appendicectomy group and 0.75% in the TULAA group). We recorded nine (3.75%) cases of intra-abdominal abscess in the laparoscopic appendicectomy group and 5 (3.8%) in the Transumbilical Laparoscopic Assisted Appendicectomy group.

Only two studies attempted to compare open appendicectomy, laparoscopic appendicectomy, and Transumbilical Laparoscopic Assisted Extracorporeal Appendicectomy. Bergholz and colleagues [24] compared 20 patients undergoing Transumbilical Laparoscopic Assisted Appendicectomy with 20 matched patients treated with laparoscopic appendicectomy and open appendicectomy, respectively. No significant difference between the three groups was found except for a slight increase in the analgesic requirements for the Transumbilical Laparoscopic Assisted Appendicectomy group. Scirè [27] and colleagues compared 46 patients treated with laparoscopic appendicectomy, 62 treated with Transumbilical Laparoscopic Assisted Appendicectomy, and 88 treated with open appendicectomy. They found an increase in wound infection rate and a reduction in length of hospital stay with Transumbilical Laparoscopic Assisted Extracorporeal Appendicectomy.

4. Discussion

The overall quality of the literature published so far is significantly limited: no prospective study analysing the outcomes of Transumbilical Laparoscopic Assisted Appendicectomy has been published. No randomised trial comparing

TABLE 1: Summary of the analysed literature including population, inclusion/exclusion criteria, and trocars and scopes used.

Author	Population number of patients, age in years	Selection criteria	Trocar(s)	Scope
Esposito 1998 [5]	51 patients 4–16 (μ 7)	Not specified	Single trocar 10 mm	Operative scope
Valla et al. 1999 [6]	200 patients 5–18 (μ 9)	No peritonitis No abscess No palpable mass	Single trocar 11 mm	Operative scope
Martino et al. 2001 [7]	40 patients, paediatric, age not specified	Not specified	Single trocar 10 mm	Operative scope
Pappalepore et al. 2002 [8]	58 patients paediatric, age not specified	Uncomplicated	Two trocars 10 mm and 5 mm	Normal scope
D'Alessio et al. 2002 [9]	150 patients 2.5–17.4	Not specified	Single trocar	Not specified
Rispoli et al. 2002 [10]	65 patients mixed population, age not specified	Not specified	Single trocar 10 mm	Operative scope
Koontz et al. 2006 [11]	111 patients μ 11 ± 3.2	All children with preoperative diagnosis of appendicitis	Single trocar 10 mm	Operative scope
Varshney et al. 2007 [12]	11 patients 12–56 y.o. (μ 34)	Not specified	Single trocar 10 mm	Operative scope
Visnjic 2008 [13]	29 patients 5–17 (μ 9.5)	Not specified	Single trocar	Not specified
Guanà et al. 2010 [14]	231 patients μ 11.6 (3–18)	Exclusion of perforated appendicitis	Single trocar 11 mm	Operative scope
Sesia et al. 2010 [15]	262 μ 11.4 (1.1–15.9)	Exclusion of perforated appendix suspected on USS	Single trocar 12 mm with 5 mm working channel	Normal scope
Saber et al. 2010 [16]	26 patients M 33 (13–64)	Exclusion of perforated appendix or abscess at USS or CT	Two trocars (12 mm and 5 mm) through the same umbilical incision	Normal scope
Shekherdimian and DeUgarte 2011 [17]	21 patients paediatric, age not specified	Not specified	Single trocar 3 or 5 mm	Normal scope, grasper inserted through wound
Stylianos et al. 2011 [18]	398 patients paediatric, age not specified	Not specified	Single trocar 12 mm	Operative scope
Ostlie 2011 [19]	180 patients μ 11.5 ± 3.47	Not specified	Single trocar 12 mm plus fascial incision	Normal scope, instruments inserted through fascial incision
Ohno et al. 2012 [20]	500 patients M 10.2 (2–16)	Not specified	Single trocar 12 mm used with 2 instruments	Normal scope, grasper inserted via the same port
Codrich et al. 2013 [21]	203 patients μ 10 (3–17)	As per study protocol	Single trocar 11 mm	Operative scope
Koizumi et al. 2015 [22]	94 patients μ 41.1 (13–89)	Exclusion of patients with peritonitis	Single trocar, triport	Normal scope
Nicola 2014 [23]	120 patients μ 9.9 (6–14)	0–14 years old, uncomplicated appendicitis	Single trocar 10 mm	Operative scope
Bergholz et al. 2014 [24]	20 patients Not reported	Not reported	Not reported	Not reported

Table 1: Continued.

Author	Population number of patients, age in years	Selection criteria	Trocar(s)	Scope
Gupta et al. 2014 [25]	58 patients μ 10.2 (3–16)	Only interval appendectomy	Single trocar 5 mm	Normal scope, second instrument inserted through facial incision
Kulaylat et al. 2014 [26]	132 patients μ 9.4 (±3.8)	Not specified	2 × 5 mm trocars inserted through two umbilical fascial incisions	30 degrees 5 mm scope
Scirè et al. 2014 [27]	62 patients Not specified	Not specified	Not specified	Not specified
Noviello et al. 2015 [28]	300 patients	Uncomplicated appendicitis	Not reported	Not reported

the outcomes of standard techniques with Transumbilical Laparoscopic Assisted Appendicectomy has been identified. It is important to highlight that a significant number of the published reports (12/24) enrolled a limited number of patients, less than 100. If we exclude those small studies, the range of surgical complications rate changes significantly (see Table 3 for details). Overall results seem to be comparable with what is reported in the literature for both a mixed population [29] (Table 3) and a paediatric population [30] (Table 4).

Inclusion and exclusion criteria as well as preoperative investigations vary significantly across the analysed studies. Valla and colleagues [6] exclude patients affected by peritonitis, with a palpable mass or abscess, but do not specify by which means such conditions are diagnosed. While peritonitis and palpable mass are both clinical diagnosis, a confirmatory ultrasound may be needed to assess the presence of an abscess. Pappalepore [8] and colleagues included only patients with uncomplicated appendicitis: again they do not specify what preoperative investigations were carried out to assess the presence or the absence of complications. Koontz and colleagues [11] excluded all patients with documented perforated appendix at computer tomography: those patients were initially treated with antibiotics and an interval Transumbilical Laparoscopic Assisted Appendicectomy was performed at 4–6 weeks. Guanà and colleagues excluded patients with evidence of perforated appendix: all patients included were evaluated on the basis of biochemical (full blood count, C reactive protein) and radiological (ultrasound of the abdomen) investigations. Sesia and colleagues [15] adopted a similar approach. Saber [16] and colleagues used ultrasound or computed tomography to exclude patients with a perforated appendix or an abscess. Codrich and colleagues [21] used ultrasound to assess the presence of an appendiceal mass and schedule patients for an immediate appendicectomy or an interval/delayed appendicectomy. Koizumi and colleagues [22] excluded patients with evidence of peritonitis. Noviello and colleagues [28], finally, excluded patients affected by complicated appendicitis based on clinical and ultrasound findings: patients affected by complicated appendicitis were treated with open appendicectomy. The heterogeneity of the preoperative protocols adopted in the management of these patients might have influenced the reported surgical outcomes. In this context, it is important to highlight that only one study [21] explicitly enrolled all patients with acute appendicitis regardless of the initial clinical, radiological, or biochemical presentation.

The techniques described in the literature are extremely different between each other and in three out of 24 analysed studies details of the technique are not reported. The most commonly used technique reported in the literature requires the use of an operative laparoscope. We analysed 24 studies, ten of which involved the use of this kind of laparoscope, which carries the invaluable advantage of allowing the surgeon to visualise and perform dissection using a single port. Alternative described techniques involve the use of two trocars: the second trocar can be positioned suprapubically [8] or directly through the same umbilical incision [16, 26]. Ostlie [19] described the use of a second instrument inserted directly via an umbilical fascial incision, without the use of an additional port. Such a variety in the surgical technique could potentially affect the quality of the surgical outcome.

The operating time reported in the literature for Transumbilical Laparoscopic Assisted Appendicectomy is extremely variable. As mentioned, this range from 10 to 223 minutes and the mean or median operating time reported ranges from 15 to 58.6 minutes. If we exclude studies including less than 100 patients, the mean or median operating time does not change significantly (see Tables 3 and 4 for details). It is important to highlight, however, that the operating time is not significantly different from what is expected to be the operating time needed for a standard open or laparoscopic appendicectomy in a mixed population [29] or in a paediatric population [30]. These results may be biased by the lack of inclusion and exclusion criteria and a comparison to standard techniques may not be reliable.

The overall hospital stay reported in the literature for Transumbilical Laparoscopic Assisted Appendicectomy ranges from 1 to 89 days. Again, if we exclude the smaller studies (less than 100 patients enrolled), the picture does not change. It is important to highlight, however, that if we exclude the unfortunate case reported by Ohno and

TABLE 2: Summary of the analysed literature including surgical time (in minutes), length of hospital stay (in days unless otherwise specified), and complications/need for additional ports.

Author	Population number of patients, age in years	Surgical time (minutes)	Hospital stay (days)	Complications/need for additional ports
Esposito 1998 [5]	51 patients 4–16 (μ 7)	M 25 (12–45)	M 2 (1–4)	None
Valla et al. 1999 [6]	200 patients 5–18 (μ 9)	M 15 (10–90)	M 2 (1–22)	16 (8%): insertion of another trocar 3 (1.5%): parietal complications 7 (3.5%): intra-abdominal complications
Martino et al. 2001 [7]	40 patients, paediatric, age not specified	M 50.9 (30–120)	Not specified	Not specified
Pappalepore et al. 2002 [8]	58 patients paediatric, age not specified	M 25	2–4	1: conversion to open (1.7%) 1: additional trocar (1.7%)
D'Alessio et al. 2002 [9]	150 patients 2.5–17.4	μ 35	μ 3.5	28: additional trocar (18.6%) 6: conversions to OA (4%)
Rispoli et al. 2002 [10]	65 patients mixed population, age not specified	M 25 (15–70)	M 2 (1–4)	5: additional trocar (7.7%) 5: conversions to OA (7.7%)
Koontz et al. 2006 [11]	111 patients μ11 ± 3.2	M 36 (9–140)	μ 1.8 (1–11)	2: additional trocar (1.8%) 2: conversions to OA (1.8%) 1: intra-abdominal abscess (0.9) 7: wound infections (6.3%)
Varshney et al.2007 [12]	11 patients 12–56 y.o. (μ 34)	M 20 (15–25)	M 1.5 (1-2)	None
Visnjic 2008 [13]	29 patients 5–17 (μ 9.5)	μ 39 (24–66)	M 3	4: wound infections (13.7%)
Guanà et al. 2010 [14]	231 patients μ 11.6 (3–18)	μ 38 (25–100)	μ 3.5 (3–7)	1: insertion of second trocar (0.43%) 1: insertion of two additional trocars (0.43%) 1: enlargement of initial incision 2: conversions to OA (8.6%)
Sesia et al. 2010 [15]	262 μ 11.4 (1.1–15.9)	Not specified	Not specified	3: intra-abdominal abscess (1.1%)
Saber et al. 2010 [16]	26 patients M 33 (13–64)	M 45.9 (30–80)	M 1.1 (0–2)	4: additional trocar (15.4%) 3: two additional trocars (11.5%)
Shekherdimian and DeUgarte 2011 [17]	21 patients paediatric, age not specified	μ 51 ± 15	μ 1.2 ± 0.8	3: conversions to OA (14.3%)
Stylianos et al. 2011 [18]	398 patients paediatric, age not specified	μ 24 (5–56)	Not reported	39: additional one or more trocars (9.8%)
Ostlie 2011 [19]	180 patients μ 11.5 ± 3.47	μ 35.2 ± 14.5	M < 1 day (22.7 ± 6.2 h)	3.3%: surgical site infection
Ohno et al. 2012 [20]	500 patients M 10.2 (2–16)	M 44.5 (10–169)	M 7.9 (1–89)	3: single additional trocar (0.6%) 11: two additional trocars (2.2%) 21: intraoperative complications (4.2%) 26: postoperative complications (5.2%)

TABLE 2: Continued.

Author	Population number of patients, age in years	Surgical time (minutes)	Hospital stay (days)	Complications/need for additional ports
Codrich et al. 2013 [21]	203 patients μ 10 (3–17)	M 52	Not reported	181: urgent operations 5: wound infections (2.5%) 5: abscess (2.5%)
Koizumi et al. 2015 [22]	94 patients μ 41.1 (13–89)	M 54 (23–223)	M 4.7 (1–33)	5: surgical site infection (5.3%) 1: abscess (1%) 2: ileus (2.1)
Nicola 2014 [23]	120 patients μ 9.9 (6–14)	μ 58.6 (14–135)	μ 3.7 (2–14)	11: additional trocar (9%) 8: conversion to LAP (6%) 5: surgical site infection (4%) 1: abscess (0.8%)
Bergholz et al. 2014 [24]	20 patients Not reported	Not reported	Not reported	Reported to be not significantly different from OA and LA group
Gupta et al. 2014 [25]	58 patients μ 10.2 (3–16)	M 52	μ 1.2 ± 0.8	3 cases converted to OA (5.2%)
Kulaylat et al. 2014 [26]	132 patients μ 9.4 (±3.8)	μ 36	M 4 (0.7–12)	1: surgical wound infection (0.75%) 5: intra-abdominal abscess (3.8%)
Scirè et al. 2014 [27]	62 patients Not specified	Not specified	Not specified	Similar complications in the three included groups (see text for details)
Noviello et al. 2015 [28]	300 patients	μ 42	Not reported	45: conversion to OA (15%) 3: conversion to LA (1%) 11: surgical site infection (3.7%)

μ: mean, M: median, and OA: open appendicectomy.

TABLE 3: Comparison of outcomes with College of Surgeons National Surgical Quality Improvement Program (NSQIP) database for 2005 to 2008, data published by Fleming et al. [29].

	Fleming et al. [29]		Range of mean/median or percentage value reported in the literature for TULAEA	
	Open appendicectomy	Laparoscopic appendicectomy	Including all studies	Including only studies with >100 patients
Operating time	49 minutes (M)	47 minutes (M)	15–58.6 minutes (M/μ)	15–58.6 minutes (M/μ)
Hospital stay	2.3 days	1.8 days	2–7.9 days (M/μ)	2–7.9 days (M/μ)
Conversion rate	N/A	1.9%	0–15%	0–15%
Surgical wound infection	5.2%	1.7%	0–13.7%	0–6.3%
Organ space infection	1.9%	1.8%	0–3.8%	0–3.8%

M: median, μ: mean, M/μ: range of median or mean values reported in the literature, and N/A: not applicable.

colleagues [20], the range drops to 1 to 22 days. The reported mean or median hospital stay ranges from 2 to 7.9 days. This is comparable with what we would expect for a standard or open laparoscopic appendicectomy in a mixed population [29] or in a paediatric population [30]. Again, the lack of clear inclusion and exclusion criteria makes the comparison difficult.

The reported need for one or more additional ports ranges from 0 to 26.9%. If we exclude the smallest reports (including less than 100 patients), this ranges from 0 to 18.6%. This is an extremely important factor to take into account: one-fifth of the cases required the use of an additional port. Unfortunately, the number of cases requiring the use of two additional ports (conversion to standard laparoscopic appendicectomy) is poorly documented in the literature.

The conversion rate reported ranges from 0 to 15%. If we exclude the smallest studies (including less than 100 patients), this does not change. These figures are not that different but still are slightly higher than the one normally reported in the literature for a laparoscopic appendicectomy in the adult

Table 4: Comparison of outcomes with meta-analysis data of open versus laparoscopic appendicectomy, data published by Aziz et al. [30].

	Aziz et al. [30]		Range of mean/median or percentage value reported in the literature for TULAEA	
	Open appendicectomy	Laparoscopic appendicectomy	Including all studies	Including only studies with >100 patients
Operating time	83 to 46 minutes (μ)	73 to 31 minutes (μ)	15–58.6 minutes (M/μ)	15–58.6 minutes (M/μ)
Hospital stay	2.4 to 6.5 days (μ)	1.70 to 7 days (μ)	2–7.9 days (M/μ)	2–7.9 days (M/μ)
Conversion rate	N/A	0 to 25.9%	0–15%	0–15%
Surgical wound infection	5%	1.5%	0–13.7%	0–6.3%
Organ space infection	3.4%	3.8%	0–3.8%	0–3.8%

M: median, μ: mean, M/μ: range of median or mean values reported in the literature, and N/A: not applicable.

and mixed population [29–32]. If we consider a paediatric population [30], however, the conversion rate is comparable.

The quality of the data related to complication rate is poor. The follow-up period is extremely variable in the published literature and often not reported (see Table 2).

Overall, we can say that wound infection rate ranges from 0 to 13.7%. If we exclude the smallest studies (less than 100 patients enrolled), this ranges from 0 to 6.3%. If we compare the data with what is reported for open appendicectomy in the adult and paediatric population, we realise that the figures are extremely similar and higher than what is reported for laparoscopic appendicectomy. The argument that performing an extracorporeal appendicectomy with the inflamed appendix going through the umbilical wound increases the infection rate compared to a laparoscopic approach seems to be true.

Organ space infection (intra-abdominal abscess) is reported in a rate variable from 0 to 3.8%. If we compare this data with what is known for a mixed adult and paediatric population [29], we realise that these figures are slightly higher. On the other hand, if we compare the data with what is reported in the literature for the paediatric population, there is basically no difference [30]. This could be due to multiple factors: first of all, the lack of inclusion and exclusion criteria, the fact that the population is mostly paediatric, and finally the fact that Transumbilical Laparoscopic Assisted Appendicectomy is a technique much less standardised compared with open and laparoscopic appendicectomy. Performing an extracorporeal appendicectomy with a purse string suture to bury the appendiceal stump seems not to reduce the risk of intra-abdominal collection.

Another very important point is related to costs: using one single port and simple instruments, the technique itself is cheaper than a standard laparoscopic appendicectomy as shown by different authors [11, 13, 18, 26]. Visnjic [13] compared their outcomes with three different appendicectomy techniques: laparoscopic appendicectomy with staplers (34), laparoscopic appendicectomy with loops (9), and Transumbilical Laparoscopic Assisted Appendicectomy (29). Considering only the cost of consumables used in the three techniques, they highlight how Transumbilical Laparoscopic Assisted Appendicectomy is cheaper as it involves the use of single multifilament absorbable suture instead of staples or endoloops. Kulaylat and colleagues [26] analysed their experience with 132 patients treated with Transumbilical Laparoscopic Assisted Appendicectomy and 240 patients treated with standard laparoscopic appendicectomy. They concluded that Transumbilical Laparoscopic Assisted Appendicectomy is comparable to laparoscopic appendicectomy in terms of surgical outcomes but is overall cheaper. They identified a statistically significant difference in favour of Transumbilical Laparoscopic Assisted Appendicectomy considering both admission and overall cost (including costs associated with readmissions for treatment of complications). It is difficult to identify what factors contributed in generating such difference, but it is overall important to highlight how both operative time and overall length of stay were shorter for patients treated with Transumbilical Laparoscopic Assisted Extracorporeal Appendicectomy. Another relevant factor to consider is that the number of patients treated with laparoscopic appendicectomy found to have a perforated appendix at operation was significantly higher, which could have contributed to increase the overall cost associated with this procedure. Stylianos and colleagues [18] reported their experience with 508 children treated with Transumbilical Laparoscopic Assisted Appendicectomy and compared their surgeon directed disposable supply costs with 17 other children's hospitals. Overall, their single port appendicectomy technique was recorded to be the cheapest. The main factor driving such difference was identified in the use of endomechanical devices which are clearly not required in Transumbilical Laparoscopic Assisted Extracorporeal Appendicectomy.

This technique seems to be particularly helpful in the paediatric population. This is especially true for few reasons. First of all, the value of a diagnostic laparoscopy is particularly significant in the paediatric population: it allows visualisation of the intra-abdominal content minimising the exposure to radiations, even when the diagnosis is in doubt. This is especially relevant if we consider that the resection of Meckel diverticulum can be performed via a single umbilical incision (Laparoscopic Assisted Resection of Meckel's Diverticulum or LATUM [33]). A second very important point is related to the mobilisation of the caecum: while on one side the relatively smaller size of the paediatric patient may represent a challenge for laparoscopic surgery, it makes it easier to externalise the appendix via the umbilical incision. A final relevant aspect to consider is related to the aesthetic impact: few authors highlighted how single port surgery has the potential of leaving a "scarless" abdomen [25, 26].

A further essential aspect to consider in this context is related to the learning curve. Again the quality of the literature available is poor: no specific learning curve study has been published so far and is difficult to identify a single surgical or clinical outcome to determine the shape of such curve. The main issue in this specific case is related to acquiring familiarity with the use of an operative laparoscope. As mentioned before, this seems to be the instrument most commonly used to perform a single port appendicectomy. Using an operative laparoscope requires the surgeon to to adapt to counterintuitive movements and tolerate a high degree of instrument conflict and frequent change in point of view. This could partly justify the high conversion rate and the need for use of further ports to perform the appendicectomy itself. Valla and colleagues [6] highlight how the number of cases that required the use of an additional port to perform the appendicectomy significantly declined following the first 100 procedures: from 7 out of 100 to 2 out of 94. Koontz and colleagues [11] highlight how the use of a procedure such as Transumbilical Laparoscopic Assisted Appendicectomy allows the surgeon to practice and maintain both laparoscopic and open surgery skills. Codrich and colleagues [21] highlight how 75% of the conversions recorded were performed by nonexpert members of the staff and 66% of the conversions to open surgery were performed in the first two years of the study. They highlight how the introduction of this procedure could help introduce less experienced surgeons to laparoscopy. Nicola [23] mentioned a specific number of procedures needed to overcome the learning curve: while for laparoscopic appendicectomy 15 procedures are needed, for Transumbilical Laparoscopic Appendicectomy 10 are deemed sufficient. Unfortunately, the author does not report a specific evidence to support such a statement. Nicola also highlight how in their experience most of the conversions to open technique or standard laparoscopic technique were performed in the first year of the study. If we compare the results reported in the literature for the learning curve for laparoscopic appendicectomy [34], we realise that the learning curve is generally comparable or even shorter. Kim and colleagues [34] report how to overcome the learning curve for laparoscopic appendicectomy; a surgical trainee would need to perform 30 procedures. Unfortunately, due to the fact that the data available in the literature is of poor quality, it is impossible to provide a reliable picture.

A final relevant aspect to consider in this context is the applicability of such technique to acute appendicitis complicated with localised abscess or mass. The approach to such condition is extremely different in the reported literature. Valla and colleagues [6], Noviello and colleagues [28], Sesia and colleagues [15], and Varshney and colleagues [12] decided not to consider Transumbilical Laparoscopic Assisted Extracorporeal Appendectomy a feasible technique in the presence of an abscess or appendiceal mass. On the other hand, Codrich and colleagues [21] and Gupta and colleagues [25] decided not to exclude such patients. Codrich and colleagues report their experience with 7 patients diagnosed with appendicular mass at admission: such patients were treated initially conservatively with antibiotics and all underwent a safe interval Transumbilical Laparoscopic Assisted Appendicectomy 8 weeks later. A similar experience is reported by Gupta and colleagues [25]: seven of the enrolled patients were identified as having an appendicular mass and were treated with antibiotics and interval Transumbilical Laparoscopic Assisted Appendicectomy 6 weeks later. According to the limited data available in the literature, Transumbilical Laparoscopic Assisted Appendicectomy should be considered as an alternative to open technique or laparoscopic technique for interval appendicectomy.

5. Conclusions

Transumbilical Laparoscopic Assisted Appendicectomy seems to be a safe and effective technique when compared with open and laparoscopic appendicectomy in a paediatric population. Wound infection rate seems to be higher with Transumbilical Laparoscopic Assisted Appendicectomy and open appendicectomy compared with laparoscopic appendicectomy. The main advantage of this approach is combining the possibility of exploring the peritoneal cavity and performing a simple and safe extracorporeal appendicectomy with a single umbilical incision. The overall quality of the published literature was found to be poor: the absence of prospective randomised trials makes the comparison with standard techniques difficult and potentially biased.

Competing Interests

The authors declare that there is no conflict of interests regarding the publication of this paper.

References

[1] C. Amyand, "Of an inguinal rupture, with a pin in the appendix coeci, incrusted with stone; and some observations on wounds in the guts," *Philosophical Transactions*, vol. 39, pp. 329–342, 1735.

[2] S. H. Yale and K. A. Musana, "Charles Heber McBurney (1845–1913)," *Clinical Medicine & Research*, vol. 3, no. 3, pp. 187–189, 2005.

[3] K. Semm, "Endoscopic appendectomy," *Endoscopy*, vol. 15, no. 2, pp. 59–64, 1983.

[4] M. A. Pelosi, "Laparoscopic appendectomy using a single umbilical puncture (minilaparoscopy)," *The Journal of Reproductive Medicine*, vol. 37, no. 7, pp. 588–594, 1992.

[5] C. Esposito, "One-trocar appendectomy in pediatric surgery," *Surgical Endoscopy*, vol. 12, no. 2, pp. 177–178, 1998.

[6] J.-S. Valla, R. M. Ordorica-Flores, H. Steyaert et al., "Umbilical one-puncture laparoscopic-assisted appendectomy in children," *Surgical Endoscopy*, vol. 13, no. 1, pp. 83–85, 1999.

[7] A. Martino, M. Zamparelli, G. Cobellis, L. Mastroianni, and G. Amici, "One-trocar surgery: a less invasive videosurgical

approach in childhood," *Journal of Pediatric Surgery*, vol. 36, no. 5, pp. 811–814, 2001.

[8] N. Pappalepore, S. Tursini, N. Marino, G. Lisi, and P. Lelli Chiesa, "Transumbilical laparoscopic-assisted appendectomy (TULAA): a safe and useful alternative for uncomplicated appendicitis," *European Journal of Pediatric Surgery*, vol. 12, no. 6, pp. 383–386, 2002.

[9] A. D'Alessio, E. Piro, B. Tadini, and F. Beretta, "One-trocar transumbilical laparoscopic-assisted appendectomy in children: our experience," *European Journal of Pediatric Surgery*, vol. 12, no. 1, pp. 24–27, 2002.

[10] G. Rispoli, M. F. Armellino, and C. Esposito, "One-trocar appendectomy: sense and nonsense," *Surgical Endoscopy and Other Interventional Techniques*, vol. 16, no. 5, pp. 833–835, 2002.

[11] C. S. Koontz, L. A. Smith, H. C. Burkholder, K. Higdon, R. Aderhold, and M. Carr, "Video-assisted transumbilical appendectomy in children," *Journal of Pediatric Surgery*, vol. 41, no. 4, pp. 710–712, 2006.

[12] S. Varshney, A. Sewkani, S. Vyas et al., "Single-port transumbilical laparoscopic-assisted appendectomy," *Indian Journal of Gastroenterology*, vol. 26, no. 4, pp. 192–198, 2007.

[13] S. Visnjic, "Transumbilical laparoscopically assisted appendectomy in children: high-tech low-budget surgery," *Surgical Endoscopy and Other Interventional Techniques*, vol. 22, no. 7, pp. 1667–1671, 2008.

[14] R. Guanà, R. Gesmundo, E. Maiullari et al., "Treatment of acute appendicitis with one-port transumbilical laparoscopic-assisted appendectomy: a six-year, single-centre experience," *African Journal of Paediatric Surgery*, vol. 7, no. 3, pp. 169–173, 2010.

[15] S. B. Sesia, F.-M. Haecker, R. Kubiak, and J. Mayr, "Laparoscopy-assisted single-port appendectomy in children: is the postoperative infectious complication rate different?" *Journal of Laparoendoscopic and Advanced Surgical Techniques*, vol. 20, no. 10, pp. 867–871, 2010.

[16] A. A. Saber, M. H. Elgamal, T. H. El-Ghazaly, A. V. Dewoolkar, and A. Akl, "Simple technique for single incision transumbilical laparoscopic appendectomy," *International Journal of Surgery*, vol. 8, no. 2, pp. 128–130, 2010.

[17] S. Shekherdimian and D. DeUgarte, "Transumbilical laparoscopic-assisted appendectomy: an extracorporeal single-incision alternative to conventional laparoscopic techniques," *The American Surgeon*, vol. 77, no. 5, pp. 557–560, 2011.

[18] S. Stylianos, L. Nichols, N. Ventura, L. Malvezzi, C. Knight, and C. Burnweit, "The "all-in-one" appendectomy: quick, scarless, and less costly," *Journal of Pediatric Surgery*, vol. 46, no. 12, pp. 2336–2341, 2011.

[19] D. J. Ostlie, "Single-site umbilical laparoscopic appendectomy," *Seminars in Pediatric Surgery*, vol. 20, no. 4, pp. 196–200, 2011.

[20] Y. Ohno, T. Morimura, and S.-I. Hayashi, "Transumbilical laparoscopically assisted appendectomy in children: the results of a single-port, single-channel procedure," *Surgical Endoscopy and Other Interventional Techniques*, vol. 26, no. 2, pp. 523–527, 2012.

[21] D. Codrich, M. G. Scarpa, M. A. Lembo et al., "Transumbilical laparo-assisted appendectomy: a safe operation for the whole spectrum of appendicitis in children—a single-centre experience," *Minimally Invasive Surgery*, vol. 2013, Article ID 216416, 4 pages, 2013.

[22] N. Koizumi, H. Kobayashi, Y. Nakase, T. Takagi, and K. Fukumoto, "Efficacy of transumbilical laparoscopic-assisted appendectomy for appendicitis: a four-year experience at a single center," *Surgery Today*, vol. 45, no. 10, pp. 1245–1249, 2015.

[23] Z. Nicola, "Transumbilical laparoscopic-assisted appendectomy in children: clinical and surgical outcomes," *World Journal of Gastrointestinal Endoscopy*, vol. 6, no. 4, pp. 101–104, 2014.

[24] R. Bergholz, T. F. Krebs, I. Klein, K. Wenke, and K. Reinshagen, "Transumbilical laparoscopic-assisted versus 3-port laparoscopic and open appendectomy: a case-control study in children," *Surgical Laparoscopy, Endoscopy and Percutaneous Techniques*, vol. 24, no. 3, pp. 244–247, 2014.

[25] R. K. Gupta, A. Gupta, P. Kothari, K. K. Kesan, V. Dixit, and R. Kamble, "Transumbilical laparoscopic-assisted appendectomy: a safe and useful technique for interval appendectomy in pediatric population," *Journal of Minimally Invasive Surgical Sciences*, vol. 3, no. 3, 2014.

[26] A. N. Kulaylat, A. B. Podany, C. S. Hollenbeak, M. C. Santos, and D. V. Rocourt, "Transumbilical laparoscopic-assisted appendectomy is associated with lower costs compared to multiport laparoscopic appendectomy," *Journal of Pediatric Surgery*, vol. 49, no. 10, pp. 1508–1512, 2014.

[27] G. Scirè, A. Mariotto, M. Peretti et al., "Laparoscopic versus open appendectomy in the management of acute appendicitis in children: a multicenter retrospective study," *Minerva Pediatrica*, vol. 66, no. 4, pp. 281–285, 2014.

[28] C. Noviello, M. Romano, A. Martino, and G. Cobellis, "Transumbilical laparoscopic-assisted appendectomy in the treatment of acute uncomplicated appendicitis in children," *Gastroenterology Research and Practice*, vol. 2015, Article ID 949162, 4 pages, 2015.

[29] F. J. Fleming, M. J. Kim, S. Messing, D. Gunzler, R. Salloum, and J. R. Monson, "Balancing the risk of postoperative surgical infections: a multivariate analysis of factors associated with laparoscopic appendectomy from the NSQIP database," *Annals of Surgery*, vol. 252, no. 6, pp. 895–900, 2010.

[30] O. Aziz, T. Athanasiou, P. P. Tekkis et al., "Laparoscopic versus open appendectomy in children: a meta-analysis," *Annals of Surgery*, vol. 243, no. 1, pp. 17–27, 2006.

[31] L. Brügger, L. Rosella, D. Candinas, and U. Güller, "Improving outcomes after laparoscopic appendectomy: a population-based, 12-year trend analysis of 7446 patients," *Annals of Surgery*, vol. 253, no. 2, pp. 309–313, 2011.

[32] S. V. Sakpal, S. S. Bindra, and R. S. Chamberlain, "Laparoscopic appendectomy conversion rates two decades later: an analysis of surgeon and patient-specific factors resulting in open conversion," *Journal of Surgical Research*, vol. 176, no. 1, pp. 42–49, 2012.

[33] T. R. S. Prasad, C. H. Chui, and A. S. Jacobsen, "Laparoscopic-assisted resection of Meckel's diverticulum in children," *Journal of the Society of Laparoendoscopic Surgeons*, vol. 10, no. 3, pp. 310–316, 2006.

[34] S. Y. Kim, S. G. Hong, H. R. Roh, S. B. Park, Y. H. Kim, and G. B. Chae, "Learning curve for a laparoscopic appendectomy by a surgical trainee," *Journal of the Korean Society of Coloproctology*, vol. 26, no. 5, pp. 324–328, 2010.

37

Strangulated Hernia Can Be a Risk Factor of Seroma following Laparoscopic Transabdominal Preperitoneal Repair

Ryu Matsumoto, Yoshio Nagahisa, Kazuki Hashida, Mitsuru Yokota, Michio Okabe, and Kazuyuki Kawamoto

Department of Surgery, Kurashiki Central Hospital 1-1-1, Miwa, Kurashiki, Okayama 710-8602, Japan

Correspondence should be addressed to Ryu Matsumoto; rm15367@kchnet.or.jp

Academic Editor: Diego Cuccurullo

Purposes. Seroma is a postoperative complication following laparoscopic transabdominal preperitoneal repair (TAPP) for inguinal hernioplasty. Seroma naturally resolves in most cases, but it can lead to an increased amount of visits to the outpatient clinic and can result in anxiety of the patient. Local inflammation of the inguinal area is etiology of seroma formation. Strangulated hernia involves severe inguinal pain and can lead to severe inflammation and subsequent seroma. There have been no reports demonstrating the links of seroma and strangulated hernia. This study aimed to retrospectively evaluate the risk of seroma after TAPP and to identify the association between strangulated hernia and seroma. *Methods.* We treated 300 inguinal hernias by TAPP between 2013 and 2016 at Kurashiki Central Hospital. We used the Chi-square test. Factors significant in each association were further examined using multiple subsequent logistic regressions. *Results.* A total of 222 hernias were eligible for analysis. The incidence of seroma was 11% (n=25). There were nine cases of strangulated hernias, and three (33%) resulted in seroma. The ratio of strangulated hernia of seroma group is significantly high ($p<0.03$). Multiple subsequent logistic regressions showed that strangulated hernia was associated with a significantly increased risk for seroma formation ($p = 0.023$; OR 6.564; 95% CI 1.29-33.3). *Conclusion.* This study shows that strangulated hernia can be a risk factor in seroma formation. This risk should be incorporated into a management plan of TAPP for strangulated hernia, with careful consideration of patients' concerns.

1. Introduction

Seroma is a postoperative complication following laparoscopic transabdominal preperitoneal repair (TAPP) for inguinal/ femoral hernioplasty. Seroma naturally resolves in most cases, but it can lead to an increased amount of visits to the outpatient clinic and can result in anxiety of the patients because they misunderstand seroma as recurrence of hernia. A remaining fluid hernia sac during the operation is a major risk of seroma. Moreover, local inflammation of the inguinal area resulting from dissection of the preperitoneal layer and the use of prosthetic materials to cover the myopectineal orifice have been reported as etiologies of seroma formation. However, the precise etiology of seroma needs to be clarified. Strangulated hernia is a common disease, which is often observed in surgery and the emergency room, and involves severe inguinal pain. Strangulated hernia can lead to severe inflammation and subsequent seroma. Consensus on the surgical approach for strangulated hernia is yet to be reached.

This study aimed to retrospectively evaluate the risk of seroma after TAPP and to identify the association between strangulated hernia and seroma. To the best of our knowledge, this is the first report to demonstrate that strangulated hernia can be a risk factor of seroma.

2. Materials and Methods

This retrospective study was conducted at one institution. We obtained written informed consent for the inclusion of data from all of the participating patients.

We perform approximately 12,000 elective surgeries and 600 emergent surgeries in our hospital per year. We treated 300 adult inguinal/ femoral hernias by TAPP between 2013 and 2016 at Kurashiki Central Hospital. We excluded patients'

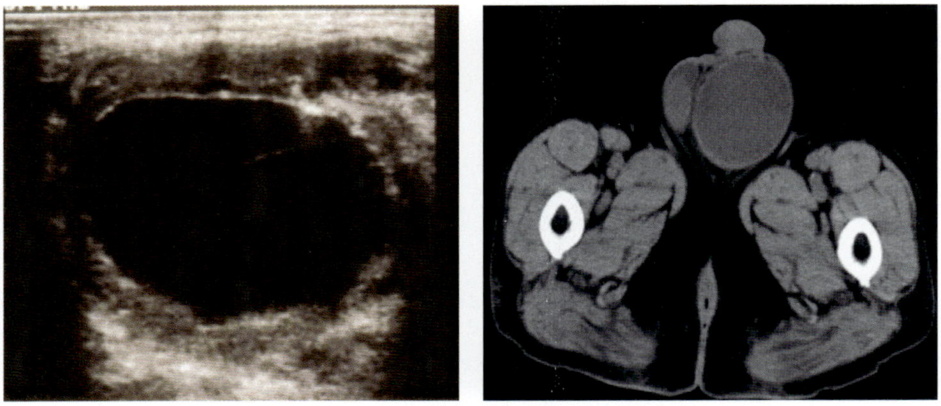

Figure 1: Seroma was diagnosed by ultrasonography (left) or computed tomography (right).

data if there was no information on the size of the hernia, which is correlated with the risk of seroma [1]. We also excluded patients with combined surgeries because we could not precisely evaluate the postoperative pain and complications after multiple surgeries. We examined all patients visually for signs of inguinal swelling, and by palpation in the outpatient clinic on postoperative day 7, and further investigation by ultrasonography or computed tomography (CT) was undertaken in patients with findings suggestive of seroma (Figure 1).

The diagnosis of strangulated hernia was based on physical examination such as painful palpable bulge and/or nonreducible mass of the inguinal region. We performed the emergent surgery for the nonreducible hernia, but for the reducible strangulated hernias we performed the early elective surgery (within 48 hours from the diagnosis) after the preoperative evaluation. Laparoscopy allowed for identification of hernia sac contents (small intestine or omentum). Strangulated hernias were reduced using a combination of manual and laparoscopic manipulation. If the resection of small intestine or omentum was required, we firstly performed inguinal repair with mesh. The hernias over 3cm in diameter were defined as large hernias and the hernias less than 3cm were defined as small hernias. The nurse at each surgical unit evaluated the postoperative pain score with the visual analogue scale (VAS) 0 and 6 hours after, and on the next day after the operation. The largest score was defined as VAS MAX. We allocated the cases to two groups (VAS MAX<0 or VAS MAX>1).

We allocated the patients into the seroma and no seroma group. The patient's demographics included gender, age, and body mass index (BMI). Hernia data was collected about position of the hernia, type of hernia, hernia anatomy, strangulated hernia, and size of hernia. Operation time, airway device, intraoperative complication, mesh type, VAS MAX, and analgesic use were examined as intraoperative and postoperative data.

2.1. Surgical Procedures. Preoperative antibiotic administration was performed to only the strangulated cases. All surgeries were undertaken through three ports using a rigid endoscope (30°) under general anesthesia. A urinary catheter was used only when required. Abdominal CO_2 pressure was established as 10 mmHg during the procedure. We dissected the preperitoneal layer using the Sandwich approach, because it is feasible for patients with prominent adhesion and is able to be safely performed by young surgeons [2]. We dissected all the hernia sac and did not retract the transversalis fascia. We used two types of mesh: L size 3DMax mesh (Bard, Cranston, RI) and M size Parietex anatomical mesh (Covidien, Mansfield, MA). In strangulated hernias, the same mesh was also used after evaluation as a clean operation. All mesh was fixed with AbsorbaTack (5-mm fixation device; Covidien) at least on the Cooper's ligament and transverse abdominal muscle. After fixation with mesh, we added dissection if needed to reduce the redundant organ incision and the operation time. The peritoneal flap was closed with 3-0 Vicryl in all cases. All surgeries were performed by surgical residents with 3–5 years of experience, and who were supervised by an experienced doctor who also operated as a scopist.

2.2. Statistical Analyses. All statistical analyses were performed with Statistical Package for Social Scientists software version 21.0. Associations between position of the hernia, type of hernia, hernia anatomy, strangulated hernia, size of hernia, airway device, mesh type, vas max, and analgesic use and seroma were calculated by Chi-square test. $P<0.05$ was considered as statistically significant. Factors significant in each association were further examined using multiple subsequent logistic regressions.

3. Results

After the exclusion, 222 hernias were eligible for analysis (Figure 2).

Table 1 showed the postoperative complications after TAPP.

The incidence of seroma was 11% (n=25) and the recurrent hernia was one (0.4%). One patient showed the peritonitis. The cause of peritonitis was unknown, but it improved with antibiotics. Four patients presented the port site infection, but they improved naturally without antibiotics. Patient clinical characteristics were similar in seroma group and no seroma group (Table 2).

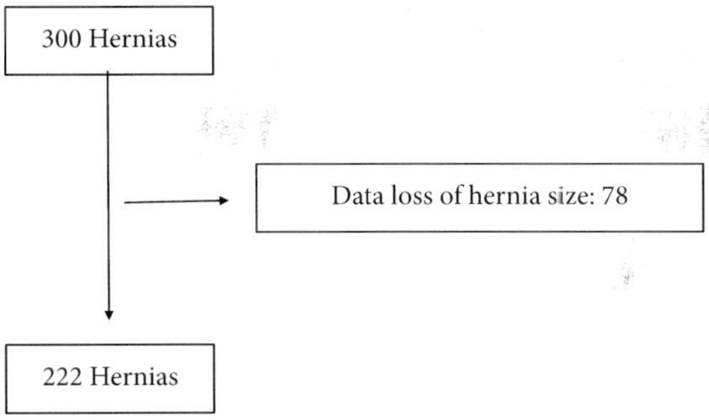

FIGURE 2: The number of eligible hernias following the exclusion criteria.

TABLE 1: Postoperative complications following TAPP.

Complications	N(%)
Seroma	25(11)
Recurrence	1(0.4)
Port site infection	4(1.6)
Subcutaneous bleeding	1(0.4)
Peritonitis	1(0.4)
Intraabdominal bleeding	1(0.4)
Total	30(13)

TABLE 2: Patients' characteristics.

	Seroma group	No seroma group
Gender		
Male (%)	24 (96)	162 (82)
Female (%)	1 (4)	35 (16)
Total	25	197
Age		
Median (range), years	72 (52-89)	73 (21-100)
BMI		
Mean (± SD), kg/m^2	22.6 (±2.83)	22.8 (±2.84)

BMI: Body Mass Index

Table 3 showed the hernia data of the two groups.

There were no significant difference with the position of the hernia, type of hernia, and hernia anatomy. There were nine cases of strangulated hernias. In all cases, there were intestine or omentum in the hernia sac. Two patients required the partial resection of the intestine because of bowel ischemia. Three strangulated hernias (33%) resulted in seromas. All cases were indirect hernias. The ratio of strangulated hernia in seroma group was significantly greater than in no seroma group ($p<0.03$). There was also a significant difference of size of hernia ($p<0.02$).

Table 4 showed the intraoperative and postoperative data in two study groups. We did not experience any intraoperative complications. There were no significant difference in airway device, mesh type, and analgesic use in two study groups. VAS MAX was significantly high in no seroma group compared to seroma group, but there was no significant difference in analgesic use in two study groups.

Multiple subsequent logistic regressions showed that strangulated hernia was associated with a significantly increased risk for seroma formation ($p = 0.023$; OR 6.564; 95% CI 1.29-33.3). The size of hernia was statistically borderline as s risk factor ($p = 0.055$; OR 3.616; 95% CI 0.97-13.4) (Table 5).

4. Discussion

We found that TAPP for strangulated hernia could cause seroma. To the best of our knowledge, this is the first study to show that strangulated hernia can be a risk factor for formation of seroma.

A seroma is an accumulation of local fluid, and the incidence of seroma is 3–11% after TAPP [3, 4].

A seroma does not affect the patient's recovery and is considered as a minor complication. However, seroma mimics the symptoms of recurrent hernia. Moreover, the incidence of seroma is higher than that of recurrent hernia following TAPP [1, 5]. Patients often mistake a seroma as a recurrent hernia, which can lead to increased visits to the outpatient clinic. This is a serious problem.

There have been several reports on formation of seroma [1, 6]. A large hernial defect space remaining during surgery plays an important role in formation of seroma. In our research, hernia size was statistically borderline as a risk factor of seroma formation. Additionally, an inflammatory response by preperitoneal preparation in surgery and from the presence of polypropylene mesh has also been reported to cause seroma [1]. However, the mechanisms of seroma formation are still unclear. There have been no reports that specifically demonstrated an association between strangulated hernia and seroma formation. In the present study, multiple subsequent logistic regressions showed that strangulated hernia was a risk factor of seroma formation.

The overall incidence of emergent inguinal hernia repair in patients undergoing watchful waiting is 2.5% over 10 years [7]. In patients with strangulated hernia, we first attempt to reduce the strangulated hernia, but if we cannot reduce the hernia, emergent surgery or an early elective surgery is necessary. These operations are performed during the occurrence of severe inflammation. Therefore, in addition to local inflammation resulting from hernial strangulation,

Table 3: Hernia data.

	Seroma group	No seroma group	*P* value
Position of the hernia			0.079
Right (%)	12 (48)	114 (58)	
Left (%)	13 (52)	83 (42)	
Total	25	197	
Type of hernia			0.87
Primary (%)	19 (76)	16 (8)	
Recurrent (%)	6 (24)	181 (92)	
Total	25	197	
Hernia anatomy			0.67
Indirect (%)	14 (56)	122 (62)	
Direct (%)	9 (36)	50 (25)	
Femoral (%)	1 (4)	15 (7)	
Other (%)	1 (4)	10 (5)	
Total	25	197	
Strangulated hernia (%)	3 (12)	6 (3)	0.036*
Size of hernia			0.022*
small (≦3cm) (%)	21 (84)	188 (95)	
Large (>3cm) (%)	4 (16)	9 (5)	
Total	25	197	

* Statistically significant

Table 4: Intraoperative and postoperative data.

	Seroma group	No seroma group	*P* value
Operation time			
Median, minute	94	93	
Airway device			0.267
SGA(%)	10 (40)	101 (51)	
ETT(%)	15 (60)	96 (49)	
Total	25	197	
Intraoperative complication	0	0	
Mesh type			0.94
Anatomical mesh (%)	14 (56)	109 (54)	
3D mesh (%)	11 (44)	88 (45)	
Total	25	197	
Vas Max			0.014*
0 (%)	9 (36)	30 (15)	
>1 (%)	16 (64)	167 (85)	
Total	25	197	
Analgesic use	6 (24)	85 (43)	0.08

* Statistically significant, ETT: Endotracheal tube, SGA: supraglottic airway
VAS: Visual Analogue Scale

Table 5: Risk factors (Odds Ratio, 95% confidence interval, and p value) for the seroma formation after laparoscopic transabdominal preperitoneal repair.

	OR	95% CI	*p* value
The size of hernia	3.616	0.97-13.4	0.055
Strangulated hernia	6.564	1.29-33.3	0.023*
VAS MAX	0.424	0.15- 1.168	0.097

* Statistically significant, VAS: Visual Analogue Scale

surgical dissection and mesh implantation may cause a further inflammatory response, which could lead to formation of seroma.

However, the incidence of seroma varies depending on each physician [8], because an objective examination, such as ultrasound and computed tomography, is generally not performed [1]. Furthermore, consensus is yet to be reached about the appropriate timing of diagnosis of seroma. A seroma is considered as a normal postoperative physiological phenomenon. Therefore, the incidence of seroma immediately following surgery is high [6, 9]. Parl et al. suggested that seroma should be diagnosed only if it is symptomatic and persistent beyond 6 weeks [10]. In our series, seroma formation was detected based on an US examination or CT for visible inguinal swelling at postoperative day 7 to ensure correct diagnosis and evaluation of its incidence.

Awareness of strangulated hernias as a risk factor of seroma and its inclusion in a management plan are important. First, consensus has yet to be reached on the best surgical approach of strangulated hernias [5, 11, 12]. Schmedt et al. showed that Lichtenstein repair resulted in a lower incidence of seroma formation than endoscopic procedures [12]. TAPP results in more seroma formation than laparoscopic total extraperitoneal repair [13]. However, these reports did not focus on formation of seroma as the primary goal. In our hospital, we usually perform TAPP for strangulated hernias because of its safety and have experienced no incidence of conversion to open repair or organ injury. Therefore, we consider TAPP as a feasible approach for repair of strangulated hernia. However, an operative approach should not be determined based on the risk of seroma alone. The best approach should be decided with the patient after a clear explanation about the risk and management of seroma. Second, minimization of the potential space of fluid collection is important. The International Endohernia Society has stated that, in indirect hernia repair, complete reduction of the hernia sac may eliminate the occurrence of chronic seroma [1, 5]. Additionally, the incidence of seroma in cases of direct hernia can be significantly reduced when the lax transversals fascia is inverted, which is performed without an increase in postoperative pain, despite being tacked to Cooper's ligament [5, 8]. Suture of the lax transversals fascia to Cooper's ligament instead of tacking is also an alternative option, which can reduce costs [5]. Third, changing the type of mesh may reduce the formation of seroma.

Macrophages, T cells, and mast cells are the main etiologies of an inflammatory response of mesh insertion. Rosch et al. compared the inflammatory response to polypropylene, prolene, and propylene/polyglactin mesh. In the polypropylene mesh group, inflammation continued for longer than 90 days postoperatively, but polypropylene/polyglactin mesh insertion resulted in lower inflammation and proliferation [14]. However, their study was experimental and conducted on mice. Additionally, a reduction in inflammatory tissue response was not directly associated with a reduction in seroma formation, and the incidence of other complications, such as recurrence and chronic pain, was unclear. Therefore, further research on this issue is necessary. Management of seroma does not always require an invasive procedure. If patients complain about inguinal discomfort and pain because of inguinal swelling, percutaneous aspiration of the fluid may be useful, but this involves a risk of infection of the region proximal to the mesh site [5]. In our series, we experienced one case of seroma aspiration, but, in all other patients, this resolved without the need for intervention. We should inform the patients about the possible seroma, especially after the strangulated hernia repair, and advise them to do self-assessment through palpation, which will resolve the insecurity.

There are some limitations of this study. First, this was a retrospective study. Second, the sample size was small and may have caused subsequent allocation bias. However, we perform many elective and emergent surgeries in our hospital and we think this study can be generalized to the hernia patients.

Third, hernia size was well-known as a risk factor of seroma formation, but this study did not show the significant difference in multiple subsequent logistic regressions. Fourth, the patients with strangulated hernia cause ascitic fluid because of local inflammation, which may accumulate in the hernia space and lead to seroma. This study did not analyze the ascites of strangulated hernia. Therefore, we think further study will be necessary.

5. Conclusion

Strangulated hernia can be a risk factor in seroma formation. This risk should be incorporated into a management plan of TAPP for strangulated hernia, with careful consideration of patients' concerns.

Acknowledgments

We would like to thank Paul Williams (Kurashiki Central Hospital) for reviewing the English used in this manuscript.

References

[1] H. Lau and F. Lee, "Seroma following endoscopic extraperitoneal inguinal hernioplasty," *Surgical Endoscopy*, vol. 17, no. 11, pp. 1773–1777, 2003.

[2] Y. Nagahisa, S. Homma, K. Chen et al., "Feasibility of a new approach for creating a preperitoneal space in transabdominal preperitoneal repair inguinal hernia repair: using a sandwich approach," *Surgery Today*, vol. 47, no. 5, pp. 595–600, 2017.

[3] D. E. Litwin, Q. N. Pham, F. H. Oleniuk, A. M. Kluftinger, and L. Rossi, "Laparoscopic groin hernia surgery: the TAPP procedure. Transabdominal preperitoneal hernia repair," *Canadian Journal of Surgery*, vol. 40, no. 3, pp. 192–198, 1997.

[4] G. S. Ferzli and T. Kiel, "The role of the endoscopic extraperitoneal approach in large inguinal scrotal hernias," *Surgical Endoscopy*, vol. 11, no. 3, pp. 299–302, 1997.

[5] R. Bittner, M. E. Arregui, T. Bisgaard et al., "Guidelines for laparoscopic (TAPP) and endoscopic (TEP) treatment of inguinal hernia [International Endohernia Society (IEHS)]," *Surgical Endoscopy*, vol. 25, no. 9, pp. 2773–2843, 2011.

[6] S. Susmallian, G. Gewurtz, T. Ezri, and I. Charuzi, "Seroma after laparoscopic repair of hernia with PTFE patch: Is it really a complication?" *Hernia*, vol. 5, no. 3, pp. 139–141, 2001.

[7] R. J. Fitzgibbons Jr., B. Ramanan, S. Arya et al., "Long-term results of a randomized controlled trial of a nonoperative strategy (watchful waiting) for men with minimally symptomatic inguinal hernias," *Annals of Surgery*, vol. 258, no. 3, pp. 508–514, 2013.

[8] V. M. Reddy, C. D. Sutton, L. Bloxham, G. Garcea, S. S. Ubhi, and G. S. Robertson, "Laparoscopic repair of direct inguinal hernia: A new technique that reduces the development of postoperative seroma," *Hernia*, vol. 11, no. 5, pp. 393–396, 2007.

[9] A. Cihan, H. Ozdemir, B. H. Uçan et al., "Fade or fate: Seroma in laparoscopic inguinal hernia repair," *Surgical Endoscopy*, vol. 20, no. 2, pp. 325–328, 2006.

[10] A. Park, D. W. Birch, and P. Lovrics, "Laparoscopic and open incisional hernia repair: A comparison study," *Surgery*, vol. 124, no. 4, pp. 816–822, 1998.

[11] J. G. Bittner, "Incarcerated/Strangulated Hernia: Open or Laparoscopic?" *Advances in Surgery*, vol. 50, no. 1, pp. 67–78, 2016.

[12] C. G. Schmedt, S. Sauerland, and R. Bittner, "Comparison of endoscopic procedures vs Lichtenstein and other open mesh techniques for inguinal hernia repair: a meta-analysis of randomized controlled trials," *Surgical Endoscopy*, vol. 19, no. 2, pp. 188–199, 2005.

[13] F. Köckerling, R. Bittner, D. A. Jacob et al., "TEP versus TAPP: comparison of the perioperative outcome in 17,587 patients with a primary unilateral inguinal hernia," *Surgical Endoscopy*, vol. 29, no. 12, pp. 3750–3760, 2015.

[14] R. Rosch, K. Junge, A. Schachtrupp, U. Klinge, B. Klosterhalfen, and V. Schumpelick, "Mesh implants in hernia repair: Inflammatory cell response in a rat model," *European Surgical Research*, vol. 35, no. 3, pp. 161–166, 2003.

Prediction of Muscle Fatigue during Minimally Invasive Surgery Using Recurrence Quantification Analysis

Ali Keshavarz Panahi and Sohyung Cho

Industrial Engineering, Southern Illinois University Edwardsville, Edwardsville, IL 62026, USA

Correspondence should be addressed to Sohyung Cho; scho@siue.edu

Academic Editor: Othmar Schöb

Due to its inherent complexity such as limited work volume and degree of freedom, minimally invasive surgery (MIS) is ergonomically challenging to surgeons compared to traditional open surgery. Specifically, MIS can expose performing surgeons to excessive ergonomic risks including muscle fatigue that may lead to critical errors in surgical procedures. Therefore, detecting the vulnerable muscles and time-to-fatigue during MIS is of great importance in order to prevent these errors. The main goal of this study is to propose and test a novel measure that can be efficiently used to detect muscle fatigue. In this study, surface electromyography was used to record muscle activations of five subjects while they performed fifteen various laparoscopic operations. The muscle activation data was then reconstructed using recurrence quantification analysis (RQA) to detect possible signs of muscle fatigue on eight muscle groups (bicep, triceps, deltoid, and trapezius). The results showed that RQA detects the fatigue sign on bilateral trapezius at 47.5 minutes (average) and bilateral deltoid at 57.5 minutes after the start of operations. No sign of fatigue was detected for bicep and triceps muscles of any subject. According to the results, the proposed novel measure can be efficiently used to detect muscle fatigue and eventually improve the quality of MIS procedures with reducing errors that may result from overlooked muscle fatigue.

1. Introduction

Since minimally invasive surgery (MIS) is performed using an endoscope and several thin instruments through small incisions made in patients, it provides patients with some advantages like shorter recovery time, less postoperative pain, earlier resumption of normal activity, and cost savings. However, it is more ergonomically challenging to performing surgeons due to its inherent complexity such as limited work volume and degree of freedom. Specifically, such complexity induces abnormal movements of arm and shoulder while holding certain body postures, for example, head and torso, for prolonged time [1–3]. Importantly, this complexity often exposes performing surgeons to increased ergonomic risks including muscle fatigue that can result in critical errors during surgical procedures [4–6]. The vulnerability to ergonomic risk is well confirmed in a literature stating that "performing laparoscopic surgery is significantly more stressful for the surgeon than open surgery" [7]. In addition, it has been reported that MIS carries more complications than open surgery [8, 9]. Therefore, it is important to quantitatively measure ergonomic risks on performing surgeons, particularly muscle fatigue during MIS procedures. Note that timely intervention with information about muscle fatigue can ensure improved quality of MIS procedures.

Some existing study for fatigue analysis has focused on quantitative measures and their applications for isometric or isotonic contractions during relatively short bouts of high-force activities. Among these studies, frequency banding analysis predicted muscle fatigue when lower frequency bands increase and higher frequency bands decrease [10]. Standard discomfort analysis was also used to detect the level of muscle fatigue on subjects, which may lack objective analysis [11]. In addition, heart rate [12] and tissue oxygen saturation [13] were used as indicators of fatigue development. Importantly, power spectral density (PSD) of transformed EMG data through Fast Fourier Transform approach was widely used to detect muscle fatigue [14–16]. In this approach, frequency and

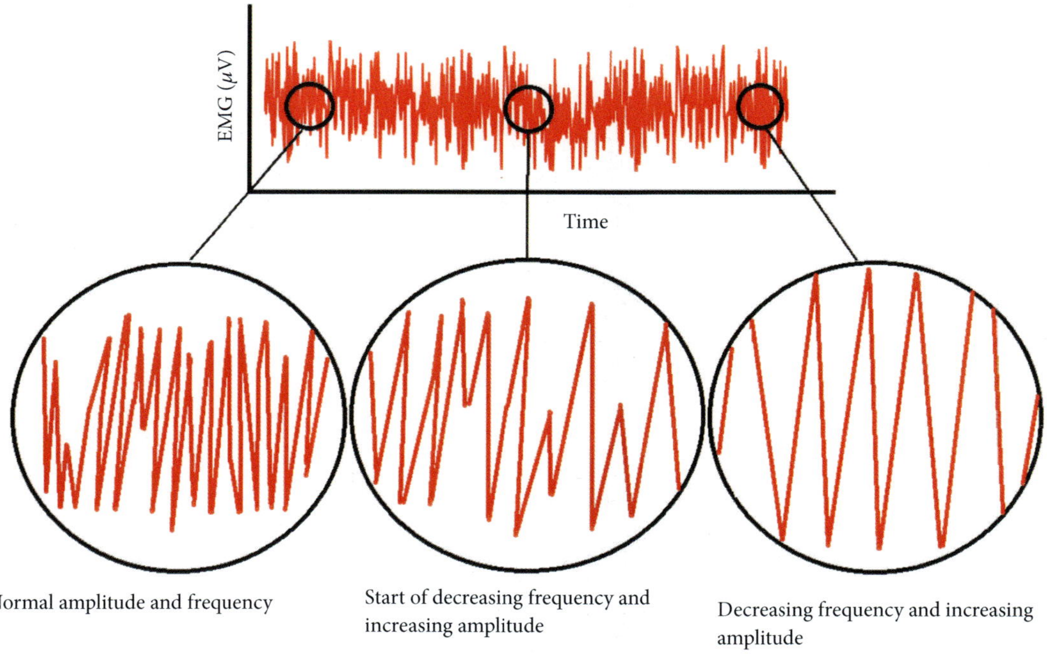

FIGURE 1: Schematic of changes in EMG data during muscle fatigue.

amplitude changes are considered as a result of a reduction in conduction velocity in the muscle fibers and larger motor unit synchronization. Figure 1 schematically depicts these changes in various stages of the muscle fatigue.

As MIS operations can be considered as prolonged light muscle activation, PSD based measure, which is mainly for static activities, may not be efficiently used to predict muscle fatigue during MIS operations. Specifically, when PSD based measures are used for light muscle activations, conflicting results and complicated relationship between subjective and objective fatigue have been reported [17, 18]. Such conflicts result from stationary data requirement for PSD based measures to be successfully used. In fact, EMG data collected from light muscle activations are nonstationary due to changing distance between muscle and EMG sensor, as well as changing muscle length. From the literature, it is noted that fatigue mechanism during these activities is not well understood in comparison to high-force (or intense) muscle activities [19]. Although there are no significant reductions in muscle force level during MIS operations, there are some physiological changes in muscles that can lead to muscle fatigue affecting the capacity of muscles and the performance of subjects [20, 21]. Uhrich et al. [22] assessed the muscle fatigue during a relatively short time during simulated laparoscopic surgery. In their study, the effects of fatigue, monitor placement, and surgical experience have been compared. After obtaining the EMG activity and muscular discomfort scores before and after a fatigue session, it was found that the EMG data and discomfort scores demonstrated a fatigue response in several muscle groups. They found minimal differences between the two monitor positions and less muscle activity and discomfort in the attending surgeons. In another study, Slack et al. [23] studied the effect of operating time on surgeon's muscular fatigue. The length of the operations varied within 1–10 hr, but only one minute period before and after operations were analyzed using frequency analysis. They found that brachioradialis was being used more and fatigued faster. In addition, the muscle fatigue increases proportional to time. On the other hand, recurrence quantification analysis (RQA) has been tested on biceps brachii and shown to be more sensitive to muscle fatigue than FFT variable spectral center frequency (fC) [24]. In another study, Filligoi and Felici [25] showed that Determinism%, which is one of the RQA variables, is more effective than median frequency to detect EMG signal changes in biceps brachii muscle. For the first time, this novel data analysis method is used in our study to quantify any possible muscle fatigue in real laparoscopic surgery operations which is known as prolonged and low-force muscle activity compared to some intense tasks which involve isometric muscle contraction throughout the whole task.

The main goal of this study is to answer the following questions:

(i) Can objective manifestations of muscle fatigue be detected from EMG data during a laparoscopic surgery as prolonged light muscle activation?

(ii) What is time-to-fatigue for the muscles experiencing fatigue during laparoscopic surgery?

(iii) Which muscle has the highest possibility level of fatigue in laparoscopic surgery among the tested muscle groups?

2. Methods

As the first step, EMG data for fatigue analysis was collected. Specifically, surface EMG electrodes were attached to upper arm muscles of participants to collect muscle activations

Table 1: MIS operations from which EMG data was collected*.

Subject	Lap #	Completion time (min)	Description
Surgeon 1	Lap 1	96	Ventral hernia repair
	Lap 2	113	Cholecystectomy
	Lap 3	132	Inguinal hernia repair
Surgeon 2	Lap 1	55	Sleeve gastrectomy
	Lap 2	66	Sleeve gastrectomy
	Lap 3	128	Sleeve gastrectomy
Surgeon 3	Lap 1	131	Heller myotomy, Dor fundoplication, and liver biopsy
	Lap 2	152	Ventral hernia repair
	Lap 3	171	Paraesophageal hernia repair
Surgeon 4	Lap 1	122	Sleeve gastrectomy
	Lap 2	101	Inguinal hernia repair
	Lap 3	88	Sleeve gastrectomy
Surgeon 5	Lap 1	71	Heller myotomy
	Lap 2	116	Ventral hernia repair
	Lap 3	144	Cholecystectomy

*Ventral hernia repair: the hernia is repaired by mesh or sutures entered through instruments placed into small incisions in the abdomen. Cholecystectomy: to remove the gallbladder using several small incisions. Inguinal hernia repair: to repair a hernia in the abdominal wall of the groin. Sleeve gastrectomy: to remove a large portion of the stomach to help with weight loss. Heller myotomy: to treat the achalasia by cutting the muscles of the cardia to allow food and liquid to pass to the stomach. Dor fundoplication: to prevent reflux from the stomach into the esophagus by partially wrapping the stomach around the esophagus. Paraesophageal hernia repair: the diaphragm at the esophageal hiatus is closed to prevent the stomach from reherniating, and then the fundoplication is performed to keep the stomach from herniating back into the chest cavity.

while performing various MIS procedures. Next, EMG data was converted into higher dimensional data using time shift and represented by recurrence plots that facilitate recurrence quantification analysis (RQA), particularly computation of determinism values. Then, moving average technique was applied for trajectories of determinism values to detect any changes as the indicator of muscle fatigue.

2.1. EMG Data Collection. Under an IRB-approved protocol, five right-hand-dominant expert laparoscopic surgeons, who have performed more than 100 laparoscopic surgeries, performed fifteen MIS procedures in a local hospital. Table 1 shows more details about those surgical operations.

On each participant, a total of eight surface EMG (sEMG) electrodes were attached to the following four bilateral muscles including bicep, triceps, deltoid, and trapezius. Note that since lower arms are scrubbed from the fingertips to the elbow, electrodes were not placed on these sterilized muscle compartments. Tricep and bicep were selected due to their high activity level during arm flexion and extension. Since the shoulder and neck are the common area of muscle fatigue, trapezius and deltoid were also included in our study. All sEMG data were collected using an 8-channel Bioradio® 150 physiologic data acquisition system (Great Lakes Neurotechnologies, Incorporated®, Cleveland, OH). After wiping skin surfaces overlying target muscle groups with rubbing alcohol and allowing the alcohol to dry, two 1″ × 1″ MVAP-II® electrodes (MVAP Medical Supplies, Incorporated, Newbury Park, CA) were placed over the muscle bellies of each muscle group and connected to the positive and negative input poles for each channel. An electrode was also attached to the right elbow and connected to the ground input on the Bioradio 150 to complete the input circuit. The Biocapture® data acquisition software package (Great Lakes Neurotechnologies, Incorporated, Cleveland, OH) was used to capture and filter sEMG data. More specifically, sEMG data was sampled at frequency of 256 Hz from each channel. Digital signal processing filters were then applied to exclude the noise that are at low (<10 Hz) and high frequency (>127 Hz) signals.

2.2. Recurrence Quantification Analysis (RQA). RQA is a time series analysis method and detects the deterministic structure of the dynamical systems. It also provides some valuable information from recurrence plots [26]. The principle of recurrence plots analysis can be summarized as follows. Let $x(i)$ be the ith point on the orbit describing a dynamical system in d-dimensional space, for $i = 1, \ldots, N$. The recurrence plot is an array of dots in a $N \times N$ square, where a dot is placed at (i, j) whenever $x(j)$ is sufficiently close to $x(i)$. In order to obtain a recurrence plot from a time series $\{u_i\}$, the following procedures are required. First, we choose an embedding dimension d and construct the d-dimensional orbit of $X(i)$ by the method of time delays: if u and i are scalar, $x_{(i)} = (u_i, u_{i+1}, \ldots, u_{i+d-1})$. Next, we choose $r_{(i)}$ such that the ball of radius $r_{(i)}$ centered at $x_{(i)}$ in R^d contains a reasonable number of other points $x_{(j)}$ of the orbit. Finally, we plot a dot at each point (i, j) for which $x_{(j)}$ is in the ball of radius $r_{(i)}$ centered at $x_{(i)}$. We call this picture a recurrence plot (RP) and an example of RPs is shown in Figure 2. Note that i and j are, in fact, times; therefore, a recurrence plot describes natural time correlation information.

Recurrence plots tend to be fairly symmetric with respect to the diagonal $i = j$ because if $x_{(i)}$ is close to $x_{(j)}$, then $x_{(j)}$ is close to $x_{(i)}$. There is, however, no complete symmetry

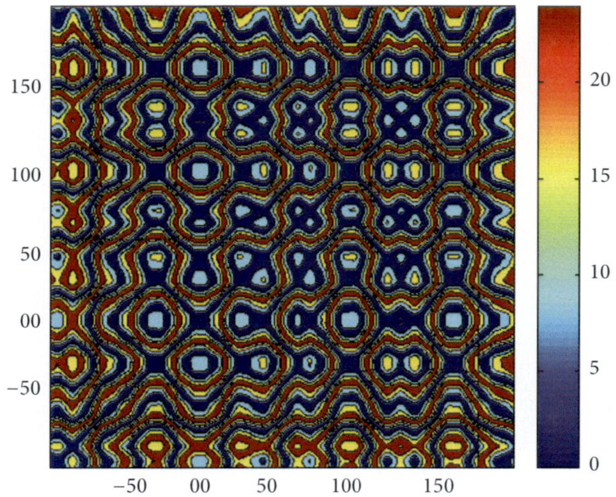

FIGURE 2: Example of a recurrence plot.

because we do not require $r_{(i)} = r_{(j)}$ [27]. When N is more than 2 dimensions in a phase space, projection is performed. Starting from the time series $s_{(t)} = \{s_1, \ldots, s_n\}$, the attractor of the underlying dynamics is reconstructed in a phase space by applying the time-delay vector method by Takens [28]. The reconstructed trajectory X can be expressed as a matrix where each row is a phase space vector:

$$X = [x_1, x_2, \ldots x_m]^T, \tag{1}$$

where $x_i = [s_1, s_{i+T}, \ldots s_{i+(D_E-1)T}]^T$, $m = n - (D_E - 1)T$, D_E is the embedding dimension, and T is the delay time. The recurrence plot is a tool that can be used to investigate higher dimensional dynamics through a two-dimensional binary plot of its recurrences. Any recurrence of state i with state j is pictured on a Boolean matrix expressed by

$$R_{i,j}^{D_E,\varepsilon} = \Theta\left(\varepsilon - \left\|x_i - x_j\right\|\right), \tag{2}$$

where $x_{i,j} \in R^{D_E}$ are the embedded vectors, $i, j \in N, \Theta(\cdot)$ is the Heaviside step function, and ε is an arbitrary threshold. In the graphical representation, each nonzero entry of $R_{i,j}$ is marked by a black dot in the position i, j. Since any state is recurrent with itself, the recurrent plot (RP) matrix fulfills $R_{i,j} = 1$ which hence contains the diagonal line of identity (LOI).

The percentage of determinism (%DET) derived from diagonal lines and related to predictability of the system is an important parameter in RQA which quantifies the ratio of the recurrence points. The following formula is typically used to calculate %DET from a recurrence plot [26]:

$$\%\text{DET} = \frac{\sum_{l=l_{\min}}^{N} lP(l)}{\sum_{l=1}^{N} lP(l)} \times 100\,(\%), \tag{3}$$

where $P(l)$ is histogram or frequency distribution of diagonal line lengths, N is the length of a data series, and $l_{\min}$ is predefined minimal length of a diagonal line. In this study, the above %DET for EMG data was used as a muscle fatigue indicator. Cross recurrence plot (CRP) toolbox available in MATLAB was used for RQA analysis [26]. In order to ensure optimized results, RQA parameters including embedding dimension (D_E), time delay (T), and threshold (ε) should be selected carefully. In the CRP toolbox, one can set the parameters of optimal embedding dimension and time delay to the obtained values from false nearest neighbors (FNN) and average mutual information (AMI) function which may lead to the optimal recurrence plots as shown in Figure 3.

Using these functions, embedding dimension and time-delay parameters were set to 10 and 4, respectively. To facilitate optimal threshold value, it has been suggested to consider the threshold value only a few percent of the maximum phase space diameter [29]. Therefore, the threshold value was chosen according to the 10% of the minimum value of maximum phase space diameter of the data. In this study, the minimum number of points constructing a deterministic diagonal line was set to two.

The whole duration of MIS operations summarized in Table 1 was analyzed by applying RQA for each minute of the operation with a window length of 15,360 data points. Then, %DET value was derived from RQA analysis and the results were plotted against operation time. Finally, a moving average analysis with the interval (or window size) of ten was applied to the %DET values to determine time-to-fatigue.

3. Results

Figure 4 shows %DET values of all eight muscles for surgeon 1 performing case 3 for 132 minutes as an example. It was observed from Figures 4(g) and 4(h) that moving average of %DET of bilateral trapezius muscles increased after 45–50 minutes of operation. In addition, moving average of %DET of bilateral deltoid increased after 55–60 minutes of operation as shown in Figures 4(e) and 4(f). Between deltoid and trapezius, bilateral trapezius became more deterministic with %DET close to 75% at the end of operation while bilateral deltoid was less deterministic with %DET value close to 50%. In this study, the increase in the moving average of %DET values is considered as the development of muscle fatigue. Thus, it is conjectured from these observations that trapezius became more fatigued than deltoid for surgeon 1 performing case 3. However, there were no changes in moving averages of %DET of bilateral bicep and triceps throughout the entire operation as shown in Figure 4.

As the next step, %DET was tested for all the MIS operations and results are summarized in Table 2. DET results did not detect any changes in any of the muscles for surgeon 2 in case number 1 which had the least completion time of 55 minutes. Also, surgeon 4 in case number 2 as well as surgeon 5 in case number 3 did not experience any fatigue in their deltoid muscle. Specifically, no fatigue signs were detected on bilateral bicep and triceps in any of the subjects. Figure 5 shows the mean of moving average values for DET% of all the operations and subjects. Table 2 also shows that fatigue signs are developed at least 45 minutes after operations begin and trapezius gets fatigue sign earlier than deltoid.

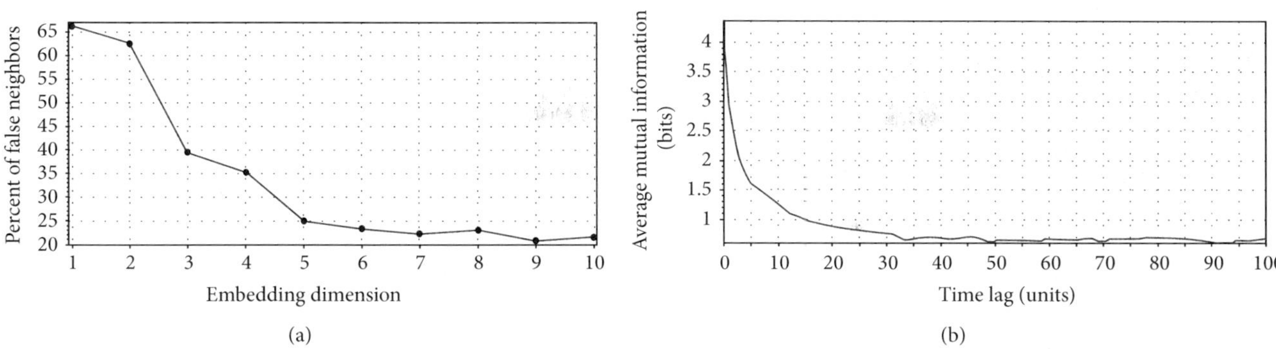

FIGURE 3: Optimal embedding dimension using FNN (a) and time delay using AMI (b).

4. Discussion

The moving average of %DET for bilateral trapezius deltoid increased after 45–50 and 55–60 minutes of operation, respectively. This might be caused due to the following nature of MIS procedures: (i) during MIS, surgeons should maintain their head positions at certain orientation to keep watching the monitor and this may impose significant stress on trapezius muscle, and (ii) as the surgeon operates thin and long instrument through a small incision, they often use excessive shoulder movements to overcome the limited degree of freedom and this may impose fatigue on deltoid muscle. In this study, higher %DET value implies that the EMG data are getting more deterministic and periodic. This deterministic and periodic pattern is the result of synchronization of motor units in fatiguing stage [30]. In order to supply necessary force to continue certain tasks, more motor units are involved during muscle fatigue. If almost all motor units have already been involved, motor unit synchronization takes place to continue task operation and prevent the failure. The fact that more motor units are recruited and synchronized during the course of muscle fatigue has been shown in literature [31]. For conventional occupational tasks, increase in synchronization of motor units has been successfully detected using %DET values through a computer simulation model [32].

On the other hand, shoulder disorder is considered as one of most important musculoskeletal disorders, especially in prolonged repetitive activations with high precision [33–35]. An increase in interstitial potassium concentrations in trapezius muscle can be the cause of decreased conduction velocity [36]. Also, the intra- and extracellular sodium and potassium concentration changes can be the main reason for changes in EMG data which are related to muscle fatigue [37]. Although the recovery of these metabolic changes is quick, in prolonged light muscle activation, muscles need longer recovery times in order to regain the primary force capacity [37, 38]. Because of orderly recruitment of motor units, low threshold fibers are vulnerable in prolonged muscle activation, which necessitates the importance of recovery time to avoid myalgic disorders in trapezius [39, 40]. It can be summarized from the literature review that fatigue analysis is highly difficult for prolonged light muscle activation tasks such as MIS procedures.

This study shows that trapezius was the first muscle to show fatigue sign in prolonged light muscle activation during MIS procedures. It is interesting to note that similar results were reported in a light assembly task in industrial operations [41]. While the existing study also suggested recovery/break time for workers at 90 minutes after the task begins, the results in this study suggest recovery/break time after 45–50 minutes after MIS operations begin. More likely, this difference results from intensity and precision level of two tasks: industrial and surgical. Bicep and triceps did not experience any muscle fatigue. This might be because of less muscle activation and less muscle contraction in laparoscopic surgery for these two muscles.

As muscles are vulnerable to fatigue during MIS operations which have prolonged and intense nature, detecting the muscle fatigue and estimation of time-to-fatigue are of great importance. To meet this need, this study proposed and tested a novel measure that can be efficiently used for detection of muscle fatigue and time-to-fatigue from EMG data. In the future study, correlation between objective and subjective results would be important. Here, objective results mean fatigue analysis using the proposed measure of this study and subjective results correspond to survey analysis to subjects asking whether they feel fatigue symptoms during MIS procedures. Also, it would be interesting to compare performance analysis with fatigue analysis in the future, since the final goal for muscle fatigue analysis is to detect any possible effect on surgeon's performance. This will emphasize the importance of quantitative muscle fatigue analysis, although it might be challenging to apply performance analysis to real surgical operations. However, performance analysis can be easily applied to dry lab experiments such as Fundamentals of Laparoscopic Surgery (FLS) tasks, since there are validated methods to analyze the performance of subjects. Therefore, the combination of RQA, as a quantitative muscle fatigue analysis method, and standard performance analysis of FLS tasks will open up new doors for future studies related to muscle fatigue and performance analysis of real MIS operations which would be very beneficial for surgical community. Also, future

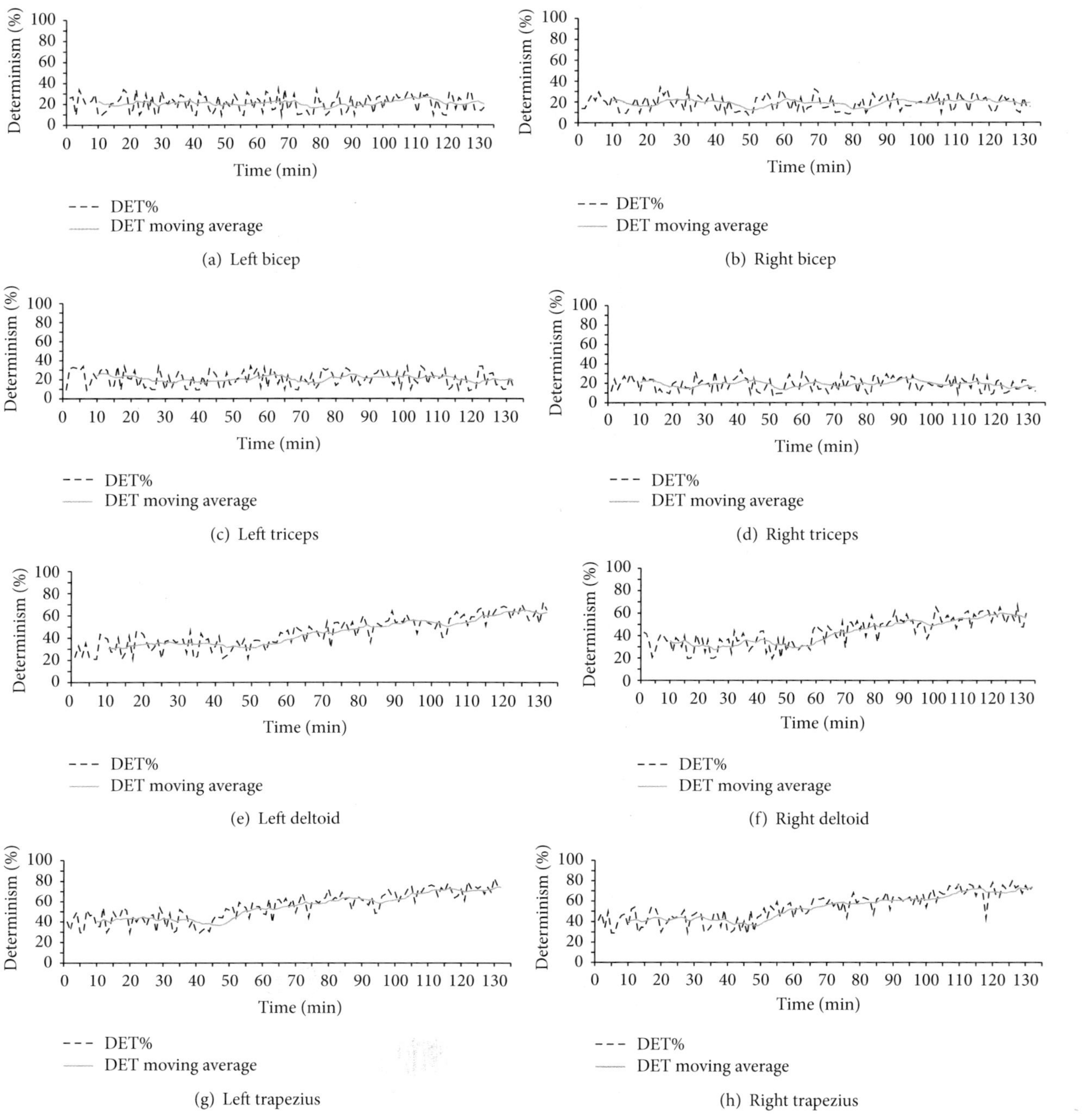

FIGURE 4: %DET value for all the muscle groups of surgeon 1, case 3. The vertical axis is Determinism % and the horizontal axis is time (min). (a) left bicep, (b) right bicep, (c) left triceps, (d) right triceps, (e) left deltoid, (f) right deltoid, (g) left trapezius, and (h) right trapezius.

studies should include larger number of subjects and more surgical operations in order to confirm findings of this study.

5. Conclusion

In this study, recurrence quantification analysis (RQA) was applied to EMG data recorded from eight muscle groups of five surgeons while doing fifteen MIS operations. The results showed that this novel measure could detect the sign of muscle fatigue on bilateral deltoid and trapezius at 45–55 minutes after operations began, and no sign of fatigue was found on other muscles. It was found from this study that trapezius and deltoid were the most vulnerable muscles among all eight muscle groups tested. Here, it is worthwhile to note the nature of MIS procedures such that surgeons manipulate long and thin instruments for the frequent changes of their orientation and position mainly using bicep and triceps and maintain their arm posture using deltoid while gazing through monitor using trapezius muscle for prolonged time. Considering this nature, deltoid and trapezius may show clear sign of fatigue

Table 2: Time-to-fatigue for all the muscle groups (minutes).

Surgeon	Case	L-bicep	R-bicep	L-tricep	R-tricep	L-deltoid	R-deltoid	L-trap	R-trap
	1	N/F	N/F	N/F	N/F	F(55–60)	F(55–60)	F(45–50)	F(45–50)
1	2	N/F	N/F	N/F	N/F	F(55–60)	F(55–60)	F(45–50)	F(45–50)
	3	N/F	N/F	N/F	N/F	F(55–60)	F(55–60)	F(45–50)	F(45–50)
	1	N/F	N/F	N/F	N/F	N/F	N/F	N/F	N/F
2	2	N/F	N/F	N/F	N/F	F(55–60)	F(55–60)	F(45–50)	F(45–50)
	3	N/F	N/F	N/F	N/F	F(55–60)	F(55–60)	F(45–50)	F(45–50)
	1	N/F	N/F	N/F	N/F	F(55–60)	F(55–60)	F(45–50)	F(45–50)
3	2	N/F	N/F	N/F	N/F	F(55–60)	F(55–60)	F(45–50)	F(45–50)
	3	N/F	N/F	N/F	N/F	F(55–60)	F(55–60)	F(45–50)	F(45–50)
	1	N/F	N/F	N/F	N/F	F(55–60)	F(55–60)	F(45–50)	F(45–50)
4	2	N/F	N/F	N/F	N/F	N/F	N/F	F(45–50)	F(45–50)
	3	N/F	N/F	N/F	N/F	F(55–60)	F(55–60)	F(55–60)	F(55–60)
	1	N/F	N/F	N/F	N/F	F(55–60)	F(55–60)	F(55–60)	F(55–60)
5	2	N/F	N/F	N/F	N/F	F(55–60)	F(55–60)	F(55–60)	F(55–60)
	3	N/F	N/F	N/F	N/F	N/F	N/F	F(55–60)	F(55–60)

Note: N/F: no fatigue.

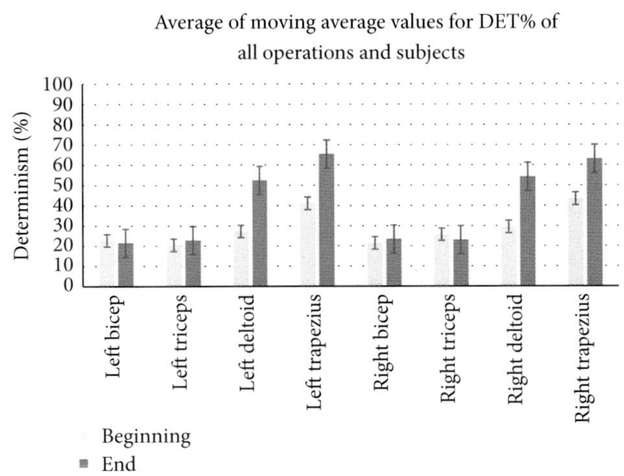

Figure 5: Average of moving average values for DET% of all the operations and subjects for the beginning and end of operations.

while other muscles do not show any sign of fatigue as tested in this study. Based on the results, it could be suggested that surgeons need to take break time at 45–50 minutes after MIS operations begin in order to minimize muscle fatigue and other possible muscle disorders. To have a better understanding about the effect of recovery time on surgeons doing such a complicated laparoscopic operation, future research might test different recovery times to find an optimum amount of time for muscle relaxation before muscles fatigue. In addition, ergonomic improvement of surgical equipment to reduce the intensity level might be efficient in reducing muscle fatigue or at least increasing time-to-fatigue.

Competing Interests

The authors declare that they have no competing interests.

References

[1] R. Berguer, J. Chen, and W. D. Smith, "A comparison of the physical effort required for laparoscopic and open surgical techniques," *Archives of Surgery*, vol. 138, no. 9, pp. 967–970, 2003.

[2] R. Berguer, D. L. Forkey, and W. D. Smith, "Ergonomic problems associated with laparoscopic surgery," *Surgical Endoscopy*, vol. 13, no. 5, pp. 466–468, 1999.

[3] U. Matern, P. Waller, C. Giebmeyer, K. D. Rückauer, and E. H. Farthmann, "Ergonomics: requirements for adjusting the height of laparoscopic operating tables," *Journal of the Society of Laparoendoscopic Surgeons*, vol. 5, no. 1, pp. 7–12, 2001.

[4] T. M. Kowalewski, *Real-time quantitative assessment of surgical skill [Ph.D. dissertation]*, University of Washington Department of Electrical Engineering, 2012.

[5] M. Riojas, C. Feng, A. Hamilton, and J. Rozenblit, "Knowledge elicitation for performance assessment in a computerized surgical training system," *Applied Soft Computing*, vol. 11, no. 4, pp. 3697–3708, 2011.

[6] E. Domany, "Protein folding in contact map space," *Physica A: Statistical Mechanics and Its Applications*, vol. 288, no. 1–4, pp. 1–9, 2000.

[7] R. Berguer, W. D. Smith, and Y. H. Chung, "Performing laparoscopic surgery is significantly more stressful for the surgeon than open surgery," *Surgical Endoscopy*, vol. 15, no. 10, pp. 1204–1207, 2001.

[8] A. G. Gallagher and R. M. Satava, "Virtual reality as a metric for the assessment of laparoscopic psychomotor skills," *Surgical Endoscopy and Other Interventional Techniques*, vol. 16, no. 12, pp. 1746–1752, 2002.

[9] J. H. Peters, G. M. Fried, L. L. Swanstrom et al., "Development and validation of a comprehensive program of education and assessment of the basic fundamentals of laparoscopic surgery," *Surgery*, vol. 135, no. 1, pp. 21–27, 2004.

[10] P. Dolan, A. F. Mannion, and M. A. Adams, "Fatigue of the erector spinae muscles-a quantitative assessment using 'frequency banding' of the surface electromyography signa," *Spine*, vol. 20, no. 2, pp. 149–159, 1995.

[11] M. P. Van der Grinten, "Test-retest reliability of a practical method for measuring body part discomfort," in *Designing for Everyone*, Y. Quéinnec and R. Daniellou, Eds., pp. 54–57, Taylor & Francis, 1991.

[12] N. Hubert, M. Gilles, K. Desbrosses, J. P. Meyer, J. Felblinger, and J. Hubert, "Ergonomic assessment of the surgeon's physical workload during standard and robotic assisted laparoscopic procedures," *The International Journal of Medical Robotics and Computer Assisted Surgery*, vol. 9, no. 2, pp. 142–147, 2013.

[13] M. Heiden, E. Lyskov, M. Djupsjöbacka, F. Hellström, and A. G. Crenshaw, "Effects of time pressure and precision demands during computer mouse work on muscle oxygenation and position sense," *European Journal of Applied Physiology*, vol. 94, no. 1-2, pp. 97–106, 2005.

[14] J. V. Basmajian and C. J. De Luca, *Muscles Alive: Their Functions Revealed by Electromyography*, Lippincott Williams & Wilkins, Baltimore, Md, USA, 5th edition, 1962.

[15] C. J. De Luca, "Myoelectrical manifestations of localized muscular fatigue in humans," *Critical Reviews in Biomedical Engineering*, vol. 11, no. 4, pp. 251–279, 1984.

[16] O. Lippold, "The tremor in fatigue," *Ciba Foundation Symposium*, vol. 82, pp. 234–248, 1981.

[17] T. Bosch, M. P. de Looze, and J. H. van Dieën, "Development of fatigue and discomfort in the upper trapezius muscle during light manual work," *Ergonomics*, vol. 50, no. 2, pp. 161–177, 2007.

[18] G. P. Y. Szeto, L. M. Straker, and P. B. O'Sullivan, "A comparison of symptomatic and asymptomatic office workers performing monotonous keyboard work–1: neck and shoulder muscle recruitment patterns," *Manual Therapy*, vol. 10, no. 4, pp. 270–280, 2005.

[19] J. T. Dennerlein, V. M. Ciriello, K. J. Kerin, and P. W. Johnson, "Fatigue in the forearm resulting from low-level repetitive ulnar deviation," *American Industrial Hygiene Association Journal*, vol. 64, no. 6, pp. 799–805, 2003.

[20] K. R. Sahlin and J. M. Ren, "Relationship of contraction capacity to metabolic changes during recovery from a fatiguing contraction," *Journal of Applied Physiology*, vol. 67, no. 2, pp. 648–654, 1989.

[21] E.-P. Takala, "Static muscular load, an increasing hazard in modern information technology," *Scandinavian Journal of Work, Environment and Health*, vol. 28, no. 4, pp. 211–213, 2002.

[22] M. L. Uhrich, R. A. Underwood, J. W. Standeven, N. J. Soper, and J. R. Engsberg, "Assessment of fatigue, monitor placement, and surgical experience during simulated laparoscopic surgery," *Surgical Endoscopy and Other Interventional Techniques*, vol. 16, no. 4, pp. 635–639, 2002.

[23] P. S. Slack, C. J. Coulson, X. Ma, K. Webster, and D. W. Proops, "The effect of operating time on surgeons' muscular fatigue," *Annals of the Royal College of Surgeons of England*, vol. 90, no. 8, pp. 651–657, 2008.

[24] C. L. Webber Jr., M. A. Schmidt, and J. M. Walsh, "Influence of isometric loading on biceps EMG dynamics as assessed by linear and nonlinear tools," *Journal of Applied Physiology*, vol. 78, no. 3, pp. 814–822, 1995.

[25] G. Filligoi and F. Felici, "Detection of hidden rhythms in surface EMG signals with a non-linear time-series tool," *Medical Engineering and Physics*, vol. 21, no. 6-7, pp. 439–448, 1999.

[26] N. Marwan, M. C. Romano, M. Thiel, and J. Kurths, "Recurrence plots for the analysis of complex systems," *Physics Reports*, vol. 438, no. 5-6, pp. 237–329, 2007.

[27] J.-P. Eckmann, S. Oliffson Kamphorst, and D. Ruelle, "Recurrence plots of dynamical systems," *EPL*, vol. 4, no. 9, pp. 973–977, 1987.

[28] F. Takens, "Detecting strange attractors in turbulence," in *Dynamical Systems and Turbulence, Warwick 1980*, D. Rand and L.-S. Young, Eds., vol. 898 of *Lecture Notes in Mathematics*, pp. 366–381, Springer, New York, NY, USA, 1981.

[29] G. B. Mindlin and R. Gilmore, "Topological analysis and synthesis of chaotic time series," *Physica D: Nonlinear Phenomena*, vol. 58, no. 1–4, pp. 229–242, 1992.

[30] Y. Liu, M. Kankaanpää, J. P. Zbilut, and C. L. Webber Jr., "EMG recurrence quantifications in dynamic exercise," *Biological Cybernetics*, vol. 90, no. 5, pp. 337–348, 2004.

[31] B. R. Jensen, M. Pilegaard, and G. Sjøgaard, "Motor unit recruitment and rate coding in response to fatiguing shoulder abductions and subsequent recovery," *European Journal of Applied Physiology*, vol. 83, no. 2-3, pp. 190–199, 2000.

[32] D. Farina, L. Fattorini, F. Felici, and G. Filligoi, "Nonlinear surface EMG analysis to detect changes of motor unit conduction velocity and synchronization," *Journal of Applied Physiology*, vol. 93, no. 5, pp. 1753–1763, 2002.

[33] K. Walker-Bone and C. Cooper, "Hard work never hurt anyone: or did it? A review of occupational associations with soft tissue musculoskeletal disorders of the neck and upper limb," *Annals of the Rheumatic Diseases*, vol. 64, no. 10, pp. 1391–1396, 2005.

[34] S. Kvarnström, "Occurrence of musculoskeletal, disorders in a manufacturing industry with special attention to occupational shoulder disorders," *Scandinavian Journal of Rehabilitation Medicine, Supplement*, vol. 8, no. 1, pp. 1–114, 1983.

[35] H. Christensen, "Muscle activity and fatigue in the shoulder muscles during repetitive work—an electromyographic study," *European Journal of Applied Physiology and Occupational Physiology*, vol. 54, no. 6, pp. 596–601, 1986.

[36] L. Rosendal, A. K. Blangsted, J. Kristiansen et al., "Interstitial muscle lactate, pyruvate and potassium dynamics in the trapezius muscle during repetitive low-force arm movements, measured with microdialysis," *Acta Physiologica Scandinavica*, vol. 182, no. 4, pp. 379–388, 2004.

[37] G. Sjøgaard, G. Savard, and C. Juel, "Muscle blood flow during isometric activity and its relation to muscle fatigue," *European Journal of Applied Physiology and Occupational Physiology*, vol. 57, no. 3, pp. 327–335, 1988.

[38] G. W. Kroon and M. Naeije, "Recovery of the human biceps electromyogram after heavy eccentric, concentric or isometric exercise," *European Journal of Applied Physiology and Occupational Physiology*, vol. 63, no. 6, pp. 444–448, 1991.

[39] E. Henneman, G. Somjen, and D. O. Carpenter, "Excitability and inhibitability of motoneurons of different sizes," *Journal of Neurophysiology*, vol. 28, no. 3, pp. 599–620, 1965.

[40] B. Rolander, D. Jonker, A. Karsznia, and T. Öberg, "Evaluation of muscular activity, local muscular fatigue, and muscular rest patterns among dentists," *Acta Odontologica Scandinavica*, vol. 63, no. 4, pp. 189–195, 2005.

[41] Santy and S. Z. Dawal, "Investigation on time to fatigue for upper limb muscle during a repetitive light assembly task," in *Proceedings of the International MultiConference of Engineers and Computer Scientists (IMECS '10)*, vol. 3, pp. 1584–1588, March 2010.

39

Routine Cysticotomy and Flushing of the Cystic Duct in Patients with Low Risk of Common Duct Stones: Can It Be Beneficial?

Piera Leon,[1] Fabiola Giudici,[1] Antonio Sciuto,[2] and Francesco Corcione[2]

[1]*Department of Medical, Surgical and Health Sciences, General Surgery Clinic, University of Trieste, Trieste, Italy*
[2]*Department of General Surgery, "Azienda Ospedaliera dei Colli", Monaldi Hospital, Naples, Italy*

Correspondence should be addressed to Piera Leon; pieraleon5@gmail.com

Academic Editor: Casey M. Calkins

Background. Gallstone disease affects 15–20% of the general population and up to 20% of these patients present common bile duct stones. *Aim.* This observational study reports our experience on routine cysticotomy and flushing of the cystic duct in patients with low risk of common duct stones. *Materials and Methods.* We analyzed 731 patients who underwent laparoscopic cholecystectomy between September 2013 and September 2015. *Results.* Patients were preoperatively stratified on the clinical risk; those presenting with low preoperative risk of common bile duct stones were referred to undergo laparoscopic cholecystectomy and routine cysticotomy with bile duct flushing. Patients presenting thick bile sludge, solid debrides, and/or increased tension of bile outflow underwent unplanned cholangiography. No intraoperative complications or conversion to open technique occurred. Average follow-up time was 22,8 months (range 12 to 37). Rate of retained ductal stones accounted for 0,3%. *Conclusions.* Routine cysticotomy and bile flushing in our experience is a valid, simple, and not time consuming manoeuvre that can help decompressing and flushing CBD. Moreover, it is a valid tool for extending selective IOC approach in a focused manner. Further evaluations have to be conducted to evaluate risks and effectiveness of this manoeuvre.

1. Introduction

Gallstone disease (GSD) is one of the most common biliary tract disorders affecting 15–20% of the general population in both Western and Eastern Countries.

Moreover, up to 20% of these patients present simultaneously common bile duct stones (CBDS) which can lead to many severe life-threatening conditions, such as acute pancreatitis, jaundice, ascending cholangitis, and hepatic abscesses [1, 2].

In the era of laparoscopic treatment for cholelithiasis (more than 80% of the cholecystectomies are laparoscopic in Western Countries), intraoperative cholangiography (IOC) and laparoscopic common bile duct exploration (LCBDE) have been advocated to diagnose and manage CBDS in a single stage [3]: this strategy shows excellent outcomes in CBD clearance, morbidity, and mortality. The single stage strategy permits shorter hospital stay and fewer procedures and is more cost-effective in comparison to the two-stage strategy provided by ERCP (endoscopic retrograde cholangiopancreatography) and surgery [4–9].

However, laparoscopic IOC and CBD exploration is technically demanding and time consuming and needs proper instrumentation for every single procedure: for all these reasons, it is far from being a commonplace in most surgical departments.

Current international guidelines provided by ASGE (American Society for Gastrointestinal Endoscopy) do not recommend routine IOC as a limited number of patients can benefit among all procedures performed [10]. Then, the accepted strategy is selective IOC based on the preoperative prediction model of risk [10, 11]. Selective IOC is nowadays performed in no more than 20% of the general surgery departments.

Therefore, the majority of the patients do not undergo intraoperative CBD evaluation during standard cholecystectomy and up to 5% of these patients presents retained ductal stones after surgery [12, 13].

Table 1: Population studied, stratified by preoperative risk of CBDS.

History of pancreatitis, cholangitis, jaundice	Altered LFTs or bilirubin level > 1,8 mg/dL	CBD > 6 mm	Probability of CBDS	*Patients (num)*	
–	–	–	Low	*486*	*486*
–	–	+	Intermediate	*83*	
–	+	–	Intermediate	*11*	*131*
+	–	–	Intermediate	*37*	
–	+	+	High	*23*	
+	+	–	High	*42*	*114*
+	–	+	High	*33*	
+	+	+	High	*16*	

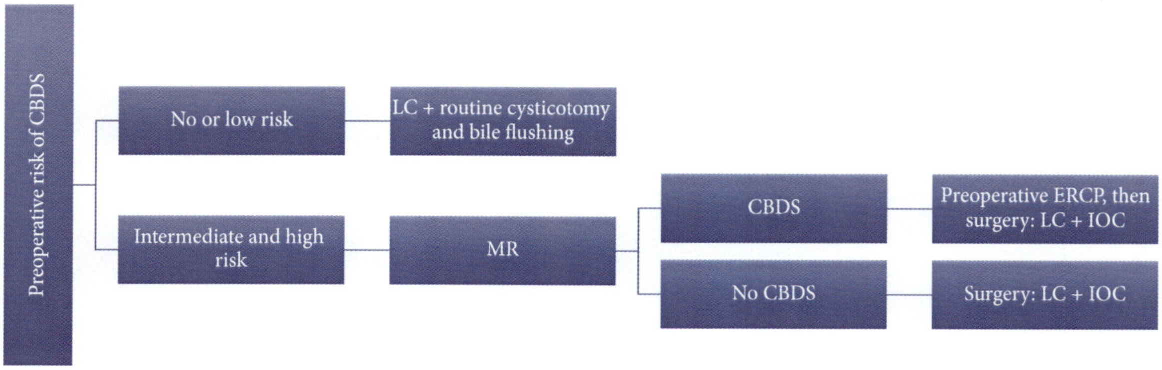

Figure 1: Flow-chart showing therapeutic strategy.

We added routine partial cysticotomy with bile duct flushing during standard laparoscopic cholecystectomy in all patients with low risk of common duct stones.

2. Materials and Methods

Over a period of two years, between September 2013 and September 2015, 776 laparoscopic cholecystectomies (LC) have been performed for symptomatic GSD in the General Surgery Department of "Monaldi" Hospital in Naples: among them, 82 LC were performed during other laparoscopic procedures as, in main part, right colectomies and gastrectomies. Urgent procedures (45 cases) have been excluded for our analysis.

All 731 patients analyzed underwent preoperative clinical evaluation, liver functional tests, and abdominal ultrasound examination. Based on these features, patients were stratified into three categories of risk for carrying CBDS.

Population studied is summarized in Table 1 and treatment strategy in Figure 1.

Surgery was performed according to the classic priority criteria, after an average of time of 104 days (range 17–379 days), taking into account the first symptomatic event. Main reason for this delay of time was the availability of the operating room for a benign disease. An abdominal ultrasound evaluation was repeated close to the operation, when the preoperative radiologic workup was older than 30 days.

All patients underwent a modified LC operative technique with routine cysticotomy and main duct bile flushing.

Patients presenting with intermediate to high risk of CBDS according to the clinical algorithm, were referred to perform intraoperative cholangiography, although part of them have already undergone ERCP.

First postoperative visit was planned one week after surgery and then after two months.

All patients were clinically reevaluated in September 2016.

3. Modified LC Operative Technique

The patient is placed in supine position with legs abducted. Surgeon stands between the legs of the patient, first assistant/cameraman stands on the left side of the patient and second assistant on the right. Pneumoperitoneum is created performing an open approach into the umbilicus. We use to place trocar as in the North-American position, which permits an easier access to the CBD, facilitating transcystic introduction of the catheter for IOC, and a safer approach to the Calot's triangle.

Operative technique has largely been described. Performing a gentle dissection of fatty-areolar tissues of the Calot triangle, two structures running parallels into the gallbladder are exposed: cystic duct and cystic artery. Once cystic duct and artery are identified, a single 5 mm titanium clip is placed on the junction between the infundibulum and the cystic duct. Others three metallic clips are placed on the

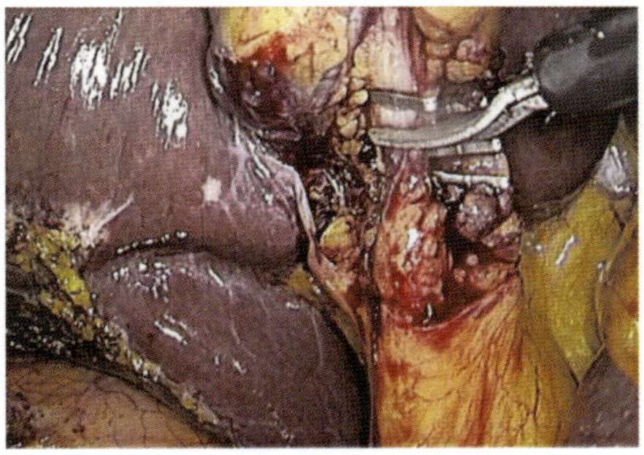

Figure 2: Partial cysticotomy.

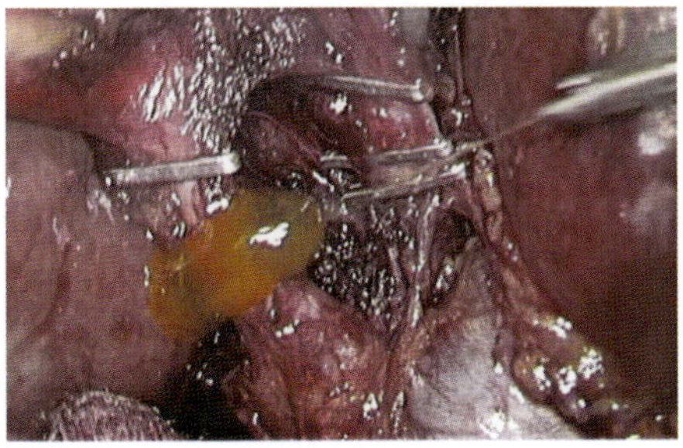

Figure 3: Flushing and bile outflow evaluation.

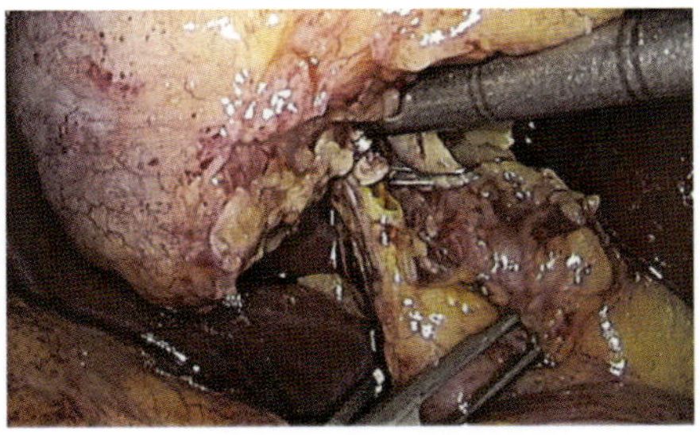

Figure 4: Gentle squeeze on the CBD and the cystic duct.

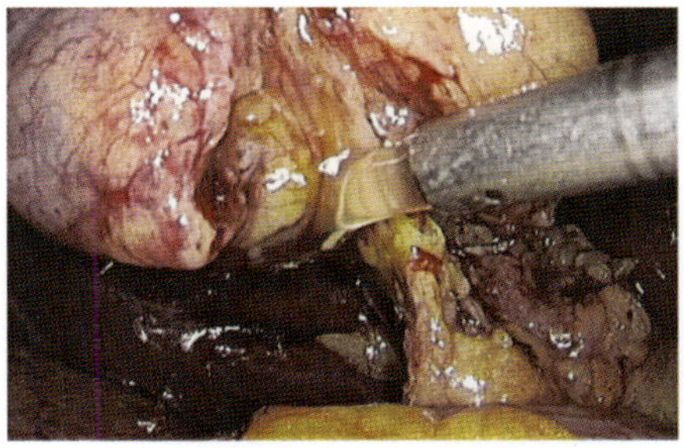

Figure 5: Bile rinsing.

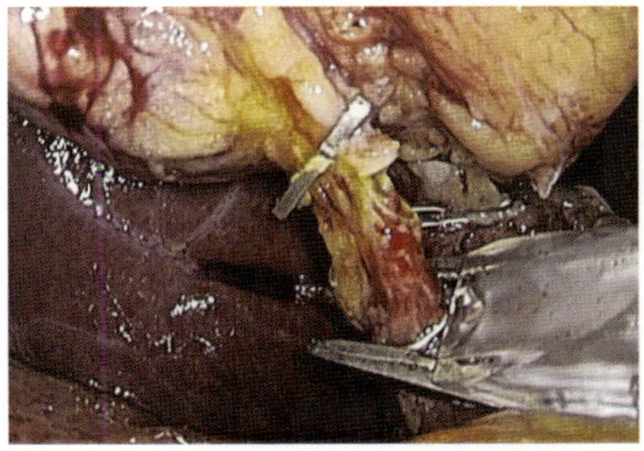

Figure 6: Clipping of the cystic duct.

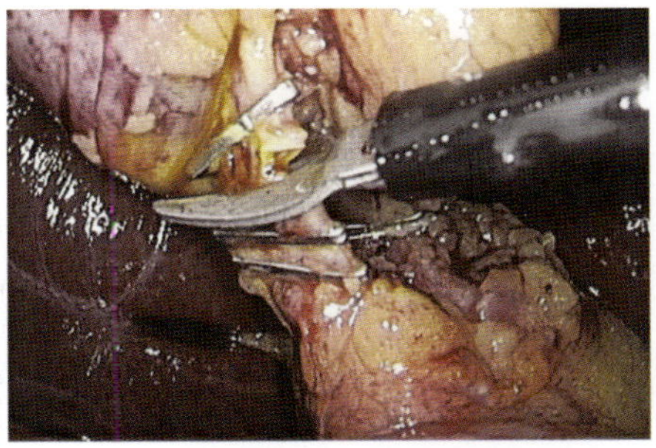

Figure 7: Cystic duct complete section.

cystic artery, two proximal and one distal. A partial section of the cystic duct is performed, allowing bile to flow out (Figure 2). Bile thickness and tension of outflowing out are important features to evaluate (Figure 3). A gentle squeezing of the hepatic peduncle (Figure 4) is repeated while multiple washings are performed with an irrigator (Figure 5): action is repeated till bile becomes yellowy clear and fluid. When bile clearance is satisfactory, two metallic clips are placed to close proximally the cystic duct (Figure 6). Once the cystic duct is clipped and divided (Figure 7), the infundibulum is retracted cephalic and the gallbladder is mobilized from the liver. Gallbladder extraction is performed using a retrieval bag, subhepatic drainage is positioned, trocars removal is undertaken under vision, and trocar sites are sutured.

4. Results

Population studied accounts for 731 patients, undergone LC per GSD over 2 years. Male to female ratio was 1 : 1,7, the average age was 59 years (range 19–82), and the average BMI was 28,2 (range 20–39,5).

Patients were preoperatively stratified on the clinical risk of CBDS: 486 presented with no or low risk for CBDS, while 245 presented with intermediate to high one. Among these 245 patients, 127 had CBDS detected by the preoperative RM and were referred to a preoperative ERCP: 96 (75,6%) presented ductal stones, while 31 (24,4%) had no CBDS detected during the endoscopic procedure.

All these 127 patients underwent LC with IOC after ERCP (average time 4,6 days, range 3 to 14 days). In three cases (2.4%) over 127 round-shaped fill-defects were detected at cholangiography. The transcystic extraction of CBDS in these three cases was provided using Dormia basket.

Patients with no evidence of CBDS at the preoperative MR but at risk for CBDS were candidate to LC with IOC. Among these 118 patients, 16 (13,5%) presented ductal fill-defects at IOC: 3, having smaller defects, were successfully

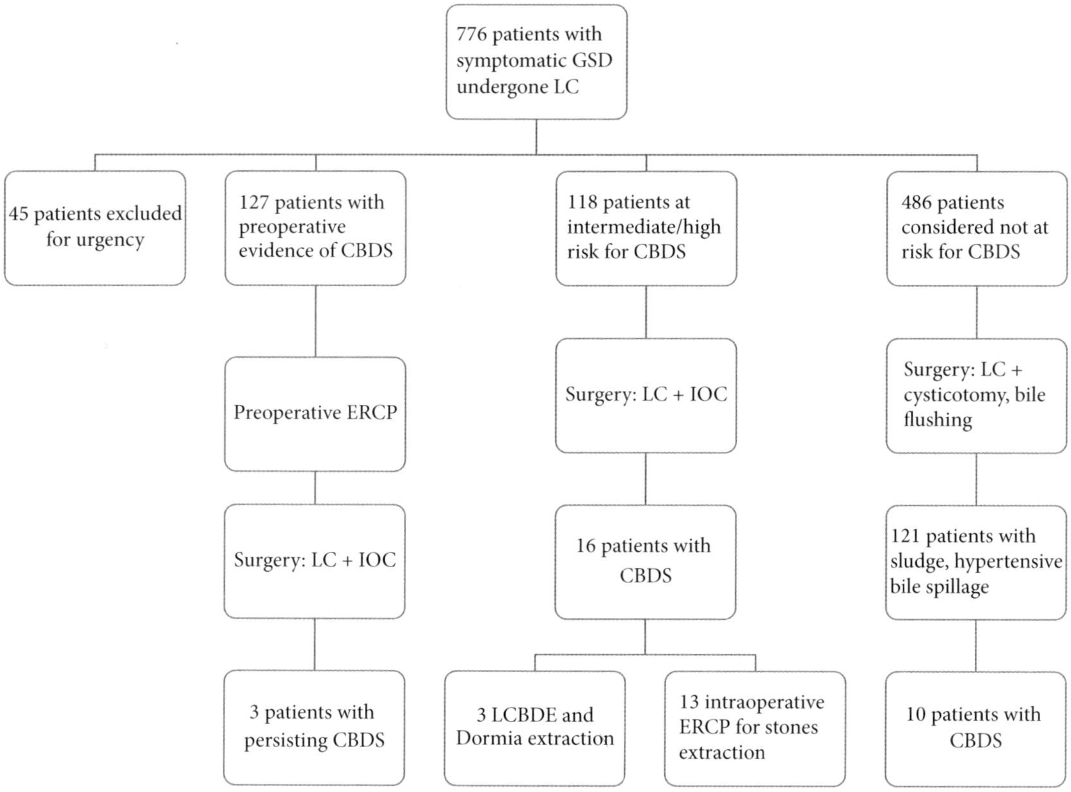

FIGURE 8: Flow-chart: population studied.

managed using a Dormia basket, while 13 underwent intraoperative ERCP for stones extraction (see Figure 8).

Patients presenting with low preoperative risk of CBDS (486 cases) were candidate to LC with routine cysticotomy and bile flushing: 121 patients among them presented thick bile sludge, solid debrides, or augmented tension of the bile outflow while performing the maneuver. In all these 121 patients we proceed to IOC, which helped in detecting 10 cases (2%) of ductal stones: clearance of the CBD was achieved using a Dormia basket in this subgroup.

No intraoperative complications or conversion to open technique occurred.

Postoperative morbidity was 4% including medical conditions and umbilical trocar site infections (2,2%). Neither cholangitis nor pancreatitis occurred in the short postoperative period.

Average follow-up time was 22,8 months (range 12 to 37).

Nonspecific abdominal symptoms as dyspepsia, flatulence, and abdominal discomfort occurred in 114 patients (15,6%) after LC.

Two patients (0,3%) were diagnosed with retained ductal stones during this follow-up: both of them had been preoperatively considered at intermediate risk of CBDS.

5. Discussion

Laparoscopic cholecystectomy (LC) has become the gold standard for the treatment of GSD, since it was introduced in the latter eighties, for its proven safety and feasibility and for short-term advantages provided compared to the open technique [14, 15].

No univocal consensus, otherwise, has been reached yet on timing and management of CBDS in the era of LC [4, 5]. Certainly, preoperative workup lacks in sensitivity [11].

Unrecognized ductal stones can lead to undertreatment and potentially frightening conditions [1, 16–18]. Postoperative complications due to retained stones are described to be as high as 5%. GSD being an endemic disease, 5% accounts for a significant part of population.

Current international guidelines recommend selective IOC based on preoperative risk of CBDS. This attitude, actually, deals well with the frequent limited availability of both the equipment and the operating room. In any case, IOC is performed in no more than 20% of the general surgery departments.

We routinely employ the selective IOC strategy for GSD since the Nighties. However, we were found to have symptomatic residual ductal stones' rate as high as in literature.

Therefore, we modified LC's operative technique introducing a systematic noninvasive exploration of the CBD in order to help in integrating standard LC.

The manoeuvre is simple and fast. No injury of the main bile tract occurred in our experience. Taking 1.8 to maximum 4.2 minutes, it aims to realize the evaluation and the clearance of the bile into the CBD in a noninvasive manner.

Our criteria to further proceed to an unplanned IOC are presence of thick bile sludge, solid debrides, and/or augmented tension of the bile outflow.

As high as one in every four low-risk patients (121 patients over 486) presented one or more of these criteria and was referred to an unplanned IOC: in 10 cases (2%) unsuspected CBDS were detected and directly cleared.

Furthermore, advantages of the manoeuvre can be postulated as it could help in reducing pressure into the CBD in the immediate postoperative time.

We did not evidence any increase on postoperatory surgical site infection's rate. Umbilical trocar site infections accounted for 2,2% in our population. Neither postoperative cholangitis nor pancreatitis occurred in the short-term period.

After a median follow-up time of 22,8 months (range 12 to 37, no routine cholangiography is undertaken), the postoperatory rate of retained CBDS in our population was 0.3%.

6. Conclusions

Routine cysticotomy and bile flushing in our experience is a valid, simple, and not time consuming manoeuvre that can help in decompressing and flushing CBD, perhaps helping in reducing postoperative intraductal tension on the surgical clips. Furthermore, it is a valid tool for extending selective IOC approach in a focused manner.

Further evaluations have to be conducted to evaluate risks and effectiveness of this manoeuvre.

Disclosure

Data were collected and study was performed in the Department of General Surgery, "Azienda Ospedaliera dei Colli", Monaldi Hospital (Naples, Italy).

References

[1] R. Costi, A. Gnocchi, F. Di Mario, and L. Sarli, "Diagnosis and management of choledocholithiasis in the golden age of imaging, endoscopy and laparoscopy," *World Journal of Gastroenterology*, vol. 20, no. 37, pp. 13382–13401, 2014.

[2] L. Bencini, C. Tommasi, and R. Manetti, "Modern approach to cholecysto-choledocholithiasis," *World Journal of Gastrointestinal Endoscopy*, vol. 6, no. 2, pp. 32–40, 2014.

[3] M. K. Li, C. N. Tang, and E. C. Lai, "Managing concomitant gallbladder stones and common bile duct stones in the laparoscopic era: a systematic review.," *Asian journal of endoscopic surgery*, vol. 4, no. 2, pp. 53–58, 2011.

[4] V. K. Bansal, M. C. Misra, K. Rajan et al., "Single-stage laparoscopic common bile duct exploration and cholecystectomy versus two-stage endoscopic stone extraction followed by laparoscopic cholecystectomy for patients with concomitant gallbladder stones and common bile duct stones: a randomized controlled trial," *Surgical Endoscopy and Other Interventional Techniques*, vol. 28, no. 3, pp. 875–885, 2014.

[5] B. V. Dasari, C. J. Tan, and K. S. Gurusamy, "Surgical versus endoscopic treatment of bile duct stones," *The Cochrane Database of Systematic Reviews*, vol. 9, article CD003327, 2013.

[6] J. Lu, Y. Cheng, X.-Z. Xiong, Y.-X. Lin, S.-J. Wu, and N.-S. Cheng, "Two-stage vs single-stage management for concomitant gallstones and common bile duct stones," *World Journal of Gastroenterology*, vol. 18, no. 24, pp. 3156–3166, 2012.

[7] K. S. Gurusamy, V. Giljaca, and Y. Takwoingi, "Endoscopic retrograde cholangiopancreatography versus intraoperative cholangiography for diagnosis of common bile duct stones," *The Cochrane Database of Systematic Reviews*, vol. 2, article CD010339, 2015.

[8] E. Naumowicz, J. Białecki, and K. Kołomecki, "Results of treatment of patients with gallstone disease and ductal calculi by single-stage laparoscopic cholecystectomy and bile duct exploration," *Wideochirurgia I Inne Techniki Maloinwazyjne*, vol. 9, no. 2, pp. 179–189, 2014.

[9] A. A. ElGeidie, "Single-session minimally invasive management of common bile duct stones," *World Journal of Gastroenterology*, vol. 20, no. 41, pp. 15144–15152, 2014.

[10] ASGE guidelines, "The role of endoscopy in the evaluation of suspected choledocolithiasis," *Gastrointestinal Endoscopy*, vol. 71, no. 1, pp. 1–9, 2010.

[11] G. Singhvi, R. Ampara, J. Baum et al., "ASGE guidelines result in cost-saving in the management of choledocolithiasis," *Ann Gastroenterol*, vol. 29, no. 1, pp. 85–90, 2016.

[12] M. R. Cox, J. P. O. Budge, and G. D. Eslick, "Timing and nature of presentation of unsuspected retained common bile duct stones after laparoscopic cholecystectomy: a retrospective study," *Surgical Endoscopy and Other Interventional Techniques*, vol. 29, no. 7, pp. 2033–2038, 2015.

[13] B. J. Ammori, K. Birbas, D. Davides, A. Vezakis, M. Larvin, and M. J. McMahon, "Routine vs 'on demand' postoperative ERCP for small bile duct calculi detected at intraoperative cholangiography. Clinical evaluation and cost analysis," *Surgical Endoscopy*, vol. 14, no. 12, pp. 1123–1126, 2000.

[14] E. Phillips, L. Daykhovsky, and B. Carroll, "Laparoscopic cholecystectomy: instrumentation and technique," *Journal of Laparoendoscopic & Advanced Surgical Techniques*, vol. 1, no. 1, pp. 3–15, 1990.

[15] S. B. Orenstein, J. M. Marks, and J. M. Hardacre, "Technical aspects of bile duct evaluation and exploration," *Surgical Clinics of North America*, vol. 94, no. 2, pp. 281–296, 2014.

[16] V. Giljiaca, K. S. Gurusamy, and Y. Takwoingi, "Endoscopic ultrasound versus magnetic resonance cholangiopancreatography for common bile duct stones," *The Cochrane Database of Systematic Reviews*, vol. 2, article CD011549, 2015.

[17] P. Li, Z. Zhang, J. Li, L. Jin, W. Han, and J. Zhang, "Diagnostic value of magnetic resonance cholangiopancreatography for secondary common bile duct stones compared with laparoscopic trans-cystic common bile duct exploration," *Medical Science Monitor*, vol. 20, pp. 920–926, 2014.

[18] M. Moller, U. Gustafsson, F. Rasmussen, G. Persson, and A. Thorell, "Natural course vs interventions to clear common bile duct stones data from the swedish registry for gallstone surgery and endoscopic retrograde cholangiopancreatography (gallriks)," *JAMA Surgery*, vol. 149, no. 10, pp. 1008–1014, 2014.

40

Instrumental Mechanoreceptoric Palpation in Gastrointestinal Surgery

Rozaliia F. Solodova,[1] Vladimir V. Galatenko,[1] Eldar R. Nakashidze,[2] Sergey G. Shapovalyants,[3] Igor L. Andreytsev,[2] Mikhail E. Sokolov,[1] and Vladimir E. Podolskii[1]

[1] *Faculty of Mechanics and Mathematics, Lomonosov Moscow State University, Moscow, Russia*
[2] *1st Surgery Department, Clinical Hospital No. 31, Moscow, Russia*
[3] *Department of Hospital Surgery No. 2, Therapeutic Faculty, N.I. Pirogov Russian National Research Medical University, Moscow, Russia*

Correspondence should be addressed to Rozaliia F. Solodova; rozaliya@solodov.org

Academic Editor: Casey M. Calkins

Background and Aims. Small gastric or colorectal tumours can be visually undetectable during laparoscopic surgeries, and available methods still do not provide a 100% localisation rate. Thus, new methods for further improvements in tumour localisation are highly desirable. In this study, we evaluated the usage of the Medical Tactile Endosurgical Complex (MTEC) in gastrointestinal surgery for localisation of tumours. The MTEC provides the possibility of instrumental mechanoreceptoric palpation, which serves as an analogue of conventional manual palpation. *Methods.* Ninety-six elective surgeries were performed, including 48 open surgeries, 43 laparoscopies, and 5 robot-assisted surgeries. The 20 mm version of the MTEC tactile mechanoreceptor was used in open surgeries, and the 10 mm version in laparoscopic and robot-assisted surgeries. *Results.* The mean time of instrumental mechanoreceptoric palpation was 3 minutes 12 seconds for open surgeries, which constituted the early stage of the learning curve, and 3 minutes 34 seconds for laparoscopic surgeries. No side effects or postoperative complications related to instrumental mechanoreceptoric palpation were observed, and this procedure provided data sufficient for tumour localisation in more than 95% of cases. *Conclusion.* Instrumental mechanoreceptoric palpation performed using MTEC is a simple, safe, and reliable method for tumour localisation in gastrointestinal laparoscopic surgery.

1. Introduction

Colorectal and gastric cancers are major causes of morbidity and mortality globally, comprising 9.7% and 6.8% of all cancers, respectively [1]. Specifically, colorectal cancer is the third most commonly diagnosed cancer [1, 2], and gastric cancer is the third mostly common cause of cancer death [1, 3]. Minimally invasive techniques for surgical treatment of these malignancies are now widespread and provide faster recovery, reduction of postoperative pain, and better cosmetic results [4–6]. However, small gastric or colorectal tumours that have not invaded the serosa can be visually undetectable during surgery [7, 8]. Precise localisation of such tumours in open surgeries is performed by palpation, especially in cases of intraluminal malignancies without surface invasion. In laparoscopic surgeries, the haptic feedback from the instrument is frequently insufficient, and localisation of a colonic lesion based solely on colonoscopy is also difficult for such tumours [8, 9]. Thus, additional methods including preoperative CT colonography, tattooing, titanium clips, double contrast barium, intraoperative gastroscopy, or ultrasound examination are used for tumour localisation [7–11]. However, achievement of a 100% localisation rate still evades surgeons [11, 12]. Furthermore, these methods have certain limitations and possible complications. For tattooing most complications are related to transmural injection, and the incidence of invisible lesions (resulting mainly from superficial injection or an injection into the mesenteric side) reaches 15% [12, 13].

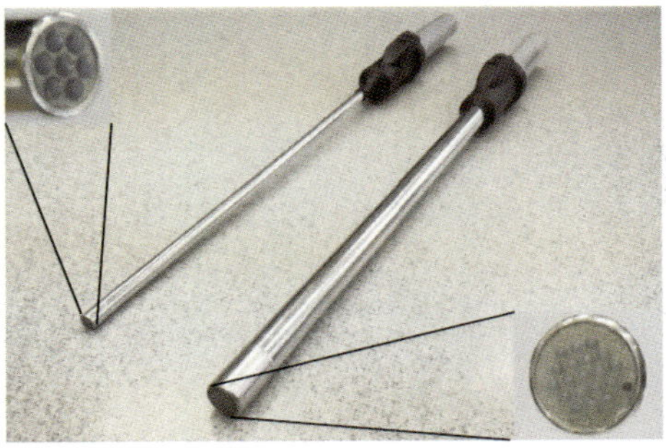

FIGURE 1: Tactile mechanoreceptors with 7 pressure sensors (left) and 19 pressure sensors (right).

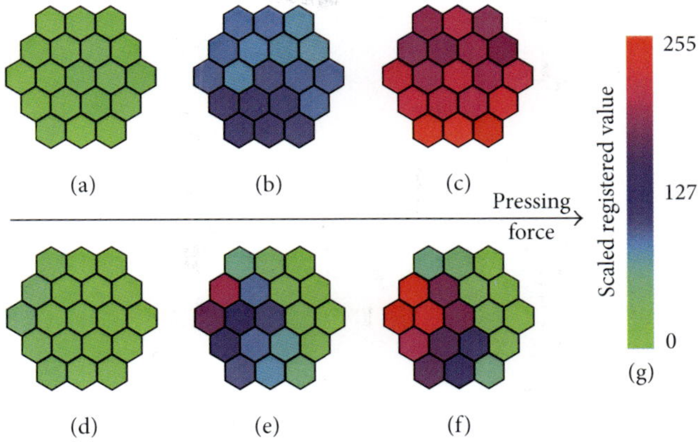

FIGURE 2: Visualisation of tactile frames registered during examination of a homogeneous area (a–c) and a heterogeneous area (d–f). Pressing force grows from left to right. Each hexagon corresponds to 1 pressure sensor. Registered values are scaled and colour-coded using a green-blue-red colour scale presented in panel (g).

Intraoperative ultrasonography or endoscopy requires a specialist at the time of surgery. Insufflation of gas during intraoperative gastroscopy or colonoscopy leads to bowel distention, which reduces the working space available to the surgeon [14].

Thus, new methods and techniques for further improvements and optimisation of localisation of small colorectal and gastric tumours during minimally invasive surgeries are highly desirable. The natural approach is to perform localisation by instrumental mechanoreceptoric palpation, which is applicable in laparoscopic surgery and serves as an analogue of conventional manual palpation in open surgery. To the best of our knowledge, the only currently available commercial device for intraoperative instrumental mechanoreceptoric palpation is the Medical Tactile Endosurgical Complex (MTEC). Results of MTEC usage in thoracoscopic surgery have been reported previously [15]. In this research, we evaluated the usage of MTEC in gastrointestinal surgery.

2. Materials and Methods

2.1. Medical Tactile Endosurgical Complex (MTEC). The MTEC is a complex consisting of tactile mechanoreceptors, a computer, and an optional tactile display [16]. A tactile mechanoreceptor registers tactile data via pressure sensors located in its operating head and wirelessly transmits the results to a computer. A computer processes raw data [17], performs real-time visualisation of tactile images [16], and reproduces tactile images on a tactile display, where images can be perceived simply with the use of a finger. Two versions of tactile mechanoreceptors are available (Figure 1). The first one performs registration via 19 pressure sensors and has a 20 mm diameter. The second one has 7 pressure sensors and a diameter of 10 mm. The 20 mm version was designed primarily for utilisation in open surgery, while the 10 mm version was developed specifically for laparoscopic surgery.

Detection and localisation of tumours using MTEC are based on identification of lesion boundaries, which produce heterogeneous tactile images. A press on a homogeneous area results in homogeneous tactile frames, while a press on a boundary results in highly contrasting tactile frames (Figure 2; see also [16, Figures 2 and 3]).

2.2. Patients and Surgeries. The MTEC was tested in Clinical Hospital No. 31 (Moscow, Russia). The study was approved by the Ethics Committee of Clinical Hospital No. 31. Each patient signed informed consent form before surgery, which included having their depersonalised data used for medical scientific study/research and presented in any medical scientific/research paper. All surgeries were comprehensively registered.

From January 2013 to December 2015, 96 elective surgeries were performed, including 48 open surgeries, 43 laparoscopies, and 5 robot-assisted surgeries with the da Vinci™ robotic system (Intuitive Surgical, Sunnyvale, CA, USA). Patients—40 males and 56 females—were aged between 30 and 91 years, with an average age of 66.9 years (standard deviation: 12.4 years). Tumour localisation and type for the patients are summarised in Table 1. T stage distribution for malignant tumours is summarised in Table 2. Tumour long diameter data is summarised in Table 3.

All surgeries were performed by surgeons familiar with the technique of instrumental mechanoreceptoric palpation.

There were no side effects or postoperative complications related to instrumental mechanoreceptoric palpation.

2.3. Medical Tactile Endosurgical Complex (MTEC) Utilisation. In open surgeries, the 20 mm version of the tactile mechanoreceptor was used. For visually detectable tumours, instrumental mechanoreceptoric palpation was performed starting from the proximal end of the lesion towards the boundary. After the boundary was reached, instrumental mechanoreceptoric palpation was continued clockwise until complete localisation of the lesion was achieved. A contact angle between the tissue and the mechanoreceptor was kept maximally close to 90°. For visually undetectable tumours, instrumental mechanoreceptoric palpation started from the supposed site of localisation (determined by the preoperative diagnostic studies) and was carried out in the same manner. A surgeon perceived mechanoreceptorically registered tactile data through visualisation and reproduction on a tactile

TABLE 1: Tumour localisation and type for patients involved in the study. GIST stands for gastrointestinal stromal tumour. "Other" tumour types included undifferentiated neoplasm (for gaster) and neuroendocrine carcinoma, hemangioma, fibroid polyp, and undifferentiated neoplasm (for intestine). Brackets contain numbers of open surgeries, laparoscopic surgeries, and robot-assisted surgeries, respectively.

Type	*Localisation* Caecum and ascending colon	Sigmoid colon	Descending colon and transversum	Rectum	Gaster	Intestine	*Total*
Adenocarcinoma	25 (13/11/1)	25 (12/13/-)	16 (11/5/-)	10 (8/2/-)	3 (-/1/2)	—	*79* (44/32/3)
Adenoma	6 (1/5/-)	1 (-/1/-)	1 (-/1/-)	—	—	—	*8* (1/7/-)
GIST	—	—	—	—	3 (-/2/1)	1 (1/0/-)	*4* (1/2/1)
Other	—	—	—	—	1 (-/-/1)	4 (2/2/-)	*5* (2/2/1)
Total number of patients	*31* (14/16/1)	*26* (12/14/-)	*17* (11/6/-)	*10* (8/2/-)	*7* (-/3/4)	*5* (3/2/-)	*96* (48/43/5)

TABLE 2: T stage distribution of malignant tumours for patients involved in the study. Brackets contain numbers of open surgeries, laparoscopic surgeries, and robot-assisted surgeries, respectively.

T stage	*Localisation* Caecum and ascending colon	Sigmoid colon	Descending colon and transversum	Rectum	Gaster	Intestine	*Total*
T1	—	1 (1/-/-)	—	1 (1/-/-)	—	—	*2* (2/-/-)
T2	2 (2/-/-)	2 (2/-/-)	1 (-/1/-)	—	4 (-/2/2)	2 (1/1/-)	*11* (5/4/2)
T3	12 (3/8/1)	14 (3/11/-)	6 (4/2/-)	4 (2/2/-)	1 (-/-/1)	1 (1/-/-)	*38* (13/23/2)
T4	11 (8/3/-)	8 (6/2/-)	9 (7/2/-)	5 (5/-/-)	2 (-/1/1)	—	*35* (26/8/1)

TABLE 3: Tumour long diameter (cm) for patients involved in the study. The mean values are presented, along with the minimum and the maximum values (where applicable).

Surgery type	*Localisation* Caecum and ascending colon	Sigmoid colon	Descending colon and transversum	Rectum	Gaster	Intestine
Open	6.14 (2–10)	4.58 (3–7)	7.77 (5–12)	6.38 (3.5–8)	—	5.00 (2–8)
Laparoscopic	3.44 (1–7)	4.00 (1–6)	3.75 (1–6)	3.50 (3-4)	3.67 (3–5)	1.40 (1.3–1.5)
Robot-assisted	5	—	—	—	5.88 (4–8.5)	—

display and collated these data with the perception provided by conventional manual palpation.

In laparoscopic surgeries, the 10 mm version of the tactile mechanoreceptor was used. The tactile mechanoreceptor was inserted through a trocar port. Instrumental mechanoreceptoric palpation was carried out in the same way as was performed in open surgeries, but in laparoscopic surgeries larger deviations of a contact angle from 90° were unavoidable. In cases of intestine tumours, instrumental mechanoreceptoric palpation was followed by ultrasound examination performed with Flex Focus Ultrasound Machine (BK Medical, Herlev, Denmark).

In robot-assisted surgeries, the 10 mm version of the tactile mechanoreceptor was used. An assistant performed tactile examination via an additional port under the guidance of a surgeon [16]. A surgeon perceived tactile data through a tactile display. An assistant controlled the force applied to the tactile mechanoreceptor based on the visualisation of tactile images.

3. Results

3.1. Open Surgeries. The study began with testing MTEC in open surgeries (Figure 3). Open surgeries constituted the early stage of the learning curve for instrumental mechanoreceptoric palpation, and surgeons collated perception of tactile properties of tissues provided by instrumental and conventional palpation. In 44 out of 48 open surgeries (91.7%), lesions were visually detectable, and all these lesions were detectable by instrumental mechanoreceptoric palpation as well. Overall, lesions were detectable by instrumental mechanoreceptoric palpation in 47 out of 48 cases (97.9%).

The undetectable case was an adenocarcinoma of the rectosigmoid region, which was also impalpable by conventional palpation. Its precise localisation was determined using intraoperative colonoscopy.

The time of instrumental mechanoreceptoric palpation varied from 1 minute 30 seconds to 5 minutes 20 seconds, with an average of 3 minutes 12 seconds (details are presented in

TABLE 4: Duration of instrumental mechanoreceptoric palpation. The mean values are presented (minutes:seconds), along with the minimum and the maximum values (where applicable).

Surgery type	*Localisation* Caecum and ascending colon	Sigmoid colon	Descending colon and transversum	Rectum	Gaster	Intestine	*Total*
Open	3:08 (1:45–4:30)	3:33 (2:00–4:45)	3:20 (1:30–5:20)	2:32 (1:35–4:05)	—	3:17 (2:20–4:15)	*3:12* (1.30–5:20)
Laparoscopic	3:21 (1:45–5:30)	3:28 (1:50–5:05)	4:24 (2:55–6:40)	2:55 (2:40–3:10)	3:10 (2:30–4:15)	4:35 (3:40–5:30)	*3:34* (1:45–6:40)
Robot-assisted	3:40	—	—	—	3:23 (2:35–4:30)	—	*3:26* (2:35–4:30)

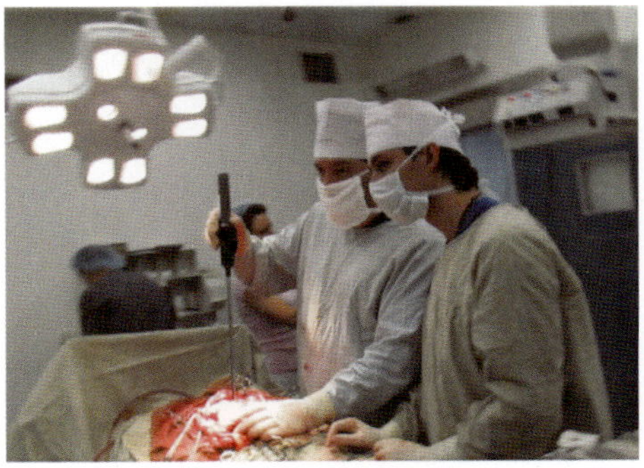

FIGURE 3: Instrumental mechanoreceptoric palpation in an open surgery.

Table 4). Certain areas were inspected multiple times by surgeons in order to improve collation of instrumental and conventional palpation. The fastest examinations corresponded to lesions with stages T3 and T4 by TNM classification. More time was required for smaller lesions (stages T1 and T2). This difference is consistent with a similar difference for conventional manual palpation.

Analysis of intraoperative mechanoreceptoric palpation in open surgeries confirmed that a deviation of the contact angle between the tactile mechanoreceptor and the examined tissue from 90° essentially affects tactile images registered by MTEC and complicates their interpretation. As these deviations are unavoidable in laparoscopic surgeries, specific algorithms aimed at suppression of contact angle artifacts were implemented, tested, and included in the MTEC software [17]. Currently, MTEC software also includes additional preprocessing methods that compensate for the excessive force applied to a mechanoreceptor [17].

3.2. Laparoscopic Surgeries. Lesion boundaries were clearly detected by instrumental mechanoreceptoric palpation in 41 out of 43 laparoscopic surgeries (95.3%) (Figure 4). The mean time of instrumental palpation—3 minutes 34 seconds—was slightly longer than that in open surgeries, but the difference was not significant. Detailed information about the time of instrumental palpation is presented in Table 4. In most of the laparoscopic surgeries, lesions were visually undetectable, despite the fact that in 5 cases, preoperative tattooing was performed.

In particular, in one case, visual localisation of the lesion was complicated despite preoperative tattooing. The patient had a polyp of the caecum opposite the ileocecal valve identified by colonoscopy. Instrumental mechanoreceptoric palpation took 5 minutes 15 seconds and provided correct localisation, which was then confirmed by intraoperative colonoscopy. The histological examination revealed tubular adenoma.

In the other case, multiple tubulovillous adenomas of the hepatic flexure colon were identified during colonoscopic examination and tattooed, but preoperative tattooing also appeared to be uninformative. Due to the soft consistency and close arrangement, instrumental mechanoreceptoric palpation provided localisation of only 1 lesion.

The remaining case in which a lesion could not be detected via instrumental mechanoreceptoric palpation was multiple neuroendocrine carcinomas of the ileum. Correct localisation in this case was achieved by intraoperative laparoscopic ultrasound examination.

3.3. Robot-Assisted Surgeries. In all 5 cases of instrumental mechanoreceptoric palpation performed in robot-assisted surgeries, lesions were correctly localised. The cases included 2 gastrectomies, 2 stomach resections, and a right hemicolectomy. These cases were described in [16], which is focused on using instrumental mechanoreceptoric palpation in robot-assisted surgery.

4. Discussion

The loss of the ability to palpate tissues and organs during laparoscopies essentially complicates localisation of visually undetectable tumours [7, 8, 18, 19]. At the same time, imprecise tumour localisation can lead to the removal of an incorrect segment of intestine [12]. Existing methods for tumour localisation still do not provide a 100% localisation rate and have specific limitations and possible complications. In up to 20% of cases, tumour locations identified by preoperative colonoscopy appear to be inconsistent with the intraoperative tumour site [9], and for preoperative tattooing, the incidence of invisible lesions reaches 15% [12, 13]. Intraoperative procedures, such as colonoscopy, gastroscopy, or ultrasonography, prolong surgical and anaesthesia time for patients. They also have their own challenges such as risk of splenic capsular tear,

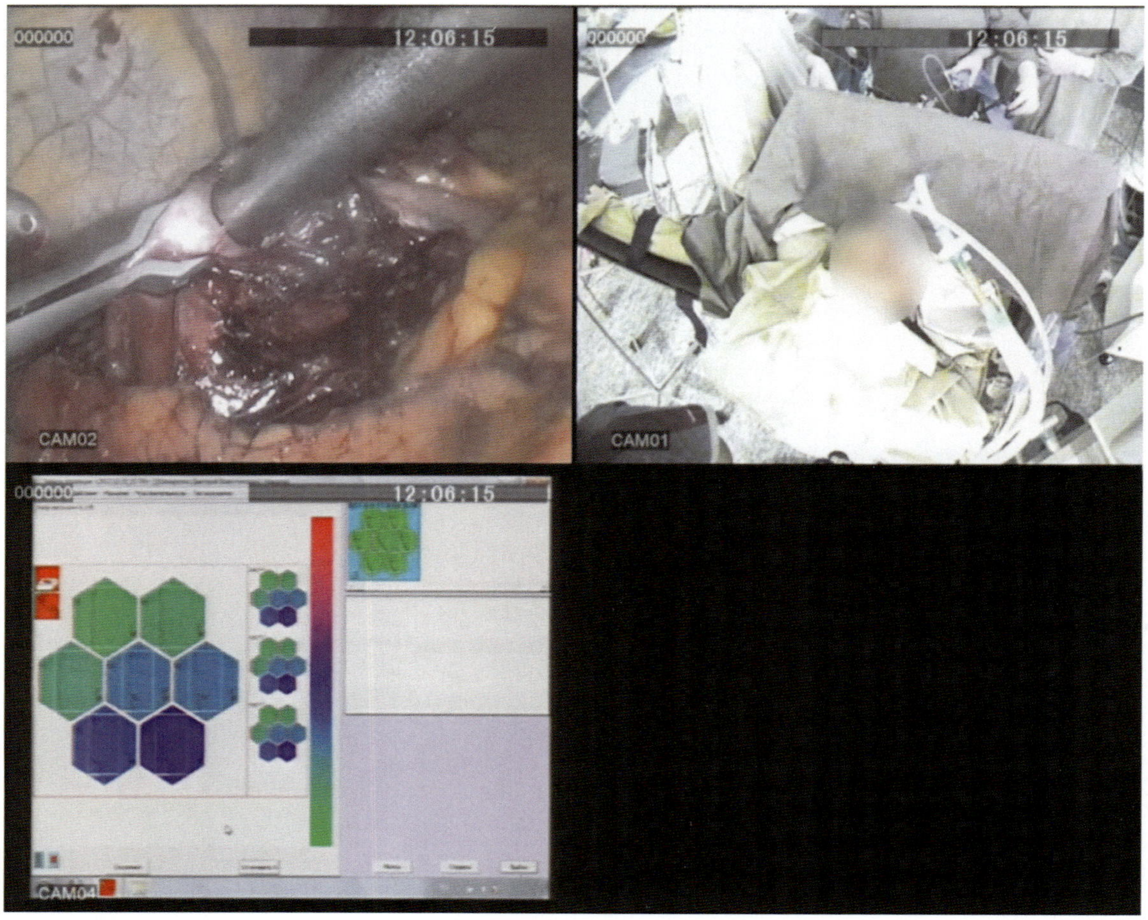

FIGURE 4: Instrumental mechanoreceptoric palpation of a stomach gastrointestinal stromal tumour (GIST) in laparoscopic surgery: simultaneously registered video streams from the external camera (CAM01), the laparoscopic camera (CAM02), and visualisation of tactile images (CAM04).

serosal tear of the colon or even perforation, and reduction of working space available to a surgeon due to bowel distention ([14, 20], [21, Ch. 3], and [22, Ch. 12]).

In this research, we evaluated the possibility of localisation of colorectal and gastric tumours via intraoperative instrumental mechanoreceptoric palpation performed using MTEC. This method is based on the fact that tactile properties of tumours are different from the tactile properties of normal adjacent tissues [16, 23] and serves as an analogue of conventional manual palpation. Our evaluation confirmed that instrumental mechanoreceptoric palpation is a simple and safe method with a short learning curve. It requires neither preoperative preparations nor presence of additional specialists at the time of surgery. The instrumental mechanoreceptoric palpation procedure is brief; furthermore, it can be used independently or in combination with other methods for lesion localisation. No side effects or postoperative complications related to this procedure were observed.

Localisation of lesions via instrumental mechanoreceptoric palpation performed using MTEC can be difficult in cases of small, soft lesions. This is consistent with the limitations for manual palpation [24–26].

Another limitation of this procedure is the requirement of only small deviations of the contact angle between the tactile mechanoreceptor and the examined tissue from 90°. This limitation was partially overcome by introducing special data processing methods into the MTEC software [17], but further improvements are desirable. They can be potentially achieved by optimisation of the construction of a tactile mechanoreceptor, particularly its operating head.

Localisation of gastrointestinal stromal tumours (GIST) via intraoperative instrumental mechanoreceptoric palpation was less apparent in comparison with other cases. It has been observed in both laparoscopic and robot-assisted surgeries [16]. In all GIST cases (including two laparoscopic and one robot-assisted surgeries) lesions were correctly localised, but due to palpatory indistinct boundaries and tactile heterogeneity of tumours it required more thorough instrumental palpation with very accurate application of MTEC mechanoreceptor.

5. Conclusion

Localisation of lesions by intraoperative instrumental mechanoreceptoric palpation performed using MTEC is a simple, safe, and reliable method which can be used either independently or in combination with other methods for tumour localisation. No side effects or postoperative complications related to instrumental mechanoreceptoric palpation were observed, and this procedure provided data sufficient for tumour localisation in 95.3% of laparoscopic surgeries.

Acknowledgments

The authors thank Dr. Alexey V. Galatenko for his valuable comments. The research was supported by the Russian Science Foundation (Project 16-11-00058: "The Development of Methods and Algorithms for Automated Analysis of Medical Tactile Information and Classification of Tactile Images").

References

[1] J. Ferlay, I. Soerjomataram, R. Dikshit et al., "Cancer incidence and mortality worldwide: sources, methods and major patterns in GLOBOCAN 2012," *International Journal of Cancer*, vol. 136, pp. E359–E386, 2014.

[2] R. L. Siegel, K. D. Miller, S. A. Fedewa et al., "Colorectal cancer statistics," *A Cancer Journal for Clinicians*, vol. 67, no. 3, pp. 177–193, 2017.

[3] B. J. Dicken, D. L. Bigam, C. Cass, J. R. Mackey, A. A. Joy, and S. M. Hamilton, "Gastric adenocarcinoma: review and considerations for future directions," *Annals of Surgery*, vol. 241, no. 1, pp. 27–39, 2005.

[4] D. Vanderpool and M. V. Westmoreland, "Laparoscopically assisted colon surgery," vol. 13, pp. 211–213, 2000.

[5] V. E. Strong, "Defining the role of laparoscopic gastrectomy for gastric cancer," *Journal of Clinical Oncology*, vol. 32, no. 7, pp. 613-614, 2014.

[6] J. M. Parker, T. F. Feldmann, and K. G. Cologne, "Advances in laparoscopic colorectal surgery," *Surgical Clinics of North America*, vol. 97, no. 3, pp. 547–560, 2017.

[7] W. J. Hyung, J. S. Lim, J. H. Cheong et al., "Intraoperative tumor localization using laparoscopic ultrasonography in laparoscopic-assisted gastrectomy," *Surgical Endoscopy*, vol. 19, no. 10, pp. 1353–1357, 2005.

[8] Q. Wang, E. Chen, Y. Cai et al., "Preoperative endoscopic localization of colorectal cancer and tracing lymph nodes by using carbon nanoparticles in laparoscopy," *World Journal of Surgical Oncology*, vol. 14, no. 1, article no. 231, 2016.

[9] N. Piscatelli, N. Hyman, and T. Osler, "Localizing colorectal cancer by colonoscopy," *JAMA Surgery*, vol. 140, no. 10, pp. 932–935, 2005.

[10] K. I. Fu, T. Fujii, S. Kato et al., "A new endoscopic tattooing technique for identifying the location of colonic lesions during laparoscopic surgery: a comparison with the conventional technique," *Endoscopy*, vol. 33, no. 8, pp. 687–691, 2001.

[11] S. A. Acuna, M. Elmi, P. S. Shah, N. G. Coburn, and F. A. Quereshy, "Preoperative localization of colorectal cancer: a systematic review and meta-analysis," *Surgical Endoscopy*, vol. 31, no. 6, pp. 2366–2379, 2016.

[12] A. Trakarnsanga and T. Akaraviputh, "Endoscopic tattooing of colorectal lesions: is it a risk-free procedure?" *World Journal of Gastrointestinal Endoscopy*, vol. 3, no. 12, pp. 256–260, 2011.

[13] P. J. Conaghan, C. A. Maxwell-Armstrong, M. V. Garrioch, L. Hong, and A. G. Acheson, "Leaving a mark: the frequency and accuracy of tattooing prior to laparoscopic colorectal surgery," *Colorectal Disease*, vol. 13, no. 10, pp. 1184–1187, 2011.

[14] K. Nakajima, S. W. Lee, T. Sonoda, and J. W. Milsom, "Intraoperative carbon dioxide colonoscopy: a safe insufflation alternative for locating colonic lesions during laparoscopic surgery," *Surgical Endoscopy*, vol. 19, no. 3, pp. 321–325, 2005.

[15] V. Barmin, V. Sadovnichy, M. Sokolov, O. Pikin, and A. Amiraliev, "An original device for intraoperative detection of small indeterminate nodules," *European Journal of Cardio-Thoracic Surgery*, vol. 46, no. 6, pp. 1027–1031, 2014.

[16] R. F. Solodova, V. V. Galatenko, E. R. Nakashidze et al., "Instrumental tactile diagnostics in robot-assisted surgery," *Medical Devices: Evidence and Research*, vol. 9, pp. 377–382, 2016.

[17] V. M. Staroverov, V. V. Galatenko, T. V. Zykova, Y. I. Rakhmatulin, D. V. Rukhovich, and V. E. Podol'skii, "Automated real-time correction of intraoperative medical tactile images: sensitivity adjustment and suppression of contact angle artifact," *Applied Mathematical Sciences*, vol. 10, pp. 2831–2842, 2016.

[18] M. D. Holzman and S. Eubanks, "Laparoscopic colectomy," *Gastrointestinal Endoscopy Clinics of North America*, vol. 7, no. 3, pp. 525–539, 1997.

[19] Y. B. Cho, W. Y. Lee, H. R. Yun, W. S. Lee, S. H. Yun, and H.-K. Chun, "Tumor localization for laparoscopic colorectal surgery," *World Journal of Surgery*, vol. 31, no. 7, pp. 1491–1495, 2007.

[20] J. L. Cohen and K. A. Forde, "Intraoperative colonoscopy," *Annals of Surgery*, vol. 207, no. 3, pp. 231–233, 1988.

[21] P. H. Gordon and S. Nivatvongs, *Principles and Practice of Surgery for the Colon, Rectum, and Anus*, CRC Press, 3rd edition, 2007.

[22] J. E. Fischer, K. I. Bland, and M. P. Callery, *Mastery of Surgery*, Wilkins, Lippincott Williams, 5th edition, 2006.

[23] G. Kharaishvili, D. Simkova, K. Bouchalova, M. Gachechiladze, N. Narsia, and J. Bouchal, "The role of cancer-associated fibroblasts, solid stress and other microenvironmental factors in tumor progression and therapy resistance," *Cancer Cell International*, vol. 14, no. 1, article no. 41, 2014.

[24] R. J. Heald and H. J. R. Bussey, "Clinical experiences at St. Mark's hospital with multiple synchronous cancers of the colon and rectum," *Diseases of the Colon & Rectum*, vol. 18, no. 1, pp. 6–10, 1975.

[25] R. M. Richter, L. Littman, and B. S. Levowitz, "Intraoperative Fiberoptic Colonoscopy: Localization of Nonpalpable Colonic Lesions," *JAMA Surgery*, vol. 106, no. 2, p. 228, 1973.

[26] J. L. Cameron and A. M. Cameron, *Current Surgical Therapy*, Elsevier, 12th edition, 2011.

Permissions

All chapters in this book were first published in MIS, by Hindawi Publishing Corporation; hereby published with permission under the Creative Commons Attribution License or equivalent. Every chapter published in this book has been scrutinized by our experts. Their significance has been extensively debated. The topics covered herein carry significant findings which will fuel the growth of the discipline. They may even be implemented as practical applications or may be referred to as a beginning point for another development.

The contributors of this book come from diverse backgrounds, making this book a truly international effort. This book will bring forth new frontiers with its revolutionizing research information and detailed analysis of the nascent developments around the world.

We would like to thank all the contributing authors for lending their expertise to make the book truly unique. They have played a crucial role in the development of this book. Without their invaluable contributions this book wouldn't have been possible. They have made vital efforts to compile up to date information on the varied aspects of this subject to make this book a valuable addition to the collection of many professionals and students.

This book was conceptualized with the vision of imparting up-to-date information and advanced data in this field. To ensure the same, a matchless editorial board was set up. Every individual on the board went through rigorous rounds of assessment to prove their worth. After which they invested a large part of their time researching and compiling the most relevant data for our readers.

The editorial board has been involved in producing this book since its inception. They have spent rigorous hours researching and exploring the diverse topics which have resulted in the successful publishing of this book. They have passed on their knowledge of decades through this book. To expedite this challenging task, the publisher supported the team at every step. A small team of assistant editors was also appointed to further simplify the editing procedure and attain best results for the readers.

Apart from the editorial board, the designing team has also invested a significant amount of their time in understanding the subject and creating the most relevant covers. They scrutinized every image to scout for the most suitable representation of the subject and create an appropriate cover for the book.

The publishing team has been an ardent support to the editorial, designing and production team. Their endless efforts to recruit the best for this project, has resulted in the accomplishment of this book. They are a veteran in the field of academics and their pool of knowledge is as vast as their experience in printing. Their expertise and guidance has proved useful at every step. Their uncompromising quality standards have made this book an exceptional effort. Their encouragement from time to time has been an inspiration for everyone.

The publisher and the editorial board hope that this book will prove to be a valuable piece of knowledge for researchers, students, practitioners and scholars across the globe.

List of Contributors

P. Grunert
Neurosurgical Department, University of Saarland, 66424 Homburg, Germany

Tamburrelli Francesco Ciro, Scaramuzzo Laura, Genitiempo Maurizio and Proietti Luca
Department of Spinal Surgery, Catholic University of Rome, lg A. Gemelli 8, 00135 Rome, Italy

Hong-Fei Nie
Department of Orthopaedic Surgery, West China Hospital, Sichuan University, Chengdu, Sichuan 610041, China

Kai-Xuan Liu
Atlantic Spine Center, 475 Prospect Avenue, Suite 110, West Orange, NJ 07052, USA

Donald A. Ross
Section of Neurological Surgery, Operative Care Division, Portland Veterans Administration Hospital, Portland, OR, USA
Department of Neurological Surgery, Oregon Health and Science University, 3303 SWBond Avenue, CH8N, Portland, OR 97239, USA

Rafik Shalaby, Refaat Ibrahem, Abdelaziz Yehya and Mohamed Abdalrazek
Pediatric Surgery Unit, Al-Azhar University Hospitals, Cairo, Egypt

Mohamed Shahin and Ibrahim Alsayaad
Pediatric Surgery Unit, Al-Azhar University Hospitals, Damietta, Egypt

Maged Ali Shouker
Diagnostic Imaging Department, Al-Azhar University Hospitals, Cairo, Egypt

Erdal Alkan, MehmetMurad BaGar, Oguz Acar, and Mevlana Derya Balbay
Department of Urology, Memorial Sisli Hospital, Okmeydani, Sisli, 34385 Istanbul, Turkey

Ali Saribacak
Department of Urology, Izmit Konak Hospital, Kocaeli, 41100 Izmit, Turkey

Ahmet Oguz Ozkanli
Department of Anesthesiology, Memorial SisliHospital, Okmeydani, Sisli, 34385 Istanbul, Turkey

Jason McMaster and SreyRam Kuy
Department of Surgery, Medical College ofWisconsin, Milwaukee, WI 53226, USA

Anahita Dua
Department of Surgery, Medical College ofWisconsin, Milwaukee, WI 53226, USA
Department of Surgery, Center for Translational Injury Research, University of Texas-Houston, Houston, TX 77030, USA

Abdul Aziz
Department of Surgery, Queens Medical Centre, Nottingham NG7 2UH, UK

Sapan S. Desai
Department of Surgery, Duke University, Durham, NC 27710, USA

Edjah Kweku-Ebura Nduom, Eric A. Sribnick and D. Ryan Ormond
Department of Neurosurgery, Emory University School of Medicine, 1365B Clifton Road NE, Suite 6200, Atlanta, GA 30322, USA
Winship Cancer Institute of Emory University, Atlanta, GA, USA

Costas G. Hadjipanayis
Department of Neurosurgery, Emory University School of Medicine, 1365B Clifton Road NE, Suite 6200, Atlanta, GA 30322, USA
Winship Cancer Institute of Emory University, Atlanta, GA, USA

Francis Ting, Richard Savdie, Sam Chopra, Carlo Yuen and Phillip Brenner
St Vincent's Hospital, Darlinghurst, Sydney, NSW2010, Australia

Jyothi Shetty and Deeksha Pandey
KMC, Manipal University, Manipal 576104, India

Asha Shanbhag
KMC, Manipal University, Mangalore 575001, India

Leen van Garsse, Mark La Meir and Jos G. Maessen
Cardiothoracic and Cardiology Department, Maastricht University, The Netherlands
Heart and Vessels Department, Careggi Hospital, Florence, Italy

Sandro Gelsomino
Cardiothoracic and Cardiology Department, Maastricht University, The Netherlands
Heart and Vessels Department, Careggi Hospital, Florence, Italy

Fabiana Lucà
Cardiothoracic and Cardiology Department, Maastricht University, The Netherlands
Heart and Vessels Department, Careggi Hospital, Florence, Italy
Cardiology Department, Paolo Borsellino Hospital, Marsala, Italy

CarmeloMassimiliano Rao, Orlando Parise, Rocco Carella, Roberto Lorusso and Gian Franco Gensini
Heart and Vessels Department, Careggi Hospital, Florence, Italy

Calogero Puntrello and Gaspare Rubino
Cardiology Department, Paolo Borsellino Hospital, Marsala, Italy

Bhuyan Ritwick, Krishanu Chaudhuri, Gareth Crouch, James R. M. Edwards, MichaelWorthington and Robert G. Stuklis
Darcy Sutherland Cardiothoracic Surgical Unit, Level 4, EastWing, Royal Adelaide Hospital, North Terrace, Adelaide, SA 5000, Australia

Mehmet Ali Yagci and Cuneyt Kayaalp
Department of Surgery, Turgut Ozal Medical Center, Inonu University, 44315 Malatya, Turkey

Tara Loux and Gavin A. Falk
Miami Children's Hospital, Miami, FL, USA

Carmen Ramos, Leopoldo Malvezzi Colin G. Knight and Cathy Burnweit
Miami Children's Hospital, Miami, FL, USA
HerbertWertheim College of Medicine, Florida International University, Miami, FL, USA
Miami Associates in Pediatric Surgery, Miami, FL, USA

Michaela Gaffley
HerbertWertheim College of Medicine, Florida International University, Miami, FL, USA

Stephanie Ortega
Florida International University, Miami, FL, USA

Nadine Di Donato and Renato Seracchioli
Minimally Invasive Gynaecological Surgery Unit, S. Orsola-Malpighi Hospital, University of Bologna, Via Massarenti 13, 40138 Bologna, Italy

Stefan K. Burgdorf and Jacob Rosenberg
Department of Surgical Gastroenterology, Herlev Hospital, University of Copenhagen, Herlev Ringvej 75, 2730 Herlev, Denmark

Pietro Gambadauro
Karolinska Institutet, LIME/NASP-C7, 17177 Stockholm, Sweden
Department of Obstetrics and Gynaecology, Catholic University of the Sacred Heart, Largo A. Gemelli 8, 00168 Rome, Italy

Vincenzo Campo and Sebastiano Campo
Department of Obstetrics and Gynaecology, Catholic University of the Sacred Heart, Largo A. Gemelli 8, 00168 Rome, Italy

Sriram Garudeswaran, Sohyung Cho and Ali K. Panahi
Industrial Engineering, Southern Illinois University Edwardsville, Edwardsville, IL 62026, USA

Ikechukwu Ohu
Industrial Engineering, Gannon University, Erie, PA 16541, USA

Shulin Guo, 1 Donghua Xie, Chuance Du, Lunfeng Zhu, Xiaolin Deng, and Zhongsheng Yang
Department of Urology, The Affiliated Ganzhou City People's Hospital of Nanchang University, Ganzhou, Jiangxi 341000, China

Xiangfei He
Linyi City People's Hospital, Linyi, Shandong 276003, China

A. Solodkyy, A. R. Hakeem, N. Oswald, F. Di Franco, S. Gergely and A. M. Harris
Department of Upper Gastrointestinal Surgery, Hinchingbrooke Hospital, Hinchingbrooke Park, Huntingdon, Cambridgeshire PE29 6NT, UK

Nyakuru Z. Ndaro and Shu-Yi Wang
Department of Biomedical Engineering, School of Medical Instrument and Food Engineering, University of Shanghai for Science and Technology, Shanghai 200093, China

Casey H. Halpern, Shih-Shan Lang and John Y. K. Lee
Department of Neurosurgery, Hospital of the University of Pennsylvania, 235 South Eighth Street, Philadelphia, PA 19106, USA

Vinay Gunnala and Nigel Pereira
The Ronald O. Perelman and Claudia Cohen Center for Reproductive Medicine, Weill Cornell Medical College, New York, NY 10021, USA

Robert Setton
Department of Obstetrics and Gynecology, Weill Cornell Medical College, New York, NY 10021, USA

Jian Qun Huang
Department of Obstetrics and Gynecology, Gynecologic Robotic Surgery, NYU Langone Medical Center, New York, NY 10016, USA

Katherine A. O'Hanlan, Margaret S. Sten, Stacey P. McCutcheon, Danielle M. Struck and Joseph K. Hoang1
Laparoscopic Institute for Gynecology and Oncology, 4370 Alpine Road, Portola Valley, CA 94028, USA

Pamela L. Emeney and Alfred Peters
University of California at San Francisco-Fresno, 155 North Fresno Street, Fresno, CA 93701, USA

Emad Mikhail, Stuart Hart and Anthony N. Imudia
Department of Obstetrics and Gynecology, University of South Florida, Morsani College of Medicine, Tampa, FL 33606, USA

Jason L. Salemi
Department of Family and Community Medicine, Baylor College of Medicine, Houston, TX 77098, USA

Ziqi Xu
Department of Neurology, The First Affiliated Hospital of College of Medicine, Zhejiang University, No. 79 QingChun Road, Hangzhou, Zhejiang 310003, China

Ning Ma, Dapeng Mo and Feng Gao
Department of Neurology, The First Affiliated Hospital of College of Medicine, Zhejiang University, No. 79 QingChun Road, Hangzhou, Zhejiang 310003, China
Department of Interventional Neuroradiology, Beijing Tiantan Hospital, Capital Medical University, No. 6 Tiantan Xili, Beijing 100050, China

Zhongrong Miao
Department of Neurology, The First Affiliated Hospital of College of Medicine, Zhejiang University, No. 79 QingChun Road, Hangzhou, Zhejiang 310003, China
Department of Interventional Neuroradiology, Beijing Tiantan Hospital, Capital Medical University, No. 6 Tiantan Xili, Beijing 100050, China
Department of Neurosurgery, Xuanwu Hospital, Capital Medical University, Beijing, China

Edward Ho chungWong,
Department of Medicine andTherapeutics, Chinese University of Hong Kong, Hong Kong

Liqun Jiao
Department of Neurosurgery, Xuanwu Hospital, Capital Medical University, Beijing, China

Meena Bedi
Department of Radiation Oncology, Medical College ofWisconsin, 8701Watertown Plank Road, Milwaukee, WI 53045, USA

David M. King
Department ofOrthopaedic Surgery, Medical College of Wisconsin, 8701 Watertown Plank Road, Milwaukee, WI 53045, USA

Sean Tutton
Department of Interventional Radiology, Medical College ofWisconsin, 8701Watertown Plank Road, Milwaukee, WI 53045, USA

Kevin Y. Chang and Wellington K. Hsu
Department of Orthopedic Surgery, Northwestern University Feinberg School of Medicine, 676 N. Saint Clair St., Suite #1350, Chicago, IL 60611, USA

Pierce D. Nunley
Spine Institute of Louisiana, Shreveport, LA, USA

Vikas V. Patel
The Spine Center, University of Colorado Hospital, Denver, CO, USA

Douglas G. Orndorff
Spine Colorado, Mercy Regional Hospital, Durango, CO, USA

William F. Lavelle
Upstate Bone and Joint Center, East Syracuse, NY, USA

Jon E. Block
San Francisco, CA, USA

Fred H. Geisler
Chicago, IL, USA

Jannah Baker and Monika Janda
Queensland University of Technology, School of Public Health, Institute of Health and Biomedical Innovation, Brisbane, QLD 4059, Australia

David Belavy
University of Queensland, School of Medicine, Brisbane, QLD 4072, Australia

Andreas Obermair
Queensland Centre for Gynaecological Cancer, Ned Hanlon Building, Butterfield St. Herston, Brisbane, QLD 4029, Australia

Vikal Chandra Shakya, Bikram Byanjankar, Rabin Pandit, Anang Pangeni and Anir RamMoh Shrestha
Department of Surgery, Civil Service Hospital of Nepal, Kathmandu, Nepal

Bishesh Poudyal
Clinical Hematology and Bone Marrow Transplant Unit, Department of Medicine, Civil Service Hospital of Nepal, Kathmandu, Nepal

Y. El Harrech, N. Abakka, J. El Anzaoui, O. Ghoundale and D. Touiti
Department of Urology, Hospital Avicenne, Marrakech 40000, Morocco

Emad Mikhail, Lauren Scott, Anthony N. Imudia and Stuart Hart
Department of Obstetrics and Gynecology, University of South Florida, Morsani College of Medicine, Tampa, FL 33606, USA

Branko Miladinovic
Center for Comparative Effectiveness Research and Evidence-Based Medicine, University of South Florida, Morsani College of Medicine, Tampa, FL 33612, USA

Eleni Papalekas and Jay Fisher
Department of Obstetrics and Gynecology, Beaumont Hospital, Royal Oak, MI, USA

Roman A. Polkin, Sergey V. Ochkal and Ivan A. Stepanov
Irkutsk State Medical University, Krasnogo Vosstaniya St. 1, Irkutsk, Russia

Vadim A. Byvaltsev
Irkutsk State Medical University, Krasnogo Vosstaniya St. 1, Irkutsk, Russia
Irkutsk Scientific Center of Surgery and Traumatology, Bortsov Revolutsii St. 1, Irkutsk, Russia
Railway Clinical Hospital, Irkutsk-Passazhirskiy of Russian Railways Ltd., Botkina St. 10, Irkutsk, Russia
Irkutsk State Medical Academy of Postgraduate Education, Jubileiniyi 100, Irkutsk, Russia

Evgenii Belykh
Irkutsk State Medical University, Krasnogo Vosstaniya St. 1, Irkutsk, Russia
Department of Neurosurgery Research, Barrow Neurological Institute, St. Joseph's Hospital and Medical Center

Yerbol T. Makhambetov, Talgat T. Kerimbayev and Serik K. Akshulakov
National Center of Neurosurgery, 34/1 Turan Av., Astana, Kazakhstan 350West Thomas Road, Phoenix, AZ 85013, USA

Michael Staren and Mark C. Preul
Department of Neurosurgery Research, Barrow Neurological Institute, St. Joseph's Hospital and Medical Center,

Giordano Perin and Maria Grazia Scarpa
Paediatric Surgery and Urology, Institute of Maternal and Child Health, IRCCS Burlo Garofolo, Trieste, Italy

RyuMatsumoto, Yoshio Nagahisa, Kazuki Hashida, Mitsuru Yokota, Michio Okabe and Kazuyuki Kawamoto
Department of Surgery, Kurashiki Central Hospital 1-1-1, Miwa, Kurashiki, Okayama 710-8602, Japan

Ali Keshavarz Panahi and Sohyung Cho
Industrial Engineering, Southern Illinois University Edwardsville, Edwardsville, IL 62026, USA

Piera Leon and Fabiola Giudici
Department of Medical, Surgical and Health Sciences, General Surgery Clinic, University of Trieste, Trieste, Italy

Antonio Sciuto and Francesco Corcione
Department of General Surgery, "Azienda Ospedaliera dei Colli", Monaldi Hospital, Naples, Italy

Rozaliia F. Solodova, Vladimir V. Galatenko, Mikhail E. Sokolov and Vladimir E. Podolskii
Faculty of Mechanics and Mathematics, Lomonosov Moscow State University, Moscow, Russia

Igor L. Andreytsev and Eldar R. Nakashidze
1st Surgery Department, Clinical Hospital No. 31, Moscow, Russia

Sergey G. Shapovalyants
Department of Hospital Surgery No. 2, Therapeutic Faculty, N.I. Pirogov Russian National Research Medical University, Moscow, Russia

Index